ISAM-GENT-1981

Proceedings of the Fourth International Symposium on Ambulatory Monitoring and the Second Gent Workshop on Blood Pressure Variability

Edited by

F.D. Stott

Division of Bioengineering
Clinical Research Centre
Harrow, Middlesex, UK

E.B. Raftery

Department of Cardiology
Northwick Park Hospital
Harrow, Middlesex, UK

D.L. Clement

Department of Cardiology
University Hospital
Gent, Belgium

S.L. Wright

Division of Bioengineering
Clinical Research Centre
Harrow, Middlesex, UK

1982

ACADEMIC PRESS

A Subsidiary of Harcourt Brace Jovanovich, Publishers

London   New York
Paris   San Diego   San Francisco   São Paulo
Sydney   Tokyo   Toronto

ACADEMIC PRESS INC. (LONDON) LTD,
24/28 Oval Road,
London NW1

United States Edition published by
ACADEMIC PRESS INC.
111 Fifth Avenue
New York, New York 10003

British Library Cataloguing in Publication Data
ISAM-GENT-1981
    1. Heart—Diseases—Diagnosis—Congresses
    2. Heart—Measurement—Congresses
    3. Ambulatory medical care—Congresses
    4. Monitoring (Hospital care)—Congresses
    I. Stott, F.D.
    616.1'20754   RC683.5
    ISBN 0-12-672360-5

LCCCN 82-45032

Printed in Great Britain by
Whitstable Litho Ltd., Whitstable, Kent.

PARTICIPANTS

AARTS, J.H.P. Inst. vor epilepsiebestijding, Achterweg 5, Heemstede, Netherlands.

ABETEL, G. 6 Place du Marche, 1350 Ombe, Switzerland.

ABRAHAM, N. Clinical Monitoring Department, Charing Cross Hospital, Fulham Palace Rd, London W6 8RF, UK.

ALLAZ, A-F. Policlinique Univ. de Medicine, Dpt. Cardiologie, 10 Vieux-Billard, 1205 Geneva, Switzerland.

ALTMAN, D.G. Div. of Comput.& Stats. CRC, Harrow, Middlesex, HA1 3UJ, UK

ANDERSSON, M. Pacemaker Dept. Huddinge Hospital, M64, Huddinge S-14186, Sweden.

ANTONIN, K-H. Humanpharmakologischs Inst. Ciba-Geigy, ob dem Himmelreich 7, D-7400 Tubingen, FRG.

ARZBAECHER, R. Pritzker Inst. Med. Eng. Illinois Inst. Technology, Chicago, Ill.60616, U.S.A.

AUBERT y TULKENS, G. Clin. Univ. St. Luc, UCL-EEG, Ave. Hippocrate 10, B-1200 Brussels, Belgium.

BALASUBRAMANIAN, V. Cardiology Dept. Northwick Park Hospital, Harrow, Middx, UK.

BAILEY, C. EEG Dept, Park Hospital, Oxford, UK.

BASHFORD, C.C. Bioeng. Dept. St.Mary's Hospital Med. School, Norfolk Place, Paddington, London W2, UK.

BASSEY, E.J. Dept. of Physiol. & Pharmacol., Univ. Hospital & Med. School, Clifton Boulevard, Nottingham, UK.

BAUSCH-GOLDBOHM, S. Dept. Environ. Health Wageningen, Netherlands Agricult. Univ., Wageningen, Netherlands.

BEHEYT, P. Hopital Mama Yemo, Dept. of Internal Med. & Cardiology, Kinshasa, BP 164, Zaire.

BEKAERT, I. Dept. of Cardiology, Akademisch Ziekenhuis, De Pintelaan 135, 9000 Gent, Belgium.

BERZEWSKI, Schering Berling FB Medizin, Zimmermannstr. 12, 1000 Berlin 41, FRG.

BINNIE, C.D. EEG Afdel. Inst. voor Epilepsiebestrijding, Achterweg 5, Heemstede, Netherlands.

BLACKBURN, J. Department of Clinical Measurement, Westminster Hospital, Page Street, London SW1, UK.

BLEICHER, W. Inst. fur Biomediz Technik, Seidenstr. 32, D-7000 Stuttgart 1, FRG.

BLUMHARDT, L. Univ. Dept. of Neurology, Radcliffe Infirmary, Oxford, UK.

BOUSQUET, J.C. Sandoz Produckte Schweiz, 62 Missionsstr. Basle, Switzerland.

BOWLES, M.J. Cardiology Dept., Northwick Park Hosp., Harrow, Middx, HA1 3UJ, UK.

BRANICKI, F.J. Dept. Surgery, Univ Hosp. Queen's Med. Centre, Nottingham, UK.

BRANKIN, P.R. Oxford Medical Systems, 39-41 Nuffield Way, Abingdon, Oxon OX14 1BZ, U.K.

BRATZLAVSKY, M. Dept. of Neurology, Akademisch Ziekenhuis, De Pintelaan 135, 9000 Gent, Belgium.

BUDWIG, G. Abt.f. Paed. Kardiologie, Univ. Kinderklinik Tuebingen, Ruemelinstr. 23, Tuebingen, FRG.

BURCH, J.R. Dept. of Engineering, Univ. of Lancaster, 1 Cork Road, Lancaster, Lancs LA1 4AJ, U.K.

BURGAT, J-M. Univ. Geneve, 4 Rue Prevost-Martin, 1205 Geneve, Switzerland.

BURKE, M. Blood Pressure Measurement Lab, Royal College of Surgeons in Ireland, 123 St. Stephens Green, Dublin 2, Ireland.

BURR, W. Univ. Nervenklinik - Epileptologie Bonn, Sigmund Freud str.

25, D-53 Bonn 1, FRG.

CAMPBELL, J.   Leith Hospital, Edinburgh, Scotland, UK.

CARRAGETA, M.   Hosp. Univ. de Santa Maria, Rua Beneficencia 203-1D, 1600 Lisboa, Portugal.

CASHMAN, P. Div. Bioengineering, CRC, Harrow, Middx, HA1 3UJ, UK.

CATTAERT, A. Dienst Cardiovasculaire revalidatie St.Barbara, Weligerveld 1, B-304 Pellenberg, Belgium.

CHADHA, T.S. Div. of Pulmonary Disease, Mount Sinai Med. Centre, 4300 Alton Road, Miami Beach, Fl.33140, USA.

CIOFFI, P. Dept. Bioingegneria, Politecnico di Milan, Milan, Italy.

CLINCKE, G. Dept. Pharmacology, Janssen Pharmaceutica, B-2340 Beerse, Belgium.

COHN, M. Div. of Pulmonary Disease, Mount Sinai Med. Center, 4300 Alton Road, Miami Beach, Fl.33140, USA.

CONTINI, C. CNR Clin. Physiology Inst., Via P.Savi 8, Pisa, Italy.

CORBEEL, L. Clinique St.Pierre, Av. Fabiola 9, 1340 Ottignies, Belgium.

COWAN, R. Computer Center U-76, Univ. of California, San Francisco, CA.94143, USA.

CREISSEN, J.   Societe BEFIC, 89 Rue d. Alpes, Silic 515, 94 623 Rungis Cedex, France.

CROSBY, P.   Biomed. Eng. Ser. Royal North Shore Hosp, Pacific Highway, St. Leonards, NSW 2065, Australia.

CUMMINGS, B.S. Oxford Med. Systems Ltd, 39-41 Nuffield Way, Abingdon, UK.

DALL'AVA, J. Dept. de Physiologie, UER Cochin Port Royal, 24 Rue d.Fg. St. Jacques, 75014 Paris, France.

DASHWOOD, S. Div. Clin. Sciences, CRC, Harrow, Middx. HA1 3UJ, UK.

DAVIES, A. Northwick Park Hosp. Harrow, Middx, HA1 3UJ, UK.

DAVIES, W. Cardiology Dept, Guy's Hosp., 84 East Dulwich Grove, London SE22, UK.

DE GROEN, G. Dept. Clin. Neurophysiology, Univ. of Limburg, Maastricht, Netherlands.

DELAGE, M.   Lab. Houde, ISH, 15 rue O.Metra, Paris 20, France.

DEN ENGELSMAN, J.W. Cardio-Logic Services B.V., Huis Ter Heideweg 42, PO Box 213, Zeist, Netherlands.

DE LEEUW, Dr.   Rotterdam, Netherlands.

DE WASSEIGE, F. I Ph.IB, c/o IRE, B-6220 Fleurus, Belgium.

DION, J.L.   Quebec, Canada.

DOUCHAMPS, J.A.S.   Clin. Pharmacology Unit, Hopital du Royal de Soleil, Route de Gazee, 61100 Montigny-le-Tilleul, Belgium.

DRAKE, B.   Medtronic Inc. Internat. Div. 3055 Old Highway Eight, Minneapolis, Minn.55418, USA.

EBM, W. Univ. Vienna, Cardio.Dept, Elisabethstr. 10, 2301 Grossenzersdorf, Austria.

EVANS, D. Dept. Surgery, Univ. Hosp, Queen's Med. Centre, Nottingham, UK.

EYRE, J.A.   Special Care Baby Unit, John Radcliffe Maternity Hospital, Headington, Oxford, UK.

FAVRE, L. Div. Endocrinology, Hopital Cantonal, 1211 Geneva, Switzerland.

FAZZINI, F.P.   Via B. Varchi 35, 50121 Florence, Italy.

FELDMAN, C. Cardio.Dept, Univ. Massachusetts Med. Sch., Lane Street, Worcester, Mass. USA.

FITZGERLAND, D. Hypertension Clinic, Jervis Street Hospital, Dublin, Ireland.

FLORAS, J.S. Canada

FORREST, G. Park Hospital for Children, Oxford, UK.

FOUILLOT, J-P.   Lab. de Physiologie, CHU Cochin, 24 rue d.Fbg St. Jacques, 75014 Paris, France.

GALASSE, R.   Squibb Labs, 130A Ave Louise, 1050 Brussels, Belgium.
GERMANO, G.   IV Med.Cal Path.Policlino Umberto I, via Pavia 124, 00161
Rome, Italy.
GIBBS, M.R.   Marketing Support Group Ltd, 67/73 Park Street, Camber-
ley, Surrey, UK.
GOLDBERG, A.D.   Cardiovas. Med. Dept, Henry Ford Hosp, 2799 W. Grand
Avenue,   Detroit, MI.48202, USA.
GOULD,B.   Dept.Cardiol., Northwick Park Hosp, Harrow, Middx, HA1 3UJ, UK.
GOULDING, L.   Cardiovas.Med., John Radcliffe Hosp., Oxford OX3 9DU, UK.
GRIFFITHS, J.W.   St. Mary's Hosp.Med.School, Norfolk Place, London W2, UK.
GRIMBURGEN, C.A.   Med. Physics Lab, Univ. of Amsterdam, Meremgracht
196, 1016 BS Amsterdam, Netherlands.
GUALTIERE, G.   Dept.Bioingegneria, Politecnico di Milan, Milan, Italy.
HAGG, G.M.   Sektion Amak, S-171 84 Solna, Sweden.
HALL,D.   Child Health, St.George's Hosp, Blackshaw Road, London SW17, UK.
HARDING, B.   Med. Sales Dept, Cambridge Medical, Rustat Road,   Cam-
bridge,   UK.
HAYWARD, R.
HESLA, P.E.,   S.I.A. 1474 Nordbyhagen, Norway.
HEYTENS, L.   Squibb Labs, Louizalaan 130A, 1050 Brussels, Belgium.
HILL, S.L.   Dept.Clin.Measurement, Westminster Hosp, 65 Romney Street,
London WC2, UK.
HOHLWECK, H.   Linder Hohe, Inst. fur Flugmedizine, 5 Cologne 90, FRG.
HORNUNG, R.S.   Cardiology Dept, Northwick Park Hosp, Harrow, Middx. HA1
3UJ,   UK.
HUNYOR, S.N.   Cardiovascular Research Unit, Royal North Shore Hosp, St.
Leonards, NSW 2065, Australia.
IRVING, J.M.   Dept. Physiol. & Pharmacol, Univ. Med. School,   Notting-
ham, UK.
IVES, J. Montreal Neurological Inst. & Hosp, 3801 University Street,
Montreal, Quebec, Canada. H3A 2B4.
IZOU, M.A.   CHU Cochin-Port Royal, 24 Rue d.Fbg St.Jacques, 75014 Paris,
France.
JACKSON, C. Oxford Medical Systems, 39-41 Nuffield Way, Abingdon, Oxon,
UK.
JACOT DES COMBES, B.   Service de Nephrologie et d'Hypertension, Centre
Hosp. Univ. Vaudois, 1011 Lausanne, Switzerland.
JAUSSI, A.   Policlinique Med. Univ. Cesar-Roux 19, CH-1005 Lausanne,
Switzerland.
JENKINS, J.M.   Dept.of Electrical and Computer Engineering, University of
Michigan, Dept ECE, 2500 East Engineering, Ann Arbour, MI 48109, USA.
JIRAK, T.L.   Medtronic, (Mail Stop A212), 3055 Old Highway Eight, Minnea-
polis, Minn.55418, USA.
JOHNSON, P.   Nuffield Inst. of Medical Research, Oxford, UK.
JONES, J.V.   Cardiac Dept, John Radcliffe Hosp, Oxford, UK.
JULIEN, D.   Hopital Laennec, 42 rue de Sevres, 75007 Paris, France.
KANEKO, Y. 2nd Dept.of Internal Med, Yokohama City Univ., Urafunecho,
Minamiku, Yokohama 232, Japan.
KASTFELT, S-O.   Medicotest A/S, Rugmarkenio, DK-3650 Olstykke, Denmark.
KELUVER, C.A.   Oxford Instruments Nederland BV, v.Gijnstraat 13, 2288
GB Rijswick (Z.H), Netherlands.
KIMMICH, H-P. Dept. of Physiology, Postbus 9101, NL-6500 HB Nijmegen,
Netherlands.
KLOSS, W.   Neurology Clinic, 3578 Schwalm-stadt, FRG.
KRAUSE, J.   Abt.Pneumologie, Med.Hochschule Hannover, Karl-Wiechert-Allee
9, 3 Hannover 61, FRG.
KUNZ, B.   Deutsche Forschungs-und Versach.f.Luft-und Reumfahrt e.V.

Inst.f.Nachrichtentechnik, Post Wessling,D-8031 Oberpfaffenhofen,FRG.

LAFFAY, J.   Centre Hospitalier A. Mignot, 177 route de Versailles, 78 Le Chesnay, France.

LAURENT, J-M.   Hopital Cardiologique, Lille, France.

LAURENTIADOU, E.   Schering Berlin, Kastanienallee 24, D-1000 Berlin 19,FRG.

LAURO, R.   Rome, Italy.

LAUWERS, P.   20 Patryzenlaan, 1950 Kraainem, Belgium.

LENDERS, J.   Dept. Int. Med., Univ. of Nijmegen, Geert Groteplein, Nijmegen, Netherlands.

LESPINASSE, P.   Medtronic, 120 Ave Charles de Gaulle, 92200 Neuilly/Seine, France.

LOVELY, D.F.   Univ. of Strathclyde, Bioengineering Unit, c/o Wolfson Centre, Rottenrow, Glasgow G4, Scotland, UK.

MALLION, J.   Medecine Interne et Cardiologie, Centre Hosp. Regional et Univ., Grenoble 38000, France.

MANN, S.   Dept. Cardiology, Bristol Royal Infirmary, Bristol BS9 1SN, UK.

MARCHESI, C.   Istituto di Fisiologia Clinica CNR, Via Savi 8, 56100 Pisa, Italy.

MARCHI, F.   Cardiology Div., Careggi Hosp, Florence, Italy.

MARTENS, W.L.J.   Epilepsy Centre "Kempenhaeghe", Dept. Neurophysiology, Sterkselseweg 65, 5591 VE Heeze, Netherlands.

MAUS, Y.   Univ. of Liege, Dept. of Medicine, Hosp. Baviere, Blvd. Constitution, B-4020 Liege, Belgium.

MATSUBAYASH, K.   Neurologischen Klinik Hepta, 3578 Schwalm-stadt, FRG.

MECHELSE, K.   Academisch Ziekenhuis Dijkzigt, Dr.Molewaterplein 40, 3015 GD Rotterdam, Netherlands.

MILES, L.   Sleep Research Center, Stanford Medical Center, Room R301, Stanford, CA 94305, USA.

MILLAR-CRAIG, M.W.   Div. of Medicine, Victoria Infirmary, Glasgow, Scotland, UK.

MILLIGAN, N.   Chalfont Centre for Epilepsy, Chalfont St. Peter, Bucks, UK.

MITCHELL, R.H.   Electrical Eng. School, Ulster Polytechnic, Jordanstown, Newtownabbey, Co. Antrim, Ireland.

MOERKERKE, F.   Upjohn N.V., Lichterstraat, 2670 Puurs, Belgium.

MORRIS, M.   EEG Dept, Park Hospital, Oxford, U K.

MONSTER, A.W.   Depts. of Neurology & Physiology, Temple Univ. Med. School, 3400 N. Broad St, Philadelphia, PA.19140, USA.

MORMINO, P.   Univ. of Padova, Istituto di Medicina Clinica, Via Giustinani 2, Padova, Italy.

MURNAGHAN, G.   Dept. of Midwifery & Gynaecology, The Queen's Univ. of Belfast, Inst. of Clinical Science, Grosvenor Road, Belfast, N.Ireland.

MURRAY, A.   Freeman Hosp., Medical Physics Dept, Newcastle Upon Tyne, UK.

NEILSON, J.M.M.   Reynolds Medical Ltd, Cawthorne House, 51 St.Andrew St, Hertford SG14 1HZ, UK.

OAKLEY, D.   Cardiothoracic Unit, Northern Gen.Hosp, Sheffield, UK.

O'BRIEN, E.   Dept. of Cardiology, The Charitable Infirmary, 9 Clifton Terrace, Monkstown, Co.Dublin, Ireland.

O'CALLAGHAN, W.   Dept. of Clin. Pharmacology, Royal College of Surgeons, Dublin 2, Ireland.

OJA, P.   Inst. of Occupational Health, Dept. of Physiology, Laajaniityntie 1, 01620 Vantaa 62, Finland.

O'KANE, M.J.   Swiss Epilepsy Clinic, Bleulerstr. 60, CH-8008 Zurich, Switzerland.

O'KANE, F.S.   Swiss Epilepsy Clinic, Bleulerstr. 60, CH-8008 Zurich, Switzerland.

OLDANO, G.   Politecnico di Milano, Piazza Leonardo Da Vinci 32, 20133 Milano, Italy.

OLDENBORG, E.   Academisch Medisch Centrum, Dept. Elektronica, Meibergdreef, Amsterdam, Netherlands.

ORBAN, L.C.   Academisch Ziekenhuis, Neurology-EEG Dept, De Pintelaan 135,   9000 Gent, Belgium.

OXLEY, J. Chalfont Centre for Epilepsy, Chalfont St. Peter, Bucks, SL9 ORJ, U.K.

PAHLM, O.   Dept. Clin. Physiology, Lasarettet, S-221 85 Lund, Sweden.

PALM, A. Pacemaker Dept, M-62, Huddinge Hosp, S-171 86 Huddinge, Sweden.

PARADA, J.   Schering A.g.,General Mola 9, 3°, Madrid 1, Spain.

PARRY, J.   21 Swynnerton Way, Widnes, Cheshire.

PATRICK, J.M.   Dept. Physiology & Pharmacology, Univ. Med. School, Clifton Boulevard, Nottingham NG7 2UH, UK.

PAUWELS, C.   Cardiologie-O.G.W.VI.1755, Hugo Verrieststr. 78, 8800 Roeselare, Belgium.

PESSINA, A.C.   Clinica Medica IIe, Univ. di Padova, Padova, Italy.

PHILLIPSON, E.A. 6355 Medical Sciences Bldg, Toronto, Ontario, Canada M55 1AT.

PEETERS, M.   Janssen Pharmaceutica n.V, Turnhoutseweg 30, B-2340 Beerse, Belgium.

PINCIROLI, F. Centro Teoria dei Sistemi del CNR, Politecnico di Milano, Piassa Leonardo da Vinci 32, 20133 Milano, Italy.

POOL, J.   Thoraxcenter, Erasmus Univ. P.O.1730, Rotterdam, Netherlands.

POPEYE, R.   St. Augustinusklinick, Iepersteenweg Veurne, Yslandvaardernstr. 18, 8460 Koksyde, Belgium.

PORCHET, M. Service Hypertension, Medecine CHUV, 1011 Lausanne, Switzerland.

RAFTERY, E.B. Cardiology Dept, Northwick Park Hospital, Harrow, Middx, HA1 3UJ, UK.

RAMSAY, E. Dept. of Neurology (127A), Univ. of Miami & Miami VA Hosp., 1201 NW 16th Street, Miami, FL.33125, USA.

RASCHKE, F.   Inst. f. Arbeitsphysiologie u. Rehabilitationschung, Ketzerbach 21, D-355 Marburg, FRG.

REDA, G.   IIa Clinica Medica, Policlinico Umberto I, Univ. di Roma, Viale del Policlinico, Rome, Italy.

REHNQUIST-AHLBERG, N.   Dept. of Medicine, Danderyds Hosp., S-18288 Danderyd, Sweden.

REICHENBERGER, H.   Siemens AG, Henkestr.127, D-8520 Erlangen, FRG.

RICH, J.   9 Walsingham Rd, Enfield, Middx, EN2 6EX, UK.

RICHALET, J-P.   Lab. de Physiologie, Faculte de Med. de Creteil, 8 rue du General Sarrail, 94010 Creteil Cedex, France.

RICHENS, A.   Dept. of Psychiatry, The Heath Hosp, Cardiff, Wales, UK.

ROCHE, P. CEA Saclay, Dept.l'Electronique, BP2, 91191 Gif sur Yvette, France.

RIEBOLD, K.   Oxford Medical Elektr., Niederwaldstr. 7,   D-6200 Wiesbaden, FRG.

DI RIENZO, M.   Centro di Bioingegneria, Via Gozzadini 7, Milano, Italy.

RODANO, R.   Centro di Bioingegneria, Via Gozzadini 7, Milano, Italy.

RODIGER, R.   Schering AG, Falkenthalersteig 92, 1 Berlin 28, FRG.

RODRIGUEZ, L.   Medtronic Europe, 120 Ave.Charles de Gaulle, 92200 Neuilly sur Seine, France.

ROGOWSKY, M.   2 Clos du Cinquantenaire, 1040 Brussels, Belgium.

ROMAN, B.E.   Medtronic Europe, 120 Ave.Charles de Gaulle, 92200 Neuilly sur Seine, France.

ROWLANDS, D.   Dept. Cardiovas. Med., East Birmingham Hosp., Bordesley Green East, Birmingham B9, UK.

ROYSTON, D.   Div. Anaesthesia, Northwick Park Hosp., Watford Road,
  Harrow, Middlesex, HA1 3UJ, UK.
SACKNER, M.   Mount Sinai Medical Center, 4300 Alton Road, Miami Beach,
  Fl.33139, U.S.A.
SAMSON-DOLLFUS, D.   Ser. Exploration Neurol., Hosp. Charles Nicolle,
  76031   Rouen Cedex, France.
SANSEN, W.   National Univ. Leuven, Elektrotechniek, 94K Mercierlaan
  B-3030 Heverlee, Belgium.
SARANUMMI, N.   Biomedical Eng. Lab., PO Box 316, 33101 Tampere 10,
  Finland.
SAYED, Z.   Dept. of Applied Neurophysiology, Tameside Gen. Hosp., Ashton
  Under Lyne, Gr. Manchester, UK.
SCHEPPOKAT, K-H. Robert Koch Krankenhuis, D-3007 Gehrden, Netherlands.
SCHEIBECHOFER, W.   Kardiologische Univ. Klinik, Garnisong 13, A-1090
  Vienna, Austria.
SCHREIBER, H.   12 Av.Mazarin, F-91380 Atilly Mazarin, France.
SCHWAB, N.A.   Univ. Frankfurt, 6000 Frankfurt, FRG.
SHORTIS, G.S.   (Heritage Fraser Assoc. Res.Lab) 1 Branksomedene Road,
  Bournemouth, Hants, UK.
SIEBEN, G.   Janssen Pharmaceutica N.V., Turnhoutseweg 30, 2360 Beerse,
  Belgium.
SIEBENBROCK gen. HEMKER, K.   Schering AG, JH-D, Mullerstr. 1 Berlin
  65, FRG.
SIX, R.   Vriye Univ. Brussels, Rucaplein 99, B-2610 Wilrijk, Brussels,
  Belgium.
SKOLDSTROM, B.   National Board of Occup. Safety & Health, 171 84 Solna,
  cSweden.
SLAGER, C.J.   Thoraxcentrum, Erasmus Univ. PO Box 1730, Rotterdam,
  Netherlands.
SMITH, E.B.O.   Barnes Unit, John Radcliffe Hosp, Headington, Oxford, UK.
SPERTI, G.   Clinica Medica 2a Univ. di Padova, Via Giustiniani 2, 35100
  Padova, Italy.
STEIN, I.M.   1371 Beacon Street, Brookline, MA 02146, USA.
STORES, G.   Park Hospital for Children, Headington, Oxford, UK.
STOTT, F.D.   Div. of Bioengineering, CRC, Harrow, Middx, HA1 3UJ, UK.
STUBBE, D.   Clinique St. Pierre, 1340 Ottignies, Belgium.
SUNDLER, M.   Reynolds Medical Ltd, Cawthorne House, 51 St.Andrews Street,
  Hertford, Herts, UK.
TALBOT, C.   Park Hosp. for Children, Old Road, Headington, Oxford, UK.
TEEDER, J.F.   Oxford Medical Systems Ltd, 39-41 Nuffield Way, Abing-
  don, Oxon OX14 1BZ, UK.
THEHU,W.   Medtronic B.V., Pastoor Petersstraat 6, Eindhoven, Netherlands.
TEKAIA F.   Lab. de Physiologie, CHU Cochin Port-Royal, 24 rue du Fg. St.
  Jacques, 75014 Paris, France.
TEMMERMAN, J.   Astra Nobel Pharma, 1001 Chaussee D'Alremberg, 1180
  Brussels, Belgium.
THIEN, T. Dept. Internal Med., St. Radhoudhospital, Univ. of Nijmegen,
  Geert Grooteplein Zuid 16, Nijmegen, Netherlands.
TJIAM, A.T.   Dept. Neurology, Eudokia Hosp., Bergsingel 215, Rotterdam,
  Netherlands.
TSCHURTSCHENTHALER, G.   Krankenhaus der Barmherziggn Schwester II, In-
  terne Abteilung, Langgasse 16, A-4020 Linz, Austria.
VAN DEN BERG, Y.Z.   Haverziekenhuis Rotterdam, Dept. of Neurology,
  Havingvliet 2, Rotterdam, Netherlands.
VAN DIEST, R.   Med. Psychology, Rijks Univ. Gimburg, PO Box 616, 6200 MD
  Maastricht, Netherlands.
VAN DUIJN, H. Valeriuskliniek, Valeriusplein 9, 1075 BG Amsterdam,

Netherlands.

VAN DURME, J.P. Cardiology Dept, University Hosp., 9000 Gent, Belgium.

VAN MAELE, G. Dept. of Med. Informatics, University Hospital, De Pintelaan 135, 9000 Gent, Belgium.

VAN MONTFRANS, G.A. Academic Hosp., Dept. Internal Med., Metbergtreef, Amsterdam, Netherlands.

VAN QUICKENBORNE, G.H. Hart Kliniek, Kortaijk, 1H Consciencestr. 8500 Kortrijk, Belgium.

VAN SPEYBROECK, W. Sonotron N.V., Onderwysstr. 58, 1930 Zaventem, Belgium.

VASTESAEGER, M. US Public Health Service, Internal Med., 163 Hitchcock Ave, Staten Island, NY 10306, USA.

WATSON, H. Mount Sinai Medical Center, 4300 Alton Road, Miami Beach, FL.33140, USA.

WATSON, R. Dept. of Cardiovas. Med., East Birmingham Hosp., Bordesley Green, Birmingham BG5 ST, UK.

WEBER, M.S. Kardiolog. Univ. Klinik Vienna, Garnisong 13, A-1050 Vienna, Austria.

WILLEMSE, P.J.A. Groene Hilledyke 315, Rotterdam 3075 EA, Netherlands.

WOLFF, H.S. Div. of Bioengineering, CRC, Harrow, Middx, HA1 3UJ, UK.

WOLLNER, J.C. Nuffield Inst. for Med. Res., Headley Way, Headington, Oxford, UK.

WONG, P-K. Univ. Dept. of Med.(I), c/o Singapore Gen. Hosp., Sepoy Lines, Singapore 0316.

WOUTERS, L. Janssen Pharmaceutica, Clin.Res., 34 Schoonhoudtstr., 9180 Belsele, Belgium.

YOUNG, J. Clin. Pharm. Unit, I.C.I. Pharmaceuticals Ltd, Alderley Park, Macclesfield, Cheshire, UK.

PREFACE

The first three ISAM meetings, in 1975, 1977 and 1979, were all held at the Clinical Research Centre in London. For the 4th meeting the venue was changed and the symposium was combined with the 2nd Gent Workshop on Blood Pressure variability, and took place at the University Hospital in Gent, Belgium. This volume contains the Proceedings of both the ISAM conference and the Gent Workshop; hence its imposing size. The volume has grown larger with each succeeding conference of the series; the next one will have to reverse this trend, perhaps by restricting the range of topics covered.

On this occasion, cardiovascular applications still represented the largest section of the proceedings; with the Gent Workshop included, the section devoted to Blood Pressure was particularly large and varied. Ischaemic Heart Disease received more attention at this conference than at any of the earlier ones, and may well become a major area of interest at the next meeting, which is planned for 1983. Respiratory monitoring and Neuropsychiatry, especially childhood epilepsy, were also important topics; the use of ambulatory monitoring techniques in those specialities is now well established. It will be noted that most of the contributions in these two sections deal primarily with clinical problems rather than with the technical problems of recording and analysing the required data.

Having waded this time through about half a million words of papers and discussion, we await with interest, not unmixed with some degree of trepidation, your contributions to the next ISAM meeting.

The editors and conference organising committee wish to thank all those who helped make this conference a success; in particular the authorities of the University of Gent and of the Academic Hospital for their hospitality. It is impossible to list all the individuals to whom we are indebted, but three people must be thanked especially for their dedicated efforts over an extended period, namely Linda Packet, Nicole Beanne and Evelyn Weston.

F.D. Stott
E.B. Raftery

D.L. Clement
S.L. Wright

CONTENTS

OPENING ADDRESS

PROFESSOR R. PANNIER

Ladies and Gentlemen,

It is a great privilege to welcome all of you to Gent to this symposium entirely devoted to ambulatory monitoring.

This meeting is organised by the joint efforts of the Clinical Research Centre (London) and the University of Gent, because it originated from the fusion of two separate entities: the International Symposium on Ambulatory Monitoring and the International Workshop on Blood Pressure Variability. I am confident that co-operation of both these groups will lead to a most rewarding experience and stimulate further research.

In our department of Cardiovascular Diseases, we have for several years been interested in the study and treatment of cardiac arrhythmias, to evaluate which the continuous recording of ECG is an absolute necessity. A section for ambulatory ECG monitoring was therefore created under the supervision of Dr. J.P. Van Durme, who will discuss some aspects of this work in the first lecture of this morning.

The idea of continuous recording has now expanded to several other disciplines such as electroencephalography (EEG) and pneumology. Many most interesting papers on these subjects will be discussed in the first part of the meeting.

The second part will be entirely devoted to continuous recording of arterial blood pressure. About 10 years ago, a section for study and treatment of arterial hypertension was created in our department of Cardiovascular Diseases, supervised by Dr. D.L. Clement. Beside the clinical care of hypertensive patients, our scientific interest is focused on two main topics; the first, the regulation of blood pressure and vascular tone by reflex mechanism, is a continuation of the ideas developed in this university by C. Heymans and J.J. Bouckaert; the second, the problem of blood pressure variability, arose from the old and simple clinical observation that, when blood pressure is repeatedly measured in a short period of time in the same patient, different readings are obtained.

The last part of this meeting will form the Second International Workshop on Blood Pressure Variability, an official satellite of the 6th meeting of the International Society for Hypertension; this workshop is also organised under the auspices of the Belgian Hypertension Committee. This meeting is devoted to the memory of Sir George Pickering, who delivered the introductory lecture at our first workshop. He was one of the pioneers of the concept of Blood Pressure Variability and his ideas will certainly stimulate many further generations of research workers in this area.

A NEW AMBULATORY MONITOR WITH PACEMAKER ANALYSIS CAPABILITY

T.L. JIRAK,* R. SMITH,* AND D.G. BENDITT,**

*Medtronic, Minneapolis, **Cardiovascular Division,
Dept. Medicine, University of Minnesota, Minneapolis, USA

Summary

We have developed a real-time ECG rhythm analyser for ambulatory arrhythmia screening applications. The device is a battery-powered, portable microcomputer programmed to analyse ECG and pacer functions while it is worn by the patient. We have conducted preliminary clinical and beat-by-beat bench testing on the device. This paper reports the beat-by-beat test methods used and discusses the preliminary results we obtained. These results indicate that the real-time ECG rhythm analyser detects pacer malfunctions and QRS complexes accurately.

Introduction

An ambulatory real-time ECG monitor can analyse ECG data as it occurs, eliminating the following practical shortcomings of conventional Holter ECG equipment (1):
1.Delays, often exceeding 24 hours, between completion of the tape recording and reception of the completed scanner report.
2.Need for a skilled scanning technician and an expensive high-speed scanner.
3.Variation in scanner report quality due to technician fatigue.
    The potential advantages of real-time ambulatory ECG monitoring are especially attractive for two clinical applications of Holter ECG that fit under the umbrella of arrhythmia screening. These applications are evaluation of patients with transient symptoms suspected to be of cardiac origin, and cardiac rhythm characterization of apparently healthy patients for epidemiological studies and industrial medicine. An effective arrhythmia screening device for these two applications must simply detect and document, but not necessarily classify abnormalities that manifest themselves as changes in R-R interval and ORS morphology (2). Since transient symptoms in a pacemaker patient may be caused by intermittent pacing system malfunctions, a pacing system function analysis capability appears to be a useful adjunct to any arrhythmia screening device (3).
    We have developed the Medtronic S3^{tm} screening system, a real-time ECG rhythm analyser for the ambulatory arrhythmia screening applications described above. The device is a battery-powered, general-purpose microcomputer with specialized peripherals, resident software and Random Access Memory (RAM) storage for statistical data and 54 eight second ECG strips. ECG and, optionally, pacer function are analysed while the patient carries the device. The analysis algorhythm operates on two channels of ECG data and the output of a pace-pulse detector circuit, all sampled at 300 Hz. The algorhythm

detects QRS complexes, analyses pacer performance, stores statistical data and saves single-or dual-channel eight-second ECG samples when user programmed criteria are met. Rhythm analysis results are retrieved via direct or telephone connection to a centralized base station that completes a report, including statistics, graphs and ECG chart strips, within ten minutes after data retrieval begins. The base station is also used to programme the rhythm analyzer operating mode and set ECG episode detection criteria.

The pacer analysis feature of the rhythm analysis algorithm measures the interval between adjacent pace-pulse artefacts, as well as the interval from pace-pulse artefact to the next QRS complex, by operating on the output of the pace-pulse artefact detector circuit. The pacer-related timing data is analyzed to determine whether the pacing system has failed to: stimulate the heart; sense ventricular contraction; or pace at the set rate. The pacer analysis feature will store summary statistics on pacer peformance and save ECG samples whenever the preset failure criteria are met.

The ECG rhythm analysis algorithm uses a single-pass feature-extraction technique to: detect QRS complexes; classify complexes as premature or non-premature; extract R-R interval data; and detect whether user-programmed ECG storage criteria have been met. Any R-R intervals contaminated by severe baseline shifts or bursts of noise with frequencies above 8 Hz are ignored and excluded from analysis. The ECG is analyzed by performing the following processing steps on a single channel of eight-bit ECG digitized data:

1. Differentiate and notch-filter the digitized ECG to reduce the effect of T-waves, baseline wander and both 50 Hz and 60 Hz power line interference.

2. Process the absolute value of the filtered and differentiated ECG to detect QRS complexes and extract the following QRS feature data: R-R interval; QS interval (QRS duration); and slope-ratio (ratio of the peak slope in the QR interval to the peak slope in the RS interval).

3. Classify QRS complexes as premature beats (PB) if their features meet any of the following criteria when the features are compared to their running averages:
    (a)   The R-R interval is at least 12.5% premature (shorter) and the sum of QS interval changes and slope-ratio changes is greater than 50%.
    (b)   The R-R interval is at least 25% premature and the following R-R interval is a compensatory pause.
    (c)   The QRS is an interpolated beat.

4. Compare PB and R-R interval pattern data to user programmed criteria and store ECG samples if criteria are met.

5. Store R-R interval data in data structures that the base station uses to generate trends, R-R interval histograms and R-R interval-difference histograms (4).

We conducted preliminary clinical studies with the rhythm analyser that indicated the potential clinical utility of the new device. However, the preliminary clinical results could not be used to quantify QRS detection and PB classification because the real-time rhythm analyser produces a summary report that does not indicate how each QRS complex is treated. Therefore, we developed the beat-by-beat bench test techniques described in the following sections of this paper to obtain detailed performance information, including sensitivity and specificity parameters.

Methods

Beat-by-beat testing of the pacer analysis feature was complicated by the need for a pace-pulse artefact with sufficient rise-time to trigger the pace-pulse detector circuit. Since none of the available analog or digital data bases was capable of developing the required waveform, we employed the "manual" beat-by-beat setup shown in Figure 1. The combination of pacer and pacer-interactive simulator provided realistic pace-pulse artefacts and permitted simulation of many types of pacer malfunction in a short time. The rhythm analyser hardware was modified to interface with an analog chart recorder that had a chart-edge printer. The rhythm analyser software was modified to output the sampled ECG signal onto the analog chart with the location of each pace-pulse artefact marked by a spike on the analog channel and each QRS complex annotated with a numeric code from the chart-edge printer. The QRS complex code signified how the pacer analysis feature interpreted each QRS. We manually interpreted the strip and compared the codes to our interpretations to determine whether the pacer analysis feature was operating correctly.

Initially, we used a variant of the "manual" beat-by-beat test setup shown in Figure 1 for evaluating ECG analysis algorithm performance. However, we abandoned the "manual" approach because the chart output from each run had to be evaluated by a trained ECG interpreter, a time-consuming process that compared algorithm performance to a single individual. In order to broaden the study, we adopted the MIT/BIH digital data base and developed the "automated" ECG analysis test setup shown in Figure 2, based on the work of Schulter et al (5). Each of the 40 tapes in the data base contains a file of digitized ECG data and a file of annotations describing each QRS complex on the tape. The annotation for each complex resulted from agreement between two out of three trained ECG interpreters (6). The study control micro-computer directed ECG data from the digital tape to the rhythm analyzer via a digital-to-analog converter. The rhythm analyzer hardware was unchanged, but the software was modified to store its own QRS classifications in RAM instead of ECG strips and to transmit the classifications to the study control microcomputer when a tape was completed. The study control micro-computer compared the rhythm analyzer's classification file to the data base annotation file and tabulated the number of QRS complexes from each data base classification that fell into each rhythm analyzer classification. Equipment malfunctions forced us to terminate the study after completing only 6 of the 40 tapes in the data base.

Results

Beat-by-beat testing of the pacer analysis feature demonstrated that the pace-pulse timing analysis can successfully determine if the heart was stimulated. The simulated pacer sensing system malfunctions were detected correctly when the pacer sensing refractory was

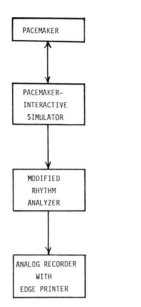

Fig. 1   Manual beat—by—beat
          study setup for
          testing pacer
          analysis feature.

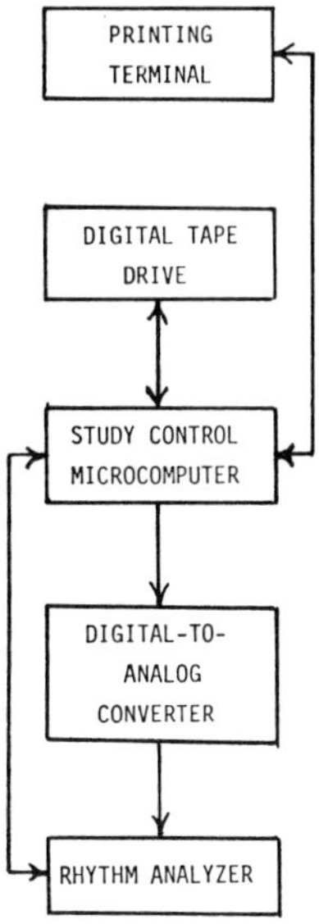

Fig. 2   'Automatic' beat—by—
          beat study setup for
          testing the ECG
          analysis algorithm.

equivalent to the preset standards in the rhythm analyser. All cases
of pace-to-pace interval decreases (rate increases) greater than 80
msec. were detected.

   The results of beat-by-beat tests on the ECG analysis algorithm
are summarized in Table 1 through 4. The six MIT/BIH data base tapes
were separated into three rhythm groups as shown in Table 1. Groups
I and III have stable background rhythms, while Group II is characterized by an unstable rhythm. The QRS complex annotation and classification codes used in the data base and by the rhythm analyser are
defined in Table 2. Table 3 contains raw data from the rhythm analyser study for all three groups; each number indicates how many QRS
complexes in each data base category the rhythm analyser classified
or missed. Detailed inspection of detection errors indicated that
QRS complexes were missed because they were either masked by noise or
were low in amplitude or slew-rate.

In order to compute the performance statistics in Table 4, we
combined the seven data base classificatgions into two categories.
The N, RBBB, SVPC, NEB and F categories in Table 2 were treated as
NPB complexes because they tend to be either "normal" in shape or
non-premature in timing. The AB and PVC categories in Table 2 were
combined into a PB category because both types tend to be premature and wide.

Table 1
Data Base Separation

Rhythm Group	Data Base Tapes	Description
I	101	Normal sinus rhythm (NSR) with rare APBs
II	201, 202 & 232	Unstable supraventricular rhythm with VPC's. Tape 201 and 202 have NSR with high-grade supraventricular ectopic activity. Tape 232 has sick sinus syndrome.
III	200 & 231	NSR with VPC's. Tape 200 has high grade ventricular ectopic activity. Tape 231 has abnormal A-V conduction with varying degrees of intermittent block.

Table 2
QRS Classification and Annotation Code

Code	Meaning
N	Normal QRS
RBBB	Right bundle-branch block beat
AB	Aberrantly-conducted beat
SVPC	Supraventricular premature contraction (includes atrial and nodal beats)
NEB	Nodal escape beat
VPC	Ventricular premature contraction
F	Fusion VPC
NQRS	Non-QRS signal (T-wave, artefact etc.)
PB	Premature beat (VPC or AB)
NPB	Any QRS that is not a PB (N, RBBB, SVPC, NEB or F)
MISS	Any undetected QRS

Table 3
Raw Data from Rhythm Analyser Beat-by-Beat Study

| Data Base QRS Classification | Rhythm Analyser Classification (Counts) | | | | | | | | |
| | Rhythm Group I | | | Rhythm Group II | | | Rhythm Group II | | |
	NPB	PB	MISS	NPB	PB	MISS	NPB	PB	MISS
N	1779	0	3	3506	27	6	2005	0	1
RBBB				374	0	0	1179	4	2
AB				35	61	19			
SVPC	1	2	0	1327	17	6	30	3	0
NEB				11	0	0			
VPC				74	141	1	159	634	6
F				3	0	0	1	0	1
NQRS	0	1	--	0	1	--	1	4	--

Table 4
Rhythm Analyser Performance Statistics

Rhythm Group	Group I	Group II	Group III	Total
QRS Detection Rate (%)	99.8	99.4	99.8	99.6
QRS Error Rate (%)	0.06	0.02	0.1	0.06
PB Sensitivity (%)	--	61.0	79.5	74.0
PB Specificity (%)	99.7	98.9	99.7	99.3
Data Base NPB Count	1,785	5,277	3,226	10,288
Data Base PB Count	0	331	798	1,129
Rhythm Analyser NPB Count	1,780	5,330	3,374	10,484
Rhythm Analyser PB Count	3	247	645	895

The performance metrics in Table 4 were calculated according to the following formulas:

$$\text{QRS Detection Rate} = \frac{\text{Number of true QRS deteced by rhythm analyser}}{\text{Number of QRS in data base}}$$

$$\text{QRS Error Rate} = \frac{\text{Number of NQRS detected as QRS by rhythm analyser}}{\text{Number of events detected as QRS by rhythm analyser}}$$

$$\text{Specificity} = \frac{\text{Number of true PB classified as PB by rhythm analyser}}{\text{Number of PB in data base}}$$

$$\text{Sensitivity} = \frac{\text{Number of true NPB classified as NPB by rhythm analyser}}{\text{Number of NPB in data base}}$$

Conclusion

Beat-by-beat testing on the pacer analysis feature demonstrated that the rhythm analyser is capable of detecting pacer malfunctions on the basis of timing data alone. The simulator-based study did not include a wide variety of QRS morphologies or the effect of large pace-pulse artefact variations. However, these issues can be resolved with a well-designed clinical study.

The ECG analysis algorithm beat-by-beat performance data in Table 4 indicates that the rhythm analyser is capable of detecting QRS complexes well. All rhythm groups have a QRS detection rate between 99.4% and 99.8% and a QRS error rate less than 0.1%. Detailed review of QRS sensing failures indicated that the rhythm analyser missed either QRS complexes masked by noise or premature contractions (AB, SVPC, or VPC) with low amplitude or slew rate. We believe that the QRS detection and error rate data indicate that the rhythm analyser can perform rhythm related tasks very well. Rate trends as well as interval and interval-difference histograms should be accurate; ECG samples saved on the basis of rate or interval data rare likely to be meaningful.

PB sensitivity and specificity data in Table 4 indicates that the rhythm analyser is more likely to classify a PB or NPB event correctly when the background rhythm is stable (Group I and Group

III). Since the PB classification parameters vary greatly from group to group, we cannot reach any meaningful conclusions about potential rhythm analyser PB classification performance until beat-by-beat studies have been performed on the full MIT/BIH data base.

References

1. Mark R.G., Moody G.B., Olson, W.H. et al (1979) Computers in Cardiology, 57-62.
2. Kennedy H.L., Caralis D.G. (1979) Annals Int. Med.**87**, 6, 729-737.
3. Ward D.E., Camm A.J. Spurrel R.A. (1979) Biotelemetry **4**, 109-114.
4. Cashman P.M.M. (1977) J. Med. Eng.and Tech. **1**, 1, 20-28.
5. Schluter P.R., Mark R.G., Moody G.B. et al (1980) Computers in Cardiology, 267-270.
6. MIT-BIH Arrhythmia Data Base: Tape Directory and Format Specifications; Biomedical Engineering Centre for Clinical Instrumentation, Technical Report No. 10, MIT (1980).

Acknowledgements

We gratefully acknowledge the work of Steven Hodges, Pan-Logic Systems, and George Moody, MIT. Their efforts produced the "automated" beat-by-beat bench test system shown in Figure 2.

Discussion

DR. MURRAY: How much ECG information will the monitor store during any one session?

MR. JIRAK: At this point, we have memory for it to store 54 single-channel tracings or 27 dual-channel. There is also a lock-out mechanism that can be programmed to set how many minutes of time must elapse between any time a sample is stored - so that there can be some control over whether this (ECG storage usage) occurs all at once or is spaced.

DR. MILES: What processor was used and how much ROM and RAM is in it? Is the programme in ROM, or is it loaded in? Can variables be defined and also data compression schemes - or is that all set?

MR. JIRAK: To start with, we are using the NSC 800, which is a Z80-type processor packaged to have some of the advantages of the 8085; it is a CMOS processor. It is very powerful and has very low current requirements. Unfortunately, it was not available until January, which has delayed us. This device has the software stored in 12K bytes of ROM and the user can programme it by setting various control points. There is about 24K bytes of RAM for data storage. Since the software is resident in ROM, and ECG storage criteria (e.g. high rate and low rate) are user-programmable, the criteria variables are entered into RAM. The system gets the variables out of RAM when it needs them to make a test against criteria.

SEARCH UNIT FOR SYMPTOMATIC EVENTS

A. MURRAY AND M.H. MAGUIRE

Regional Medical Physics Dept., Freeman Hospital,
Newcastle-upon-Tyne, UK

Summary

Many patients who experience intermittent symptoms, such as palpitations or dizziness, have their ambulatory ECG recorded in an attempt to discover the cause of the symptoms. If symptoms are infrequent, recordings may be taken over several days in an attempt to capture a symptomatic period. It may be necessary to examine only a single symptomatic period. Such an approach must be considered when a large number of recordings have to be analysed and the analysis time must be kept as short as possible.

A search unit has been developed which will find patient-activated "event" marks or times of day dialled via thumbwheel switches into the unit. The unit is connected to a Medilog PB-2 replay unit so that searches can be undertaken on one recording while another is being analysed using the main replay unit.

The time required to analyse some symptomatic recordings has thus been greatly reduced and re-analysis of selected sections when required has been greatly speeded up.

Introduction

One of the most important clinical uses of ambulatory ECG recording techniques is to assess the relationship between a patient's symptoms and the ECG at the time of these symptoms (1-4). By such means recordings have been made of arrhythmias such as ventricular tachycardia and asystolic pauses during symptoms. Many of these arrhythmias, although perhaps suspected, would not previously have been documented in any other way. In addition, if the ECG reveals no arrhythmia during the time of symptoms an arrhythmic cause can be ruled out and other possible sources investigated.

If symptoms are being investigated, it is much more effective to examine the symptomatic periods than the non-symptomatic periods. At a time when the cost-effectiveness of any service has to be considered, it must be more worthwhile to analyse a limited but selected portion of recording on more patients than analyse the whole recording on fewer patients.

Symptoms, however, are not frequently related to arrhythmias. In a study by Ward et al (3), only 7.5% of 531 patients had symptoms and an arrhythmia during the symptoms, which could be classed as diagnostic. A further 9.2% had an arrhythmia which could not be classed as diagnostic and 9.7% had no arrhythmia during indicated symptom. In spite of these low yields, only 7.5% of the rest of the recordings yielded important ECG information. Hence, examining a

selected portion of the recordings would have an arrhythmia incidence
yield of 16.7% and a useful information yield of 26.4% while analysing all 24-hours of the other recordings would have had an arrhythmia
incidence yield of only 7.5%.

Although equipment is available which can search for pre-
selected patients' symptom-times, such equipment frequently has three
specific limitations. The first is that it ties up analysis equipment during the time of the search. The second is that on older
equipment which record elapsed time-pulses, still the most common
type in use, facilities are not available for fast searches. The
third is that patient-activated "event" signals cannot normally be
detected during fast search speeds.

A search unit has been developed to overcome the above problems
with the frequently used Medilog equipment.

Search Unit

ECGs or EEGs recorded on Medilog equipment are played back on a PB-2
Medilog replay unit. This replay unit is normally always connected
to the search unit, but is sometimes used for analysis when the
analysis replay unit is undergoing maintenance. Hence this search
unit is provided as an independent facility, which can be operated in
parallel with normal ECG analysis and so does not tie up the analysis
equipment when searches are required. After the appropriate position
on the recording has been found, the tape is transferred to the
analysis system.

The replay unit reads the elapsed time pulses in the normal
way, so the recording must be run from the start of the tape. This
start time is set up on the replay unit before commencing a search.
To enable searches to be achieved quickly, the search unit, when
connected, changes the PB-2 replay speed to approximately 120 times
the recording speed, allowing events at the end of the tape to be
found within 12 minutes. Speed of search, however, is not considered
important as the search unit is preparing one tape for analysis while
another tape is actually being analysed.

The "event" signal is decoded along with the elapsed time markers, and hence searches can also be made for patient-activated
"event" signals.

A simplified block diagram illustrating the control and signal
connections between the replay and search unit is shown in Figure 1.
A functional diagram is given in Figure 2.

Time from the PB-2 replay is multiplexed serially through each
of the four digits (hours and minutes). These digits are loaded into
digital logic, which enables the tape-time to be compared with the
stop-time set up on the search unit. When this time is found or an
event detected, a signal is sent to stop the replay unit. The tape
is then ready for analysis.

Conclusion

When a patient's symptom-time is given, the ECG recording will be
searched not just at that time, but from some time before, usually up
to an hour before. This allows for any uncertainty over a patient's
symptom times. If the unit stops on an event, the tape is rewound

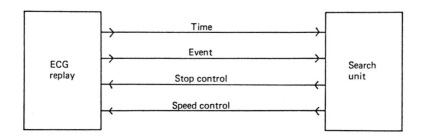

Fig. 1   Signal and control connections.

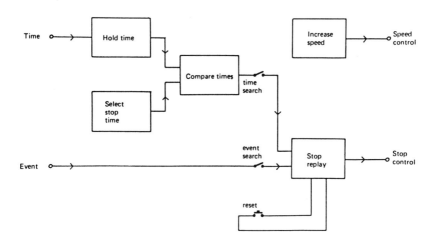

Fig. 2   Block diagram of search unit.

for several minutes to enable the symptomatic period to be analysed.

In addition to symptom and event searches, the unit has been useful in allowing previously documented arrhythmias to be found easily so that they can be written-out again for further closer scrutiny.

We can confirm that the frequency of patient-reported symptoms is low and that patients do not always, for a variety of reasons, manage to activate the "event" push button control. Nevertheless, on those patients who do report symptoms, this search unit has been a most useful addition to the facilities of the ambulatory ECG analysis laboratory.

References

1.   Goldberg A.D., Raftery E.B., Cashman P.M.M. (1975) Br. Med. J. 4, 569-71.
2.   Johansson B.W. (1977) Eur. J. Cardiol 5, 39-48.

3.   Ward D.E., Camm A.J., Darby N. (1980) Biotelemetry Pat.
     Montg 7, 57-66.
4.   Shenasa M., Curry P.V.L., Sowton E. In: ISAM 1979 Stott
     F.D., Raftery E.B., Goulding L. eds. London: Academic Press
     1980: 39-48.

Discussion

DR. BALASUBRAMANIAN: Dr. Murray is recording 24 hours of information
to identify very brief periods of symptomatic activity. What advantage does he gain in time-effectiveness, and even cost-effectiveness
over modulator recorders, like the cassette recorder which records in
real time and requires only an ordinary ECG machine to play back, and
which costs much less than a complete system?

DR. MURRAY: Some patients are not at all clear about whether or when
they have had symptomatic events recorded and the decision to use
this approach is based on discussions with the patients about their
symptoms, and whether they are clear that they had those symptoms.
Another point associated with event recorders is that there is not
often much information obtained before the event. The longest memory
available at the moment is about 8 sec, but many of the event recorders in use have no memory at all and only record the event after it
has been actuated. Although in cases where the event - perhaps a
tachycardia - is long, an event recorder is very useful, it is useless if we are trying to discover very short arrhythmias. The majority of our symptom-related arrhythmias are short, perhaps even just
palpitations, which are single ventricular events, ventricular tachycardia which may only be a few beats long, or an asystolic pause,
which may be only 2 or 3 seconds long.

DR. CASHMAN: Am I right in thinking that when the search unit has
stopped the tape at the first event that has been requested, the tape
has then to be taken off and put into the only analyser, playing
around that area to see if there is anything recorded?

DR. MURRAY: That is right - it is only used for searching.

DR. SOUTHALL: From our experience with the Medilog, Channel 4, on
which Dr. Murray had his clock and event is often lost on replay for
short periods of time due to tracking errors. How would that affect
his system?

DR. MURRAY: If we were to lose a signal, it would obviously decode
the time wrongly, but that is not a big problem. We find that it
usually occurs because the tape does not sit correctly in the guides
on either side of the head. If it is ensured that the tape fits in
between the guides, there should not be many problems.

DR. SOUTHALL: We have analysed about 6000 recordings in the past
year, in a large proportion of which we see the loss of clock signal
at some time during the 24-hour period. We monitor the clock signal
on replay using a Reynolds tape check and we see the light flashing
regularly on large numbers of our tapes. So, if Dr. Murray was
relying on that clock signal to find the events, he might be in
trouble.

DR. MURRAY: All I can say is that we have not found it to be a
significant problem.

DR. BALASUBRAMANIAN: I agree with Dr. Southall that time is a big
problem in the Medilog recorders. Even with Medilog Mark II, which
we have been using extensively, there are timing problems in more

than 50% of the tapes at some time. The timing signals, which come
out in the Mark I and Mark II are still imperfect for various reasons.

DR. MURRAY: I can only repeat that we do not find that it is a
significant problem.   In those cases where it has been found to be a
problem, an attempt is made to rectify it.   Perhaps in a later discussion somebody from the manufacturers might like to give a technical comment.

DR. CASHMAN: In general, though, you are not searching specifically
for times, but for event marks near the times.   Usually, if the clock
comes back somewhere near the time that is wanted, you will still get
the event mark.

SYMPTOM-CORRELATED ECG-REGISTRATION USING LONGTERM ECG AND ECG TELEPHONE TELEMETRY

W. SCHEIBELHOFER, H.S. WEBER, G. JOSKOWICZ, D. GLOGAR,
P. PROBST, K. STEINBACH, F. KAINDL

Kardiologische Universitäts-Klinik, Wien, Austria

Summary

Ambulatory 24-hours longterm EGC (HM) and ECG-telephone-telemetry
(TTM) were used to achieve a symptom-synchronous ECG registration in
53 patients, with symptoms in their history, possibly related to
arrhythmias (dizzy spells, palpitations, syncopes etc.). HM alone
led in 50%, TTM in 60%, both methods together in 75% to a full
success. In 71% out of these 42 patients, arrhythmias, commonly of
negligible severity, could be found as explanation for their symptoms
and in the remainder, could be excluded. Only in 5 patients (9%)
with a symptomatic history neither did symptoms occur during HM
and/or TTM, nor could asymptomatic arrhythmias be recognized in HM.

Introduction

In daily practice physicians are often confronted with the question
whether symptoms like dizziness, palpitations etc. are caused by
arrhythmias or not (1). 12-lead ECG alone is not able to answer this
question in many patients (1). But there exist two methods, which can
be helpful in solving this problem: Holter monitoring (HM) and ECG-
telephone-telemetry (TTM) (2).
So the purpose of this study was to achieve an ECG registration
during such a symptomatic period using both methods.

Methods and Materials

53 patients, 27 women and 26 men, aged 18-73 years ($\bar{m}$ 51),were
introduced into the study. In their history, symptoms occurred which
were possibly related to arrhythmias: paroxysmal pulse irregularities (53%), dizzy spells (42%), palpitations (42%), syncopes (20%),
angina (20%), intermittent bradycardia (4%) and dyspnoea (4%). 43%
had only one symptom, 42% two symptoms, 15% more than two symptoms.
During physical examination, the following underlying diseases
could be found: Coronary heart disease and congestive cardiomyopathy
in 11% each, WPW, HOCM and suspected pacemaker malfunction in 4%
each. Other reasons could be found in 8% including one patient with
mitral valve replacement, arterial hypertension and a stenosis of the
left carotid artery. In the majority of the patients (58%) no underlying disease could be found.
The patients underwent 24-hours continuous longterm ECG recording (HM) under ambulatory conditions and ECG telephone telemetry
(TTM) with a mean duration of three weeks (1-6 weeks)

Routine ECG:
No symptomatic period could be captured during routine ECG registration. Routine 12-lead ECG was normal in 68%. 24% demonstrated premature ventricular contractions (PVC's), 6% supraventricular premature contractions (SVP's) and one patient AV-block of first degree. No complex ventricular arrhythmias could be found in any patient.

Longterm ECG (HM) Analyis:
Using the computer (PDP 11/60) supported "Multipass-Scanning" analysis system, the ECG is played back at 60 x recording speed and, after data reduction using the linear segmentation technique (3), stored in digital form on random access medium (e.g. magnetic disc). During multiple passes primitive parameters of each QRS complex are generated and put together to obtain clinically relevant diagnoses including further multi-stage artefact detection algorithms. The data can be further worked up statistically or stored in a data base at choice as mentioned in another paper during that Congress (4).

ECG-Telephone-Telemetry (TTM)
The transmitter unit of the TTM consists of an amplifier to which the electrodes were connected by the telephone handset. The ECG signals (0.5-150 Hz) are encoded as frequency modulation of the carrie frequency of 1700 ± 200 Hz. Then the carrier tone is fed into the mouthpiece of the transmitter telephone. In the receiving unit, the acoustic signal was picked up by the earpiece microphone and underwent a frequency demodulation process after amplification. The ECG was strip-chart-recorded maintaining a permanent acoustic patient-physician contact. The patients could have a telephone connection to the receiving unit placed in the CCU each time they wanted.

Results

Arrhythmias during HM (Figure 1)
In 18 patients, arrhythmias could be detected during HM (Figure 1). In 11 patients, these arrhythmias could be correlated to symptoms, whereas in 7 patients, the rhythm disturbances occurred asymptomatically. On the other hand, 16 out of 35 patients with no disturbances of the heart rhythm during HM complained about various symptoms and described them in their diaries (Figure 1).

Symptoms during HM (Figure 2)
On the other hand, 27 patients developed typical symptoms during HM. In 21%, these symptoms were caused by arrhythmias and in 30%, arrhythmias could be excluded as reason for the mentioned symptoms. Among asymptomatic patients (26 patients), in seven patients, arrhythmias like supraventricular tachycardia (> 120 bpm), sinus bradycardia (< 45 bpm) frequent and complex PVC's and paroxysmal atrial fibrillation could be recognized during HM.

ECG-Telephone-Telemetry (TTM, Figure 3)
32 patients experienced symptoms while they had the possibility to transmit their ECG per telephone and called up the clinic successfully. In 24 of these patients, arrhythmias could be recognized and in 8 patients practically excluded.

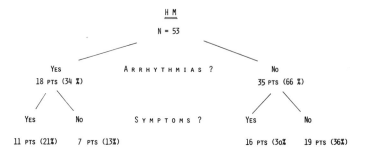

Fig. 1   **Arrythmias during HM.**

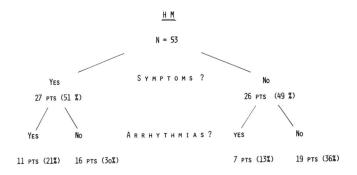

Fig. 2   **Symptoms during HM.**

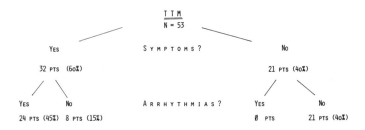

Fig. 3   **Symptoms and arrythmias during TTM.**

21 patients did not develop symptoms during TTM, so that only scheduled routine calls were done without any recognizable rhythm disturbance.

Arrhythmias transmitted during ECG–TTM were sinus tachycardia (100–150 bpm) in 9 patients, 5 episodes of symptomatic SVPC's, 7 episodes of PVC's; sinus bradycardia (< 50 bpm) occurred in 2 patients; also in 2 patients, paroxysmal atrial fibrillation and in one patient, a supraventricular tachycardia > 150 bpm were present. Three patients suffered from more than one arrhythmia.

Discussion

HM is the method of choice for discovering arrhythmias, which occur at least once during the monitoring period of one day (Figure 4). In 34% of our group, arrhythmias could be recognized during HM, in 13%, they occurred asymptomatically.

The application of TTM depends on the patient's symptoms and their duration (6). They have to be so long-lasting that a telephone connection could be established (Figure 4). 51% of our patients used the TTM successfully during their typical symptomatic period. It seems evident that minor rhythm disturbances like sinus bradycardia etc. may lead to severe patient-irritating symptoms in 22%. Having achieved a symptom-synchronous-ECG registration with TTM, arrhythmias could be excluded in 29% as the reason for the patient's symptoms.

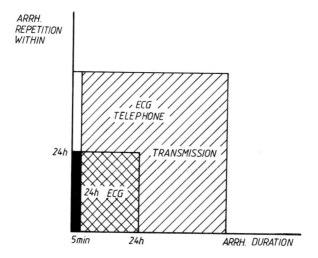

Fig. 4   Diagram illustrating the overlapping coverage of symptomatic arrhythmias provided by the use of TTM and 24-hour-Holter monitoring. Short-lasting, symptomatic arrhythmias (<5 min., i.e. mean TTM-connection time) of a high reoccurence frequency (min. one phenomenon/day) could only be captured using HM (pure black field), whereas rare arrhythmias (<1/day) will remain undiscovered despite the application of both methods used (pure white field) (6)

This group, and the 30% of the patients who developed symptoms during HM, but without simultaneous arrhythmias, point out the importance of psychological factors in the genesis of symptoms, which could be also demonstrated in 12 patients (22%), who never developed typical symptoms either during HM or TTM.

The aim, a symptom-synchronous-ECG-registration, could be obtained in 17% with HM only and in 27% with TTM only, whereas the complementary method failed.

In 34% of the patients, each method led to success, but with conflicting results in 17%: once arrhythmias could be found as reason for their symptoms, once no arrhythmias could be detected during typical symptoms.

In 12 patients, (23%), both methods failed to reach our diagnostic aim.

But only in 5 patients (9%) with a symptomatic history, neither did symptoms occur during HM and/or TTM, nor could asymptomatic arrhythmias be found during HM.

So the application of both methods reduced the white field (Figure 4) of undiscovered symptomatic arrhythmias (6).

Conclusions

In patients with symptoms in their history possibly related to arrhythmias, HM alone was successful in 50% and TTM in 2/3 to obtain a synchronous ECG/symptom registration. The combined application of both methods led in 3/4 to a full success. In 29 patients, 71% of this group, the reasons for symptoms were arrhythmias, whereas in the remaining 29% rhythm disturbances could be excluded. In only 9% of the total with a symptomatic history did both methods fail, because of absent symptoms and failure to detect asymptomatic arrhythmias in HM.

The value of HM depends on the frequeny of arrhythmias, the value of TTM on the duration of symptoms. Both methods are useful tools to reduce the white field of undiscovered, symptomatic arrhythmias.

Acknowledgements

We are indebted to Mrs. Marina Vukovic, Mrs. Trude Haagen, Mrs. Ulrike Grojer and Mrs. Angela Reich for their assistance in analysing the records. This work was supported, in part, by the Austrian Heart Foundation and the Austrian "Fonds zur Förderung der Wissenschaften".

References

1.   Grodman R.S., Capone R.J., Most A.S. (1979) Am. Heart J. **98**,459.
2.   Abdon N.J., Lecerof H., Johansson D.D. (1980) Pace **2**, 94.
3.   Joskowicz G., Balatka H., Glogar D., Weber H., Steinbach K. In: IEEE-Proc. of Comp. in Card. p. 277, Geneva, 1979.
4.   Weber HJ., Joskowicz G., Glogar D., Steinbach K. Probst P., Kaindl F. Continuous quality control in longterm ECG evaluation, ISAM 1981. (In press).

5.   Weber H., Glogar D., Joskowicz G., Pfundner P., Steinbach
      K.(1979) In: Telemetry of the Cardiovascular System; Ed. J.
      Bachmann, Erlangen   (In press).
6.   Weber H., Steinbach K., Joskowicz G., Glogar D., Kaindl F.(1980)
      Am. Heart. J. **100**, 764.

Discussion

DR. van DURME: What symptoms were found in these 53 patients?

DR. SCHEIBELHOFER: They had mostly palpitations and dizziness. One
patient complained of syncope, but did not have any cause during
monitoring.

DR. van DURME: When the ECG information reaches you, how is it
possible to decide whether there was causal relationship?

DR. SCHEIBELHOFER: The patients are given a diary which they are
obliged to keep, and they write down the symptoms they experience and
the time is on the tape so we can correlate symptom and ECG to the
minute.

DR. OAKLEY: Is there a system by which the patient can talk down the
telephone at the time he has the symptoms? That would be a very
simple way of correlating symptoms with the time.

DR. SCHEIBELHOFER: I understood that the first question related to
the Holter monitoring. In telephone transmission, it is very easy;
the patient dials our number, talks with us, tells us that he has a
symptom and asks us to record it. We push a button, he puts the
electrodes on his chest and this gives the ECG. If the quality is
bad, we can tell him not to press so hard, or to put some jelly on
the electrodes and so on. He can talk to us on the telephone.

DR. BLUMHARDT: I am not clear about the symptoms. Dr. Scheibelhofer
put up a list of symptoms that the 53 patients had, all together.
But is it possible to correlate negative findings on the recording
with the type of symptoms experienced by the patient. Is there any
predictive value of the symptoms? Other studies have shown that
there is no predictive value in palpitations, for example, and that
they do not correlate with the results found. It might be expected to
find an increase, say, in the non-specific vague dizzy symptoms in
the 29% - were they looked at?

DR. SCHEIBELHOFER: We could have looked at that, but it has not yet
been done.

DR. DAVIES: I do not think that Dr. Scheibelhofer is justified in
calling sinus tachycardia an arrhythmia. It could, after all, be a
normal response to anxiety.

DR. SCHEIBELHOFER: These were patients who were at rest. There was
no occasion on which somebody was running, had symptoms and tele-
phoned us. These were events experienced when a patient was watching
television, for instance, and they were the kind of symptoms that the
patient always had. When a patient called us, we were able to say,
perhaps, that this is only sinus tachycardia - but for such a patient, this is a symptom, and this is an arrhythmia, if it occurs at
rest. It is very irritating for the patient, and the sinus tachycardia explains his symptoms.

PROF. FELDMAN: Are there any plans to use more permanent electrodes
and some kind of a memory unit?

DR. SCHEIBELHOFER: Yes, that would be wonderful - but at the moment, we do not have the technology to do it.

DR. RICH: Since most patients have periods of dysrhythmia that last for less than five minutes, surely it must be impossible to record most of the periods of dysrhythmia experienced by these patients.

DR. SCHEIBELHOFER: That was not our impression. There were only two instances of arrhythmia, which was already over. This did not happen with most of the patients, who said that they had the arrhythmia at that moment and could we please record it.

PROF. DR. POOL: One of our problems is patient education. More than half our patients are over 65 - or even over 70. It is very difficult to teach them even to press a simple button, such as an event marker. Probably about half the patients over 65 or 70 cannot do that, and information is obtained only by taking a history when they bring back their Holter monitor. What is Dr. Scheibelhofer's experience?

DR. SCHEIBELHOFER: Our mean age was 51, but the range was 18 to 73. It is quite easy to carry out the telephone transmission because all the patients have to do is to dial our number, take an electrode mounted on a piece of plastic and put it on their bare chest. They are motivated to do it, because they are so troubled by their symptoms.

PANEL DISCUSSION

DR. MILES: I would be very interested in comments about electrodes.
Dr. van Durme mentioned that that is one of the critical aspects of
long-term recording. We have an interest in recording patients for
several weeks at a time and have found only one electrode was tolerated for more than a few days, a relatively new electrode which was
developed in Japan by Lectec and is made of the sort of gum arabic
that used to be put around colostomy bags. It is a totally different
proposition from any other electrode that I have ever tried. They get
rather messy but there is no need to abrade the skin - one lady we
had was able to wear one of these electrodes continuously for three
months.
DR. MURRAY: I do not know this electrode, but I am sure part of the
reason for having so few problems with it is that there is no need to
abrade the skin. Could Dr. Miles comment on the quality of the
signal?
DR. MILES: It has been used by many of the cardiologists at Stanford, who are rather impressed with it, particularly over long periods of time. The skin does not have to be prepared - and the signal
becomes better when a patient perspires.
DR. SOUTHALL: For babies and young children, whose skin is very
sensitive, we are looking at the moment, at a carbon electrode made
in the United States which can be sewn into a vest, and which con-
tacts the skin using only water. This seems to work and may be one
answer to long-term ECG monitoring.
        Dr. van Durme mentioned that in the clinical evaluation of
therapy for arrhythmias, Holter monitoring is not very important in
older patients. But Holter monitoring is valuable in infants and very
small children, who obviously cannot describe their symptoms
DR. van DURME: I fully agree. I did not mean to say that it was
useless. The message I wanted to get across is that it is a mistake
to believe that one needs Holter recording to assess the efficacy of
antiarrhythmic therapy in most symptomatic patients. I agree that
some of the patients either cannot describe their symptoms, or may
even have the arrhythmia without having any symptoms. Coronary
patients are very prone to that type of event. But in most patients
with symptomatic arrhythmias, the efficacy [of treatment] can be
assessed directly from the patients themselves. Let us take the
example of someone who shows paroxysmal atrial fibrillation - a
Holter recording is carried out, the diagnosis is established, the
patient is treated and he becomes asymptomatic. Then another Holter
recording is carried out, and there are still episodes of premature
atrial contractions - is the therapy going to be changed? Most
clinicians would say that they would not, but I would like to hear
what other people have to say about that.
DR. SOUTHALL: I completely agree with Dr. van Durme, but all this
fundamentally comes down to what is normal in the ambulatory recording of an adult, and where do normal or harmless arrhythmias overlap
with those arrhythmias that are harmful and which cause symptoms.

DR. van DURME: Would you not agree that in clinical practice a
normal arrythmia could be defined as one that does not induce symptoms and is not dangerous for the patient? There we come back to the
example of the sinus tachycardia. In some patients, it will induce
symptoms, but if it is asymptomatic its relevance becomes a matter
for clinical research.
DR. SOUTHALL: I would agree that if it is asymptomatic, it is perhaps not necessary to treat it. To answer the question whether it is
dangerous, prospective studies are needed - which have not been done.
DR. BALASUBRAMANIAN: The whole concept of whether to treat asymptomatic or symptomatic arrhythmias is in a state of turmoil. I do not
think that most people would now agree about treating asymptomatic
arrhythmias in ambulant patients. The whole concept of what is
dangerous and what is not has been developed from coronary care data.
There is very little epidemiological data based entirely on asymptomatic patients, even with ventricular tachycardia or ectopics. What
is the long-term prognosis, and is it changed by giving antiarrhythmic therapy? We still do not have the answer, and more work is
needed to produce it.
DR. SCHEPPOKAT: With regard to the paper by Mr.J. Jirak on real-time
analysis of ECG, if I understand correctly, there is an urgent need
for data reduction using this method at the earliest possible moment.
The 24-hour ECG contains at least two sets of information, one about
the arrhythmias as they are known in the textbooks (the Lown classification and so on), and the other about heart-rate behaviour. This
is not in the textbooks. This information is displayed by
conventional methods of processing by histograms, trend recordings
and so on, and we do not know much about that.
     Later in this symposium, there is a long session on blood
pressure variability. In the future, it might be very interesting to
have a symposium on heart-rate variability. The data on this subset
of information should not be omitted before rather more is known
about it. I would hesitate to use a system in which everything
possible has to be done for arrhythmia detection, while all other
data contained in the 24-hour ECG recording is ignored.
MR. T. JIRAK: The real-time system also stores trends of heart-rates
(although I did not show the relevant slides) in so far as it gives
the average, in this instance over 10 minute intervals, the minimum
and the maximum of the 4-beat averages of the rate. Histograms of
that are also given. I agree with Dr. Scheppokat; there is information to be found, both in the trends and in the stability of the
rate, that is not shown in samples alone.
DR. BALASUBRAMANIAN: It is extremely important to study the heart-
rate variability and the heart-rate itself. This has not been done
in the great detail with which blood pressure variability has been
investigated. If there is a place for ambulatory monitoring in a
patient with chronic stable angina, one is the study of the heart
rates. We have clearly demonstrated (and have presented the data)
that in the early morning (6.00 a.m. to 8.00 a.m.) the heart-rate
increases so much that most of the patients have early morning
angina. Thus, if the information is to be used clinically, a 24-hour
heart rate pattern is extremely important.
DR. MILES: Heart rate has certainly been very useful and interesting
to us in a sleep disorders' clinic because the R-R interval histogram

is one of the best ways of screening for obstructive sleep apnoea, a potentially lethal disorder. But there are many other applications too. Workers with whom we are collaborating at Stanford have calibrated patients on treadmills for their change in pulse rate with physical activity, as monitored by a motion sensor at different levels of activity. They have been able to derive a formula by which people can be categorised into different states throughout 24 hours or a week of monitoring - states such as anxiety, exercise, down-time and artefacts.

DR. SOUTHALL: Surely, the question [by Dr. Scheppokat] was pointing towards the suggestion that we should be collecting 24 hours of data, but perhaps trying to analyse it in two ways: first, automatically to relieve pressure on the operator and, second, semi-automatically, leaving the doctor or the operator only a small amount to look at. In other words, we are talking about a combination of event and of scanning-recordings.

DR. van DURME: Along the same line of thought, what Dr. Murray is presenting agrees with that idea. Does Dr. Murray have data on the performance of such a system in his unit?

DR. MURRAY: No, we do not - it is all qualitative feeling. It has had to be introduced because of pressure, and so there has not been the chance to do the assessment. We are trying now to collect some figures. It is being introduced very gradually; probably less than 20% of our recordings are looked at in this way.

DR. van DURME: But did I understand correctly, that it is not an all-or-none system? It is not either the search unit system or the regular Holter unit system?

DR. MURRAY: The patients are selected whom we want to analyse purely for search events. Once it has been decided that we want to look at a particular event or time, we will find that event and once it is found, it will be analysed - so it is back to the Holter system to do the analysis of a selected portion of the recording. Normally, we try to find the time, perhaps one hour before the event,and then scan through for that hour and the hour after the event. This is about 2-minutes' worth of scanning.

Dr. van DURME: What about the other situation in which the patient is selected for the search unit on the basis of the information available about him, and who does not have any symptom during the recording? Is that tape not analysed?

DR. MURRAY: It depends on how sure we are that we have got the patient information correct. If there is any doubt, if it is possible that the patient has been given the wrong time or seems uncertain [about it], the whole recording is analysed.

DR. van DURME: If you are sure that the information given by the patient is correct and that he had no symptom during the recording, the tape would not be analysed?

DR. MURRAY:That is right. That would be reported as the patient saying that he had symptoms at this particular time, that the tape had been analysed from a time preceding to a time after [the symptoms], and that there were no arrhythmias. It is then a clinical decision whether further analysis is needed.

DR. van DURME: That is a very interesting approach. There are pros and cons to it, but from a clinical point of view it might help to solve some problems - also the problems of the cost of personnel, the

limitations in the numbers of ECG recorders available and so on.
DR. MURRAY: We are introducing it very cautiously and would like to
hear comments from people at this meeting.
PROF. FELDMAN: It is a problem which we all have. The other side of
it, of course, is that often symptomatic patients do not have those
symptoms during the 24 hours of recording. There is a lot of data in
this recording which can be used inferentially, maybe incorrectly.
The person might not have his paroxysmal atrial fibrillation, but he
may well have a great number of supraventricular premature beats - so
it can be inferred that it is probably supraventricular rather than
ventricular, or vice-versa. I do not know how true this might be.
The method described is useful, but I wonder whether information in
those cases is not being thrown away which is perhaps 75% reliable
anyway?
DR. MURRAY: Certainly, information is being thrown away, but I think
a lot of what is thrown away is not used anyway.

COMPUTER ASSISTED LONGTERM ECG ANALYSIS IN PATIENTS WITH MITRAL VALVE PROLAPSE SYNDROME

W. EBM, H. WEBER. M. KLICPERA, D. GLOGAR, G. JOSKOWICZ,
P. PROBST, K. STEINBACH AND F. KAINDL

Kardiologische Universitats-Klinik Wien, Austria

Summary

Twenty-nine patients with mitral valve prolapse (MVP) were compared to a sex and age-matched group consisting of twenty-one healthy people. Both groups underwent on the one hand, M-mode and 2D-echocardiography to exclude or confirm MVP with special regard to the prolapsing leaflet (anterior, posterior or both). On the other hand 24-hours' ambulatory longterm ECG recordings with computer assisted analysis were performed with qualitative and quantitative description of arrhythmias present.

MVP patients demonstrated in 76% a significantly higher incidence in the occurrence of single premature ventricular contractions ($p < 0.005$) and complex ventricular arrhythmias ($p < 0.02$) independent of age. A tendency of a higher frequency of arrhythmias could be found in patients with MVP of the posterior mitral leaflet compared to the prolapsing anterior or both leaflets.

Introduction

During the past decade, idiopathic mitral valve prolapse (MVP) has emerged as the "most common valvular disorder" probably affecting about 4% of the population (1-4). The prognosis in BVP is generally favourable. However, the course of this syndrome can infrequently be complicated by malignant arrhythmias and sudden death (5, 6). In familial studies sudden death has been reported in relatives of the propositi (5, 6). Besides ventricular fibrillation and tachycardias, extreme bradycardias were documented in rare cases. However, the reasons of these arrhythmias are still unknown. Myocardial or mechanical courses will be discussed (7, 8).

The routine use of echocardiography (ECHO) and ambulatory longterm ECG recordings (HM) facilitated substantially the diagnosis of MVP and the evaluation of accompanying arrhythmias.

The aim of this study was to investigate the frequency and quality of ventricular arrhythmias using a computer-supported HM-analysis and to test a probable dependency of arrhythmias from the quality of MVP in 2D-Echo.

Patients and Methods

29 patients (19 females, 10 males) with a mean age of 41 ± 14 years (18-68 years) with an echocardiographic and/or angiographic documented MVP introduced the study.

These patients were compared with a respective age and sex-

matched collective of 21 healthy people (13 females and 8 males) with
an age range from 12 - 52 years (m 35 ± 12 years). In the latter
group MVP was excluded by 2D-Echo.

Thus both groups underwent M-mode and 2D-echocardiography and
also one 24-hour ambulatory longterm ECG recording.

Echocardiography

Echocardiograms were performed with a commercially available dynamically focused phased sector scanner. The two-dimensional studies were
done in ventricular long axis with careful examination of the entire
mitral valve by sweeping the echo plane laterally to medially so that
all abnormalities may be detected.

The following sonographic criteria have been referred to the
diagnosis of mitral valve prolapse as described by Gilbert et al
(14):

1.   Displaced posterior coaptation of the mitral leaflets.
2.   Superior motion of either one, or both, mitral leaflets above
the level of the mitral ring in systole, and
3.   Abnormal systolic curling motion of the posterior mitral ring on
its adjacent myocardium.

On the basis of the two-dimensional echo studies, the patients
have been divided into three sub-groups:

Patients with systolic prolapse of both mitral leaflets and
patients with prolapse of the anterior or posterior leaflet only.

Long-Term-ECG (LT-ECG)-Analysis with "Multipass-Scanning":

Using Oxford Medilog recorders and playback units, the tape-
recorded ECG is played back at 60x recording speed. After digitisation and data reduction, using the linear segmentation technique (9),
clinically relevant rhythm diagnoses are built up through multiple
passes of computer processing.

The data presentation includes a summarized printout, histograms and a detailed description of severe arrhythmias with the
possibility of resynthesizing the ECG from the digital data stored on
magnetic disc (10).

Statistics:

The statistical evaluation was done using the Mann-Whitney-
Wilcoxon rank correlation test (11). Complex ventricular arrhythmias
were calculated using the Xi or Chi-square Test (12).

Complex ventricular arrhythmias were defined as couplets,
triplets and ventricular tachycardias.

Results

1.   Heart rate (Figure 1).
No difference could be found in the mean heart rate of hourly
segments between both groups. To exclude age-related arrhythmias, we
divided the populations into two groups, younger than 40 years of age
and older. Despite the separation no difference could be found in
heart rate behaviour.

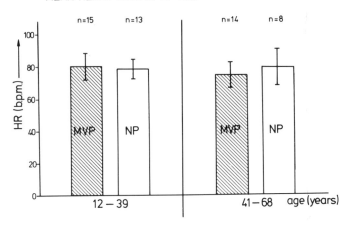

Fig. 1   No significant differences in the mean heart rate (±
           standard deviations) occurred between normal person (NP)
           and the MVP-group independent from the age (12–39 vs.
           41–68).

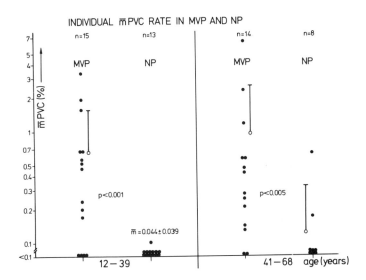

Fig. 2   m PVC rate (%) is the mean percentage on the total amount
           of detected heart beats during the total 24 hours LT-ECG
           period.

2.   Premature ventricular contractions (Figure 2)
      The mean PVC rate is defined as the percentage of PVC's on the
total amount of detected heart beats during 24-hour LT-ECG. No PVC's
could be found in 86% of the normals, but only in 26% of patients
with MVP. The mean PVC rate did not exceed 1%/24 hours (13) in the
normal group, whereas 6 patients with MVP had a PVC rate of more than
1%/24 hours. The mean PVC rates were statistically significantly (p
<0.005) lower in normal persons than in patients with MVP (Figure 2).
      Considering relationship with age, the younger normal persons
were quasi-completely free from PVC's. In the rank correlation test,
a highly significant difference between both younger groups occurred
(p < 0.001). A similar behaviour of the PVC rate could be found also
in the older groups (p < 0.005) (Figure 3). So in MVP-patients, more
PVC's could be found in LT-ECG than in normals (p < 0.005).

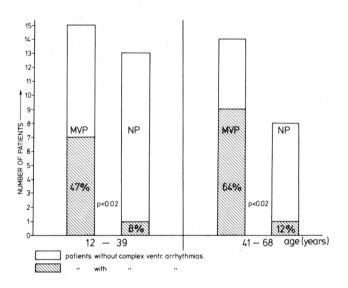

Fig. 3   Complex ventricular arrhythmias in MVP and NP.

3.   Complex ventricular arrhythmias (Figure 3)
      Ventricular couplets, triplets and other complex ventricular
arrhythmias occurred significantly (p < 0.02) more often in MVP
patients, i.e. in 47% of the younger MVP, against only one patient
of the NP (p < 0.02) group, and in 64% of the older patients with
MVP, also against only one normal patient (p < 0.02).

4.   Quality of MVP (Figure 4)
      Two-dimensional echo enables a qualitative classification of MVP
with higher specificity and accuracy than the M-mode technique (14).
In 21% of MVP patients the anterior, in 27% the posterior, and in the
remaining 52% both leaflets could be found prolapsing into the left

atrium. The PVC rates did not differ significantly between those
groups, but a tendency to higher PVC rates could be found in patients
with a prolapsing posterior leaflet. A further distribution relating
complex ventricular arrhythmias and the quality of MVP failed because
of a too small number of MVP's.

Conclusion

Using a computer-assisted analysis system, we could confirm the
higher incidence of PVC's in patients with MVP during 24-hours LT-ECG
(1,5,6). In comparison to an age and sex-matched healthy group, 22
patients with MVP (76%) demonstrated an increased PVC rate. Considering the higher PVC incidence in elderly persons, we could not find
significant PVC-differences between the younger and older people as
within NP as MVP. So, the PVC rate seems age independent, but depends on the presence or absence of a MVP.

Complex ventricular arrhythmias demonstrate a similar behaviour
and occur in our MVP group more frequently. They are well-known as
precursors of sudden death (7). Patients with MVP and late or pan-
systolic murmur are at higher risk of sudden death during longterm
follow up (8).

The question, if patients with a prolapsing posterior leaflet,
who demonstrate a tendency to more frequent ventricular and complex
arrhythmias compared with isolated anterior or both-leaflet prolapse,
have a higher incidence of sudden arrhythmogenic death, will be
examined in future investigations.

Acknowledgement

We are indebted to Mrs. Angela Reich, Mrs. Ulrike Grojer, Mrs. Ingrid
Teufelhart, Mrs. Trude Haagen and Mrs. Marina Vukovic, for their
assistance in analysing the records. This work was supported in part
by the Austrian Heart Foundation and the Austrian "Fonds zur
Forderung der Wissenschaften".

References

1.   Jeresaty R.M. (1973) Progress. Cardiovasc. Dis. **15**, 623-652.
2.   Malcolm A.D., Bonghauer D.R. Kostuk W.J. et al (1976) Br. Heart
     J. **38**, 244-256.
3.   Scampardonis G., Yong, S.S. Maranhaw V. et al (1973) Circulation
     48, 287-297.
4.   Cohen M., Pocock W.A., Lackier J.B.,McLaren M.J., Lachmann A.S.,
     Barlow J.B. (1978) Am. Heart J. **95**, 697.
5.   Kock F.H., Hancock E.W. (1976) Am. J. Cardiol. (Abstr.) **37**,149.
6.   Shell W.E., Walton J.A., Clifford M.E. et al (1969) Circulation
     39, 327-337.
7.   Gulotta S.J., Gulco L., Padmanabhan V., Miller S. (1974) Circu-
     lation **49** 717.
8.   Cobbs B.W., King S.B. (1977) Am. Heart J. **93**, 741.
9.   Joskowicz G., Balatka H., Glogar D., Weber H., Steinbach K. A
     high speed Holter-Tape analysis with full editing capability.
     In: IEEE-Proc. Comp. in Card., 277, Geneva, 1979.
10. Weber H., Joskowicz G., Glogar D., Steinbach K., Probst P.,

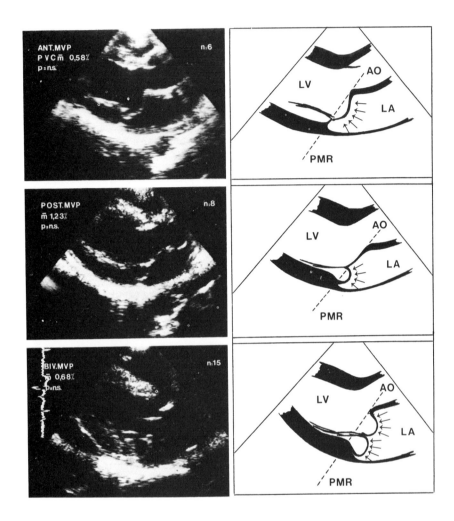

Fig. 4   2D-Echo of MVP.

Leg: Ant.MVP = prolapse of the anterior leaflet of the mitral
           valve.
           Post. MVP = prolapsing posterior leaflet.
           BIV. MVP = both leaflets are prolapsing.
           PVCm = mean rate of premature ventricular contractions
                   during LT-ECG, no statistical significant
                   difference (p=n.s.) between the MVP quality could
                   be found.
           LV = left ventricle, AO = aortic root, LA = left atrium.
           PMR = plain of the mitral ring.

Kaindle F.: Continuous quality control in longterm ECG evaluation. ISAM 1981. In press.
11. Mann H.B., Whitney D.R. (1947) Ann. Math. Statist. **18**, 60-60.
12. Sachs L. Angewandte Statistik p. 269, Springer-Verlag 1975
13. Weber H., Glogar D., Joskowicz G., Steinbach K. (1981) Z.Kardiol. **70**, 13.
14. Gilbert B.W., Schatz R.A., Von Ramm O.T., Behar V.S., Kisslo J.A. (1976) Circulation **54**, 716-1723.
15. Bluschke W., Kohler E., Seipel L., Lenner Ch. (1979) Z. Kardiol. 396-403.
16. Yahini J.H., Vered Zvi, Atlas P., Neufeld H.N.(1980) Selected Topics in Card. Arrhythmias **26** 323-329.
17. Jeresaty R.M.: Mitral valve prolapse, Raven Press (1979).
18. Mills P., Rose J., Hollingsworth B.A. et al.(1977) New England Med. J. **297**, 13-18.

Discussion

PROF. CONTINI: Have any ST segment alterations been found in these patients with mitral valve prolapse?
DR. EBM: Some ST segment variations were found in the normal ECG, but they were not looked for in the long-term ECG.
DR. DAVIES: Were the ventricles all normal? The two-dimensional echocardiograms (it was presumably a systolic frame) looked as though the ventricle was not contracting very well, with a large end-systolic volume.
DR. EBM: The slide that I showed was not from any particular patient in the programme.
PROF. FELDMAN: There is certainly an interesting question about the cause of the PVC's in this case. One of the clues might be the anatomical origin. Has Dr. Ebm the ability to measure vectors with his system? I think that Lichlin has a publication on vectorcardiogram and mitral valve prolapse. (Dr. Ebm was able to do that with his system).
DR. van DURME: Are you able to record orthogonal leads with your system?
PROF. FELDMAN It is certainly possible to deal with two orthogonal leads. About 5 or 6 years ago, we showed that this is sufficient to distinguish left from right, or apical from outflow trace ectopics.
DR. HORNUNG: I think that Dr. Ebm said that there was no difference in supraventricular ectopics - I was surprised by that statement.
DR. EBM: In the long-term ECG it is not easy to detect supraventricular beats. In our study, when we looked at the supraventricular beats, there was no difference.
DR. van DURME: There were no episodes of supraventricular tachycardia or atrial fibrillation in any of the patients?
DR. EBM: No, in none of them.
DR. BLEICHER: Has the variability of the heart rate been investigated in these patients? We have found that mitral valve prolapse patients show significantly more variability than normal patients.
DR. EBM: That is right - but in this study we looked only at the average heart rate over the 24 hours.

LONG-TERM OESOPHAEGEAL RECORDING IN THE ANALYSIS OF SUPRAVENTRICULAR ARRHYTHMIA

R. ARZBAECHER*, S. COLLINS*, M. MIRRO*, J. JENKINS**

*University of Iowa, **University of Michigan, USA

Introduction

Existing systems for ambulatory ECG recording focus on ventricular arrhythmias. This paper describes our system for long-term monitoring of supraventricular arrhythmias. Obviously, finding the P-wave is the key to the technique. Five years ago, we reported a swallowable electrode for recording the electrocardiogram from the oesophagus, just behind the left atrium. This electrode produces very sharp, well-defined P-waves and thus makes possible the recognition of supraventricular arrhythmias in ambulatory monitoring.

Method

The pill electrode consists of two metal pieces separated by an insulator and attached to a pair of thread-like wires. It is enclosed in an ordinary pharmaceutical capsule for swallowing. The patient is told to ignore the wire and swallow the pill, with water, in the usual way. In a few minutes, the electrode descends to the level of the atrium, the capsule dissolves, and the technician tapes the wire to the face to keep it from descending further. The wire is then connected to the electrocardiograph and the technician pulls the wire through the tape to raise the electrode, while observing the tracing. When the P-wave is 3 or 4 times bigger than QRS, the wire is taped more securely and a surface lead is connected for recording a second channel. Figure 1 shows a typical recording with the oesophageal lead at the top, and the surface lead at the bottom. Large P-waves and small QRS complexes are evident in the oesophageal trace.

Results

We have recently undertaken two studies, using this technique: the determination of the number of atrial premature beats, each hour, in patients being treated with a new anti-arrhythmic drug, and capturing the onset of supraventricular tachycardia. In the first study, patients are recorded for 5 to 7 days, with the pill-electrode being replaced each day. The patients eat, drink, sleep, shower and are completely ambulatory. Each day, the 24-hour tape is removed and loaded onto the hospital scanner and copied at high speed onto an FM tape for off-line computer analysis.

Figure 2 shows a hardware trigger circuit we have developed to detect P-waves from the oesophageal channel played back at 60 times real time. The ECG is bandpass filtered from 16-40 Hz (with respect to real time) with attentuation outside this range of 60 dB/decade. The signal is then differentiated and passed through an absolute value circuit and a dead space circuit, which is set to eliminate 60

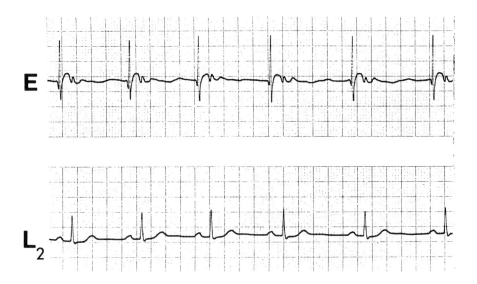

Fig. 1 Recording from the pill–electrode (top) and Lead II, showing large, distinct P–waves in the esophageal trace.

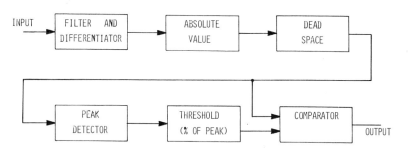

Fig. 2 Block diagram of circuit used to detect P–waves in the oesophageal channel.

Hz noise and the other high frequency, low amplitude signals. Some or all of the ventricular activity in the oesophageal ECG is also eliminated. The signal then passes through a peak detector, which follows the peak value of the incoming P–waves. The output of this circuit decays with a time constant of 2/3 seconds. The output of the threshold circuit is simply an adjustable fraction of the peak detector output and is compared to the current ECG. When the current signal crosses the threshold, an output pulse is produced, indicating a detected P–wave. As can be seen in the figure, the threshold depends upon the amplitude of the previous P–wave. This variable threshold provides an automatic gain control mechanism, which allows compensation for the changes in P–wave amplitude, which occur as the electrode moves about the oesophagus.

During the computer scan a strip chart recording is automatically produced whenever a PAC is detected on the oesophageal channel. Since we have a short delay loop, this allows us to capture the event about four beats before it occurs. Figure 3 shows a case, where the chart recorder was speeded up when a PAC was detected (5th P-wave from the left). In this case, the PAC was conducted, but when conduction to the ventricles is blocked, the technique still permits the PAC to be detected and counted, which is not possible, with surface recordings alone.

Our PAC study revealed cases of ventricular tachycardia, which prompted us to begin our second study: capturing on tape the onset of a tachycardia in the hope of deducing the underlying electrophysiology, without full electrophysiological workup in the catheterization laboratory.

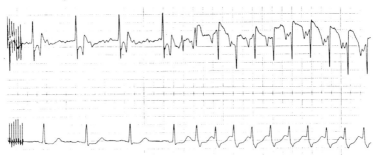

Fig. 3   Recording produced during tape playback upon computer detection of a premature atrial contraction (PAC), the fifth complex in the esophageal trace at the top.

Figure 4 shows a patient suffering from recurrent episodes of syncope. After two normal sinus beats, the patient has a slightly shortened PR interval, indicating a junctional beat: i.e. depolarization begins in the atrio-ventricular junction and spreads down to the ventricles through the usual conduction system, thus producing a normal QRS in the surface lead. An accelerated junctional rhythm is then maintained and at the seventh beat, the P-wave changes dramatically and appears after QRS. This indicates that the atria are no longer being depolarized from the sinus node, but from the A-V node, in a retrograde fashion. During electrophysiological study in the catheterization laboratory, the rhythm was indeed shown to originate in the A-V node.

In Figure 5, the oesophageal lead is seen on the lower channel and the surface lead on the upper. After 3 normal beats, a run of four fast atrial beats develops, only two of which are conducted to the ventricles. A diagnosis from the surface lead is difficult, but from the oesophagus, it is clearly atrial flutter, following which the sinus node recovers, and then another paroxysm of atrial flutter occurs. This patient's brief bouts of flutter, with variable conduction to the ventricles and, therefore, an irregular heart rate, had been called atrial fibrillation for years, but on the oesophageal trace it is clear that atrial depolarization is highly organized and no fibrillation is present.

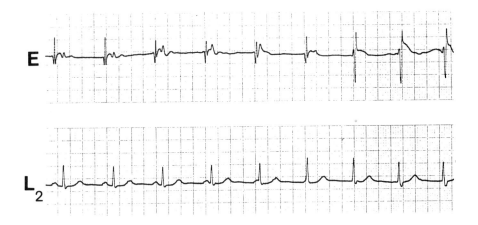

Fig. 4   Recording made during an episode of accelerated A–V junctional rhythm.

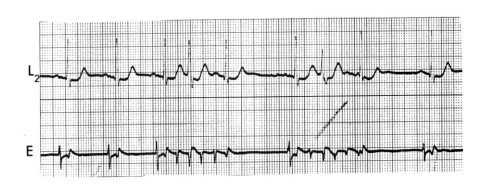

Fig. 5   Paroxysmal atrial flutter, evident on the lower (oesophageal) channel.

Figure 6 is an example of a supraventricular tachycardia in which the onset has been easily located on the Holter tape. After 3 normal beats, a PAC occurs and the tachycardia begins with an RP interval exceeding 100 msec. In the catheterization laboratory, a left-sided tract was found, which only conducted in the retrograde direction.

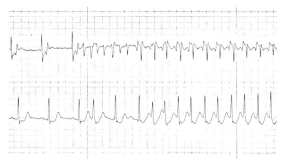

Fig. 6   The onset of a supraventricular tachycardia as viewed from the esophagus (top trace).

Figure 7 shows an accelerated idio-ventricular rhythm with retrograde conduction to the atria. After 3 beats, the sinus node takes over the atria and the ventricles are dissociated. Then in the last three beats, the sinus beats are conducted, though aberrantly. In particular, the first conducted QRS is almost imperceptible.

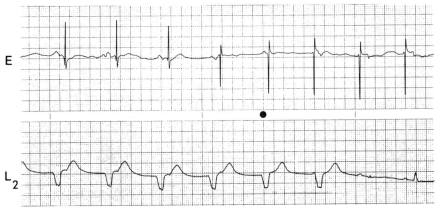

Fig. 7   Idioventricular rhythm in which the esophageal lead shows retrograde conduction to the atria at the left, giving way to sinus node takeover at the right.

Figure 8 is an example of the onset of a wide QRS tachycardia. From the surface lead alone, one might diagnose the arrhythmia as ventricular tachycardia. However, observing the oesophageal lead as well, one would be more cautious and diagnose wide QRS tachycardia

with 1:1 AV relationship, which could be either ventricular tachycardia with retrograde conduction to the atria or atrial tachycardia
with aberrant conduction to the ventricles. The left side of the
figure shows a PVC at beat 3, which clearly kicks off the tachycardia, and the atria simply follow. Thus, the diagnosis of ventricular tachycardia is proven, without going into the catheterization
laboratory to look for a His spike in front of QRS. Long-term oesophageal recording, in which the onset of the tachycardia can be
studied, thus may provide a convenient alternative to catheterization
for the diagnosis of some arrhythmias.

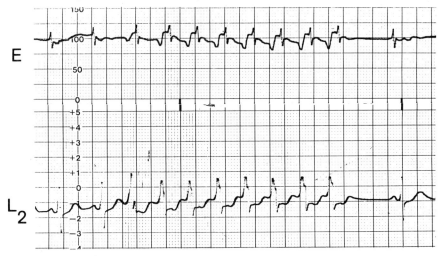

Fig. 8   Ventricular tachycardia with 1:1 V—A conduction, initiated
          by a PVC.

Conclusions

We have developed a simple, painless way of recording atrial ECG's
from the oesphagus. Instead of a bulky and uncomfortable naso-
gastric tube, we use a tiny electrode suspended from a pair of very
thin wires. This technique allows, for the first time, long-term ECG
monitoring with prominent P-waves. Techniques based on surface recordings alone cannot give conclusive data about atrial and nodal
arrhythmias. Thus, we think our method is a practical answer to the
problem of analysis of supraventricular arrhythmias in drug studies
or in routine diagnosis.
      Because of peristalsis, some movement of the electrode occurs
during long-term studies, and thus the amplitude of the oesophageal
ECG varies. This paper presents a trigger circuit, which helps to
detect P-waves as amplitude changes and when artefact corrupts the
signal. However, this still remains a difficult problem and our PAC
detector cannot operate automatically over long periods, without
false or failed triggers. But when manual over-read is added, the
system is quite capable of quantifying supraventricular arrhythmias
and provides unambiguous diagnosis of some rather difficult cases,
without catheterization.

Discussion

DR. SCHEPPOKAT: Dr. Jenkins presented one patient with bursts of atrial flutter. Has she seen only one such case? Has this patient been treated with anti-arrhythmic drugs and, if so, was the treatment successful?

DR. JENKINS: The patient was undergoing double-blind placebo-Norpace drug study for supraventricular arrhythmias. The treatment was a failure.

MR. ARZBAECHER: The diagnosis was a success!

DR. van DURME: What other drug was this patient treated with?

MR. ARZBAECHER: Following the study, he was sent home on a combination of quinidine and digitalis, but the side effects of quinidine, which prompted him to enrol in the disopyramide study initially, recurred. He, therefore, remains a treatment failure. For long-term episodes of atrial flutter, he is routinely cardioverted.

DR. van DURME: This type of arrhythmia might very well respond to amiodarone.

DR. SOUTHALL: Has there been the opportunity of using this oesophageal electrode in babies or in young children, in whom on long-term Holter monitoring, there are marked changes in the P-wave during the entire 24 hours? It would be very interesting to know what they mean.

DR. JENKINS: To my knowledge, the youngest child to swallow it was a 10-year old, but I do not believe that any younger chldren have swallowed it. It is very small, so it is possible to use in in young children.

DR. OAKLEY: Is it possible, by careful analysis of the morphology of the P waves, to distinguish between left-sided and right-sided bypasses?

DR. JENKINS: Not necessarily. The morphology will frequently change when there is retrograde activity, but not always - it often depends upon anatomical considerations as well as the direction of the activation.

DR. SCHEIBELHOFER: How many patients could not swallow the electrode? Were there any complications?

DR. JENKINS: There were no complications. I recorded patients in coronary intensive care over a period of about 2 years, and in that time, there was only one failure, who was unable to comprehend the instructions.

DR. van DURME: Was there an opportunity to see how the anti-arrhythmic action of disopyramide, for instance, spreads outwards from the oesophageal lead?...

DR. JENKINS (intervening): I presume that would be possible, but we do not know whether the four patients I studied at Northwestern, were on placebo or Norpace.

DR. van DURME: Among patients with overt atrial fibrillation, paroxysmal atrial flutter and so on, did you have any patients in whom the anti-arrhythmic treatment suppressed the sustained episodes, but in whom there were still short bursts?

DR. JENKINS: In my four patients at Northwestern University, there was absolutely no change observed. We wondered whether they were all on placebo.

DR. van DURME: Did you have the opportunity, Mr.Arzbaecher?

MR. ARZBAECHER: Of my two patients, one was a treatment failure and the other, a treatment success. Both were on disopyramide. The success was a patient, who was bothered by very frequent atrial premature contractions in the absence of sustained tachycardia. I am sorry that I have no information about the persistent tachycardia.

MR. JIRAK: How well has this electrode worked as a pacing electrode in the cases in which it has been tried?

DR. JENKINS: At the University of Michigan, where I am presently working, we are using it for atrial pacing during radionuclide ventriculography. We have done 4 patients, with Wolff-Parkinson-White syndrome trying to find the site of the bypass accessory tract and have been successful with all four. Three normal subjects were investigated in this way, prior to beginning the study, again successfully. At the University of Iowa, 10 patients have been studied, doing atrial pacing with oesophageal electrode.

CARDIAC ARRHYTHMIAS IN PULMONARY SARCOIDOSIS

R. HAYWARD AND N. McI. JOHNSON

Dept. Cardiology and Thoracic Medicine, Middlesex Hospital
London, W1, UK

Introduction

Sarcoidosis is a systemic disease, characterized by the potential for multi-system involvement. Biopsy techniques have provided evidence of occult sarcoid infiltration of organs such as the spleen and liver in cases where other evidence of such involvement has been lacking. Deposition of sarcoid tissue in the heart has been found in between 20% and 30% of cases of sarcoid disease examined at autopsy, a significant proportion of these being unsuspected during life.

In-vivo, diagnosis of cardiac sarcoidosis is important since treatment with corticosteroids, though of uncertain effectiveness, is available and because of prognostic implications. These include recognition of the possible development of one or more of the following major presenting cardiac features of sarcoidosis: major arrhythmias, sudden death, cardiac failure, conducting system damage, myocardial infarction, aneurysm and pericardial disease.

Abnormalities on resting scalar ECG have been observed in cardiac sarcoidosis, and have to some extent been correlated with disease activity. Brief examinations of this kind are not, however, likely to detect significant intermittent disturbances of rhythm, though it is possible that such disturbances may reflect intracardiac sarcoidosis in the absence of significant resting ECG abnormalities, possibly where sarcoid infiltration is either not extensive, or is actually microscopic. Sensitivity of diagnostic techniques available in cardiac sarcoidosis, though not precisely quantified, is plainly limited. It has thus seemed possible that detection of intermittent rhythm disturbance in patients with sarcoidosis not evidently involving the heart, may represent a pointer to the presence of occult cardiac infiltration.

Study Design

We have studied 3 populations of subjects, using 24-hour ambulatory ECG recording and computerised analysis (Pathfinder System) supported by direct analysis by cardiologists of arrhythmias detected, to review this possibility.

Group A consisted of 21 patients with previous pulmonary sarcoidosis, histologically documented, currently judged to be in remission.

Group B consisted of 12 patients with pulmonary sarcoidosis and histological confirmation in whom disease activity persisted.

In both groups of patients, resting 12-lead ECG's were within

normal limits. Ages ranged from 20-59 years, sex ratio was F:M 19:4.
Major disturbances of renal function, calcium and electrolyte balance
were excluded.

Group C consisted of 10 apparently healthy control subjects with
normal resting ECG's with ages spanning approximately the same range
(24-52 years), male:female ratio 6:4.

Findings

Intermittent arrhythmias were detected on 24-hour recording as shown:

Group A   -   Normal 24 hour record : 20
                Arrhythmias : 1 (intermittent 1st degree A-V block)
Group B   -   Normal record : 8
                Arrhythmias : 4 (intermittent sinus arrest, 1.)
                               APB's and paroxysmal AF, 1.
                               Bradycardia-tachycardia syndrome, 1.
                               Multifocal VPB's, 1)
Group C   -   Normal record : 11
                Arrhythmias : 1 (isolated VPB's).

Statistical significance, using X^2 test with Yates correction applied
to the inter-group variation in arrhythmia incidence, is not quite
achieved (greatest X^2 value attained = 2.88), when compared to the
control population, in whom discovery of some rhythm disturbance is
to be expected.

Conclusion

In the light of our current knowledge of myocardial sarcoidosis, it
is clear that microscopic disease may exist without overt expression.
It is also clear that one or two small localised deposits may escape
detection by standard means. Such lesions may, however, be capable
of producing potent materials such as angiotensin converting enzyme,
plasminogen activator, lysozyme, collagenase etc. It is thus not
difficult to envisage circumstances in which small foci of disease
may initiate enough local reaction within the adjacent myocardium to
trigger intermittent rhythm disturbances of the type observed here,
and may if sited near to components of the intracardiac conducting
system produce significant conducution impairment.

Results of this pilot study thus suggest that there may be an
association between arrhythmias and sarcoid disease activity, although it remains possible that inactivated disease may engender
fibrosis over a long time period, ultimately also finding expression
as cardiac arrhythmias. It is clear that precise in-vivo diagnosis
cannot always be made, though radio-isotope and endomyocardial biopsy
techniques do offer some future promise in this regard.

Plainly prolonged monitoring of rhythm provides more information than the static 12-lead ECG. The precise significance of
arrhythmias detected in this way in patients with active and inactive
non cardiac sarcoidosis, who are at risk of granulomatous or fibrotic
cardiac damage, remains to be clarified. Discovery of such arrhythmias can be regarded as an indication for closer supervision in view

of the possible prognostic implications.

Additional data are being gathered from three sources. A larger patient and normal population is being included in the study. Follow up information is being accumulated. Additional diagnostic techniques are being deployed. It is hoped that this will permit evaluation of the question of whether ambulatory ECG recording to detect intermittent arrhythmias represents a valuable additional diagnostic technique in the difficult area of detection of sarcoidosis of the heart.

NEW POSSIBILITIES IN AMBULATORY ECG-MONITORING DURING CHILDHOOD

G. BUDWIG, W. BLEICHER, R. FREY, F.FIDERER, E. EPPLE,
J. APITZ

Department of Cardiology and Institute
of Anaesthesiology,
University of Tuebingen Inst. Biomed. Technik,
Stuttgart, W.Germany

Summary

Most children with arrythmia problems suffer from congenital heart diseases or defects in the polarisation and conduction systems following inflammation or surgery. To indicate and control drug therapy and pacemaker treatment a suitable monitoring system is necessary.

Methods

We use a 2-channel radio telemetry system in order to transmit the original ECG signal and the mean heart rate. For further use only those signals are chosen which show a satisfactory quality. The signals, which are technically indisputable are now treated in two different ways as follows:

1.   The cardiotachogram recording is done with a self-developed arrythmia-detector (1, 2) and a tachogram programme (3). In the course of this process, each RR-interval is measured and recorded beat-to-beat from the ECG. Every two hours a paper output is provided, either as frequency representation (size 15 by 24 cm), or as histogram of the RR-intervals.
2.   As there is no arrhythmia computer which is adapted to the constitution of children, the original signal is aditionally recorded on commercial C120 cassettes. The ECG evaluation is done with a Holter system. We set the alarm limits on 50% prematurity of the mean RR-intervals, for asystolies on 1.5 seconds and for increasing QRS duration on a selectable value.

Thus, the chronological correlation between the original ECG and the course of the instantaneous heart rate pattern in the cardiotachogram can be obtained on a long-term basis. So the cardiotachogram is used as a directory in order to find meaningful changes in heart rhythm.

Results

(A) Babies and infants with supraventricular tachycardia are handicapped in relation to the size and duration of the tachycardia by the sudden possibility of a life-threatening heart insufficiency (4).

Occasionally, tachycardiac phases are followed by phases with

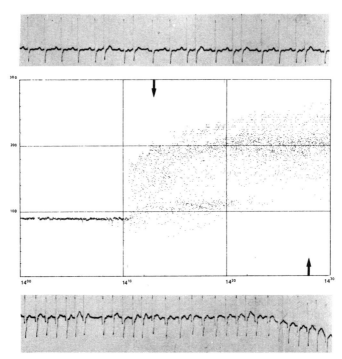

Fig. 1   Development of a premature supraventricular tachycardia.
The cardiotachogram (middle) shows the RR-distances in frequency presentation which arises up from the baseline.   The
ECG evaluates the cloud of tachycardic beats as   premature
and supraventricular.

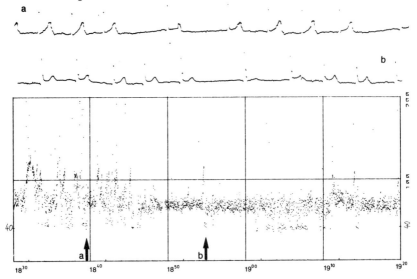

Fig. 2   Sick sinus syndrome in a 16 year old boy: the   cardiotachogram shows a group of bradycardic beats around 40 per minute.   The long term ECG at these times indicates the sinus
bradycardia that needs pacemaker therapy.

chaotic arrhythmias, which can hardly be handled by therapy. The main object of therapy is mostly the decrease in heart rate, which induces the intended increase in stroke volume.

Figure 1 shows a section of a cardiotachogram; the horizontal axis shows the time, the vertical axis, the so-called "instantaneous heart rate". Every point represents one heart action. At 14:10h (2.10 p.m.), we see a sudden strong increase in heart rate variability. In the ECG at 14:13h (2.13 p.m.) premature supraventricular beats can be seen, which are accompanied by a compensatory pause. At 14:28h (2.28 p.m.) the supraventricular tachycardia is completely developed. In this case, the patient was treated successfully with propafenon (Rhythmonorm R).

(B) Bradycardias often show clinical signs (short term Adam-Stokes-syndromes), but they are hard to verify by diagnostic means. However, an exact diagnosis must be given, and the question of therapy by drugs or pacemaker must be answered.

In Figure 2, the cardiotachogram of a 16-year old boy with possible Adam-Stokes-syndrome is demonstrated. In the past, the boy was treated by Orciprenalin-depot tablets (Alupent R-d.-depot 2 x 1 tablet/day) without the reappearance of collapses. A fall from the bicycle forced him to the hospital again.

We recognized a group of low-frequency beats below 40/min between 18:20h (6.20 p.m.) and 19:20h (7:20 p.m.).

Figure 3 shows the histogram representation of the same time interval. It is obvious that 64 beats below 40/min occurred between 18.00h (6.0 p.m.) and 20.00 h (8.0 p.m.) This is equivalent to an RR-interval of more than 1.5 sec. Because of these drops of sinus node activity in a sick sinus syndrome, even under drug-treatment, the boy was equipped with a pacemaker.

(C) To control demand-pacemakers, all of our possible forms of presentation are used. The pacemaker pulses with myocardial answer and the so-called "normal" complexes, which are recognized by our arrhythmia detector, are sampled by the data management system and are plotted in the patient chart together with the overall heart rate (5).

Figure 4 presents an arrhythmia chart in which pacemaker actions per minute are marked with asterisks. The dotted line gives the normal complexes per minute. In absence of other arrhythmic beats, the sum of these two signals gives the solid line of the heart rate. This small patient underwent open heart surgery of a congenital heart defect, and a demand-pacemaker has been implanted. In the post-operative phase, expected drops of the sinus node rhythm occurred, whereby the child remained in good condition. Each drop of sinus node rhythm under 65/min was answered by pacemaker activity, so that heart rate never fell down below 65/min.

The tachogram of one of these events shows in Figure 5 sudden decreases of sinus node rhythm falling down to 65/min., which are followed by a slight over-reaction. In the histogram of the same time span (Figure 6), a second maximum at a heart rate of 65/min - the start rate of the pacemaker - can be recognised.

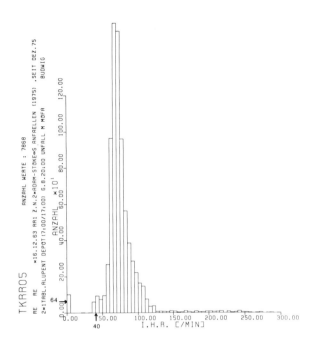

Fig. 3 The histogram of the 2 hour tachogram just shown above reveals that 0.8% of all beats are located below 40/min.

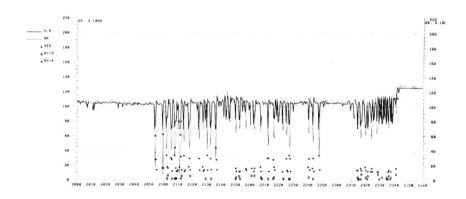

Fig. 4 Arrhythmia chart of pacemaker activity in a postsurgical patient with implanted demand pacemaker: Each drop in sinus node activity (dotted line) is answered by fire of pacemaker (asterisks), so that a normal heart rate is maintained.

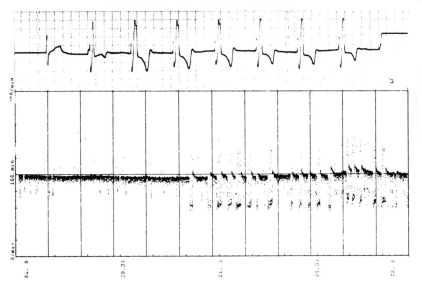

Fig. 5   The tachogram of the same case shows again sudden sinus
          node drops (down) up to 65/min.   In long term ECG we recog-
          nise pacemaker activity at these occasions.

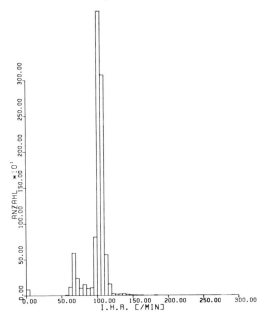

Fig. 6   The corresponding histogram presents beside a main peak at
          a heart rate of 105/min (sinus mode rhythm), a smaller peak
          at 65/min that belongs to pacemaker activity.

Conclusion

In addition to short-term diagnostic ECG interpretation, a long-term control of the heart rhythm is necessary in critically-ill children, especially in those children with heart defects. In parallel to Holter long-term storage, we write simultaneously a cardiotachogram in these cases, which registers every RR-interval on line. This is easy to survey, and we extract from it any special rhythm events and the times corresponding to them, which enables us to inspect the original ECG at this time. In some cases, for example, in pacemaker diagnostic, in bradycardia and tachycardia control, and their quant-itative aspects, the original ECG is not absolutely necessary, while the histogram representation is very useful.

References

1.   Bleicher, W.U. et al.   (1978) Biomed. Technik, **23** Ergaen-
     zungsband 18.1-18.2.
2.   Fiderer F. et al. (1980) Biomed. Technik, **25** Ergaenszungsband,
     124-126.
3.   Hiesinger E. et al. (1977) Biomed. Technik. **22** ,279.
4.   Frey R. et al. Intensive Care Medicine, **6** 83 (229).
5.   Bleicher W. et al. (1977) **22**, 229.

Discussion

DR. SOUTHALL: What Dr. Bleicher is presenting is valid, provided that it is known what is the normal pattern of heart variability in children. Has the technique been used to study a randomly-selected population of children of the age group in which the diagnosis is being made. (Dr. Bleicher had not done so). For example, a per-fectly normal child of 16 can have a heart rate below 40 beat/min with a sinus pause greater than 1.5 sec. What is more, 10% of normal children faint.

DR. BLEICHER: We looked at the boy's normal frequency, then looked at the points, where the heart rate had decreased, and then at the summary of points. It is not a fixed limit of 40 beat/min.

DR. SOUTHALL: You mean that the amount of time that the child is below 40 beat/min is important? (Dr. Bleicher assented) But it is necessary to know the amount of time that a normal 16-year old boy is below 40 beat/min before that test can be interpreted, pacemakers put in, or anti-arrhythmic drugs given.

DR.van DURME: That point is well-taken. There indeed remains a lack of data on "normal" children. All we know is that the heart rate in children is sometimes very variable, especially if the day/night variation is included. I fully agree with Dr. Southall.

DR. SOUTHALL: We now have data on children which shows, I think, that the child could fall within the normal range.

DR. BLEICHER: If there is a normal frequency of, say, 100 beat/min, and the frequency suddenly decreases to 40 beat/min, there is some-thing wrong with the patient.

DR. SOUTHALL: I see that all the time in normal children.

DR. Van DURME: How does Dr.Southall define normality in children?

DR. SOUTHALL: We have looked at over 100 children randomly-selected from schools and maternity hospitals, aged 7 to 11, aged 4 to 7 and 2 days to 14 days, and have performed ambulatory 24-hour tape recordings. These data have been analysed. they are not matched with hospital-based children, who have illness; they are normal children undergoing normal activity.

DR. Van DURME: Were any episodes of supraventricular tachycardia found? I am not talking about sinus tachycardia going up to 180, but paroxysms.

DR. SOUTHALL: In 7 to 11 year-old children, we did not find any supraventricular or ventricular tachycardias. Supraventricular and ventricular premature beats were found, but less than one per hour. Three of the 100-odd children had atrioventricular block, first and second degree. Bradycardias, (sudden falls in heart rate to between 40 and 50 beats/min) were frequent, and some children had less than 40 beats/min. The variability in children is so wide that the normal situation must be known before treatment is given.

DR. MILES: Has Dr.Southall time-of-day data and, if so, what did it show?

DR. SOUTHALL: During the night, there is a much slower heart rate. We have looked purely at the difference between day and night so far. Not all atrioventricular block is confined to the night-time period. Some chldren show first and second-degree atrioventricular block during the day-time with normal activity.

PANEL DISCUSSION

DR. BOWLES: Arrhythnias are known to increase with age and Dr. Hayward's two groups of normals and patients were not exactly age-matched.

DR. HAYWARD: If I remember rightly, there was one patient at the top of the age range and then a considerable gap. It would be necessary for all the arrhythmias to occur in that one patient to show the effect.

DR. BALASUBRAMANIAN: Was the respiratory function measured in Dr. Hayward's patients with active sarcoidosis? Was any exercise testing performed and did any of the patients show ST segment changes?

DR. HAYWARD: The full gamut of lung function tests were done in all the patients. Those with inactive disease were reckoned to be returning to normal - although, in fact, not all of them were entirely normal with regard to transfer factor, even at that time. These patients were not exercised and this should be done. Dr. Balasubramanian may know more about the literature than I do, but I find it surprising not to have seen a previous communication of this type. There is a lot on static ECG, but not much on dynamic ECG and nothing at all (as far as I am aware) on exercise testing in these patients.

DR. BALASUBRAMANIAN: The reason for asking about the respiratory function is that they may not have cardiac sarcoidosis. Even in cor pulmonale and in chronic bronchitis, there is a very marked increase in the incidence of arrhythmias.

DR. HAYWARD: Particularly on effort, There was no major lung disease in the people with either active or inactive disease. Certainly, they were not hypoxic.

DR. SOUTHALL: Did the autopsies performed on the patients with sarcoidosis include a detailed examination of the conducting system. This is available now in one or two centres, notably Prof. Anderson's group. If any of these patients die, he may well be able to help.

DR. HAYWARD: A major study has been done on this topic by an expert histopathologist. They have been examined in great detail.

DR. SOUTHALL: What about in regard to the conducting system, which is a highly specialised examination?

DR. HAYWARD: Perhaps not necessarily in terms of what Prof. Anderson would regard as adequate, but it has been examined as a specific heading of a communication in the American Heart Journal in 1977, but again, perhaps not infinitesimally detailed.

DR. SOUTHALL: Looking at the results in active disease, the impression is that some of those arrhythmias are unusual in normal subjects. Are you planning to go ahead and do a proper controlled study?

DR. HAYWARD: Yes, it is going on now.

DR. SOUTHALL: So this is just the beginning of the study. How many controls do you to intend to use?

DR. HAYWARD: Controls are difficult to find. The whole Department has been volunteered, and any more are very welcome.

DR. SOUTHALL: They are not necessarily appropriate, are they?

DR. HAYWARD: That is a major problem, to get appropriate controls.

DR. CONTINI: Has any correlation been found between the amount of arrhythmias on Lown classification, for example, and impairment of pulmonary function in sarcoidosis?

DR. HAYWARD: We have not found any such correlation so far, but this may become clear as we proceed.

DR. CASHMAN: As I understood it, the validation shown at the end by Dr. Contini had 2118 normal complexes and 18,000 SVC's (supraventricular complexes) and 18,000 ventricular complexes. But the sensitivity of abnormal beat detection was given on the basis of rejection of normals, i.e. of false-positive ectopic detections. 2000 normal beats would therefore be a rather small sample, compared to the large numbers of abnormal beats. Would Dr. Contini please clarify what exactly the validation slide tells us?

DR. MARCHESI: I will answer the question because I am responsible for the slide. It is a quite complicated method of validation because, first, there has to be reduction from a 24-hour period, selecting on a random basis some representative records. Those beats are beats selected from 24-hour patient recordings and the 30 second records describe all the 24 hours. A comparison was made, observer against computer, and we performed sensitivity and specificirty analysis where false positives and false negatives were all involved in the relationship. I do not understand what information is missing from the slide.

AMBULATORY ST SEGMENT MONITORING WITH FREQUENCY MODULATED TAPE RECORDERS - A REVIEW

V. BALASUBRAMANIAN, A.B. DAVIES, M.J. BOWLES, E.B. RAFTERY

Cardiac Department and Division of Clinical Sciences,
Northwick Park Hospital and Clinical Research Centre,
Harrow, Middlesex, UK

Summary

Continuous 24-hour ambulatory monitoring of the ST segment changes in patients with angina has been performed using a frequency modulated recorder. New methods of data analysis have been evolved. A number of commonly encountered problems, artefacts and limitations have been defined, and their solutions indicated. The clinical application and utility has been demonstrated with illustrative case reports.

Introduction

Alteration in the ST segment morphology is considered a hallmark of exertional or vasospastic angina. (1, 2). Normally, the ST segment changes in patients with ischaemic heart disease are evaluated by formal exercise testing under controlled conditions (3). The behaviour of the ST segment during normal daily activity when patients are exposed to environmental stimuli and during sleep can be obtained only by continuous ambulatory monitoring of the electrocardiogram. Conventional direct recording and playback systems do not have an adequate low frequency response and waveforms are distorted by phase shift (4). The limitations of the direct recording systems as compared to a frequency modulated recording system were reported by us in previous communications (5, 6). Based on the results of our validation data, we proceeded to use a frequency modulated recorder capable of 24-hours' monitoring on a standard cassette tape and have obtained 1021 tapes in the last two years. This review deals with the details of the equipment used for data acquisition and analysis and some of the artefacts associated with the use of FM recording systems.

Patients

A total of 1021 tapes were obtained in 303 patients attending the ischaemic clinic with either suspected or confirmed ischaemic heart disease. There were 242 males and 61 females, with age ranging from 18-81 years.

Methods

All patients were clinically assessed in the out-patient clinic and then performed a maximal exercise test on a motor-driven treadmill, (Quinton Instruments Limited). During this period, two bipolar ECG leads were continuously monitored before, during and after exercise

by an on-line digital computer (Marquette CASE). The computer analysed the electrocardiogram, identified the isoelectric line (most
horizontal part of the PR segment), located the J point and calculated the difference betweeen these two points to an accuracy of 0.1
mm and expressed the values as continuous analogue trend plots and as
one-minute-mean digital values (7). The 24-hour ambulatory monitoring was then commenced using identical electrode locations and bipolar leads (CM5 and CC5).

Ambulatory ECG Monitoring

Recorder
     The Oxford Medilog Mark II recorder (Oxford Medical Systems,
Oxon. England) was used during the entire study, using the TDK-ADC
120 tape and Mallory 9 volts alkaline battery or equivalent as the
power source. All recordings were preceded by a series of 1 m.v.
square wave calibration signals, which were used as standard values
for future data anlysis.

Electrodes
     We previously reported good results using electrodes made by
Roussell Medical Ltd. The Company stopped production due to an
inability to produce consistently good batches. The initial recordings of the series were made by Marquette Electrodes (Marquette
Electronics, Milwaukee, U.S..), which were standard silver-chloride
type and the later ones with NDM diaphoretic electrodes (01-3610)
with a very aggressive adhesive (NDM Corporation, Dayton, Ohio).

Signal Acquisition
     Proper electrode application was considered an absolute require-
ment to achieve good ECG signals free from artefacts and base line
shifts. The sites of electrode application were chosen over bony
surfaces free from major muscle masses. The hair was shaved if
necessary and the skin cleansed with isopropyl alcohol. The electrode site was identified by a felt marker and the skin lightly
abraded by a battery operated dental burr. The electrodes were
applied and the cables connected. The electrodes and cable junctions
were fixed with adhesive tape and the recorder was worn over the
chest in a cloth pouch. The recorder and cables were snugly fixed
with an elastic vest to the chest to eliminate movement.

Tape Analysis

Tape analysis was performed in three stages.

Visual Inspection
     The tape was run from an Oxford PB4 replay unit into a Reynolds
Medical Pathfinder (Reynolds Medicals, Hertford, U.K.). The quality
of the tape recording and any gross abnormalities were appraised
during this phase.

Analogue Write-out
     This was done by a combination of Oxford PB4 replay unit, Rey-
nolds Medical Pathfinder and ST trend system, and a linear recorder.

The RME trend system generated two bright spots, one of which was
located at the PR segment to identify the isoelectric line and the
other at the J point to measure the changes. The ECG was continuously monitored and the trend system measured the voltage difference between these two points averaged for 10 beats excluding artefacts and ectopic beats. The ST segment changes along with the heart
rate were written out as an analogue trend in two channels of a
linear recorder and the changes related to standard calibration
signals. Varying the speed of the recorder enabled compression or
expansion of the 24-hour trace to suit the requirements. (Figure 1A
and 1B). This method permitted rapid visual assessment of ST depression or elevation and a semi-quantitative analysis. The variables
which could be calculated from this graph were the number of episodes
of ST depression or elevation and the maximal ST segment change in 24
hours. It was also possible to calculate the area of ST change
which, however, was extremely tedious and time consuming.

Digital Analysis
     This was considered essential for accurate quantitation of ST
segment changes and to facilitate rapid access to stored data for
further detailed analysis.
     The digital analysis was designed to work with the Reynolds
Medical ST trend system. An interfacing module was designed to pick
up the heart rate and ST segment changes from the trend system and
feed it into a commercially available microcomputer with twin 5.1/4"
floppy disc drives. The programme provides an on-line data analysis
option and an off-line data retrieval and analysis option.
     The initial menu consisted of the patient details, recorder
details, ECG lead recorded, time of starting the recording, times of
symptoms and date of recording tape. The next step was feeding the
zero reference point into the computer and then calibrating the
system. Calibration was performed by feeding 1 mv square wave pulses
recorded on each tape into the computer. The computer was programmed
to reject noisy or distorted calibration signals and produce an
average of 15 complexes. If satisfactory calibration signal was not
obtainable, a standard internal calibration could be utilized. The
tape was then started and signals fed into the computer. Under
normal circumstances, the time signals from the PB4 playback were
used for timing and the computer took over if the tape time failed.
This safety feature was incorporated due to the high rate of failure
of time signals in the tape recordings. The computer had built in
noise rejection and artefact sensing circuitry. Once the tape was
run through, the data was stored in the floppy diskette, for future
analysis and retrieval. The entire procedure of digitizing took
about one hour per tape with two channels of ECG.
     All data was stored in a floppy disc, with clock-time as the
reference marker. The data stored included, for each minute, maximum
minimum and mean heart rates, and maximum, minimum and mean ST depression. The programme enabled the operator to recall any period
either as one-minute values or as averaged values. The operator
could preset appropriate limits of normality, and the total duration
and the mean ST change were also available at the end to calculate
the area of ST depression in a given time. In addition, the out-of-
limits ST values or heart rate values could be edited out or included

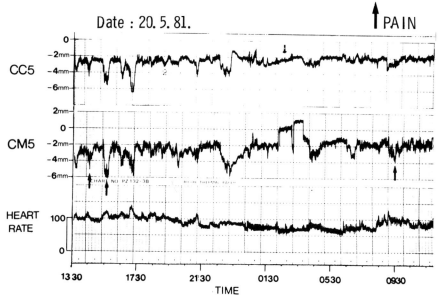

Fig. 1A   24 hr   ambulatory ST segment and heart rate trend.   Episodes of angina and clock time are marked.   Note the combination of ST elevation and depression in   the same lead and prolonged duration of the ST segment changes at 2230 hours which lasts about 2 hours.

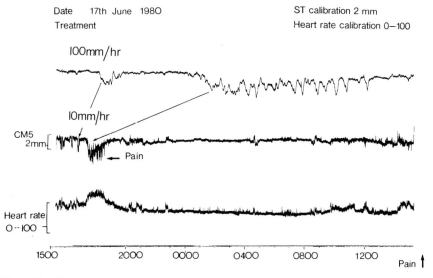

Fig. 1B   The 24 hour trend of a patient with repeated episodes   of ST depression in one hour.   The patient noted only one   episode of pain in his diary but the trend at a speed of 100 mm/hour (top panel) clearly shows episodes of ST depression.

and identified by distinct markers. Using this programme digital
analysis required less than a minute per sequence after the data has
been stored in the diskettes.

Clinical Applications

Variant Angina
     This probably represents the most important application of
ambulatory monitoring of the ST segment (ASTM). This is identified
by episodes of anginal pain, usually at rest associated with ST
segment elevation. Exercise testing is usually normal and some
patients may even have normal coronary arteries with spontaneous or
provoked spasm. The following two case-reports highlight the role of
ASTM in such cases.

     Case 1:   A 47-year old athletic female was repeatedly complain-
ing of chest pain associated with syncopal episodes for the last 5
years. Investigations in other hospitals were normal. Exercise
testing showed an excellent exercise tolerance and normal ST segment
response. ASTM revealed multiple episodes of ST segment elevation,
some of them associated with ventricular tachycardia and returning to
normal within a few minutes. Treatment was commenced with Verapamil,
a calcium ion antagonist, and the patient became totally asymptomatic. Repeated ASTM were within normal limits. During a routine
ASTM, she overslept and forgot to take one dose of the drug at the
right time. She was woken up with pain and the tape showed ST
elevation with tall peaked P and T waves, which returned to normal
after the next dose (Figure 2) This case clearly illustrated the

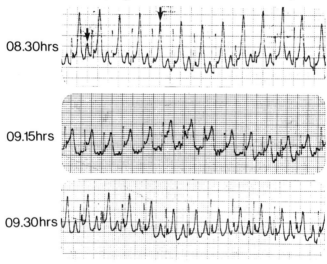

Verapamil   withdrawal

Fig. 2   The effect of inadvertent treatment withdrawal. Note the
          tall peaked P and T waves and ST elevation. The tracing
          returned to normal after starting therapy.

role of ASTM in the diagnosis, following up the course of treatment and demonstrating the harmful effects of acute withdrawal (7).

Case No. 2: This 70-year old male was admitted with episodes of chest pain occurring at rest. ASTM revealed multiple episodes of ST elevation with no marked change in heart rate (Figure 3A). There was a total of 37 distinct episodes of ST elevation in 24 hours, the shortest lasting for 2 minutes and the longest over 20 minutes. Only three episodes were associated with chest pain. The patient was started on Verapamil 120 mg every six hours and became asymptomatic. Repeated ASTM showed normal ST segments over 24 hours (Figure 3B) This case demonstrates that even ST elevation can occur without pain and effective treatment should abolish symptoms as well as ECG changes (7).

Case No. 3: This 71-year old male was seen in the ischaemic clinic with repeated attacks of exertional angina. Maximal exercise testing showed an exercise tolerance of 8.0 minutes and peak ST depression of -2.1 mm in lead CM5. These were interpreted to show a moderate ischaemic heart disease. Routine ASTM, however, revealed an entirely different profile (Figure 4). The patient had at least 8 episodes of chest pain and 28 episodes ST depression most of them not

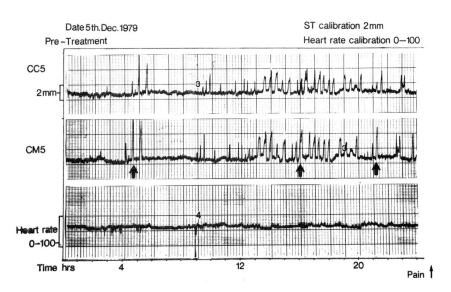

Fig. 3A   Repeated episodes of ST elevation in leads CM5 and CC5 with hardly any change in heart rate. There were 37 episodes of ST elevation but patient complained of pain   only thrice.

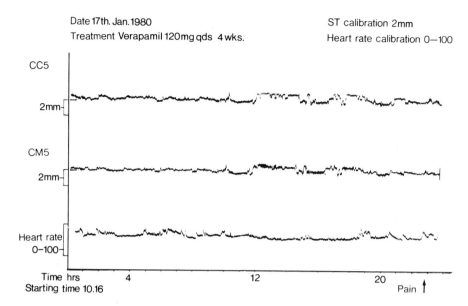

Date 17th. Jan. 1980   ST calibration 2mm

Treatment Verapamil 120mg qds 4 wks.   Heart rate calibration 0—100

Fig. 3B   ST segment trend after four weeks of treatment with   calcium channel blockers.   The tracing is now   completely   normal.

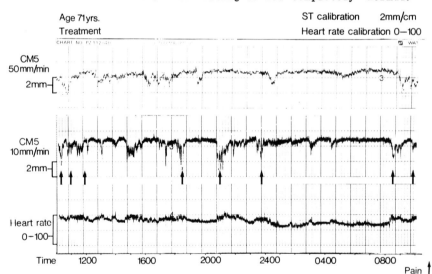

Age 71yrs.   ST calibration   2mm/cm

Treatment   Heart rate calibration 0—100

Fig. 4   The ST segment trend of a patient with a good exercise tolerance. He develops multiple episodes of pain with marked ST depression. There are no marked changes in the heart rate during angina. This dissociation between ambulatory monitoring and exercise testing suggests   coronary artery vasospasm.

associated with significant tachycardia. This dissociation between
exercise testing and ASTM was unusual and based on this, the patient
was treated with a calcium blocker with an excellent therapeutic
response. This case clearly illustrated the role of ASTM in identifying the severity of ischaemic heat disease and the underlying physiological mechanism enabling the clinician to choose the right management.

Artefacts, reliability and technical problems

ASTM using the Oxford Medilog Mark 2 FM recorder has been proved to
be a viable method to quantify accurately ST segment changes. However, we encountered a number of problems during our routine work and
enumerate some of the most common and their probable causes and
remedies.
     For purposes of this analysis, we defined a successful ASTM, if
both channels of ECG were free from artefacts and DC shifts for a
minimum of 95 per cent of time. This stringent criterion was not
difficult to obtain if meticulous care was taken in electrode application, and other technical aspects. We achieved an overall success
rate of 89 per cent. Defective electrode application or poor anchoring of lead wires were a major source of loss of data and accounted
for the failure in 70 tapes. The recorder failed during a recording
session in 30 tapes. The causes of the recorder failure were attributed to battery failure (3), head and amplifier failure (10), drive
belt (10), and the rest due to other causes. On an average the
recorder started producing problems after about 40 ASTM sessions and
after this, we could identify problems in almost every one of our 17
recorders, when checked carefully before being given to a patient.
Even though the recorders were the first few off the production line,
we considered that the reliability is still below normal. At one
stage, all our recorders were either undergoing maintenance or service, leaving us without any means of ASTM. This aspect has to be
kept in mind and workers planning ASTM should cater for at least a 50
per cent reserve to account for recorder malfunction. Careful checking before a session is mandatory to avoid failure during a recording.
     Clock failure accounted for the loss of heart rate data in 110
tapes. Some clock malfunction such as spontaneous resetting of time,
wrong starting time and 'jumping' occurred in almost 30 per cent of
all tapes, so that we had to include an alternative method of time
analysis in our digital analysis programme. This has been found by
the manufacturers to be due to residual magnetisation sometimes
present even in new tapes, and they now recommend demagnetising all
tapes before an ASTM session. We have now recorded over 100 tapes
after initial demagnetisation and there is an apparent reduction in
time problems.
     Some of the common artefacts with FM systems have now been
identified and corrected. The noisy baseline seen in our earlier
recordings were attributed to a gearbox problem by the manufacturers;
however, we subsequently identified it due to flutter in the playback
system and this was easily corrected. In some of our tapes, we found
the signals suddenly becoming very noisy at the last 6-8 hours and
this was identified to a recorder and playback head mismatch and

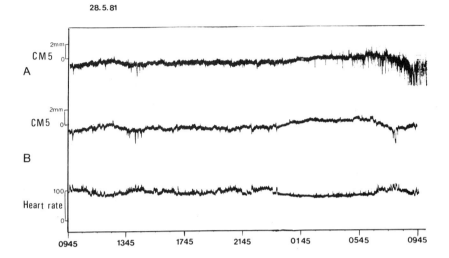

28.5.81

Fig. 5   Panels A and B are the trends from the same tape. Panel A
was played back with improperly aligned play-back head.
Panel B shows the improvement with a properly aligned playback head.

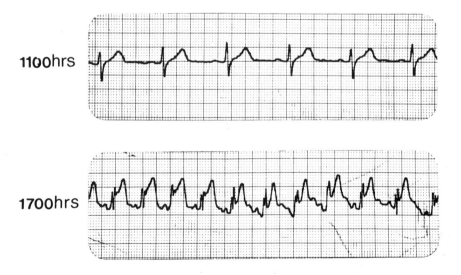

Fig. 6   Artefactual ST elevation. The tracing never returned to
normal, the clock channel was not working and a simultaneous
recording with a real time FM recorder was normal.

could easily be corrected (Figure 5). Recently we encountered six tapes in which ST segment elevation very closely resembling Prinzmetal's angina, occurred during ASTM (Figure 6). After careful analysis of the tapes, and parallel recording with another system, we found that these were artefacts, and could be caused by head misalignment or battery failure. The artefact is identified by the following events:

(a) Sudden 50 Hz artefacts of a short duration preceding the ST elevation.
(b) Loss of time signal
(c) Marked variation in QRS amplitude
(d) Failure of ST elevation to return to normal and the signal gradually degenerating into total garbage.

The combination of these four events have been noted in all our six tapes.

Conclusion

Ambulatory ST segment monitoring using Oxford Medilog Mark II frequency modulated recorder has been successfully performed in 89 per cent of 1021 tapes. We have evolved simple and effective methods of electrode site preparation, leadwire and tape recorder anchoring to reduce artefacts. We have evolved a method for digital analysis of ambulatory ST segment changes. We have been disturbed by the poor reliability of the recorders and frequent problems with the time signals. Certain artefacts, which could mimic clinical syndromes have been identified and most of them corrected. Ambulatory ST segment monitoring is definitely a viable and valuable clinical and research tool, once the common facts, artefacts and fallacies are kept in mind.

References

1. Feil H, Siegel M.L. (1928) Amer. J. Med. Sci. **175**, 255.
2. Prinzmetal M., Kennamer R., Merliss R. et al. (1959) Amer. J. Med. **27**, 375.
3. Kattus A.A., MacAlpin R.N., (1969) Cardiovas. Clin. **1**, 255.
4. Balasubramanian V., Raftery E.B., Stott F.D. (1979) (Letter) Br. Med. J. i **198**.
5. Balasubramanian V., Lahiri A., Raftery E.B. Proceedings of Third International Symposium on Ambulatory Monitoring, Harrow, 1979. Ed. Stott F.D., Raftery E.B. et al. Academic Press, London, 1980. 69.
6. Balasubramanian V., Lahiri A., Raftery E.B. et al. (1980) Br. Heart J. **44**, 419.
7. Balasubramanian V., Millar-Craig M., Davies A.B. et al (1981) Am. Heart J. **101**, 849.

AMBULATORY ECG MONITORING IN EFFORT ANGINA

P.F. FAZZINI, E.V. DOVELLINI, F. MARCHI, P. PUCCI, G.M. SANTORO

Division of Cardiology, Careggi Hospital, Florence, Italy

Summary

Stress testing is the most used diagnostic tool employed to ascertain effort angina (1, 2). Ambulatory ECG monitoring (AEM) has been utilized less. The two tests have often been compared in terms of diagnostic sensitivity (3, 4, 5).

In order to verify if the methods offer complementary information, 20 patients affected by chronic stable effort angina underwent both 24-hour AEM and stress testing (bicycle ergometer conventional).

Methods

ECG leads monitored during exercise and AEM were the same. A CM-5 lead explored the anterior wall of the heart and an A lead (6, 7) explored the inferior one. Flat or downsloping ST depression of at least 0.15 mV > 0.8 sec. after J point was considered diagnostic criterion of ischemia (8, 7).

Results

During AEM, 5 patients had no ischemic episodes. The other 15 patients experienced ischemic episodes totalling 80 attacks: 34 episodes were symptomatic for pain, 46 episodes were asymptomatic. All symptomatic episodes occurred during some physical activity. The same can be said for 44 asymptomatic episodes. 2 painless episodes occurred at rest. There were no attacks during sleep.

Of the 15 patients who experienced ischemic episodes:
- 4 had only attacks (16) with pain
- 9 had attacks with (18) and without pain (41)
- 2 had only attacks (5) without pain

Mean duration of ischemic episodes without pain was 5 min $\pm$ 8; mean duration of episodes with pain was 8 min $\pm$ 7' (P > 0.05). Maximum mean ST depression was 0.265 mV $\pm$ 0.088 in painless episodes and 0.362 mV $\pm$ 0.110 in episodes with pain (P < 0.01).

In the group of 9 patients who experienced both ischemic episodes with and without pain, painless episodes had a mean duration of 5 min $\pm$ 7', while episodes with pain had a mean duration of 10.5 min $\pm$ 8' (P < 0.05). Maximum mean ST depression in painless episodes was 0.271 mV $\pm$ 0.099 and maximum mean ST depression in episodes with pain was 0.443 mV $\pm$ 0.161 (P < 0.001).

Stress testing was positive in all 20 patients. On the basis of the temporal relationship between the appearance of ischemic ECG features and pain during stress testing, we identified 4 different

situations:
   simultaneous appearance of ST segment alterations and pain (5
      patients)
   onset of pain delayed 10 - 30 sec. (6 patients)
   onset of pain delayed more than 30 sec. (4 patients)
   absence of pain (5 patients).
(In these last patients, stress testing was stopped either because ST
segment depression had reached 3 mm or because ST ischemic alterations persisted for 3' without pain).
   These data from stress testing were compared to the data from
AEM. In the group of patients who during stress testing manifested a
simultaneous onset of ST alterations and pain, the ratio between
symptomatic and asymptomatic episodes registered during AEM was
0.18:1. In patients, who presented pain with a delay from 10 to 30
seconds, the ratio was 0.85:1.   The proportion between asymptomatic
and symptomatic episodes was 2.5:1 when the onset of pain at stress
testing was delayed by more than 30 seconds; the ratio was 3.5:1
when the pain did not occur at all. Statistical elaboration of these
findings (X^2) confirmed a significant relationship ($P < 0.05$) between
patient reactions during stress testing and the prevalence of asymptomatic or symptomatic episodes of ischemia as detected by AEM.

Conclusion

From all our data we concluded:
1. Patients with chronic stable effort angina undergo painless
episodes of ischemia.
2. Painless episodes of ischemia are more frequent than episodes
with pain.
3. Painless episodes are generally characterized by shorter duration and reduced magnitude of ST segment shift.
4. Painless episodes are particularly frequent in patients who
during stress testing show ischemic ECG features without pain, or in
patients where pain appears with noticeable delay in comparison to
ECG ischemic alterations.

References

1.   Schang S.J., Pepine C.J. (1977) Am. J. Cardiol. **39,** 396.
2.   Stern S., Tzivoni D. (1974) Br. Heart J. **36,** 481.
3.   Boucher C., Crawford M., White D., Mendoza C., O'Rourke R.
      (1978) Am. J. Cardiol.**41.** 400.
4.   Tamura K., Ozowa T., Arai U., Aizawa K. (1978) World Congress of
      Cardiology, Tokyo.
5.   Wolf E., Tzivoni D., Stern S. (1974) Br. Heart J. **36,** 90.
6.   Blackburn H., Taylor M.L., Okamoto N., Rautaharjh P., Mithell
      P.L., Kerkoof A.C. In: Karnoven M.J., Barry A. (eds) Physical
      activity and the heart, Thomas Springfield, 1967.
7.   Fazzini P.F., Marchi F., Pucci P., Santoro G.M., In: Angelino
      P.F. (eds): Il monitoraggio ambulatoriale dell'elettrocardio-
      gramma. Centro Scientifico Torinese, Torino, 1980.
8.   Ellestad H.M. Stress testing principles and practice, F.A. Davis
      Co., Philadelphia, 1975.

CARDIAC LOAD IN MIDDLE-AGED ROWERS DURING TRAINING AND COMPETITION

J. POOL, *R. ODINK, A.J. DOLMANS, J.W.M. THOEN,
S.L.A. REICHERT, H.J. RITSEMA VAN ECK, J. LUBSEN

Thorax Centre, Erasmus University Rotterdam
*Dutch Rowing Association

Summary

Cardiac load was studied in 88 middle-aged competitive rowers during training while rowing different distances. Sixteen of these were also studied during boat-races. The ECG was recorded with a portable tape-recorder. The cardiac load as measured by heart-rate was higher during long distances than during short ones. Higher heart-rates were measured during races than during training. Complex ventricular arrhythmias were observed frequently during training (13%) and particularly during the races (> 62%). Significant ST depression was seen in a considerable number of subjects (13%).

Introduction

Rowing by middle-aged people is increasingly popular, at least in the Netherlands. Many boat-races are organised for these age-groups. The organizers and the national and international rowing associations are concerned about risks, proper distances and precautionary measures. To determine the cardiac load, middle-aged competitive rowers were studied during training and boat-races, while rowing various distances.
    Objectives of the study were:
1.   To estimate the cardiac load during training and boat-races by measurement of heart-rates.
2.   To determine the relation between the distance rowed and the heart rate.
3.   To study the occurrence of electrocardiographic abnormalities during training and races.

Subjects and Methods

Eighty-eight middle-aged rowers were studied during training at distances of 250, 1000 and 5000 m. Their ages ranged from 30 to 67 years. Sixteen of them were also studied during boat-races of 250, 750, 2000 and 5000m.
    All men were healthy, had a yearly medical check up and had already rowed for years.
    Medilog II portable tape-recorders and a Medilog II replay unit and analyser (Oxford Medical Systems) were used for recording and replaying the electrocardiogram. This frequency modulated system

allows for reliable ST segment analysis. ECG strips were written out
at the end of each distance rowed and at the end of the intervening
recovery periods. From these ECG strips, heart-rates were calculated. ST segments were interpreted independently by three experienced cardiologists. To detect arrhythmias, the recordings were
analysed semi-automatically by a trained technician.

Results

The heart-rates during training are presented in Figure 1.

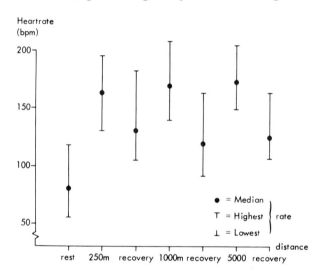

Fig. 1   Heart rates measured in 88 subjects during training at
          different distances at maximal speed.

Median, lowest and highest heart-rates are indicated at rest, at
the end of 250, 1000 and 5000 m. at maximal speed and at the end of
the intervening recovery periods.
    The highest heart-rates were observed at the end of 5000 m.
This is at variance with the subjective impression of the rowers, who
indicated that the workload during the long sprint (1000m.) was the
heaviest.
    During recovery, some rowers showed remarkably high heart-rates
(up to 180 b.p.m.).
    Figure 2 shows a comparison of the heart-rates during training
and races. The heartrates during the races were higher in nearly all
subjects, probably reflecting more stress and heavier exertion.   In
Table 1, the ventricular arrhythmias observed during training in 88
subjects and during races in 16 subjects are listed. Both during
training and races complex ventricular arrhythmias such as bigeminy,
multiform premature beats, doublets and runs were seen quite frequently. It appears that in apparently healthy men many complex
ventricular arrhythmias occur, probably due to physical and emotional

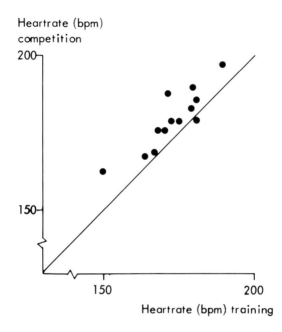

Fig. 2　　Comparison of maximal heart rates during training and competition at 5000 m.

Table 1

Premature Ventricular Complexes during Training and Competition

	Training		Competition	
	N	%	N	%
Subjects	85	100	16	100
No PVCs	46	54	2	12
Occasional uniform PVCs	20	24	4	25
Minutes with > 5 PVCs	11	13	4	25
Bigeminy	4	5	2	12
Multiform PVCs	10	12	10	62
Doublets	8	9	6	38
Runs	1	1	2	12

stress. Since the incidence of sudden death during exercise is extremely low in athletes, these arrhythmias are probably benign. ST depressions (>1mm) were seen in 11 out of 84 subjects during training. No relation was found with age and distance rowed. None of the rowers had angina pectoris or chestpain. When training and races are compared, no difference in incidence of ST depressions was seen (Table 2).

Table 2

ST Depression During Training and Competition

N	ST > 1 mm		
	Tr. only	Comp. only	Comp. + Tr.
15	2	2	4

We were unable extensively to carry out an extensive medical examination of these subjects. However, it is unlkely that they had serious ischemic heart disease, since they had no symptoms and were able to endure heavy exercise repeatedly. The exact meaning of these findings remains to be determined. However, our results indicate that middle-aged well-trained rowers are able to attain high heart-rates during exertion and that both ventricular arrhythmias and transient ST depressions are frequently observed.

Acknowledgements

The Study was supported by The Netherlands Heart Foundation.

ACCURATE AND SIMULTANEOUS RECORDING OF ST SEGMENT HEART RATE AND BLOOD PRESSURE IN PATIENTS WITH ISCHAEMIC HEART DISEASE

A.B. DAVIES, V. BALASUBRAMANIAN, P.M.M. CASHMAN
F.D. STOTT, E.B. RAFTERY

Department of Cardiology and Division of Bioengineering,
Northwick Park Hospital and Clinical Research Centre,
Watford Road, Harrow, Middlesex, UK

Summary

Accurate quantitation of ST segment changes in the ambulant patient is now possible using frequency modulated tape recording systems. We describe modifications to such a system, which enables simultaneous accurate recording of intra-arterial blood pressure along with ST segment and heart rate in the exercise laboratory or outside hospital.

Validation of the modified recorder and playback system is discussed along with examples of its clinical application in patients with ischaemic heart disease.

Introduction

Exertional chest pain has long been considered as the hallmark of angina pectoris (1). Recently, it has been recognised that pain is a crude indicator of ischaemia (2, 3) and ST segment elevation or depression, with or without pain has been demonstrated to be more consistently related to ischaemic episodes (4).

The relationship of heart rate and blood pressure to pain and ST segment changes has been extensively investigated in controlled situations, such as the catheter or exercise laboratory, but there is only one relevant report of simultaneous ECG and intra-arterial blood pressure recordings in ambulant subjects (5). In this study of eight patients with angina pectoris, pain was found to occur at the same level of cardiac work (within patient) irrespective of activity, where cardiac work was indirectly determined as the product of heart rate and systolic blood pressure; also, importantly, it was stated that there was no consistent pattern in the time-relationship between circulatory changes and ST segment changes, although the ST depression tended to occur coincident with, or after, the onset of pain.

The data was based on Medilog Mark I recordings, which had no time codes and the accuracy of the changes in ST segment level is debatable.

We undertook a study, in which accurate time marking, and ST segment reproduction, were combined with continuous intra-arterial blood pressure recordings in freely ambulant subjects with angina pectoris, using isometric and dynamic exercise as the control. This paper describes the modification to and validation of the equipment along with methods of data analysis illustrated by case reports.

Technical Considerations

The ability of the Oxford Medilog Mark II system to reproduce ST
segment changes accurately has been validated (6). The recorder has
four channels, two for flutter compensation and timing/event recording, and two for data recording.

The following modifications were made to the recorder for blood
pressure recording:
(a) One input was modified to D.C. coupling (the B.P channel).
(b) The Akers transducer in the Stott transducer/perfusion unit
      was powered from the internal voltage regulator of the
      recorder.
(c) The recorder was hard-wired to the the transducer/perfusion
      unit to reduce connector and cable artefacts.
(d) A low-pass filter was added to the PB4 playback deck to
      optimise frequency response.

Recording

The manufacturers' recommended TDK ADC 120 cassettes were used
for all recordings. Both channels were calibrated, the ECG channel
with a series of 1 mV square waves, and the blood pressure channel
with 50mmHg steps (0-250mmHg) using a mercury manometer. A minimum
of three blood pressure calibrations were performed during one recording session of 24-hours.

Data Analysis

Tapes were played back at 60 times recording speed, using the
modified Oxford BP4 replay deck. The ECG signal was analysed using a
Reynolds Pathfinder system, the ST values being continuously extracted by the ST segment trend processor. Trends of ST segment
along with heart rate were then played out on a multi-channel pen
recorder. Digitial values of these parameters were also stored on
floppy disc (7).

The blood pressure signal was evaluated in two ways:
(a) A purpose built optimally damped peak-follower allowed the
systolic and diastolic trends to be simultaneously played out with ST
segment and heart rate trends on the multi-channel recorder. This
provided the initial visual analysis from which areas of interest
could be identified for detailed evaluation.
(b) The blood pressure signal was played out using a fibre-optic
recorder with paper speed of 170 mm/sec which allowed beat-to-beat
analysis.

Averaging the last 10 beats in each minute was found to produce
values not significantly different from averaging of all beats.

Accurate timing of the blood pressure changes was ensured by
simultaneous playback of ST segment trend.

Measurement and averaging of the blood pressure signals was
facilitated by a purpose-built chart digitiser linked to a microcomputer.

The physical characteristics of the recorder/playback system
(blood pressure channel) were as follows:

1. Frequency Response: A sinusoidal pressure signal of variable frequency was applied to the recording system via the Teflon cannula and manometer tubing. The overall response of the recorder-playback system was examined by playing out onto a fibreoptic recorder (MEDE-LEC F.O.R. 4) (Figure 1).

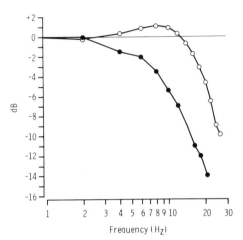

Fig. 1   Frequency response of the whole Medilog Mark II system (in open circles), compared with results obtained using the Oxford Medilog Mark I system (Millar-Craig et al 1978) (closed circles)

The response to 18 Hz is uniform (± 2 db), therefore freeing the blood pressure data from the limitations imposed by the Mark I recording system (8).

2. Signal to noise ratio: The results from 21 separate calibration series from 0-250mmHg were averaged. The S/N ratio was found to vary with the pressure level, being best at centre scale (peak-to-peak amplitude at 150mmHg was 4mmHg) and at worst always better than 25 dB.

3. Linearity: The results from the 21 calibration series were pooled. The worst deviation from linearity within the range 0-250mmHg was 6.6mmHg.

4. Temperature stability: The overall effect of an increase in temperature between $10^\circ-40^\circ$ was to change the span rather than the zero point. The worst temperature coefficient was -0.5% per $^\circ$C. A 24-hour continuous temperature recording confirmed that if the recorder and transducer/perfusion unit were both worn on the chest a maximum of 2.5 % change in span could be expected in use.

5. Battery depletion: The transducer is energised from the stabilised supply devised from a manganese-alkaline battery whose voltage falls substantially over the period of recording (approximately 1.8 volts in 21 hours). The effect of this is to change the span rather than the offset, the worst coefficient being -3% per volt. For this reason it was felt that several calibrations were required throughout each 24-hour period of recording.

Patients and Methods

We have studied 22 male patients (ages 50-74) who had exhibited
stable angina for at least three months. During maximal treadmill
exercise a diagnostic ST segment depression of at least 1 mm beyond
the resting level, measured at the J point, was present in all patients. Coronary angiography revealed at least a 70% stenosis in one
or more major vessels in all cases.

For at least two weeks prior to study, no patient was taking
medication apart from short-acting nitrates for relief of angina.

The non-dominant brachial artery was cannulated using a modified
Seldinger technique and a 10 cm long 0.8 mm internal diamter Teflon
cannula (VYGON) introduced into the artery. The cannula was connected to a Stott transducer-perfusion unit via an 80 cm length of
polythene tubing, which allowed simultaneous perfusion with heparin-
ised saline and pressure recording (8). The whole system was worn in
a pouch placed on the patient's chest, which reduced discomfort and
cable length, while ensuring optimum temperature stability. Two ECG
electrodes were applied to the patient's chest after meticulous
preparation of the electrode sites. The electrodes were positioned
at the manubrium sterni and V5 position to produce a bipolar CM5
lead.

All patients underwent a formal programme of isometric handgrip
(50% maximal for 3 minutes) and maximal symptom limited treadmill
testing (Table 1) with simultaneous electrocardiographic monitoring
using a computer assisted exercise system (Marquette C.A.S.E.)

TABLE 1
Treadmill Protocol

Stage	Time (min)	Speed (mph)	Gradient per cent
1	3	2	0
2	3	3	4
3	3	3	8
4	3	3	12
5	3	3	16
6	3	3	20
7	3	4.5	20

Following this exercise programme, patients were allowed to
return to their normal activities for a period of ambulatory monitoring varying between 20 and 24 hours, returning only for intermittent
transducer calibration.

Case Reports

Case No. 1: A 71-year old retired engineer, with a history of mild
essential hypertension had a three-and-a-half month history of severe
angina with attacks of pain every day, limiting his exercise tolerance to approximately 3/4 mile. Invasive investigation revealed
marked antero-apical left ventricular dyskenesia, a totally occluded

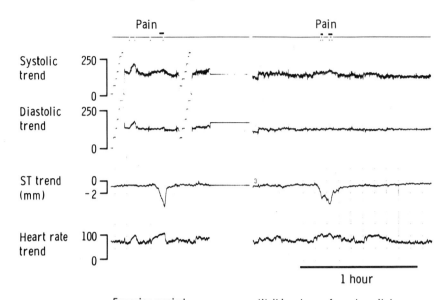

Fig. 2a   Simultaneous trend of systolic, diastolic blood pressures (scales 0–250 mmHg), ST segment and heart rate in Case No.1. Despite a marked increase in blood pressure and heart rate, isometric exercise produces no pain nor ST segment change. Later, while walking, 2 attacks of pain are associated with what is seemingly one episode of ST segment depression

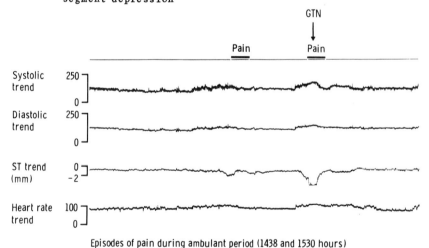

Episodes of pain during ambulant period (1438 and 1530 hours)

Fig. 2b   At the onset of pain there is a slight increase in heart rate and blood pressure; however, these changes have disappeared approximately 10 minutes before the pain abates

left anterior descending, and severely stenosed circumflex coronary artery. Isometric exercise produced a marked increase in blood pressure 140/87 to 206/123mmHg with a heart rate change of 71 to 94 bpm. There was again no ST segment change unlike dynamic exercise, which was associated with a 3mm depression, a blood pressure rise from 136/80 to 161/85 and increase in heart rate from 69 to 102 bpm. Numerous episodes of pain were experienced in the period of ambulant monitoring, which were associated with varying magnitude of ST segment heart rate and blood pressure change. Figure 3(a) and (b).

Case No. 2: A 69-year old electrical engineer had a three-year history of angina of effort and at the time of study, claimed to have mild attacks of pain approximately once a week. Investigation revealed some mild anterior left ventricular dyskinesia, with a mid-left anterior descending coronary aetery stenosis compromising its diagonal branch. Isometric exercise produced a rise in blood pressure from 111/64 to 164/93mmHg heart rate increased from 75 to 90 bpm. Dynamic exercise, however, produced a marked tachycardia from 65 to 139 bpm while blood pressure rose from 104/64 to 176/97. Isometric exercise was not accompanied by any ST segment depression, while dynamic exercise was associated with a depression of 2.7mm.

Almost immediately he left the hospital, he experienced three attacks of angina, which were associated with significant ST segment depression, but of differing magnitude. The heart rate gain was atypical of our group of patients in that it was greater than that achieved during formal dynamic exercise. (Figure 4).

Case No. 3: A 64-year old university lecturer, with a history of an inferior infarction in 1979 and a twelve months' history of mild angina, approximately 2 to 3 times a week was found to have diffuse left ventricular dyskinesia with inferior wall akinesion. Coronary angiography revealed severe triple vessel disease and in addition, a critical left main artery stenosis. Isometric exercise produced an increase in blood pressure from 178/86 to 223/128mmHg with a heart rate gain from 92 to 100 bpm with no change in ST segment, contrasting strongly with dynamic exercise, which was terminated with pain at 14 minutes. There had been a consistent fall in blood pressure throughout exercise 169/87, falling to 114/66mmHg (Figure 5).

Discussion

The modified Mark II system offers considerable advantages over the Mark I system. It is more compact and more acceptable for the patient and gives accurate ST segment reproduction and timing. However, in its present form, the system is not able consistently to record a full 24-hours and although in all cases over 20-hours of good quality recording was obtained, frequently premature battery failure was recognised by increase in noise and span, and for this reason more frequent calibrations were recorded towards the end of the recording period.

Despite the improvement in timing facility, we found considerable difficulty in relating symptoms to objective changes in ST segment, heart rate or blood pressure. Some patients kept meticulous records, noting precise times and using the event marker to the beginning and end of pain, while other patients either forgot to use the event marker or tended to 'round off' times to the nearest 15

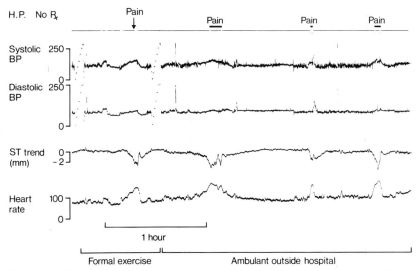

Fig. 3   Trend plots from Case No.2. As in the previous figures, calibrations are performed at the beginning and end of the formal exercise period. Event marks denote the beginning and end of exercise and the onset and relief of pain

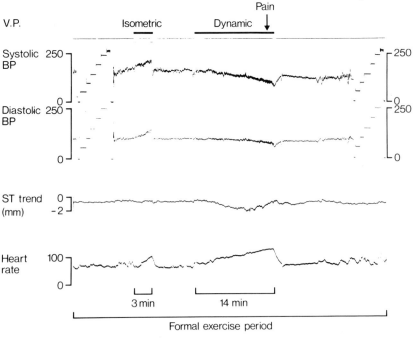

Fig. 4   Case No.3 responds to isometric exercise by elevation of systolic and diastolic pressures. The fall in pressures during dynamic exercise suggests that left ventricular failure occurs long before the onset of angina

minutes i.e. 16.12 would become 16.15. However, we were able accurately to time and quantitate ST segment changes and note whether or
not they were associated with pain. It was even more difficult to be
sure about reports and episodes of pain, where no dramatic ST segment
shifts occurred. Fortunately, such episodes were infrequent, possibly because of patient selection.

Asymptomatic ST segment depression was approximately three times
as frequent as symptomatic episodes and both types tended to occur in
relation to the journeys to and from hospital, most patients walking.

Pain was associated with a wide spectrum of ST segment depression, but none with ST segment elevation. In all cases, except Case
1, the ST segment depression and heart rate changes tended to be less
than those produced by formal dynamic exercise.

The blood pressure response, from patient to patient, was variable; in 12 cases, dynamic exercise produced an actual fall of blood
pressure prior to termination of exercise, in four of these cases,
the double product also fell prior to the onset of pain. Outside
hospital, the relationship of blood pressure to ST segment change and
pain was inconsistent; in addition, there was a wide scatter of
maximal rate-pressure products associated with pain. A further indicator that blood pressure is a relatively unimportant determinant
of ST segment change was the response to isometric exercise, where a
marked increase in blood pressure associated with a modest heart rate
gain produced no pain and significant ST segment depression in only 4
cases.

The relationship of heart rate and blood pressure to angina has
been extensively investigated in the exercise and catheter laboratories and studies have found that the product of heart rate and
systolic blood pressure have a consistent within-patient relationship
to pain, independent of the provocation (10, 11). There is a surprising paucity of data on the response of intra-arterial pressure to
upright dynamic exercise in patients with ischaemic heart disease and
even less information on patients unrestricted outside hospital.
Littler et al (5) provides the one report in the literature and his
conclusions were essentially that the relationship of the rate-
pressure product to pain, held true.

We conclude from these preliminary results that ST segment
depression tends to be most consistently associated with changes in
heart rate rather than in other variables, but this relationship does
not hold true all the time. These findings are in accordinace with
those of others (12, 13) that myocartdial ischaemia is not solely
determined by changes in myocardial demand.

Acknowledgements

We would like to thank Mr. F. Bew and Mr. R.T. Wloch, for their help
with the validation of the recording system.

References

1.   Friedberg C.K. (1966) Diseases of the Heart, 3rd ed. New York,
      Saunders
2.   Master A.M., Geller, A.J. (1969) Am. J. Cardiol. 23, 2, 173-179
3.   Cohn P.F. (1980) Am. J. Cardiol 45, 697-702.

4. Maseri A., Mimmo R., Chierchia S., Marchesi C., Pesola A.,
    L'Abbate A., (1975) Chest 68, 625-233.
5. Littler W.A., Honour A.J., Sleight P., Stott F.D. (1973)
    Circulation 48, 125-134.
6. Balasubramanian V., Lahiri A., Green H.L., Stott F.D., Raftery
    E.B., (1980) Br. Heart J. 44, 419-25.
7. Balasubramanmian V., Davies, A.B., Bowles M.J., Raftery E.B.
    (Cross Ref. ISAM 1981).
8. Millar-Craig M.W., Hawes D., Whittington J. (1978) Med. & Biol.
    Eng. & Comput. 727-731.
9. Goldberg A.D., Raftery E.B., Green H.L. (1976) Postgrad. Med. J.
    52, (Suppl. 7) 104-109.
10. Robinson B.F. (1967) Circulation 35, 1073-1083,
11. Gobel F.L., Norstrom L.A., Nelson R.R., Jorgensen C.R., Wang Y.,
    (1978) Circulation 57, No. 3 549-556.
12. Guazzi M., Polese A., Fiorentini C., Magrini F., Olivari M.T.,
    Bartorelli G. (1975) Brt. Heart J. 37, 401-413.
13. Chierchia A., Brunelli C., Simonetti I., Lazzari M., Maseri A.,
    (1980) Circulation 61, No. 4 759-768.

PANEL DISCUSSION

DR. RAFTERY: In his presentation, Dr. Marchi seemed to me to be making two very important assumptions: first, that there is a quantitative relationship between ST segment depression and the amount of myocardial ischaemia present at any one time; second, that that relationship is linear over a definite range - in other words, the more ST segment depression, the more ischaemia there is and the relationship stays the same, not altering in any way. Would Dr. Marchi like to defend that statement, or perhaps elaborate upon it?

DR. MARCHI: We have some reservations about that statement: I agree that my statement was too strong. In our experience, episodes in the same patient which were characterized by a lot of ST segment depression were symptomatic, while episodes with less ST segment depression were more likely to be painless. This is in the same patient and it is not always true, but generally that is our experience.

DR. RAFTERY: Would anyone else like to comment on that relationship between ST segment and total degree of myocardial ischaemia?

DR. MARCHI: Using only two leads, it is not possible to have a strong correlation, but if it is possible to judge from those two leads when the ST segment depression is more advanced, it is more likely that pain will be present in the same patient, but sometimes there are exceptions, also in the same patient.

DR. BALASUBRAMANIAN: What was the recording system used by Dr. Marchi, how was the ST segment depression quantitated in depth and duration, and did the patients take sublingual trinitroglycerine during attacks of pain, or were they left untreated? That could quite markedly influence the ST changes in symptomatic attacks.

DR. MARCHI: The recording system used was Avionics. Patients did not take sublingual nitrate, so the ST segment changes were not influenced by their taking sublingual nitrate.

DR. POOL: From exercise-testing, there is a lot of experience in ST segment depression and external workload. When exercise-testing is done, there is a gradually increasing ST depression and at some particular moment, the patient develops pain when either a continuously or stepwise increasing load is used. There may, therefore, be some relationship between ST depression and ischaemia. I do not think it is a linear relationship - but I do not know for sure.

DR. RAFTERY: We have some data which suggest that on exercise-testing certainly there may well be a linear relationship - it looks like a very good one, too. It may well be that the ST segment is a true indicator of the amount of myocardial ischaemia present at any one time, in those circumstances. But it certainly cannot apply with ambulatory recordings because the pattern of ST segment changes is so wildly different from the pattern observed on exercise-testing.

DR. BOWLES: When Dr. Marchi compared the exercise-testing with the Holter monitoring, he made a form of classification of angina on stress-testing in respect of the development of ST changes, as compared with the onset of pain. How is the point of development of ST changes defined and related with any accuracy to the onset of pain?

DR. MARCHI: We consider it to be diagnostic of ischaemia when the ST is flat or down-sloping 1.5 mm, 80 msec. after the J point.

DR. BOWLES: Dr. Marchi spoke of the possibility of a defective anginal warning system. What does he think constitutes the normal anginal warning system?

DR. MARCHI: It was my intention to emphasis that, in my opinion, stress-testing is useful to identify patients in whom the ratio between asymptomatic and symptomatic episodes is higher. The possibilities of defective anginal warning systems are many..

DR. RAFTERY: I suspect that Dr. Bowles is trying to say that Dr. Marchi would be better advised to use the word "ischaemia" rather than "angina". Angina, by definition, is pain, so it would be more meaningful to talk about an ischaemia warning system.

DR. MARCHESI: Firstly, about Dr. Balasubramanian's method of quantitating ST depression or elevation. We have tried to use some measurement of amplitude using the J point, but we found that this is unreliable because it is an unstable zone from which to take measurements, particularly during episodes of ST changes.

Secondly, about the time resolution he used in his trend plots. Some authors have said that 1 min. resolution is not adequate in all cases and that, in some instances, higher resolution is better.

Thirdly, with regard to the artefact problem, I remember a sentence at the end of a famous article by McFie, where he stated that the main problem with electrocardiography is whether or not it is useful. If electrocardiography is not 100% sensitive or 100% specific, then ambulatory monitoring is even less sensitive and specific, in which case, many artefacts can be expected to occur. For that reason, we must use the best possible methods of measurement, and that is why I do not agree with measurement using the J point and such high resolution. Our experience is that many artefacts are detected with high-resolution plots.

DR. BALASUBRAMANIAN: We are fully aware of that point about the resolution. The slides were made in that way because it is possible to have the entire 24 hours in one slide, but it can be written 500 times faster. The resolution that appears on the digital analysis is now final to 1-minute, which still gives both the lowest and the highest ST segment in that minute. As we are averaging 10 beats, our resolution is now 10 beats. Lower than that is not possible with the current computing techniques.

With regard to the J point, we performed considerable experimentation about where to place the reference spot. Out of all the possibilities, the J point was found to be the easiest to identify visually and was the most stable in our experience. The J point could quite easily also be identified by the computer and that is why we used it. Slope cannot be measured by this technique - it is still not possible to do so. But in all our exercise systems, we measure the slope and assume that the same slope changes occur during ambulatory monitoring.

In answer to the comment about artefacts, the resolution observed is only for visual information because it is compressed. We can go 500 times faster when artefacts can quite easily be taken out.

DR. van DURME: First, if I may repeat a question which has been asked already, how much ST segment depression is considered as significant in indicating that a patient has had an ischaemic episode?

Secondly, at what time after the end of the QRS is the ST

segment depression measured?

Thirdly, are the conclusions different according to whether or not the change is associated with symptoms?

Fourthly - this is also important, I think - is it considered important for the ST segment change to be present on a certain number of consecutive beats and, if so, how many?

DR. RAFTERY: The questions, in essence, are what is an episode, how is an episode defined and what is its significance?

DR. BALASUBRAMANIAN: First, 1 mm or more ST segment depression beyond the resting values immediately preceding the attack is considered to be significant. However, we believe that this could be changed in the future with digital analysis - so far, there has been no way of digitally analysing the ambulatory tracing.

Secondly, the ST segment is measured exactly at the J point - we measure from the isoelectric line to the J point.

Correlation with symptoms is going on now. In our initial publication, based on only 640 hours of recording, about 3 attacks of asymptomatic ST segment depression occurred to one attack of symptomatic ST segment depression.

The definition of an attack at the moment is that it should last for at least two minutes, mainly to avoid artefactual ST depressions that may occur due to electrode movements. Again, at present, this is arbitrary. As both the resolution and recorder quality increases, giving better tracings, we may change this definition. But at present, we take two minutes as one episode.

DR. MARCHI: We consider the diagnostic criterion of ischaemia, a flat or down-sloping ST depression of at least 1.5 mm, 80 msec. after the J point. I agree about the duration - but perhaps there are also shorter ischaemic episodes.

DR. POOL: As a definition of significant ST segment depression, we used: at least 1 mm depression, visually observed at about 80 msec. after the J point, and a flat or down-sloping ST segment, which must occur in at least 10 consecutive beats. But if there is marked ST depression at the 80 msec. point, there may also be a little up-sloping - it is a matter of clinical feeling. That was our definition - but I wonder whether in our study it was real ischaemia.

DR. BALASUBRAMANIAN: I beg to differ from Dr. Marchi. The flat and down-sloping ST segment depression was considered diagnostic of ischaemia - and nothing else - about 5 years ago. At least three well-documented studies during exercise-testing in which the slope was carefully measured have been published since then, and they show that if it is not sharply up-sloping (i.e. less than 2 mV/sec slope), it is still diagnostic of ischaemia. But these data are from exercise-testing only. There is still no way of measuring slope on ambulatory monitoring. That is why we exercise all our patients and calculate the slope by computer, taking that information as a parallel, assuming it to be right, until it becomes possible to measure slope.

DR. MARCHI: I agree. It is possible that ischaemic attacks can be accompanied by only small ECG changes. In 'Circulation' for September 1980, there is an article by Maseri and Chierchia, in which they document ischaemic attacks showing only changes of the T wave. We did not want to have too many false positives, so restricted our criteria - but we are sure that there are ischaemic attacks that are

accompanied by only small ECG changes - in many cases only of the T
wave and not of the ST segment.
DR. RAFTERY: If I may summarize the discussion on this topic, the
brutal truth of the matter is that very little is known about the ST
segment and, by and large, what people measure is a matter of
personal fancy, as is the way in which they interpret whatever literature there is on the subject.
DR. DAVIES: How representative does Dr. Balasubramanian think one
24-hour period of ST segment monitoring is compared with a much
longer period, say, 72 hours or even longer?
DR. BALASUBRAMANIAN: We have still not sorted out the problems of ST
segment monitoring for 24 hrs., so we have not attempted it for 72.
DR. SOUTHALL: Dr. Pool was comparing in-training with in-competition
athletes' tapes with regard to ventricular premature beats, but the
numbers in each group were completely different. There were only 16
in training, whereas there were 85 in competition. I am not sure
that if chi-squared tests were done on the differences that they
would be significant at every level. Has that been done?
DR. POOL: That is quite right - it was an incorrect picture, but it
made it easier for the audience. The arrhythmias in the 16 subjects
measured during training were compared with their arrhythmias during competition, and it gives the same picture as here. I think the
numbers are too small to do a chi-squared test.
DR. SOUTHALL: I am not sure about that - there probably are some
differences if they were looked for formally. I am not sure that the
numbers are too small. It could be quite interesting to do.
DR. POOL: We have not done it in any case. The tracings of the same
16 were compared and there is the same trend.
DR. SOUTHALL: I have done similar work to Dr. Balasubramanian, but
in a slightly different direction, using Medilog recorders. His
figures for artefact problems and failure are very similar to mine.
There are one or two minor things which we found helpful, which he
might like to consider. First, battery failure: the XM2 monitor
was used to test battery function, but we soon realised that it is
very inefficient and does not measure battery function under load,
and that battery function has to be measured using a very complicated
system to be sure that it will last 24 hours.
    Secondly, a simple lead tester is used to test our leads before
every recording, particularly to test where the 'popper' fits on to
the electrode.
    In summary, we totally agree with Dr. Balasubramanian that the
failure rate is about 10%, no matter how well the equipment is used
and how many safeguards are taken to obtain good recordings.
DR. BALASUBRAMANIAN: Both those points are well taken. One thing
that concerned us was that at one time all of our recorders were in
the Oxford workshop. The normal minimum transit for recorder repair
is 15 days and the normal maximum is two-and-a-half months - if the
workshop is left unprodded. And we are only 40 miles from Oxford!

CONTINUOUS ECG MONITORING BY A NEW DYNAMIC DISPLAY CLINICAL VALIDATION

C. CONTINI, G. BONGIORNI, G. MAZZOCCA

CNR Clinical Physiology Institute, University of Pisa,
Italy

Ambulatory ECG monitoring is one of the aspects of cardiology in which computer application may provide a valuable contribution both in speeding up diagnostic procedures and in improving the reliability and duration of the analysis.

Several approaches have been tried for continuous ECG computerization (1). Out of these, we have chosen two different ways (2), (3).

The first way, which is the object of this paper, is intended to obtain a new presentation of the ECG signal, which attracts the operator's attention, allowing him to obtain several types of information and document them immediately.

The Contourograph technique has been applied to the ECG since 1965 (1). However, due to the complexity of the original procedures, this technique has not been widely employed. On the other hand, the AVSEP system is the main principle of all devices for ECG ambulatory monitoring even of the present generation (1).

Thanks to recent technological progress, and particularly to the use of microprocessors, the idea of the Contourograph system has been revived in our Institute. Our system improves the general principle of Contourography, with a variable perspective effect, and 60 times real time speed capability (Figure 1). Principles of operation have been previously published (2), (3); a commercial series of this device is about to be produced by Remco Italia (CARDIOLINE).

When the device is working, QRS cycles run on the screen in such a way that they seem to slide away from the operator. Therefore, in any instant, he sees on the screen about 2.5 or 5.0 minutes of cardiac cycles, but rather than being superimposed one on another, such as in AVSEP system, they appear as distinct so that it is possible to make a comparison between one cycle and another or between different areas of the ECG tracings.

QRS complexes, which have not been recognized are not lined up, but they do appear on the screen in a randomly variable position (Figure 2)

Clinical validation of this system presented several problems. First, because the prototype does not have any counting device, and qualitative analysis is entirely dependent on the operator; he may use paper recordings selected by increased lightening of a tracing zone. Furthermore, it is impossible to perform any processing of the visualized signal, or trends, or other presentations.

Comparison can, therefore, be made only taking note of all al-

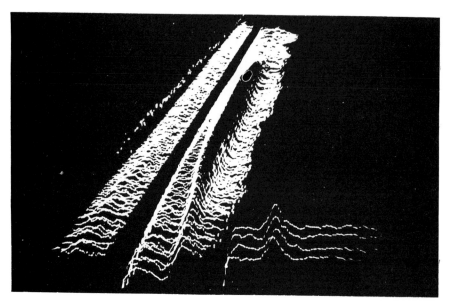

Fig. 1   This picture show a short episode of T wave elevation. The
         QRS complexes runs from bottom to top.   The episode begins
         and finishes gradually.

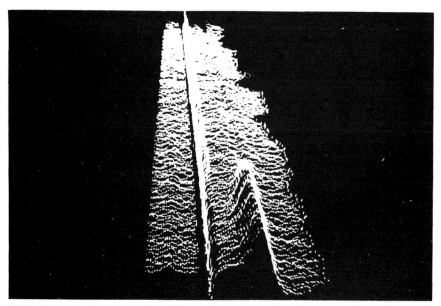

Fig. 2   Another example of the T wave elevation

terations seen and documented by the operator; a global evaluation
of the monitoring is then compared with a report on the same case
derived from the previous analysis with the ASTRI System (4). Obviously, operators were different for the two analyses and did not
know the content of tapes being analysed.

It may be useful to present the results of the initial phase of
validation; apart from a fairly good accordance as to rhythm
disturbances and a lower accordance as to ST segment, it is possible
to see (Table 1) how discordance is all to the advantage of the
Contourograph.

Table 1

Early Clinical Validation of Contourograph System

	St Segment	Rhythm
Accordance	4/10	6/10
Discordance	6/10	4/10
ASTRI ± / Cont -	0/10	0/10
ASTRI - / Cont +	6/10	4/10

This confirms that the human brain is still one of the best computers! However, the four episodes detected only by Contourograph are
all extremely short (few cardiac cycles).

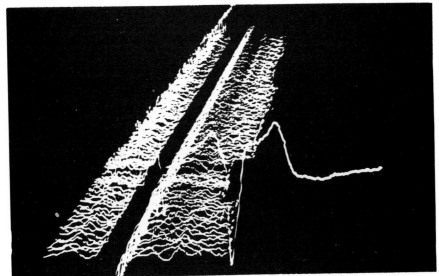

Fig. 3   Recognised QRS complexes are lined up, while a couplet of
           PVC is enhanced because of its different morphology and
           position

In conclusion, we believe that improved Contourography, and particularly variable perspective, will be a useful tool for recognition of
ST segment elevation or depression episodes; also ventricular arrhythmias can be easily recognized and their morphology analysed.
These are, in our opinion, the present aims of ECG ambulatory monitoring.

References
1.   Webb G.N. Rogers R.E. (1966) IEEE Spectrum, Vol 3, N.6, 77-78,
     83-87.
2.   Macerata A., Taddei A., Marchesi C., Mancini P. (1980) From
     Electronics to Microelectronics, Kaiser and Proebster Edit.,
     North Holland Publishing Company, 534-536.
3.   Marchesi C., Macerata A., Taddei A., Mancini P. (1980) Computers
     in Cardiologu, Williamsburg, Oct. 22-24 (In press).
4.   Biella M., Contini C., Kraft G., Marchesi C., Mazzocca G.,
     Taddei A. (1979) Computers in Cardiol. 201 IEEE.

CLINICAL APPLICATIONS OF A NEW MINICOMPUTER BASED FOR ECG AMBULATORY MONITORING

C. CONTINI, G. MAZZOCCA, G. BONGIORNI

CNR   Clinical Physiology Institute, University of Pisa,
Italy

The second way we have chosen is the full computerized analysis of magnetic tapes for Holter monitoring with a maximum of reliability of data and various modes of presentation, such as trends, histograms, hourly and total report of abnormal beats etc.

Our system, ASTRI (Analysis ST and Rhythm) has been developed to compensatew for the faults of commercially available dedicated devices, most widely used in recent years.

For a long time, since about 1970, we have been accustomed to hearing that ECG ambulatory monitoring is the ideal system for the study of arrhythmias, whereas it is of no use in diagnosis and functional evaluation of ischaemic heart disease. This seemed to be due to technical problems, almost impossible to solve, in ST measurements, and to scarcity of available leads.

The idea of a computerized system for ECG ambulatory monitoring originated in an automatic system (SOTER), devised for the monitoring of ECG and haemodynamic parameters acquired on line from CCU patients; original algorhythms for QRS detection and measurement for positive and negative ST surface area have been introduced. The system has been set up by Clinical Physiology Institute, CNR, Pisa, by the Elaboration Data Group.

This programme analysis, tested on the first 200 cases, underent several changes, especially in the phase of data presentation; one of the main changes is expansion of trends: their resolution has been increased from 7 minutes to 30 seconds, in order to recognize even low amplitude ST segment alterations, which could scarcely affect mean values, if averaged for 7 minutes (Figure 1).

Among a total of 900 tapes so far analysed, the first series evaluated with the present version is made up by 73 healed infarction patients, in which ECG ambulatory monitoring were performed at various times from the acute episode, on the average at 30, 60, 90, 180 days. In 85% of the cases, both arrhythmias and ST changes have been documented. The most surprising finding has been the high incidence of asymptomatic severe arrhythmias and ST segment elevation and depression.

Only 15% of patients were without abnormal findings. Twelve patients have been followed with at least 3 analyses, and in all 103 analyses have been performed. There have been 5 sudden deaths, or more precisely unexpected deaths, out of the Holter examination.

In a clinical correlation performed in the same group of patients, it seems possible to identify three groups. The first is formed by the 15% of patients with negative Holter monitoring, under preventive vasodilator treatment, without impairment of left ventri-

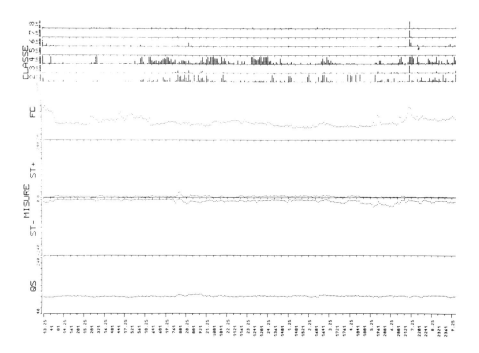

Fig. 1   The new presentation of trends with 30 seconds of resolution. On the top the classification of abnormal beats is
displayed.

cular function and good clinical condition. The second group is
represented by patients with either arrhythmias or ST segment alterations and with impairment of contractile function. A third group is
formed by patients with both severe ventricular arrhythmias and ST
segment elevation or depression and with greatly compromised left
ventricular function, responding only partially to digitalis and
diuretics (Class III - IV NYHA).

Some demonstrative examples are presented in order to illustrate
the wide possibilities of this method, especially in identifying
episodes of ST segment changes (Figures 3, 4, and 5).

Furthermore, a validation of the system has been peformed by a
comparison, cardiologist versus computer, which gave very good results both as to QRS detection and to classification of abnormal QRS
complexes (Table 1).

Our studies are becoming more and more oriented towards the
evaluation of the clinical significance of arrhythmias, either occurring in ischaemic heart disease for their relationship with ischaemic
episodes, or occurring in other pathological conditions, such as
cardiomyopathies, valvular diseases, collagen disease (scleroderma).

Our aim is to distinguish pathological arrhythmias from functional arrhythmias, as a risk factor of sudden or unexpected death.

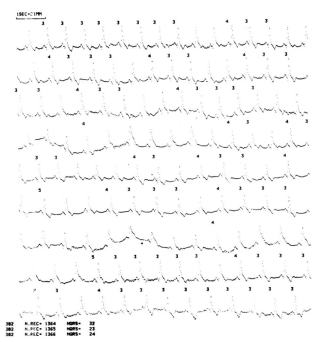

N.CASO= 382   N.REC= 1364   NQRS= 32
N.CASO= 382   N.PFC= 1365   NQRS= 23
N.CASO= 382   N.REC= 1366   NQRS= 24

Fig. 2   This picture shows the maximum of sensitivity of Astri
System   in the fourth strip it is possible to see a short
episode of ST elevation, which involves five heart beats.

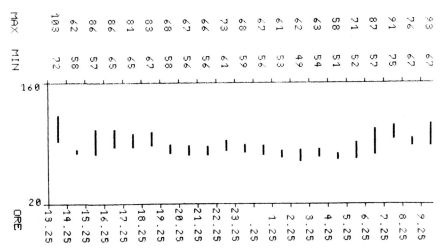

Fig. 3   This picture shows the trend of heart rate, with maximum
and minimum value per hour. This presentation is particularly useful for chronobiological studies.

```
CLASSE 1  =  NORMALI
CLASSE 2  =  PREMATURI A QS NORMALE
CLASSE 3  =  PREMATURI A QS ANORMALE
CLASSE 4  =  RITARDATI
CLASSE 5  =  FORMA VARIATA
CLASSE 6  =  FORMA VARIATA E ALLARGATO
CLASSE 7  =  TACHICARDIE A QS VARIATO
CLASSE 8  =  GEMINISMI
```

CARATTERISTICHE DELLA REGISTRAZIONE

DATA: 19-2-80   ORA INIZIO: 13.25   ORA FINE: 11.50

CARATTERISTICHE DELL'ANALISI

DURATA DEL TRACCIATO: 1348. MIN   NUM. COMPLESSI ELABORATI: 85650.
FREQUENZA MEDIA DEL COMPLESSO: 67   DISP.: 13.22
DURATA MEDIA DEL COMPLESSO: 100   DISP.: 7.04

INTERVALLO TEMPO	C1	C2	C3	C4	C5	C6	C7	C8
13.25 - 14.25	4593	7	1	56	0	0	0	2
14.25 - 15.25	3534	3	0	2	0	0	0	0
15.25 - 16.25	3832	3	0	140	0	0	0	4
16.25 - 17.25	4233	1	1	3	0	0	0	2
17.25 - 18.25	4444	11	1	35	0	0	0	0
18.25 - 19.25	3524	22	0	68	0	0	0	4
19.25 - 20.25	3527	64	5	71	0	0	1	2
20.25 - 21.25	3303	66	9	42	0	0	0	5
21.25 - 22.25	3492	39	1	117	0	0	0	1
22.25 - 23.25	3853	5	0	24	0	0	0	1
23.25 - .25	3476	15	1	142	0	0	0	2
.25 - 1.25	3262	40	0	42	0	0	0	4
1.25 - 2.25	3000	30	1	8	0	0	0	3
2.25 - 3.25	3211	62	1	43	0	0	0	4
3.25 - 4.25	3107	41	1	19	0	0	0	0
4.25 - 5.25	3054	57	0	3	0	0	0	0
5.25 - 6.25	3562	30	3	19	0	0	1	1
6.25 - 7.25	3916	37	72	62	0	0	14	12
7.25 - 8.25	4234	25	1	72	0	0	0	2
8.25 - 9.25	4008	38	3	41	0	0	0	0
9.25 - 10.25	4348	80	3	120	0	0	1	6
10.25 - 11.25	3923	20	0	15	0	0	0	0

TOTALE	81436.	696.	104.	1144.	0.	161.	17.	55.
PERCENTUALE	95.080	.813	.121	1.336	0.000	.188	.020	.064

Fig. 4   Final report of data analysed, showing different types of
             abnormal heart-beats occurring in each hourly period

TABLE 1

Results of the Validation of the Astri System

	T.B.	N.P	SENS	SPEC
QRS Detection	22933	7	99.89	99.95
C I (Normal)	2118	1	98.91	91.99
C 2 (SVE)	10267	3	96.21	98.20
C 3 (PVC)	10548	3	95.54	99.97
C 4 (Delayed)	8316	2	75.68	99.69

T.B. = Total beats; N.P. = Number of Patients; SENS = Sensitivity;
SPEC = Specificity.

In conclusion, it is possible to summarize a series of indications to the use of the computerized ECG ambulatory monitosing system, which provides more meaningful information than commercial available systems.

Indications for Astri System use:
Spontaneous angina
Conduction disturbances
Evaluation of new anti-arrhythmic and anti-anginal agents
Healed infarction follow-up
Chronobiological studies
Physiological studies.

Advantages of Astri System:
Shorter man/machine interaction time
Better detection of normal QRS
Qualitative evaluation of abnormal beats
Objective measurements of St segments and T wave
Presentation of more complete trends for a full and unusal evaluation of electric cardiac signal.

References

1. Nolle F.M. (1980) In: Continuous Electgrocardiographic Recordings. N.Wenger, I. Rinqvist, Mock M.B. Future Publishing Co.
2. Contini C., Marchesi C., Mazzocca G. (1978) VIII World Congress Cardiology, **533.**
3. Marchesi C., Chierchia S., Maseri A. (1977) Computers in Cardiology, IEEE, Rotterdam Spt. 29-Oct 1, 1977.
4. Contini C., Mazzocca G., Marchesi C., Biella M. (1978) Proc. CEE Seminar on "Perspectives of Coronary Care Units." Dec. 1-2 (1978)
5. Contini C., Mazzocca G., Marchesi C. (1979) Proc. Florence International Meeting on Myocardial Infarction, Florence.

ECG WORKSHOP

Chairman : J.P. Van Durme

Introduction

We had it in mind to deal with two topics in this workshop, starting with problems related to automated analysis of arrhythmias and ST segments, and discussing during the second part of the workshop the value, significance, detection and so on of ST segmernt changes. I propose therefore that we start with automatic analysis.

A HIGH SPEED ARRHYTHMIA ANALYSER USING PATTERN MATCHING TECHNIQUES

J.W. GRIFFITHS, and C.C. BASHFORD
Bioengineering Department, St.Mary's Hospital Medical School,
Paddington, London W2 1PG, UK

Abstract

There are still serious problems in the reliable, high speed analysis of cardiac arrhythmias from 24 hr ECG tapes. Poor quality recordings due to a variety of artefacts can lead to an unacceptably high false positive count or because of the inability to recognise arrhythmias in the presence of 'noise', a high false negative count. A pattern matching technique similar to that of Cashman(1) has been developed. The major feature of our hard-wired logic system is the independence from the need for accurate R-wave triggering. The pattern matching technique theoretically precludes false positive recognition of arrhythmias. Steps have also been taken to reduce the amount of false negatives, by attempting to overcome some of the causes, such as labile morphology by updating pattern matching and normalisation of the incoming signal and timing errors due to recording and playback instrumentation by synchronous recording of a tape clock.

Description and performance of the system

Introduction

Greater reliability of 24 hour magnetic tape recording analysis systems is still needed.

All existing automatic analysis systems rely on the detection of the R-waves of the ECG complexes by a method of differentiation which detects the rising or falling edge of complexes. In most analysis systems the detection of the complex is followed by an estimation of its area, which is carried out in a predetermined period after detection. The result of this estimation is compared with a value derived from the normal R-wave, any significant variation from this value being deemed 'ectopic'.

However during any recording period artefactual disturbances upset the analysis. Patient activity, variation of electrode contact resistance, skin tone change and fat movement can all combine to give differing disturbances at random. Sharp spikes, due to patient movement, will erroneously trigger conventional R-wave detectors.

This type of disturbance together with other artefacts are regularly found in 24 hour traces. Indeed, virtually no tape is free of at least one type of artefact

Tape speed variation either during recording or replay will cause artefactual distortion of complexes. We have corrected for this recording a time signal with the data and using it to control the analysis.

We decided to develop a system which can be programmed to pick out wanted ECG complexes from traces containing large amounts of artefact. The circuit operates continuously at a rate of 10,000

attempted correlations per second to identify an event by its shape
alone. It is in effect a continuous correlation technique. No R-
wave triggering is employed for the analysis (but it is used just for
detecting the occurrence of events).

Method

In principle the ECG is replayed from the tape a 100 x real time. A
100 Hz clock pulse recorded on the tape for timing error correctin is
also replayed, at a frequency of 10 kHz. An event of interest, a
normal complex or a specific type of ectopic complex, which has
automatically been loaded into a memory store for visual inspection
is retained. Unwanted events are rejected. Each time a timing pulse
occurs the memory store recirculates and displays all its contents
(at a clocking rate of 1.7 MHz). The free running ECG complex is fed
into a similar store. This store also recirculates and displays its
data, but in this case it continuously takes in a sample at the
beginning and rejects one at the end. Each time the free running
memory increments in this way, both memories, stored and free-
running, simultaneously play out their contents through digital to
analogue converters to an analogue division unit in which the free
running store is divided into the stored store. The resultant is
rectified, and when it gives a low value the two complexes match. A
separate trigger circuit gives an output pulse when this occurs.
        The operation is best illustrated by a series of photographs.
(Figs. 1 to 6).

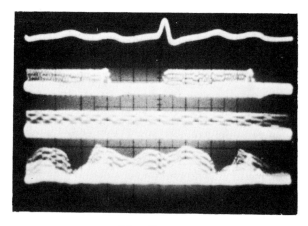

Fig. 1

Figure 1 illustrates the operation of the data flow through the
stores, and the high speed of the analysis.
        In the <u>top trace</u> is a normal ECG complex replaying at 100 x real
time.
        In the <u>second trace</u> is the disply of the entire contents of the
'free running' memory store being recirculated after each increment

enters the store.

   The <u>third trace</u>, which appears unchanging, is the stored complex being recirculated after eery increment of the free running complex.

   The <u>bottom trace</u> is the rectified resultant of the subtraction of the free running complex from the stored complex.

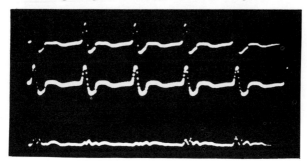

Fig. 2.

In Figure 2 the minimum resultant occurs on the centre complexes and the product is very small.

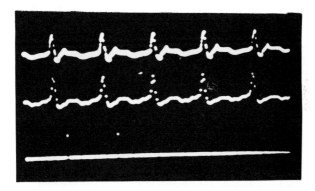

Fig. 3

In Figure 3, the <u>top trace</u> is the free running complex, the <u>second trace</u> is the stored complex, the <u>third trace</u> has pulses derived from the minimum detector circuit, showing the pulses derived from the minimum detector circuit a the complexes match. In this case the minimum has occurred twice as the complexes pass through match.

In Figure 4, the <u>top trace</u> is a free running ECG with an ectopic passing through the store, the <u>second trace</u> is a stored ectopic complex, the <u>bottom trace</u> is a 'matched' pulse.

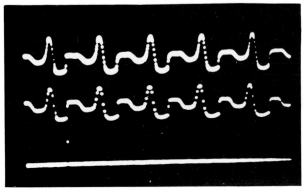

Fig. 4

In Figure 5, the <u>top trace</u> is the ECG replaying at 100 x real time, the <u>second trace</u> is the resultant of the subtraction of the free running and stored complexes, the minimum corresponding to correlation, the <u>bottom trace</u> is a 'stretched' pulse derived from the 'match' pulse or pulses as in Fig.2.

The stretched pulse on the bottom trace indicates that the complex above and ahead in time, has been recognised as a normal complex.

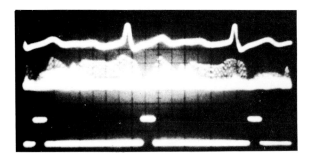

Fig. 5

In Figure 6, the <u>top trace</u> is the recognition pulses for normal complexes and the <u>second trace</u> has recognifition pulses for the ventricular ectopics present in the trace below, the <u>bottom trace</u> is the ECG replayed at 100 x real time with normals and ectopics present.

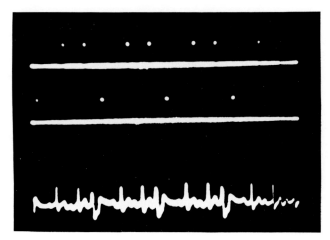

Fig. 6

References

1. Cashmen P.M.M. (1978) Computers and Medical Research, **11**(4), 311-23.
2. Griffiths J.W., Bashford C.C. (1979) Journal of Medical Engineering and Technology, **3**(3), 123-124.

Acknowledgement

This work was supported by the British Heart Foundation Grant No. 754.

DR.ENG. MARCHESI: With regard to Mr. Griffiths' definition of normality, first, is it selected by the operator and, secondly, how many normalities - or how many abnormalities - can be differentiated?
MR. GRIFFITHS: This is a prototype machine in which only two channels are in operation. First, it is loaded with a normal complex which is determined as normal by the operator. Subsequent events are loaded into a second store, and also inspected by the operator. We hope to develop a machine which has about 8 of these stores, so that one after the other will automatically load and the operator can decide what he wants to keep.
DR. MURRAY: When the word "correlation" is used, is it meant loosely? Are the characteristics of the input signal filtered or modified before putting them into the registers?
MR. GRIFFITHS: The answer to the first question is yes. The only modification is to clamp the baseline before an event occurs.
DR. MONSTER: At what speed can this correlation be done at present, and has the possibility been investigated of using standard commercially available components to do this correlation?

MR. GRIFFITHS: We cannot use any standard commercially available components at the moment, although standard shift registers and clocking components are used. The correlator Dr. Monster has in mind operates in a digital fashion and has to be converted back to an analog form for a fast subtraction. Because the samples of the ECG complex are not synchronised with the complex itself, and the sampling rate is low compared with the complex samples taken on identical complexes at different levels, and so a digital correlation could miss completely outside the threshold.

DR. MONSTER: That could be overcome by using some kind of synchronously-gated clock.

MR. GRIFFITHS: The clock cannot be synchronised to the ECG complex.

DR.MONSTER: But you are already detecting the trigger, are you not?

MR. GRIFFITHS: The whole point of this is that we are not detecting every complex as it occurs, but looking at the whole trace as it passes through in sample increments of 100 - an equivalent of 100 times a second.

DR. MONSTER: That is correct, but I suggest that that may not be so efficient.

MR. GRIFFITHS: That is possible - but this is just a new technique with which we are experimenting.

DR. SOUTHALL: What happens if the clock signal on the tape is lost?

MR. GRIFFITHS: We used a phase-locked loop which keep the last tape rate, and if a drop-out occurs it automatically fills in after a drop-out of one pulse.

A COMPUTER SYSTEM FOR INTERACTIVE ANALYSIS OF LONG-TERM ECG RECORDINGS

O. PAHLM, B. JONSON, AND K. PETERSSON

Department of Clinical Physiology, University Hospital
S-221 85 LUND, Sweden

Summary

A computer system for analysis of long-term ECG recordings has been
in routine use at our laboratory for five years. The whole ECG is
compressed, stored on disc and analysed by the computer, which locates episodes of arrhythmia and indicates them on a graphic computer
report. The diagnosis is established by the interpreter, who can
select any episode for instant demonstration or recording on paper.
Clinical experience with the system has been gained from analysis of
more than 2000 recordings.

Introduction

In Sweden long-term ECG recording (LECG) is mainly used in the
investigation of patients with dizziness, fainting spells,
palpitations and other symptoms, which may be due to cardiac
arrhythmia. The value of LECG as a diagnostic tool in these patients
is well established (1-3). Other applications, such as routine
follow-up of patients after myocardial infarction has attracted much
less attention.

Since symptoms are usually associated with tachy- or
bradycardia, R-R interval measurements and detection of abnormal R-R
interval patterns are the most important elements of automated LECG
analysis. Classification of QRS shape is of secondary importance.
This facilitates the use of small and cheap computers for the
analysis.

The variability of P-QRS patterns and the occurrence of artefacts during the recording period makes it difficult to programme a
computer for completely automatic analysis. The approach described
in this paper accepts the unique human ability for pattern recognition. The physician - not the computer - should make the final
diagnosis of arrhythmia and relate it to the clinical problem at
hand.

Methods

The system is based on an LSI-11/23 microcomputer (Digital Equipment
Corp.). The computer, an ink-jet recorder (Siemens-Elema AB) and a
floppy disc drive (RX01, Digital Equipent Corp.) are all in one unit.
The unit is also used for other signal processing applications in the
laboratory.

The sampling rate is 100 Hz. Sample data (8 bits/sample) are
compressed by linear prediction and entropy encoding (4) and are

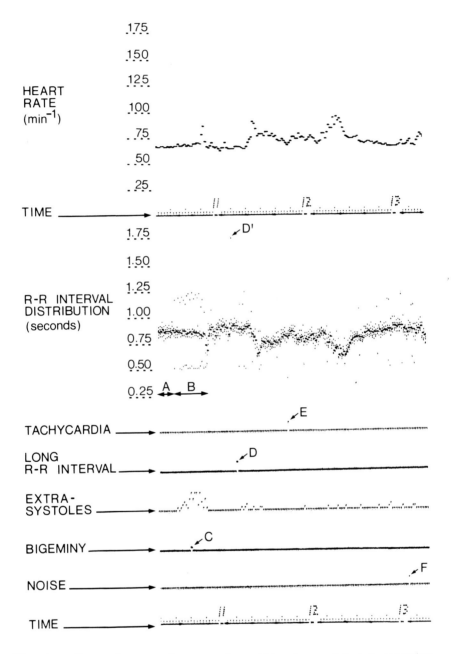

Fig. 1   Part of a computer report, written by an ink–jet recorder.
The computer report gives the operator an overview of
heart rate and rhythm. Episodes marked with letters A–F
are discussed in the text.

stored on an exchangeable cartridge disc (RL01), Digital Equipment
Corp.). Computer processing (sampling and compression, QRS-detection, R-R interval analysis and print-out of computer report) is
unsupervised.

Computer Report

At the end of computer analysis (which takes about 1 hour 15
min. for 24-hours of ECG), the computer writes a graphic report on
the ink-jet recorder (Figure 1) The figure shows:
- The heart rate each minute
- The distribution of R-R intervales each minute. The
  median is denoted by heavy dots; the 15:th and 85:th
  percentiles and the extreme values by small dots.
- The occurrence of tachycardia, long R-R intervals, extrasystoles, bigeminy and episodes with noise.
- The time scales (each hour printed, 10-minute and
  2-minute intervals indicated by vertical bars).
The ink-jet recorder also writes the name of the patient and his
ID number on each strip (omitted from the Figure).
The computer report gives the operator an overview of the rhythm
as can be seen in Figure 1. During the initial period (A), the
distribution of R-R intervals is narrow, which suggests undisturbed
sinus rhythm. During period B, some much shorter and longer R-R
intervals appear. These are indicated as extrasystoles, on one
occasion, (C) creating a bigeminal pattern. Extrasystoles also appear later during the recording. A long R-R interval is indicated at
D. The same episode also appears in the R-R interval distribution as
an "outlier" at D'. An episode of tachycardia is suggested at E.
Finally at F, the computer has detected a noisy episode.
It should be emphasized that the computer report does not, in
itself, allow a final diagnosis. The indicated episodes should be
evaluated during the ensuing phase of computer-aided analysis at
which the actual ECG is inspected.

Visual Analysis

Guided by the diary, kept by the patient during the recording,
and by the computer report, the operator locates, inspects and puts
on record, interesting segments of the LECG. For that purpose, he
takes advantage of a set of computer facilities. They are all based
on the fact that the computer can, within a fraction of a second,
time and display any indicated arrhythmia episode or time segment of
the LECG stored on the disc. If the patient has had symptoms, the
operator often chooses to enter the time of those on the keyboard and
demands a display of the ECG on the screen, at 20 or 60 times real
speed. At the most common speed - 20 times - 20 s of ECG will be
shown at a time. The picture may be frozen on the screen. The
operator can go backwards or forwards, screen by screen, or in a
running mode in his scrutiny of interesting segments of the LECG. A
digital display indicates the time of the segment shown on the
screen.
The most powerful tool of the visual analysis is the selective
automated display. The operator selects one of the following items

for display on screen:

R-R intervals > X s	}	(X and Y are operator-
	}	specified R-R interval
R-R intervals < Y s	}	durations)

Tachycardia	}	
Long R-R interval	}	
Extrasystoles	}	As indicated in the computer
Bygeminy	}	report
Noise	}	

The computer immediately displays the first episode of a desired kind on the screen, with the detected event in the middle. At a stroke of a key, the next episode of the same kind is displayed. Of course, one may also go backwards and forwards to look at segments adjacent to the episode.

The automatic display allows fast scanning of episodes indicated as arrhythmia. As an example, 10 episodes may be reviewed in less than half-a-minute even if they are distributed throughout 24-hours of ECG. Therefore, many false positive indications are acceptable, since they are easily rejected at this stage.

At any time during the analysis, a permanent ECG record of important segments may be obtained. The record is marked with patient identity, exact time of the episodes and marks for QRS complexes round by the computer.

A Clinical Example

Figure 2 shows part of the computer report of an LECG recorded from a 60-year-old woman, who complained of "uncomfortable palpitations". The report reveals several prolonged R-R intervals during the evening (about 8 hours from the start of recording). Automatic display of prolonged intervals revealed episodes of A-V block (Figure 3). The interactive analysis of this recording demanded about 1 minute of the operator's time.

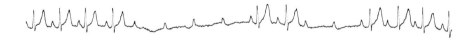

Fig. 3   Long R-R intervals indicated in the computer report of Fig. 2 were due to episodes of A-V block.

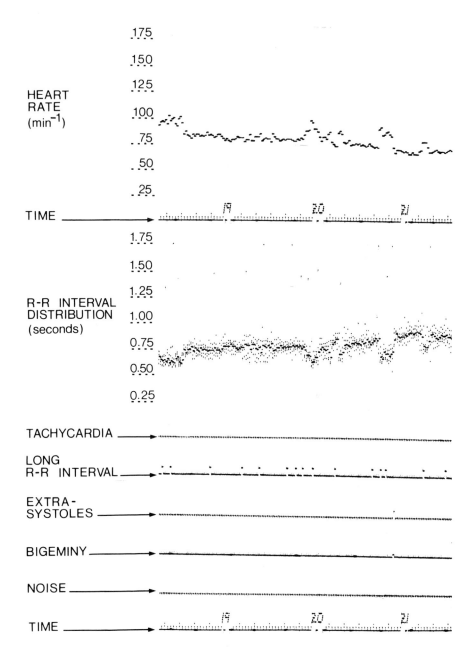

Fig. 2   Computer report of LECG from a 60-year old women with un-
          comfortable palpitations.   Note 'outliers' in R-R interval
          distribution, also indicated as long R-R intervals.

Discussion

Our approach to computer-aided LECG analysis has been to let the computer display a graphic report, which gives the operator a detailed, but still easily assimilated overview of the rhythm (Figure 1). Our way of presenting the distribution of R-R intervals, minute by minute, is of particular value. A diagram of heart rate and graphs, that suggest the types of possible arrhythmic episodes supplement the information in the R-R interval distribution. The present model was worked out during 3.5 years on about 1000 LECG's. A further 1000 recordings have been analysed by the present version of the programme.

It should be emphasized that the computer report does not allow an accurate diagnosis of cardiac rhythm. In fact, computers are as yet far inferior to a trained physician as regards the detailed analysis of arrhythmia. The final interpretation is often based on features which are difficult to analyse by computer, such as low amplitude P waves, findings in other parts of the recording or other recordings, the patient's history etc. The specific human ability to recognize a pattern is of utmost importance, especially in the presence of recording artefacts, which are common in LECG. We believe that achievement of fast and accurate analysis is possible only by efficient interaction between man and computer.

Efficient computer-man interaction requires prompt display of interesting episodes. The whole LECG must obviously be available on rapid memories. A previous publication (4) describes how far this purpose we have tried to optimize:

(1)   The amplitude of recording on tape
(2)   The analogue filtering
(3)   The sampling frequency and resolution
(4)   The system for digital data compression.

Another prerequisite for instant display is an efficient system for retrieval of events. The operator may request display of a particular episode indicated in the computer report, or of the ECG at a certain time. In both cases, the ECG segment in question is displayed within one second, regardless of when it was recorded. Details of the retrieval system are presented elsewhere (5).

A long afterglow wide screen oscilloscope has been chosen for the display. This allows fast presentation of ECG curves. It is also a cheap solution. Further, we believe that this mode of presentation is well-suited for perception by the human eye of events passing by at 20-60 times real speeds. The ink-jet recorder is also cheap and rapid, and allows generation of text by software (6), so tracings may be labelled properly.

The performance of a 12-hour version of the system has been studied with respect to speed and accuracy of analysis. Analysis of 12 hours of LECG took about 9 minutes on the average (7). Although the system may miss some episodes of arrhythmia accompanied by only a small change in R-R interval, very few arrhythmias of possible clinical significance escape detection. Little training is needed to run the system. The present system has been found efficient for the type of clinical problems that are most relevant today.

In order to evaluate the clinical impact of LECG, we made a retrospective study of 150 consecutive patients from our clinical routine (3). Seventeen of these patients were treated with permanent pacemakers and 13 patients were given anti-arrhythmic drugs as a direct result of LECG. Thirteen patients, who experienced symptoms with concomitant cardiac arrhythmia during the time of recording were considered not to require treatment. A further 17 patients experienced symptoms without concomitant arrhythmia during monitoring. In these patients cardiac arrhythmia could be ruled out as the cause of the symptoms. In 9 more patients LECG was considered to have contributed "valuable clinical information" (which could not be obtained by other diagnostic methods) to the referring physician. Thus LECG was considerd to have affected the referring physician's management of the patient in 69 cases (46%).

Acknowledgements

This study was supported by the Swedish Medical Research Council, Grant No. 14X-02872, by the Swedish National Association against Heart and Chest Diseases, by the Swedish Board for Technical Development and by Siemens-Elema AB.

References

1. Johannsson B.W. (1977) Eur. J. Cardiol. **5**, 39.
2. Tzivoni D. and Stern S. (1975) Chest. **67**, 274.
3. Eriksson L. and Pahlm O. (1980) Acta Med. Scand. **208**, 355.
4. Pahlm O., Börjesson P.O. and Werner O. (1979) Comput. Programs. Biomed. **9**, 293.
5. Pahlm O. (1980) Thesis. University of Lund, Sweden.
6. Jonson B., Werner O., Jansson L., Johansson K., Olsson L.G. and Westling H. (1976) Scand. J. Clin. Lab. Invest. **35** (suppl. 145) 7.
7. Pahlm O., Jonson B., Lukes M. and Ringqvist I. Clinical Physiology. (In press).

Discussion

DR. PALM: What kind of noise is detected in the noise channel printout?

DR. PAHLM: The detector is for high frequency, fairly high amplitude noise, so of course there is no detection of isolated base line shifts or anything like that. In most cases the QRS detector will not trigger on a pure base line shift; if it does, there will be indications in the R plot.

DR. SCHEIBELHOFER: Dr. Pahlm showed some instances of atrial fibrillation, but I did not understand what the system does with tapes containing atrial fibrillation. Are they just referred to the observer or can atrial fibrillation be diagnosed?

DR. PAHLM: No, it does not make any specific diagnosis like that. The pattern in the R interval distribution can be seen; it is up to the technician or the physician (whoever runs the system) to investigate that more closely. The whole signal is on the large disk, so the signal itself can be recalled and looked at.

DR. SCHEIBELHOFER: But if there is a 24 hour record which contains instances of atrial fibrillation, say, for 20 minutes here and 10 minutes there, each instance can only be checked by hand.

DR. PAHLM: I agree that to check up each instance like that, and really investigate it, has to be done by hand. Of course, whether that is relevant depends on the clinical question.

DR. MONSTER: It is possible to come up with a measure of rhythm regularity which would take care of that particular problem; in other words, irregularity could be defined such that atrial fibrillation would come up as a very large number, a perfectly regular rhythm as zero, something with lots of bigeminy and trigeminy coming somewhere in between. We have used such a measure, and it really is fairly easy.

CONTINUOUS QUALITY CONTROL IN LONGTERM ECG EVALUATION

H. WEBER, G. JOSKOWICZ, D. GLOGAR, K. STEINBACH,
P. PROBST, F. KAINDL

Kardiologischen Universitats-Klinik, Wien, Austria

Summary

The analysis of longterm ECG recordings deals with a large amount of serial data, which have to be analysed as fast as possible consistent with a constant quality of performance. Continuous quality control of the computer assisted system "Multipass-Scanning" has to be based on automatic methods which are integrated in each part of the analysis: statistical analysis of coupling intervals, automatic and manual edit of beat descriptors, automatic selection of representative arrhythmias during data presentation and multistage artefact detection. Such strategies are conditions for testing the reliability of the system. Beat-by-beat scanning demonstrated a specificity of 97.7% and a sensitivity of 99.7% in QRS-detection and of 99.8% versus 96.5% in PVC recognition. These data were high reproducible. The reproducibility ranged between $\pm$ 1.7% in PVC detection. Using the "dumb operator" test, it could be demonstrated that over a wide range, the variation of QRS-detection parameters cannot influence the results.

So the evaluation of performance could demonstrate that an operator-independent, constant quality can be maintained using methods to achieve redundant results as above mentioned in automatic longterm ECG analysis.

Introduction

The performance of automatic arrhythmia-detectors is usually evaluated with a set of annotated reference tapes, like those from the AHA data base (1). Such reference tapes may help in describing the properties of any analysis system and for the comparison of different systems in use, but are certainly not suitable to assess the influence of different operators and artefacts.

The main problem in daily routine analysis is the maintenance of constant quality.

This paper reviews the automatic methods we have used to assure constant quality of he computer assisted analysis system, "Multipass-Scanning" (2).

(A) Strategies for continuous quality control:

All strategies are based on the fact that ECG data are highly "redundant". That means, that most phenomena detected during the LT-ECG analysis are not single phenomena, but can be found many times during the analysis duration. The plausibility of detected arrhythmias is directly related to their quantity. The methods we used are specially suitable for a computer supported system, which is charact-

erized by the fact that the raw data are stored on random access
media and (Figure 1) that each decision made by the programme can be
checked with the actual ECG-wave form.

The data are analysed in multipe passes using contex informa-
tions acquired in the former pass.

We applied basically four methods related to our quality control:
1. Statistical analysis of coupling intervals (CI) for each beat
      family.
2. Automatic and manual edit of the beat descriptors.
3. Automatic selection of representative arrhythmias.
4. Multistage artefact detection.

1. Statistical analysis of coupling intervals for each beat family:
In our system (Figure 1) a beat family is defined by all those
beats with a similar shape independent of the actual CI. The shapes
are defined in feature space. The separation of shape and CI gives
the possibility for a consistency check. The relative CI is defined
as the ratio betwen the actual and the mean RR-Interval of the surrounding 15 beats.

$$R_I = \frac{RR_I}{RR_M} \; 100$$

$$RR_M = \left\{ \sum_{j=-7}^{+7} RR_{I+j} \right\} / 15$$

For each beat family a histogram in log. scale of the relative CI is
displayed (Figure 2). The degree of prematurity of a beat family is
shown by this method. The operator decides about the strength of the
prematurity criteria to be used for the specific beat family (Figure
2) and can also check with a selection of representative beats from
this family. The selected parameters are used during the automatic
editing process. Figure 2 demonstrates two histograms from the same
raw data set: Left, a correct discrimination between normal beats
and premature ventricular contractions (PVC's). Right, there is a
completely erroneous situation due to a false learning phase; the
two beat families are mixed.

The basic principle of this method is a comparison between the
statistical features of a beat family and selected members of this
family.

2. Automatic and manual edit of the beat descriptors:
The editing of the beat descriptors consists of a correction of
all descriptors which are not consistent with the respective beat
family (3). The editing is partly manual and partly automatic. The
process deals with 3 cases:

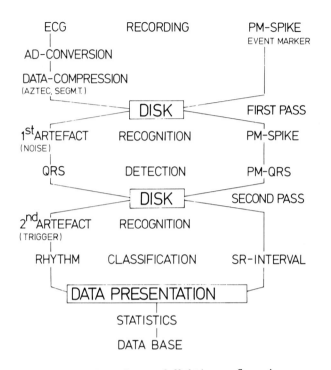

Fig. 1   Flow-chart of Multipass-Scanning

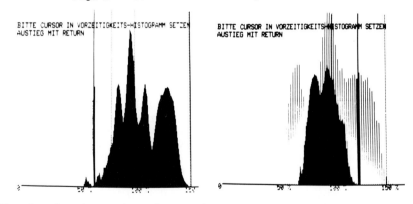

Fig. 2   Statistical analysis of coupling intervals for each beat
family. The relative c oupling interval (abscissa) is
plotted against the number of detected beats. Left: a
correct discrimination between normal beats and PVCs with a
relative CI of more than 60% of the RRm followed by a com-
pen-satory pause. The operator himself decides about the
strength of the prematurity criteria setting a cursor (dotted vertical line) between both beat families. Right: a
completely erroneous situation.

(a) False positive normal beats.
(b) False positive ventricular beats.
(c) Missed beats.

The process starts initially in automatic mode, trying to recognize these three cases and correcting automatically. If more than five corrections are needed per minute, the system reverts to manual mode, displaying each suspicious beat (Figure 3). During manual mode, the system is self-learning. Each correction made by the operator influences also the time-windows used by the consistency checks.

The following example illustrates the mechanism of the editing:

A 30-minute segment with 2319 normal beats and 299 PVC's was analysed; 2298 normal beats were recognized and 21 beats missed. 298 PVC's were also recognized and 1 PVC detected as normal. The PVC's were premature (>20% RRm) and compensated. From the 299 PVC's, 8% had a coupling interval longer than 0,8 RRm. During editing all missed beats were recognized due to their double RR interval and the small variance of the normal RRs. Three true positive PVC's with long CI were presented to the operator. After confirmation by the operator, the system changed the prematurity criteria and the remaining 21 PVC's were accepted. An unrecognized PVC was also presented as a suspicious normal beat and corrected manually (Figure 3).

3.   Automatic selection of representative arrhythmias:

Because of the clinical orientation of the system there is need to document the recognized arrhythmias. The selection of clinically important arrhythmias is automatic and is also a plausibility check. The selection algorithm works as follows :

For each arrhythmia (bradycardia , 50 bpm, tachycardias . 100 bpm, supraventricular tachycardia, ventricular couplets and tachycardias etc), a set of parameters governing the selection algorithm is defined (4). Similar arrhythmias are summarized into one description because of the reports readability without loss of information. The summary is done over a limited number of detected phenomena (e.g. one for ventricular runs, 10 for supraventricular runs etc.) and a limited time-window (e.g. 10 min. for ventricular couplets, 60 minutes for supraventricular tachycardia) in accordance with their clinical importance. Together with this summary, one representative example is stored in a data base for subsequent control (Figure 4). This means that each annotated ventricular run is checked for false positive diagnoses and that only every tenth supraventricular run needs to be checked. The stored ECG can be resynthesized on the terminal screen and strip chart recorded on choice (Figure 4). The algorithm selects the example with the most extreme coupling intervals out of all summarized arrhythmias, e.g. the fastest tachycardia within a 10 minute window and the slowest bradycardia. Therefore, this system prevents the diagnosis of false positive arrhythmias with higher reliability especially for clinically important rhythm disturbances (5).

4.   Multistage artefact detection:

The main problem of hard-ware oriented systems is the false positive recognition due to artefacts (6). On every processing stage artefacts are detected in the computer supported "Multipass Scanning" system:

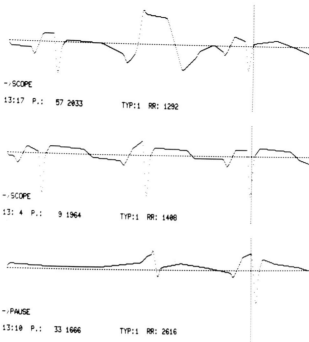

-/SCOPE

13:17 P.: 57 2033   TYP:1 RR: 1292

-/SCOPE

13: 4 P.: 9 1964   TYP:1 RR: 1408

-/PAUSE

13:10 P.: 33 1666   TYP:1 RR: 2616

Fig. 3   Automatic and normal edit of beat descriptors. Upper tracing: The actual RR interval of 1292 msec. demonstrates either a pause or a missed beat, e.g. a missed PVC. Middle tracing: A normal beat is missed (RR 1408 msec). Lower tracing: Are there a asytole, a pause a missed beat. Amplitude-artefact led on the one hand to a trigger fault, on the other hand to asytole.

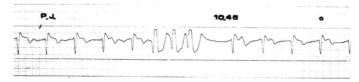

VENTRIKULAERE SALVEN - VENTRIKULAERE TACHYKARDIEN
VON   BIS   EREIGN. SCHLAEGS MITTL.PR.   KUPL.1 KUPL.2 KUPL.3
10:46   10:46   1   3   500   544   520   1208
1 EINTRAGUNGEN   GESAMTDAUER: 2. SEK.

ERLAEUTERUNGEN:
KUPL1....INTERVALL ZWISCHEN LETZTEN NORMALEN UND ERSTEN PATHOLOGISCHEN SCHLAG
KUPL2....INTERVALL ZWISCHEN ERSTEN UND ZWEITEN PATHOLOGISCHEN SCHLAG
KUPL3....INTERVALL ZWISCHEN LETZTEN PATHOLOGISCHEN UND ERSTEN NORMALEN SCHLAG

ENDE DER STANDARD - ANALYSE

Fig. 4   Automatic selection of representative arrhythmias. 10.46 a.m. one event occurred, consisting of 3 consecutive PVCs with a RRm of 500 msec, a coupling interval of the first PVC of 544 msec, second PVC of 520 msec and a compensatory pause of 1208 msec. The lower tracing does not demonstrate the original ECG-strip, but the ECG resynthesised from the digital data, stored on magnetic disk using the linear-segmentation technique(5).

(a) Artefact detection during data acquisition:
The spectral density of >35 Hz is averaged and compared with the density <35 Hz. If the ratio of these densities changes in favour of the high frequency band, a noise mark is inserted in the raw data stream instructing the QRS-detector about tape noise. During QRS-detection, the delay of the filter is compensated.
(b) Artefact-detection during QRS detection:
The QRS detector is of the finite-state type using a list of deflections from the baseline. If during the processing of this list a meaningful QRS-complex is not detectable (e.g. too many deflections within a short interval) an artefact is detected.
(c) Artefact detection during automatic edit:
A suspicious beat with an extremely shortened or prolonged CI is always presented on the operator's screen. The window is operator adjustable. The operator himself is able to wipe out portions of the ECG (Figure 4).
The strategies discussed above and included in the analysis process are conditions for the reliability of such a system. These will be checked by systematic performance-testing.

(B) Evaluation of Performance
To evaluate the system, we used three different methods:
1. Beat-by-beat scanning.
2. Tests of reproducibility.
3. Dumb operator testing.

1. Beat-by-beat scanning: The principle of beat-by-beat scanning is based on the ability to compare each result achieved by the analysis system simultaneously with the operator's visual control (strip-chart-record or screen display) (7). The operator decides whether an annotated beat is true or false positive detected (artefact), or a single beat is missed by the analysis system (missed beat, false negative).
Using 35 different tapes with different arrhythmias, artefact rates and QRS features, we performed beat-by-beat scanning over 776 randomly selected one-hundred-beat segments (Table 1). The operator evaluated among 77,305 annotated normal beats (NB in Table 1) 98% as true positive (NM, T. in Table 1) and 2,3% as artefacts (false positive) with a too close similarity to the automatic feature of the NB. On the other hand, the QRS-detector failed to recognize, 0,34% of true NB (FN). The detection raio T/A ranged from 0,84-1,00. Using the average detection ratio (AVG) or the gross detection ratio (T_n/ A_n) an estimate of the detection probability of 0,97 can be demonstrated in MP-SC. The probability that an annotated NB is true reaches a predictive value (PV) of 0,977 (Table 1).
PVC's were also scanned beat-by-beat: Out of 1805 automatic annotated (A) PVC's with different QRS-shapes, the operator classified visually 95% as true positive (T). In 8% of A-PVC's, the ventricular arrhythmia detector (VAD) was too sensitive and artefacts or normal-beats were recognized as PVC's (FP). On the other hand, in 3,5% of visually scanned PVC's the VAD failed (FN). The VAD's detection ratio ranged from 0,33 in tapes with low PVC rates up to 1,33 in tapes with a higher artefact rate. The gross detection ratio of 0,95 was much higher than the AVG. It weights the total

BEAT EVALUATION
(N= 35 TAPES)

(A)	A	T	FN	FP	TN
NB	77.3o5	75.5o2	255	1763	75542
PVC	1.8o5	1.715	63	144	73787

(B)	AVG	$\frac{T}{A}$	SPEC.	SENS.	PV	ACC.
NB	0.973	0.978	0.977	0.997	0.977	0.974
PVC	0.881	0.95o	0.998	0.965	0.922	0.892

Table 1. A = annotated beats, T = visually as true positive recognised beats, FN = overlooked beats by the computer (false negatives), TN = time negatives. NB = normal beats, PVC = premature ventricular contractions. AVG = average detection ratio of each tape. T/A = gross detection ratio of all tapes (8). Spec.= Specificity, Sens.= Sensitivity, PV = predictive value, Acc.= Accuracy.

number of annotated and detected PVC's, disregarding their distribution between the tape-segments. The gross detection ratio overestimates and the average detection ratio of 0,88 under-estimates the evaluation probability in VAD. Therefore, we should either use a larger amount of PVC's or a stochastic model should be used to achieve a greater statistical significance of VAD in MP-SC (8).

Using reference tapes, you can only point out whether the total amount of detected NB or PVC's is identical to the number counted with the user's system or not. But you cannot declare exactly whether a single beat is overlooked (false negative) or whether an artefact leads to a beat-detection (false positive). So it is impossible to evaluate the accuracy of a system with such reference tapes only. The results are too close to the identical line dependent on the scale used and over-estimates the system's quality.

2. Tests of reproducibility: Another step towards objective test procedures will be the test for reproducibility of the results achieved in the routine use of a system (9). Results of different operators are compared to each other. They should demonstrate a high agreement within a small margin of variation dependent on the number and significance of variables such as analysis time and artefact rate.

Four operators with different levels of skill in the use of MP-SC had to analyse five different tapes independently. They did not

REPRODUCIBILITY OF NORMAL-BEATS

TAPE	M̄ An.-Time		NUMBER OF DETECTED NORMAL BEATS					
	HR.	V(±%)	A	B	C	D	M̄	V (±%)
1.	23	0.0	64.034	64.189	64.157	64.022	64.100	0.1
2.	22	0.4	101.865	102.043	101.780	(95.437)'	(100.287)'	(3.2)'
						-	101.896	0.4
3.	23	0.7	116.672	-	115.518	114.124	115.438	1.1
4.	22	0.4	95.231	95.958	95.940	-	95.710	0.4
5.	23	(5.5)"	102.861	92.004	(89.651)"	98.432	(95.737)"	(6.3)"
		0.0			-		97.766	0.5
5	113	0.3	-	-	-	-	-	0.5

Table 2.   Mean.Time = mean analysis time in hours ± variability
between the operators, (A,B,C,D).   M = mean value between A-D of
detected HB ± variability (V±%). A much higher artefact rate of 6% of
operator D led to a less amount of detected QRS. Too high sensitivity
analysing tape 5 led to a signal overflow and stopped the tape 150
min.prior.

know the results obtained by the others.   On 475.000 heart beats a
mean variability of < 0,5% (0,1-1,1%) Could be achieved (Table 2).
The probability of reproducing the detection of a single beat through
computer analysis was 99,5%, with two exceptions: Operator D
performed the analysis of tape 2 (Table 2), with a much higher mean
artefact rate of 6%/23 hours than the others (1,1-1,7%), so that a
less amount of QRS complexes were detected.   Their variability increased.   To obtain a comparable result either an artefact-
correction-model would be necessary or the result had to be skipped.
On the other hand, a too high data rate, (because of too many artefacts and too high sensitivity of the system) led to stop tape no. 5,
when Operator C performed his reproducibility test, 150 min. prior to
the others.   Different analysis time led also to a less number of
detected heart beats and to an increase in ARS-variability.   So the
result once again should either be time-corrected or cancelled.
     The reproducibility in VAD depends from the artefact rate, from
the length of analysis duration, but also from the quantity of PVC's.
After time-correction, the variability of VAD decreasd from 14% in
tape 1 with rare occurring PVC's (mPVC < 1%/23 hours) over V ± 4%
(mPVC 1,5%/23 hours) to V ± 1,9% in frequent PVC's (mPVC 6%/23
hours) (Table 3).   The gross reproducibility rate in VAD was 1,7%
(Table 4) over 6400 PVC's disregarding the results of each analysed
tape.   That means, that only 2 out of 100 detected PVC's were not
reproducible using a mPVC rate of 2,5%/23 hours in MP.-SC. This
result seems consistent with beat-by-beat scanning (Table 1).

3.   Dumb operator test: The recognition and importance of the
influence of the software on obtained results should be also of
interest in a computer-supported soft-ware oriented analysis system
like MP.-SC. Therefore, we varied flexible analysis parameters
systematically, like maximal and minimal QRS-width, amplitude etc.

Op	Tape I Anal.T. (Min.)	PVC (N)	PVC (%)	Artef. (%)	Tape II Anal.T. (Min.)	PVC (N)	PVC (%)	Artef. (%)	Tape III Anal.T. (Min.)	PVC (N)	PVC (%)	Artef. (Min.)
A	1370	89	0.076	0.7	1370	1320	1.56	5.5	1400	5129	6.09	2.3
B	1370	101	0.087	0.5	1370	1058	1.27	5.9	1400	5117	6.09	2.4
	1370	95±14 V ± 14 %			1370	1189±49, V±4%			1400	5123±101, V±1.9 %		

Table 3   PVC Reproducibility in relation to mPVC-rate.

OVERALL PVC - REPRODUCIBILITY
(N = 3 TAPES)

Op	An.T. (HR)	PVC (N)	PVC (%)	Art. (%)
A	68	6,538	2,6	2,8
B	68	6,276	2,5	2,9
	68	6,407 ± 113;		V ± 1,7%

Table 4   An.-T – Analysis time   Art.= mean artefact rate over the whole tape. V = variability of the PVC-rate between the operators A and B.

The operator himself could not influence the analysis ("dumb-operator") (10). In MP-SC, it could be demonstrated that over a wide range, the variation of QRS-detection parameters cannot influence the result obtained. Extreme abnormal parameters led to an increase of the missed beats detection rate. False positive results can be avoided (10).

Conclusions

Including strategies for data-redundancy as mentioned above, like statistical CI analysis, beat descriptor's edit or selection of representative arrhythmias and multistage artefact detection algorithms, results of high plausibility and reproducibility can be achieved without disregarding the clinical standard.
   The physician needs the true result as a basis for his further patient oriented decisions. The computer can only offer the logical, most plausible result. But this has to be as close as possible to the truth, operator-independent and of a constant quality obtained within an acceptable time.

Acknowledgements

We are indebted to Mrs. Ulrike Grojer, Mrs. Angela Reich and Mrs. Trude Haagen for their assistance in analysing the records. This work was supported in part by the Austrian Heart Foundation and the Austrian "Fonds zur Forderung der Wissenschaften".

References

1. Hermes R.E., Oliver G.Ch. In: Ambulatory Electrocardiographic Recording, p.165. Ed: Kass Wenger N, Mock M.B., Rinquivist I., YearBook Med. Publ. Inc., Chicago, London 1980.
2. Weber H., Joskowicz G., Steinbach K., Glogar D. In: Modern Electrocardiography, Proc. of IVth Int. Congr. on Electrocardiology, Balatonfured 1977, Ed: Antaloczy Z., p.249, Excerpta Medica 1978.
3. Mead C.N., Clark, K.W., Oliver G.C. Thomas, L.T. In: IEEE Proc. Comp. in Card. 440, 1976.
4. Joskowicz G., Weber H., Glogar D., Steinbach K. IEEE Comp. in Card. 401, Stanford 1978.
5. Joskowicz G., Balatka H., Glogar D., Weber H., Steinbach K. In: IEEE Comp. Card p. 277, Genf, 1979.
6. Mark R.H., Moody G.B., Olson W.H., Peterson S.K. In: Ambulatory electrocardiographic recording, p.113: Ed: Kass Wenger N., Mock M.B.,Rinquist J. Year Book Med. Publ. Inc. Chicago, London, 1980.
7. Bailey J.J., Horton M., Itscoitz S. (1974) Circ. **50**, 88.
8. Cox J.R., Hermes R.E., Ripley K.L. In: Ambulatory Electrocardiographic Recording, p. 165. Ed: Kass Wenger N., Mock R.H., Rinquist J. Year Book Med. Publ.Inc. Chicago, London 1980.
9. Pipberger H.V., Cornfield J. (1973) Circ. **47**, 918.
10. Weber H., Glogar D., Joskowicz G., Steinbach K., Kaindl F. In: Management of Ventricular Tachycardia - Role of Mexiletine. Ed: Julian D., Bell W. p.358, Excerpta Medica 1978.

Discussion

DR.van DURME: How were the 5 tapes which were given to each of the technicians selected?
DR. WEBER: They were routine tapes.
DR. van DURME: So they were randomly selected?
DR. WEBER: Yes, but they differed with regard to their artefact rates, the QRS configurations and the duration.
DR. van DURME: Can any clue be given about the percentage of artefact present?
DR. WEBER: That depends on the analysis system being used. We decided that we were dealing with an excellent quality tape if the artefact rate during 24 hours was below 5%. If the artefact rate was over 10%, the tape was of a much poorer quality. Clearly, the output depends upon the input, and can never be better than the input signal.
DR. van DURME: So these selected 5 tapes had less than 5% artefact?
DR. WEBER: No, between 1 and 10%. I do not know exactly the percentage, but it is given in the Table.

SOME REMARKS ON DATA PRESENTATION OF RR-INTERVALS AS APPLIED TO THE ECG OF PATIENTS WITH FUNCTIONAL HEART DISEASE

R. RICHTER, B. DAHME, K.D. SCHEPPOKAT, G. STEMMLER
AND H. WAND

Universitatskrankenhaus Eppendorf, Pav. H23 D 2000 Hamburg
and Robert Koch Krankenhaus Gehrden, Germany

Summary

Our method of computer analysis of the RR-interval data derived from a 24-hour ECG has essentially the following characteristics:
- signal enhancing filters using an averaged P-QRS-T-pattern as a template;
- dialogue and graphic display of questionable signals initiated by the programme;
- adaptation of programme criteria for R-wave detection;
- automatic plausibility-check of computed RR-intervals and simultaneous graphic display of their time course for manual correction.

Data from the RR-interval file computed by this method can be presented in various ways, e.g. interval-time-curves, scatter plots and histograms. They then give quantitative information concerning the behaviour of cardiac rate, its time-dependence and variability.

When this method of data processing is applied to the clinical problems of studying heart rate in patients with functional heart disorders as compared to normal controls, our preliminary results seem to indicate that there are differences between the two groups: as regards beat-to-beat variability during day and night.

Methods

The 24-hour-ECG contains information on cardiac arrhythmias, on alterations of the ST-segment, and on cardiac rate. In the clinical application of the ambulatory ECG monitoring techniques, the detection and quantification of arrhythmias and of deviations from the normal QRST-pattern has received generous attention in the past. Data related to cardiac rate, however, have found much less interest.

The quantitative analysis of continuous electrocardiographic recordings poses a technical problem making great demands on soft- and hardware properties of the computer system used. The first problem to be solved is the detection of the R-wave as a basis for the exact computation of RR-intervals.

24-hour-ECG were recorded on a Medilog-recorder, and played back at 60 times recording speed and fed into a Data General Computer system Eclipse S240. An interactive Fortran-programme to determine successive RR-intervals in ECG-recordings distorted by artefacts has been developed by our group (1). The programme starts with the computation of the average of 10 typical P-QRS-T-patterns, having

been inspected and selected by the operator using a graphic display.
This intra-individual average serves as a template for the following
filtering procedure. For signal-optimizing, we use a specific filter, which includes cross-correlation and inverse filtering as special cases (details see (1)).

Figure 1 shows distorted ECG-signals of two original recordings
(upper trace) and the signals optimized by the filtering procedure,
which results in an augmentation of the R-waves and suppression of
artefacts, P- and T-waves. If the automatic detection procedure
should fail to identify a R-wave within a pre-determined interval,
the programme interrupts the processing of the ECG, and the interval
in question is displayed on the screen. The operator has then to
decide which one of different artefact-reducing strategies should be
applied to that interval (alteration of the detection criteria, de-
letion of artefactual data points, interpolation between adjacent RR-

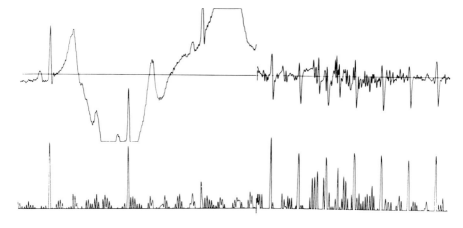

Fig. 1   Effect of filtering on badly distorted ECG signal

intervals etc). The entire data-file of successive RR-interval, computed and corrected for artefact, is stored on magnetic tape and can
be used in various ways for further statistical analysis.

Figure 2 exemplifies one possible method to present RR-interval
data. Various parameters derived from one 24-hour-ECG recording are
given as 10-minutes-averages:

Curve A represents the time course of RR-intervals, Curve B that
of the standard deviations of the RR-intervals (multiplied by 3),
Curve C gives the minimum and Curve D the maximum RR-intervals,
within each 10-minute-period. The range represented by Curves C and
D can be considered as an index for mental and physical activation,
respectively. Curve E shows the time course of the auto-correlation
lag 1, which is a measure of the serial inter-dependence of the RR-
intervals. The mean RR-interval varies betweeen 520 and 960 msec

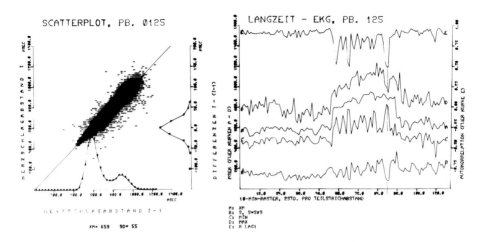

Fig. 2   **Scatterplot of 24 hr ECG, and trend plot of derived measure-ments (see text for key)**

over the entire 24-hour period. The night- and day-values differ markedly. During night/sleep, the auto-correlation lag 1 sometimes decreases to 0.5., testifying to diminishing beat-to-beat inter-dependence during sleep.

Another graphic method of presenting RR-interval data derived from a 24-hour-ECG is the scatter plot, shown in the left-hand side of Figure 2.

On the abscissa, the RR-interval histogram is plotted. It shows a bimodal distribution, as can be expected from a compilation of day and night data. Along the ordinate, the histogram of the RR-interval-differences is plotted. It shows the distribution of the differences between adjacent RR-intervals and signifies beat-to-beat variability of the heart rate. It is symmetric to 0, which means that there is no difference between the beat-to-beat variability during acceleration and deceleration of the heart rate.

The same information concerning RR-interval differences and some additional information relating to their time dependence, is con-tained in the scatter plot along the 45°-axis. It displays the auto-correlation lag 1 of the RR-intervals: each of the scattered symbols represents the relation betwen a certain RR-interval, on the ordin-ate, and its preceding RR-interval, on the abcissa. If there is ac-celeration of the heart rate, i.e. a certain RR-interval is smaller than the preceding one, the symbol is plotted below the 45°-axis. If, however, the heart rate decelerates, the symbol will be above the 45°-axis. The greater the difference between adjacent RR-intervals, the greater is the distance between the data point and the 45° axis, i.e. a great beat-to-beat variability leads to a wide scatter of symbols and vice versa. The different symbols signify frequency classes of RR-intervals, their graphic density corresponds to the frequency of data related to the x and y co-ordinates. Whereas the

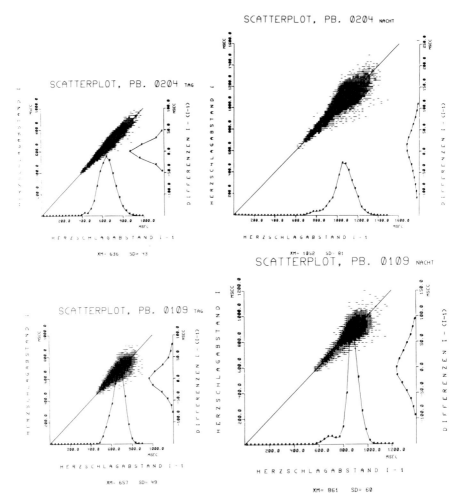

Fig. 3   (above) and 4 (below) present clinical applications of this
          method of RR-interval data analysis. Scatter plots are used
          to compare the behaviour of cardiac rate of a healthy volun-
          teer to that of a patient with functional heart disease.

width of the scatter plot represents the auto-correlation lag 1, the
length of the scatter plot displays the overall range of RR-
intervals.
     For this purpose, the 4-hour samples representing day and night,
were selected randomly from the 24-hour recordings of one subject and
one patient.   In the healthy subject, there is a greater beat-to-beat
variability during the night.   And the mean of the subject's RR-
intervals during sleep is greater than the patient's.   A similar
trend is seen when one compares small samples of 3 subjects and 3
patients each.   The preliminary conclusion would be that patients

with functional cardiac disturbances do not increase their heart rate variability during night-sleep, i.e. they do not relax during sleep to the same extent as normal subjects do.

References

1.   Stemmler G. and Thom E. (1979) EDV in Med. and Biol., **10**, 122-127.

Discussion

MR. ARMSTRONG: What resolution in msec is required on the axes to give what Dr. Richter regards as significance?
DR. RICHTER: Each data point is the average of the 10 periods, but the original resolution is about 0.1 msec.
MR. ARMSTRONG: That is a high resolution.
PROF. PINCIROLI: Dr. Richter made a distinction between night and day. What is the minimum length to the minimum time of observation necessary in order to give confidence to this kind of data presentation?
PROF. SCHEPPOKAT: I think that there should be at least 2 hours' time interval around that. We are not sure which hour of the 7 or 8 eights of sleep should be taken as representative. In general, it is felt that the second half of the night's rest is representative of the individual's sleep. In ambulatory patients, it is rather difficult to decide what time of the day is representative of the day as a time for comparison with the night. For instance, in their professional activities, people might have a tachycardia of 100 or 110, even office workers. Perhaps the time best used for comparison is in the evening.
       The clinical purpose of this study is to see whether it is possible to pinpoint differences in heart rate behaviour in patients with anxiety neurosis. It is known that the physiological part of the anxiety reaction is an increase in heart rate, an increase in the resting blood flow to the striated muscle and an increase in cardiac output. In some respects, people with anxiety neurosis react to certain stimuli with an increased heart rate response. The question being asked of this method, therefore, is whether it is possible to pinpoint certain aberrations of the heart rate behaviour in the direction of higher sympathetic tone.
DR. SOUTHALL: Has this been looked at with relationship to breathing, that is to sinus arrhythmia?
DR. RICHTER: No, we have not done that.
DR. SOUTHALL: I think this could well be very well worth doing.

A SATELLITE PRINTING STATION FOR USE WITH COMPUTER-BASED TAPE ANALYSIS SYSTEMS

C.L. FELDMAN, M. HUBELBANK, V. VALVO, AND B. LANE

University of Massachusetts Medical Centre,
Worcester, MA 01605, USA

Summary

Increasingly, sophisticated computer-based systems are used for the analysis of tape-recorded ambulatory monitoring data. These systems generally perform more accurate and comprehensive analyses than is possible with more conventional systems. Because of their high speed, such systems are often economically attractive if the load factor can be kept high. Except in very densely populated areas, maintaining a high load factor means drawing from a large geographic area and suffering the long turn-around that results from gathering the tapes and distributing the results. This report describes the design of a remote printing station, which receives the final report transtelephonically from the central analysis system, reformats the data, and prints reports containing analog, graphic and alphanumeric data on an electrostatic printer.

Introduction

For nearly 10 years, we have been engaged in the on-going development of a computer-based Holter monitor analysing system. During various phases of its development, the system has been used in a number of epidemiologic and drug studies and for a relatively small amount of clinical work.

At the present time, the system's exceptional accuracy - which has made it ideal for epidemiologic and drug research - has become increasingly important in the clinical environment. The availability of new anti-arrhythmic agents, each with an unique mode of action and a different set of side-effects, now argues for the accurate quantitative measurement of ventricular ectopic activity for purposes of titration. With a processing speed of 60 times real time, the system is sufficiently fast to be economically suited for processing clinical tapes. However, the relatively high initial cost of the equipment makes it mandatory that it be used more than the standard 40 hour work week properly to amortize its first cost. Although such utilization is perfectly practical in population dense urban areas, it seems that the less dense outlying areas might not be able to support such equipment. The way this problem has been dealt with without undue turn-around time has been to design remote printing station for use in the smaller suburbs. With this system, tapes are mailed to the central processing facility from a large "catch area" and the reports are transmitted transtelephonically to the remote printing stations located in suburban hospitals and similar facil-

Processing and Editing

The main tape processor is implemented on a PDP-11/34 with 64 KW of memory, a 7.5 MB Winchester disc and an industry-compatible floppy disc. QRS and artefact detection are implemented in hardware. Playbacks (reel and cassette) are under computer control. To permit flexibiity in processing a variety of tapes with different amounts of ectopic activity and different accuracy requirements, a display screen, a button box and a keyboard are added to the system.

Conceptually, computer processing is a two-pass system. During the first pass, A/D conversion is performed, all QRS complexes are located and the ECG is transferred from the tape on which it was recorded to a magnetic disc. During the second pass, only those areas near each complex of the stored ECG are examined. In practice, the system uses two, one-hour buffers on the disc and executes both passes concurrently, starting or stopping the tape playback unit as needed.

In the multi-template version of the WPI algorithm currently in use, room is allotted for eight separate templates. The most common template, the normal one, is always Template 1. Other templates may be normal or abnormal. Correlation of each test beat is performed first on Template 1 and then on other templates in sequence. If no match in correlation coefficient of 0.79 or above is reached, a new template is established and the old template is abandoned based on a combination of a number of occurrences and the time since last occurrence.

To achieve the required flexibility, the algorithm is capable of detecting the following events: all ventricular ectopic depolarizations (VED's), VED couplets, ventricular tachycardia (VT), early VED's, VED couplets, all supraventricular ectopic depolarizations (SVED's), early SVED's, missed beat, sudden rate increase, high rate, irregular rate, S-T segment change, new template, bradycardia, all QRS's and artefact.

Each of these events can be displayed in one of several operator-selectable and changeable modes. Whenever the system encounters an abnormality for which DISPLAY mode has been selected, it stops and presents the operator with an annotated static display. The operator can modify the annotation if it is wrong, reject it if the event was only artefact, and/or direct the system to store the event on floppy discs for future editing and/or as an example to be returned to the referring physician.

Between occurrences of DISPLAY EVENTS, the system displays all events in a segmented superimposed display. In this display, sinus beats are presented on the top third of the screen, SVED's in the middle third, and VED's on the lower third. If the operator detects a system error, he/she can back up the system and modify annotations as needed. At the conclusion of processing, the floppy disc contains sample annotated strips and all tables and is available for overreading.

In one configuration, there is a separate over-reading station consisting of an LSI-11 microcomputer with 32 KW of memory, a 19 MB rigid disc, dual floppy discs, a display made up of a Matrox 256 by 512 memory board and a standard television monitor, and either a modem for remote transmission or a Versatec V80 graphic electrostatic

printer. In the preferred alternative, the editor and processor are
combined, eliminating redundant hardware. From the over-reading
station, the operator can review the sample strips, modify the annotations as required, and delete redundant strips. The review can be
either sequential or by selective search and either time or amplitude
measurements, can be made with operator-controlled cursors. Although
only a single ECG is processed, the over-reading station presents
both channels to the operator simultaneously. Any changes in com-
puter-generated annotations are reflected by the editor in the tables
that it will finally produce. At the conclusion of the editing
process, the report is generated by formatting the edited data in
customized report modules. The report may than be printed on a
Versatec V80 graphic/alphanumeric printer or may be transmitted via
modem to report stations.

Accuracy

As is well-known, a totally satisfactory analysis of Holter analysis
systems is extremely hard to perform. However, to get some idea of
the system's performance, the standard quality control data from a
commercial use of the system were analysed. The test consisted of
"recycling", in a blinded fashion, 34 separate 12- or 24-hour tapes,
each of which had been ready beat-by-beat by a cardiologist on a
compressed, complete write-out. Because of the random selection
process, some tapes were read as many as four times, while others
were read only once. Throughout the test, analysts strove for speed
as well as accuracy, achieving a throughput of eight tapes per eight-
hour shift, including editing and transmission.

The results as evaluated in the usual linear fashion are shown
in Table 1. Although the slopes of the regression lines and the
coefficients are very close to unity, we feel that this linear model
is a poor one because tapes with large numbers of VED's contribute
disproportionately to linear coefficients. Accordingly, we have also
analysed these tapes by a logarithmic model in which we fit a best
curve of the form

$$Y = a\ x^c \qquad (1)$$

by finding the best straight line for the curve of log y vs. log x.
In this analysis, fractional errors have the same weight irrespective
of the number of VED's in a given test. The results of this analysis
are shown in Table 2. The correlation coefficient is the correlation
co-efficient of the scatter diagram of the logarithms of the data
points.

Remote Station Design

The remote station consiists of an LSI-11 microcomputer with 16 KW of
memory, a V80 Versatec printer and a 1200 baud modem. Because the
remote station programme is down-loaded from the over-reading station, no mass storage is required. The system runs under Digital
Equipment Corp.'s RT-11 operating system.

Design of the software focused on achieving an optimum combination of accuracy and speed. All data is transmitted as blocks of 512
bytes with a check sum. At the end of each block, transmission of

TABLE 1

Accuracy of Computer VED Detection System (1980)
Linear Evaluation

	N	b(intercept)	m(slope)	P_2(correlation coefficient)
VED (total)	55	−45.47	1.018	.9987
Paired VED's	39	6.75	1.003	.9926
VT Beats	38	− .17	1.030	.9881

TABLE 2

Accuracy of Computer VED Detection System (1980)
Logarithmic Evaluation

	N	a(multiplier)	c(exponent)	P_2(correlation coefficient)
VED Total	55	.994	1.0019	.9991
Paired VED's	39	1.014	.9988	.9982
VT Beats	38	.952	1.0043	.9986

the single duplex circuit is reversed to receive an acknowledge character from the remote printer. In the absence of an acknowledgement, the block is re-transmitted. As a result of this error detection scheme, the effective transmission rate is reduced to approximately 100 characters per second.

Alphanumeric characters are transmitted from the main processor to the remote station in essentially normal ASCII format. The only variation from usual practice is to compress spaces, which are then uncompressed by the remote station. Graphical data is transmitted in the same manner as characters. To achieve graphical output, special characters have been defined with arbitrary patterns within the space usually used by a character. These special characters are interpreted by the remote printer programme and used to produce graphs such as those in Figure 1. Waveforms are transmitted as data in two's complement form at 70 samples per second for each channel. The remote printer programme interpolates between points to produce a smooth graph on a grid which it prints. To minimize the usefulness of the waveforms, characters are used to indicate the time of occurrence type of event, etc.

The typical tabular and graphical output consists of eight to twelve blocks requiring approximately one minute for transmission. The number of waveforms transmitted depends on the complexity of the patient's arrhythmias, requiring approximately 10 seconds per strip. In practice, the majority of reports take between five to eight minutes.

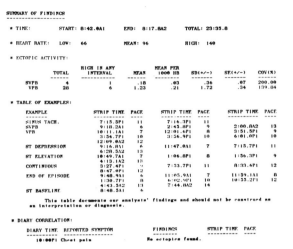
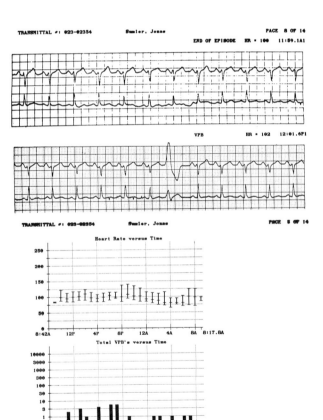

Fig. 1   Report samples.

Results and Conclusions

The editing and report generating equipment described above has been in routine use since January, 1980. During this time, it has easily achieved our primary goal of around-the-clock utilization of the basic processing equipment without degradation of turn-around time to outlying areas. Additionally, we found its data handling capability has brought a number of other benefits, including the following:

1.   Better personnel utilization through the minimization of clerical tasks.
2.   Ability to concentrate several machines in a single central location. Thus achieving the better quality control and supervision than would be possible otherwise.
3.   The ability to add easily or delete separate report sections - modules - to accommodate the needs of different drug study protocols.
4.   The ability to output all report data on magnetic tape for efficient entry into the data bases of large drug studies.

The only major miscalculation in the original design seems to have been in over-estimating the value of separate editing stations. As originally conceived, the separate editing station would enable a specialized over-reader efficiently to review each report without tying up the processing equipment. In practice, it has been found much more efficient to have the person who processes the tape perform the first review. Further, it seems preferable to do this review immediately upon completion of the scan at the processor itself. The over-reader, on the other hand, seems to work most efficiently from a hardcopy of the report using the editor station only for making relatively rare corrections to the report and transmitting the data to remote stations.

Discussion

DR. CASHMAN: Does the system analyse both channels at the same time, or do you analyse one and then look at the other?
PROF. FELDMAN: Only one channel is analysed. The superimposed display is just one channel; all the other displays are two channels. Any time it stops, the operator has both, but the machine is using only one channel.
DR. CASHMAN: If the operator wants to back up, does it back up the counts too?
PROF. FELDMAN: Yes, of course it backs up, and she can hand-step through it, or change a template and say that it is ventricular and not supraventricular, and it will re-do it as it goes forward. Likewise, in the editing phase, basically all of that can also be changed.
DR. MONSTER: Did Prof. Feldman say that the different records that have abnormalities on them are stored on floppy disks?
PROF. FELDMAN: The floppy is used as an intermediate medium. Initially, the operator goes through and decides that she wants to store a whole batch of them. On editing them she looks at them again, and usually decides that she has stored too many of any

particular focus. Then she prints out just those she really wants.
DR. WEBER: If I understood correctly, Prof. Feldman compared hand-counted tapes with the computer printout, or did he achieve a beat-to-beat analysis?
PROF. FELDMAN: It is not a beat-to-beat analysis, it is hand counts - and clearly there are compensating errors, which is a problem. There was no practical way of dealing with it.
DR. WEBER: We had the same problem.
DR. van DURME: This once again emphasises the fact that everyone should not keep his own data bank, but should gather them together as it is done. I am not sure whether it is available for different systems in the United States?
PROF. FELDMAN: The AHA database is now available from ECRI, which is a non-profit making organisation in Philadelphia. ECRI has contracted with the AHA to seel the AHA database tapes.
DR. van DURME: This is a point which returns again and again. Everyone is using his own counts and normals. I find it very difficult to compare, discuss and assess without having the same tapes on the same patients, with the same number of artefacts which have exactly the same appearance, going through these different systems. Until something like that has been done, we will continue to go round in circles and keep having long workshops (which I enjoy very much). Everyone of us should do this once the databank is available. The question is whether it will fit any type of equipment.
PROF. FELDMAN: I do not know. The databank itself is available on digital tape. I am not sure what ECRI is doing about making it available in an analog format - I hope they will do that - or in other digital formats.
DR. MONSTER: The tapes from the AHA are available in a digital form. They have then to be converted back to analog form before putting them on the scanner. Something else that ECRI has done recently is to take a standard set of tapes that has been collected inviting different manufacturers of scanners to make their scanning available and to scan this collection of tapes on their scanners. This has been published in their monthly journal. However, the person who did the work told me that he did not receive much co-operation from the various manufacturers.
DR. FELDMAN: There is another smaller - and probably less well-known - database which is available, from Prof. Mark, at MIT and the Beth-Israel Hospital, Boston. It is also a perfectly useful databse.
DR.ENG. MARCHESI: I am interested in this second MIT database. It is curious that at the moment when we look for a common reference, there are two of them in the United States. Why two databases, when we need only one? A common effort must be put into the development and dissemination of one.
PROF. FELDMAN: In fact, the MIT database does not pretend to be what the AHA database is. It was gathered informally and Prof. Mark then said that all this work had been done, and maybe somebody else could use it. It was not officially supported by anybody, and has no sort of official sanction. But it is convenient and I think it is particularly useful if a new system is being developed.
DR.ENG. MARCHESI: Are the manufacturers involved with database use sensitive to this very serious approach to validation?

PROF. FELDMAN: I am not in a position to answer that because I do
not know, but my impression is that the manufacturers of real-time
arrhythmia monitors are extremely sensitive to the issue, and are
more or less prepared to put their system through its paces as soon
as the tapes are available. As a rule, the Holter scanner
manufacturers are perhaps not quite as in tune with it as are the
real-time manufacturers. That is only an impression.
DR. van DURME: This is the problem - let's face it. The implications
of the final outcome of such a databank running through a system are
so high, and so important that it should be done by an independent
group or organisation which would be recognised by all of us and by
all the manufacturers, and from which they would accept the results.

THE NEWCASTLE 2-CHANNEL DYNAMIC ECG ANALYSIS SYSTEM

A. MURRAY, R.S. JORDAN, R.W.F. CAMPBELL, D.G. JULIAN

Regional Medical Physics Department and
Academic Cardiology Unit, Freeman Hospital,
Newcastle-upon-Tyne, UK

Summary

A dynamic ECG analysis system has been developed in Newcastle to
enable 2-channel ECG write-outs of frequent arrhythmias to be obtained, enable highly complex ECG recordings to be analysed with
ease, produce accurate analysis, reduce operator fatigue and allow
fast single-pass non-stop analysis.

All arrhythmias of interest are extracted during a single non-
stop replay of the recording and, after editing, are written-out
automatically on standard A4 paper,ready for direct inclusion in the
patient's hospital notes or research folder. Each ECG is identified
with its time of occurrence and automatically detected arrhythmias
are clearly identified.

This paper describes the way the numerous computer files are
organized so as to achieve versatility and ease of operation. The 2-
channel analysis system is a direct development from the single-
channel system, which has now been in constant use for over two years
analysing ECG recordings from the coronary care unit as well as from
out-patients.

Introduction

Many systems now exist for the analysis of dynamic ECGs. The majority are commercial systems which enable detected ECGs to be written-
out on standard ECG paper. Other systems have been specially developed on mini- or micro-computers to enable more advanced techniques
to be developed. More development effort has gone into improving the
accuracy of automatic arrhythmia detectors than into enabling detected arrhythmias to be edited and clearly presented with simple
manual intervention. The Newcastle system concentrates on these
latter features.

System Overview

A description of the first version of the system has already been
given (1) and only a brief overview will be included here. The main
aim of the system is to enable frequent complex arrhythmias to be
extracted reliably and easily from ECG recordings, during a single
high-speed replay and clearly written-out in a format that can be
easily studied. Using the initial system, it has been confirmed that
complex arrhythmias in patients with an acute myocardial infarction
do not appear randomly, but are grouped together (2) and as a consequence, are more difficult to write-out on paper using conventional

analysers. Over 60% of 1580 ECG write-outs containing complex arrhythmias (VEC pairs, VT, R-on-T VEC's) in 38 patients with a recent
acute infarction were separated by 1 minute or less, equivalent to 1s
during replay at 60 times the recording speed.

In the Newcastle analysis system, arrhythmias are stored during
analysis on a computer disc. This selective storage is activated
automatically or manually. Automatic activation is achieved using
the Pathfinder analyser (3) as a preprocessor to detect arrhythmias.
Any other type of preprocessor could, however, be used if necessary.
Arrhythmias of interest are pre-selected before analysis on a series
of switches on the computer interface. When an arrhythmia is detected a continuous 10s ECG sample is stored with the arrhythmia in the
centre. The time of occurrence is also stored. If manual storage is
used 80s of ECG preceding the operator's push-button activation is
stored. At a replay speed of 60 times the recording speed this
amounts to a 1.33s maximum permissible reaction time. A total
storage of three hours of 2-channel ECG is possible during any one
analysis session. This is usually adequate for the analysis of
several patients.

Computer-stored ECG's are retrieved for editing onto a display
screen using a hand-held control unit. Separate push buttons on this
control are used to enable the stored arrhythmias to be labelled on
the computer disc. This label is read by the plotting part of the
programme. These selected ECG's are then automatically written-out
onto standard A4 size paper, ready for direct inclusion into the
patient's notes. Any relevant patient data is written automatically
at the top of each page and each ECG is marked with the time of its
occurrence (Figure 1.) Five 10s 2-channel ECG's are plotted on one
sheet of paper.

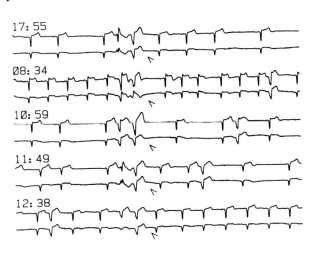

Fig. 1   Two-channel ECG write-out obtained from analysis system.

In this version of the analysis system, the quality of the final write-out has been greatly improved by using a high resolution plotter and by drawing a vector (straight line) between the sample points rather than a step. In addition, to aid a review of the system's performance, arrhythmias which have been automatically detected are marked clearly on the display and on the paper write-out.

Equipment

The computer system used is a DEC PDP-11/34 with RK05 discs. Only one disc unit is used for ECG storage. ECG's are sampled with two analogue-to-digital converters. Two digital-to-analogue converters drive the storage display (Tektronix 611) on which ECG's are viewed for editing. ECG times, and edit and manual storage command logic are fed to the system via a standard digital 16 bit interface. Arrhythmia detection logic is input via a second 16 bit interface. ECG write-outs are obtained on a Hewlett Packard plotter. Arrhythmia counts and artefact times are typed on a standard printer.

Functional Structure of Analysis System

Figure 2 diagramatically shows all the file structures used within the analysis programme. Each section is explained in turn below.

ECG
 ECG's are filtered so that frequencies above 40Hz are removed before they are presented to the analogue-to-digital convertor. Any required alteration in gain is done manually at this stage.

Digitise
 When ECG's are digitised, a sample from each of the two ECG channels is stored in one sixteen bit word. The first eight bits are used to store the ECG of channel 1. The next seven bits store the ECG of channel 2; with half the the amplitude resolution of channel 1. The final bit stores the presence of a logical signal which currently identifies the time arrhythmias are detected.

Buffer
 A circular buffer of ten-thousand words is continuously up-dated with ECG samples during the running of the analysis programme. A sampling rate of 6kHz is used, which is equivalent to 100 samples/s at real time. The length of this ring buffer is chosen to enable, under the worst case conditions, 8000 prevous samples to be stored to disc. This holds 80s (real time) of ECG for storage on manual activation.

Store
 If ECG storage is activated automatically, a file is formed in the computer memory which contains 500 sample words before the activation trigger and 500 words after. This information is stored in a 1024 word file equivalent to 4 disc blocks. The remaining 24 words,

which are retained at the beginning of the file, are used to store
information associated with the 10s ECG's. The following are stored:
ECG time, patient number and logical information associated with
automatic/manual store, ECG continuous with previous ECG, ECG to be
plotted. Most of this information is stored when the original ECG is
stored, but the information on whether it has to be plotted is obviously stored during editing. If manual storage is used 8 consecutive 10s ECG's are stored.

File
    Next, this file is stored on disc in a much larger file which
can hold over 1100 10s ECG's, equivalent to over 3h of ECG. At the
beginning of this file, space is allocated to hold patient information which has to be written on the top of each ECG report page.
This information is accessed via the patient number associated with
each ECG and is fed to the computer system via a keyboard before
analysis of a new patient is started. Three pointers are associated
with this longer file. A store pointer indicates where the next ECG
sample is to be stored on disc, an edit pointer indicates the next
ECG to be edited and the plot pointer the next ECG to be formatted
for plotting.

Edit
    During the editing procedure, ECG's are retrieved under operator
control from the disc file and both channels are displayed. If a
write-out of this ECG is wanted, the operator indicates this with one
of the push-buttons on the hand-control. This causes the edit file
to be labelled and written back, with this change, to the main disc
file.

Retrieve
    The part of the programme concerned with ECG write-outs works in
parallel with the other sections and lags behind the edit section.
All ECG's are retrieved from the disc file and checked to see if a
write-out is required. If it is, the file is passed to be formatted
for plotting on a page of ECG's.

Page
    Each page file contains an initial section which holds informa-
tion associated with the page heading. This is followed by five
sections each containing a 10s 2-channel ECG. The page file is made
up of a series of ASCII characters which are decoded by the plotter.
All page files are terminated with a character sequence which causes
the plotter to advance automatically to a new page and cut off the
previous page from the roll of paper.

Pages
    Each page is sent as a separate file to be plotted but page
files are retained so that, if required, duplication of selected
pages can be achieved.

Write out
    Finally the complete, suitably formatted pages of ECG write-outs
are obtained. An example is shown in Figure 1.

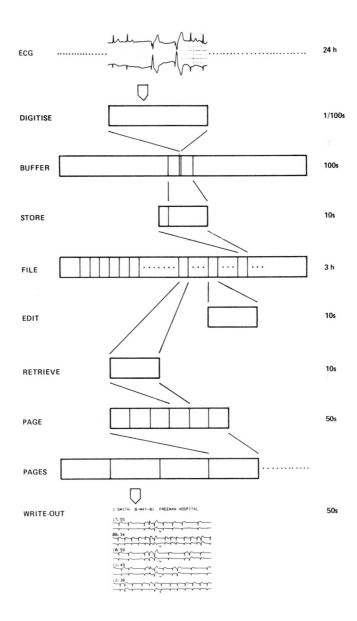

Fig. 2 Block diagram illustrating functional structure of the
        system.

Discussion

System Flexibility
     The system is designed to be highly flexible. Changing any of
the arrhythmia input switches will immediately alter the arrhythmias
to be stored. Other external trigger inputs can also be supplied if
required. The system can, if required, be asked to sample continuously. In addition to the hardware flexibility, the programme is
structured so as to enable modifications in the overall system performance to be made easily.

Interaction
     The system is designed to allow immediate interaction with the
system at all times. The ring buffer is always maintained and manual
or automatic inputs can be achieved at any time. Likewise, editing
can be undertaken simultaneously with ECG analysis. Our preferred
technique is to use a second operator to edit while the first operator analyses or, if only one operator is available, editing is
undertaken after analysis is complete. This is to ensure that a high
standard of accuracy is maintained. During analysis the operator
views the ECG and monitors the overall performance of the pre-
processor analyser.

Ease of Use
     All too often in computer systems, simple changes in function
can only be achieved through a question and answer dialogue, with the
system. No such dialogue is required with this system. Although it
is preferred that each patient is identified this is not necessary as
long as only one patient is being analysed during any one analysis
session. The operator is under total control of the system using only
a few logic switches (e.g. select VEC, VEC pairs, or VT) or push-
button controls (e.g. manual-store, edit, plot). Hence even complex
ECG recordings can be analysed accurately, with ease and with low
operator fatigue.

Conclusions

A versatile and easy-to-use operator-controlled analysis system has
been developed. The system has been in use for two years and has
become an indispensable aid to the analysis of dynamic ECG recordings, from both ambulant out-patients and coronary care unit in-
patients.

References

1.   Murray A., Campbell R.W.F., Julian D.G. In: Ripley K.L., Ostrow
     H.G., Eds. Computers in Cardiology. Long Beach, California:
     IEEE Computer Society, 1979: 197-9.
2.   Murray A., Campbell R.W.F., Julian D.G. In: Ripley K.L., Ostrow
     H.G., eds. Computers in Cardiology. Long Beach, California:
     IEEE Computer Society, 1980:379-82..
3.   Neilson J.M. In: Computers in Cardiology. Long Beach, Califor-
     nia: IEEE Computer Society, 1974: 55-9.

Discussion

DR. MONSTER: One disadvantage of this method is that it is
impossible to determine ahead of time what is going to be stored; in
other words, it is impossible to be very selective.   There is not
much sense in storing 10 periods of bigeminy if, in fact, there are
5000 on the tape, and that cannot be known until the tape has been
analysed.

DR. MURRAY: That is very true.   The analysis is not done that way,
but by an operator sitting in front of the system, ensuring that the
system performs the way she wants it to.   As I have said, the pre-
processor is the Pathfinder, which can determine whether it is a
single ventricular beat, pairs or ventricular tachycardia.   The
operator, if she chooses, can select different groups.   In research,
we operate at the moment according to the Lown criteria, and it is
the higher Lown grades that we are interested in.   If it is part of a
standard protocol, the operator knows what the protocol is and will
'output' all those events on to paper so that they can be looked at
in detail later.   But if for any reason we want to change the criteria, they can be changed instantaneously as the analysis proceeds.

PROF. PINCIROLI: Having come to the end of the day, I would like to
make a general comment, not one specifically directed to Dr. Murray.
During the whole day we have heard about systems and efforts devoted
to the singling out of arrhythmias.   I completely agree that this is
an important field, but I have the feeling that with the instruments
now available we could find out some more information about the ECG
that has not so far been investigated very much.

For instance, let me outline the problem of variability existing
between cycles.   I have in mind those analytical systems that build
the mean cycle.   In general, I do not agree with this technique.
Building the mean cycle means assuming that the only difference
between one cycle and another is the noise, and this is not true.

I would like to stress that in the future we need to study the
variability not directly connected to arrhythmias.

DR. MURRAY: The question that Prof. Pinciroli is really asking is
what should we analyse?   This is back to asking a clinical question.
We are analysing things on the basis of 'this is what the literature
says should be analysed', but not doing it blindly.   I have presented
the technical part.   We are looking at the evaluation of these
arrhythmias to see whether they are important.   One thing that has
been studied is arrhythmias preceding ventricular fibrillation.

To take up Prof. Pinciroli's general comment, I do not think
that makers of equipment should build into their equipment everything
and anything that we can dream up.   It is up to a few selected groups
to decide that something is their speciality, and that they will
investigate it, be it interval or interval variation or R-on-T, and
follow it through.   After they have followed it through, they should
then report back to the scientific audience what they have found, and
if they believe their findings to be important.   If they believe it
to be important, other people will adopt these procedures; if they
say that something is not important, other people might forget it.

DR. van DURME: This is very true, and I fully agree with what has
been said.   I will not say any more about it, although it is one of
the topics that I like.

A MINICOMPUTER BASED SYSTEM FOR ECG AMBULATORY MONITORING: DATA PRESENTATION AND STATISTICAL EVALUATION*

C. MARCHESI, G. KRAFT, L. LANDUCCI, A. TADDEI, C. CONTINI,
G.F. MAZZOCCA, M.G. BONGIORNI

CNR Institute of Clinical Physiology and Institute of
Medical Pathology of Pisa University, Italy

Summary

The Programme ASTRI (Analisi ST RItmo) represents an attempt to overcome the major limitations of commercially available systems for ECG
ambulatory monitoring.
 After a 60 times real time speed A/D conversion from the playback unit to computer tape, the operator adjusts a number of thresholds for the particular case. Thresholds are entered into an automatic analysis programme, which performs: QRS detection, feature
extraction (RR interval, QRS duration, QRS morphology factor, positive and negative areas), QRS classification based on the features,
report-printing including histograms and plots. During processing,
all relevant information is stored on disc for physician verification. The method has been successfully used in about 900 patients
showing the followng major advantages: greater reliability than
commercial systems, easily understandable data presentation and comprehensive statistical evaluation of results.
 After testing and intensive use in a routine clinical environment, the most successful features of ASTRI proved to be the self-
adjusting QRS detector algorithm and the combined graphical presentation of both rhythm classification and time plots of ST-T changes,
which allow a care-free identification of acute episodes.

Introduction

The presently available methods for ECG long-term monitoring can be
divided in four classes, according to the level of interaction between operator and system.
 Systems requiring the continuous presence of the operator during
the analysis can be classified at level 1, since no automatic procedure is implemented; level 2 includes systems allowing some automatic
analysis in combination with visual inspection; level 3 accounts for
software-based systems, where the interaction is very limited. Level
4 systems are fully automated and operate in real-time, hosted by the
portable unit; they are at development phase (1).
 In our Institutes, we developed monitoring systems belonging to
level 1 (2) and to level 3 (3). We have considered these two approaches assuming that the line of commercially available systems

*Supported by CNR, Italian National Research Council, Special Project
on Biomedical TEchnology (BM-CARD 2)

(usually at level 2) are not adequate for the real needs. In fact, when an accurate analysis on a beat-by-beat basis is required, only direct visual inspection is appropriate. A method for enhancing the visual perception of the observer has been developed. When the physician time-saving is a crucial parameter, we think that an un-supervised automatic analysis provides an adequate solution.

In our approach to level 3 system development, the features implemented with particular attention are the algorithm for the QRS detection, which can self-adjust to slow changes of ECG morphology and recover possible missed beats, and a verification. Moreover, the system, implemented on a general purpose mini-computer, can be easily tailored on any single patient.

Materials and Methods

The Programme ASTRI (3), developed for the automatic analysis of ST-T interval and rhythm disturbances, has been used so far to analyse almost 900 24-hour ECG's.

This intensive use allowed the identification of two crucial points to be improved: QRS detection and graphical presentation of results.

ASTRI is implemented on a Hewlett Packard 1000/45 system, under the supervision of the RTE IV B executive, equipped with a HP 2313 A/D converter, HP2648 video terminal HP7970 mag tape, HP7920 disc unit and HP2608 alpha-numeric-graphic printer.

The acquisition from analog tape is of course possible from any playback unit (REMCO Italia, Oxford, Avionics have been used). It is executed at 60 times the real-time speed with a sampling rate of 6 Ks/sec corresponding to 100 s/sec real-time, which is adequate for the bandwidth characteristics of the portable recorders.

An interactive procedure, limited to a few minutes, is required to select the classification thresholds for the particular patient. This is accomplished through a visual presentation of a number of records (Figure 1).

The 24-hour ECG processing is performed in about 30 minutes and it repeats, record-by-record, a sequence of 4 operations: QRS detection, feature extraction, pattern-classification, and upgrading of results.

QRS Detection

The previous algorithm (4), although extensively tested, has shown some drawback where slow ECG morphologic changes occur during the 24 hours, or in the presence of very wide or very small ectopic beats. In these cases, the specificity remained high, while the number of missed beats increased. A two-step algorithm is used to improve sensitivity.

The first pass, highly specific, is nearly the algorithm adopted in the first version (4). The absolute value of the time-derivative of the ECG is continuously compared to a threshold (Figure 2A) Each crossing instant initiates the measurement of the time, To_n, in which the derivative remains higher than the threshold, and of the time in which it remains lower, To_{ff}, within a time window T_w. The detection is based on the comparison between To_n and To_{ff}.

The second pass, intended to increase the sensitivity, is exe-

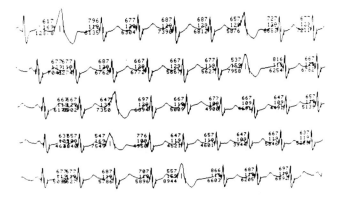

Fig. 1   The visual presentation

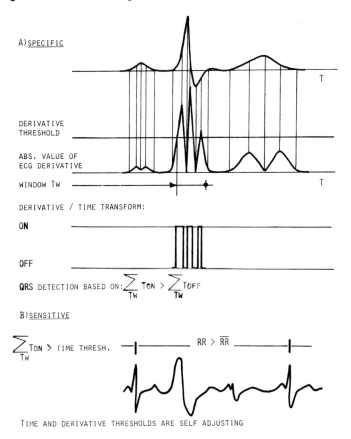

Fig. 2   A & B.   The QRS Detection Algorithm

cuted when a RR interval is found higher than a continuously updated
expectation limit. In this case To_n, which is continuously measured
within the RR intervals, is compared to an updated less restrictive
time threshold (Figure 2B), to detect possible missed beats. The
algorithm depends on many parameters; part of them are measured on
every detected beat, to allow a continuously self-adjusting process.
The second group of parameters has been fixed after a statistical
evaluation intended to evaluate their actual values. A test population of 2000 beats has been selected and the algorithm has been
applied, using many possible combinations of the values of parameters
to be fixed. The false positive (FP) and true postitive (TP) rates
have been plotted on the ROC (receiver operating characteristics)
plane (Figure 3). The fixed parameters, which correspond to the
optimal value of the ROC curve (high TP and acceptable FP), have been
adopted (5).

Feature extraction
        The features considered for the ECG cycles classification are:
RR interval, QRS duration and a shape factor based on an integral
comparison between the current beat and a typical beat assumed as
reference (6). Moreover the ST-T interval deflections are measured
by the positive and negative areas (ST+, ST-) relative to the baseline.

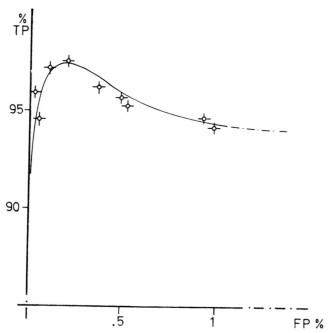

Fig. 3   Plot of false positive rate vs. true positive rate as a
          function of operating characteristics.

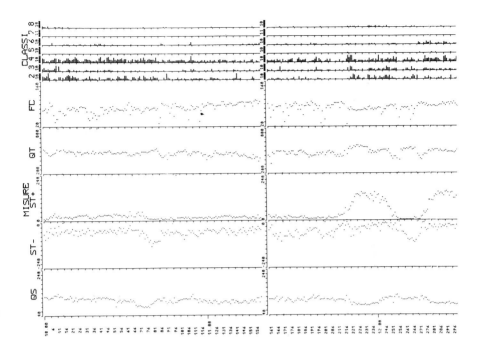

Fig. 4   Multi-parameter trend presentation

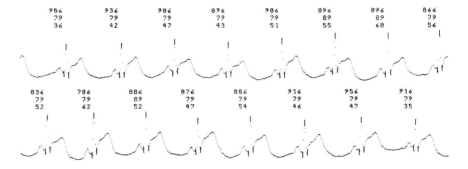

Fig. 5   Hard copy sample showing ST segment changes

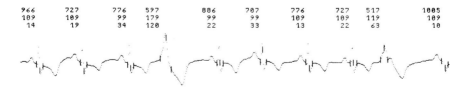

Fig. 6   Hard copy sample of disrhythmic event

Classification

The features are entered as inputs to a system of logical equations able to generate 6 classes of single beat abnormality and 2 classes of sequence abnormality, following the schema:

Class 1 = normal; Class 2 = premature with normal QS; Class 3 = premature with abnormal QS; Class 4 = delayed; Class 5 = abnormal shape; Class 6 = abnormal shape and wide QS; Class 7 = tachycardia; Class 8 = bigeminy.

Disc-updating

During processing all the relevant information is updated. Histograms of the parameters extracted are accumulated and stored on disc, and also their mean values over 30 seconds for the generation of time plots, together with beats classification.

At the end of this automatic unsupervised analysis, the results are reported in a number of ways. The most useful data presentation consists of a compact combination of rhythm analysis and time plots of the parameters, including particularly the ST+ and ST- time-courses (Figure 4). In the upper part of the figure, the number of beats belonging to the different classes in each records, are presented in a bar graph. Heart rate (HR), the QT duration (QT),the ST+ and ST- and the QRS duration (QS) are reported in the same time-scale. It is easy for the physician to identify the record(s) where are rhythm disturbances and/or episodes of ST changes and to obtain their visual (Figure 1) or hard copy (Figures 5, 6) presentation.

Conclusion

The evaluation of ASTRI and its performance have been reported in part elsewhere (3) and in part on a different paper at this Conference. We think that level 3 systems should always offer the physician the possibility to access and verify raw data, since the recordings are very often affected by artefacts and the QRS detection and classification algorithms are liable to fail.

A second remark on this class of systems is related to the validation. The use of a standardized data base and of commonly accepted quality figures are probably the most convenient technique for validation. The data available in any single institution are probably biased and, therefore, not adequate as a common reference data-base. A co-operative effort among different institutions, including manufacturers, should be stimulated towards the implementation of such a data base.

A last comment refers to the features usually employed for classification. Preliminary investigations, both from clinical (7) and technical (8, 9) sides, are showing that classification of beats, based mostly on morphology expressed through integral parameters, allows a more reliable discrimination respect to heuristic commonly used criteria.

References

1. Mark R.G., Moody G. B., Olsen W.H., Peterson S.K. et al (1979) Computers in Cardiology, pp 57-62. Long Beach, California: IEEE Computer Society.
2. Marchesi C., Macerata A., Taddei A., Mancini P. (1980) Computers in Cardiology, in Press. Long Beach,California: IEEE Computer Society.
3. Biella M., Contini C., Kraft G., Marchesi C. et al. (1979) Computers in Cardiology, pp. 201-204. Long Beach, California: IEEE Computer Society.
4. Landucci, L., Macerata A., Marchesi C., Chierchia S. et al (1978) Medical Informatics, pp. 325-339, Berlin, Springer Verlag.
5. Ripley K.L., Arthur R.M. (1975) Computers in Cardiology, pp. 27-32. Long Beach, California: IEEE Computer Society.
6. Neilson J.M. (1974) Computers in Cardiology, pp 55-59. Long Beach, California: IEEE Computer Society.
7. Schamroth L. (1979) Florence International Meeting on Miocardial Infarction, Vol. II, p. 916. Excerpta Medica.
8. Kao R., Wolson W.H. (1980) Computers in Cardiology, in Press. Long Beach, California: IEEE Computer Society.
9. Marchesi C., Giovani L., Landucci L. (1980) Computers Applications in Medical Care, pp. 1128-1132. Long Beach, California: IEEE Computer Society.

Discussion

DR. van DURME: Was the system validated with tapes?
DR. MARCHESI: (Slide) The problem of data-base validation was discussed previously, but unfortunately such a data-base is not available. The main problem is to reduce data from 24-hours to a reasonable number of records for comparison with the manual classification. To make this selection, we used a binomial statistical model, fixing a figure which would ensure that a reasonably reliable number would be collected. A correction was also made for cluster sampling because there are 30-second records, and there is no one-to-one correspondence between beat-validated and beat-recorded.

The QRS detection was validated on about 40,000 beats in 12 patients and figures were found for sensitivity and specificity.

On the same population of 12 patients, the classification of normal and various kinds of abnormality was also validated. I think we have taken a logical, scientifically valid approach. When we go into the figures in depth, it can be shown that a high percentage of the small portion of missed beats were PVC's.
DR. WEBER: I am glad that Dr. Marchesi is using an artefact detection algorithm. The double-mean R-R interval is more often an overlooked beat than a pause. It is being used as the second criterion, after the noise signal.
DR. MARCHESI: Exactly your considerations apply.

PROLONGED ELECTROENCEPHALOGRAPHIC
RECORDING IN NEONATES

J. EYRE AND C. CRAWFORD

Department of Paediatrics, John Radcliffe Hospital, Oxford

Summary

A continuous two-channel EEG with an ECG has been recorded from fourteen neonates, with neurological abnormalities. The recordings have been useful in the clinical assessment of the severity and the prognosis of cerebral damage, and in the differential diagnosis of abnormal behaviour.

Introduction

This is a preliminary report of work in progress at the Oxford Neonatal Intensive Care Unit. It is a collaborative project with the EEG Department at the Park Hospital, Oxford.

In the Oxford Neonatal Intensive Care Unit, the sixteen channel EEG, recorded over a period of up to one hour, has been used most frequently in two situations. Firstly, in the differential diagnosis of repeated abnormal behaviour, and secondly, in the assessment of the severity and prognosis of cerebral damage in the seriously ill neonate. The most frequent indication for EEG was to exclude seizure as the cause for repeated abnormal behaviour. Most common seizures in the neonate are atypical; clinical manifestations include jerking of the eyes, tonic posturing of the limbs, sucking, apnoea and respiratory pattern abnormalities. The exclusion of seizure in repeated abnormal behaviour often depends on the absence of electrographic seizure activity during an episode. The value of the standard EEG is limited by its brevity and thus the improbability of recording during an episode. In the year November 1979 to November 1980, thirty neonates in the Special Care Unit had an EEG at least once. For twelve of these neonates the indication for EEG was for the assessment of abnormal behaviour, and a total of eighteen EEG's were recorded (Table 1). Only two EEG's were recorded over the period of an episode, of these one record was uninterpretable because of artefact and the other recorded seizure activity. Fourteen EEG's were reported as normal, and two others had abnormalities not specifically related to the abnormal behaviour. These results emphasise that to be useful in the differential diagnosis of abnormal behaviour EEG recordings must be prolonged .

The second clinical situation for which EEG's are requested is for the assessment of cerebral damage. EEG abnormalities in the neonatal period reflect severity more than etiology, and the grave prognostic significance of certain EEG patterns in the first week of

TABLE 1

Standard EEG's recorded during November 1979 to November 1980
to aid the Diagnosis of Abnormal Behaviour

	Normal	Seizure activity seen	Artefact	Abnmormality unrelated to episodes
Episode occured during recording (2)	0	1	1	0
No episode occurred during recording (16)	14	0	0	2

life has now been established.

Many authors (1, 2, 3, 4, 5, 6, 7, 8) have reported the grave prognostic significance of the paroxysmal pattern (See Figure 3B). These records, characterized by periods of inactivity, interrupted by bursts of activity, must be differentiated from the discontinuous record seen in normal preterm neonates and in term infants in quiet sleep.

The prolonged inactive EEG has been established to have a poor prognosis (1, 4, 9, 10), and seizure activity with interictal flat, paroxysmal or slow backgrounds carries a poor prognosis (See Figures 4A & 4B) (1, 3, 5, 7, 8).

Of more importance, normal EEG's in the first week of life have been correlated with normal development (7) and a normal or minimally abnormal EEG in a comatosed infant indicates a good chance for normal survival.

Continuous recording of the EEG of seriously ill neonates might alert the clinician to a neurological insult, by the appearance of a severely abnormal pattern, and by recording the evolution and time course of more moderate abnormalities, the clinical significance of these may be elucidated.

Methods

There are many problems in recording a standard EEG in a neonatal intensive care unit, which make continuous or prolonged recording difficult and necessitate the continuous presence of a technician. The problems include lack of space, electrical interference, body movement and physiological artefact, and the need not to interfere with ongoing intensive care.

It was, therefore, decided to use a compact four-channel recorder which records onto a cassette tape utilising two channels for EEG.

Conventional EEG electrodes were used, sited at F_3-P_3 and F_4-P4 with reference electrodes sited on the frontal region. The preamplifiers were fixed to the scalp using collodion thereby reducing movement and electrical artefact. ECG was recorded on the third channel

and the fourth channel used for time signal and event marker. The
subjects were either newborns, with abnormal behaviour recorded at
the time of onset of these episodes, or seriously ill neonates receiving intensive care recorded during the first five days of life.
All tapes were reviewed on a page mode display (PMD 12). Relevant
sections of the tape were printed out.
     Accepting that any clearly focal abnormality may be missed by
only recording two channels, all neonates also had at least one
standard EEG recorded.

Results

We have successfully recorded from fourteen babies for periods varying from twenty-four hours to eleven days, with a total of 35 days or
820 hours of recording. We have encountered no complications and
have obtained adequate records on all neonates.
     The primary indication for recording the EEG of nine of the
subjects was the differential diagnosis of abnormal behaviour (Table
2). In seven out of the nine, the prolonged EEG was recorded during
an episode, in the other two, we could be criticised for ceasing
recording too soon. Three subjects had normal EEG's during an episode of abnormal behaviour. Two had seizure activity during an
episode of abnormal behaviour. One had EEG pattern abnormality
secondary to hypoxia during apnoea, one had prolonged periods of
abnormality not related to episodes of abnormal behaviour. The
remaining records were normal. In contrast, none of the standard EEG
were recorded during an episode; all were normal except for the
subject who had an abnormality unrelated to abnormal behaviour.

TABLE 2

Results of Standard and Prolonged EEG Tests

	Standard EEG		Results	Prolonged EEG		Results
	No of EEG's	Recorded during an episode		Hours of recording	Recorded during an episode	
1	1	–	normal	48	yes	normal
2	1	–	normal	24	yes	normal
3	1	–	normal	24	yes	2° abnormal
4	1	–	normal	24	yes	seizure activity unmarked
5	4	–	all normal	72 24x2	yes	seizure marked
6	1	–	abnormality unrelated to event	24	yes	abnormality unrelated to event
7	1		normal	24	yes	normal
8	1	–	normal	24	no	normal
9	1	–	normal	24	no	normal

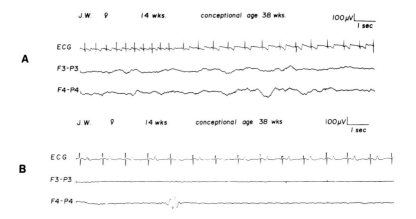

Fig. 1   A. Bradycardia with normal EEG
               B. Bradycarfdia with bilateral suppression of EEG

Case Reports

No.3. Baby J.W., born at 24 weeks gestation, wt. 675 gms, after an unevental pregnancy. No asphyxia at birth; only moderate respiratory distress; no significant metabolic acidosis or periods of hypoxia; ventilated for 38 days. Profound apnoea first noted at 14 week post partum. The apnoea was associated with unresponsiveness, but neurological examination between episodes was normal. She had one 24-hour period of recording, during which several episodes of apnoea occurred. Between and prior to marked events, the EEG pattern was normal; in association with marked events, a progressive bradycardia was noted first (See Figure 1A), followed by progresive suppression bilaterally of the EEG (See Figure 1B). On return of a normal heart rate, the normal EEG patterns returned. These findings were interpreted as an abnormality secondary to hypoxia and not supporting a diagnosis of seizure as the cause for apnoea. Obstructive apnoea was later diagnosed following polygraphic recordings of respiratory function.

No.5. Baby B.H., born at 27 week gestation wt. 990 gms, after an uneventful pregnancy. No asphyxia at birth, but a stormy neonatal period with very severe hyaline membrane disease, complicated by bilateral pneumothoracies and severe acidosis. During this period, he had a documented septicaemia, without CSF involvement, and later had a patent ductus arteriosus with heart failure. He was ventilated for 36 days in total. At 11 weeks post partum, he was noted to have episodes of abnormal behaviour, predominantly apnoea in association with tonic posturing of the limbs and occasionally with twitching of the left face and arm. Neurological examination revealed increased tone and reflexes on the left with clonus of the left ankle. CT scan showed cerebral atrophy with no focal lesion. Four standard EEG's,

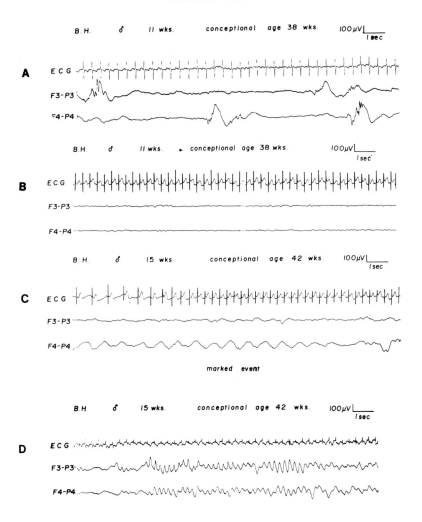

Fig. 2   A. Asynchrony of episodic EEG
          B. Low voltage EEG
          C. Right-sided semi-rhythmic slow wave
          D. Paroxysmal bilateral theta activity

not recorded over an episode of abnormal behaviour were all normal.
A total of 120 hours of continuous two-channel EEG and ECG were
recorded. All tapes had periods of moderate EEG abnormality, not
associated with marked events or ECG changes. The most frequent
abnormalities were persistent asynchrony in periods of episodic EEG
activity (See Figure 2A) and repeated periods of prolonged low voltage activity, not occurring in episodic periods of the recording (See
Figure 2B). In all marked events the EEG became abnormal prior to or
in association with an unstable heart rate. The pattern most frequ-

ently seen was the appearance of a right-sided semi-rhythmical slow
wave in association with low voltage left-sided activity (See Figure
2C), and bursts of bilateral rhythmical theta activity (See Figure
2D). These findings were interpreted as supporting seizure as the
probable cause for the abnormal behaviour.

These two cases illustrate the clinical usefulness of prolonged
EEG recording in the differential diagnosis of abnormal behaviour.

In the remaining five subjects, the primary indication for EEG
was the assessment of the severity of neurological abnormality and
prognosis. It is still too soon to report on the long-term outcome
of these infants who survived. However, I can report on the EEG
findings in two infants who died secondary to cerebral insult.

a) Baby C.G. born at term, wt. 3230 gms, after an uneventful
pregnancy. Labour was complicated by a long second stage and two
hours of documented fetal distress. She was apgar 0 at birth, the

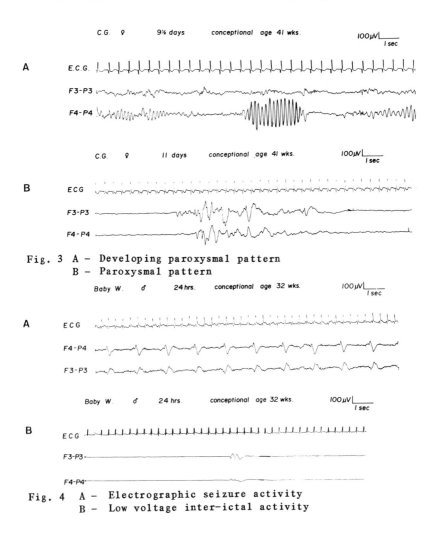

Fig. 3 A – Developing paroxysmal pattern
        B – Paroxysmal pattern

Fig. 4 A – Electrographic seizure activity
        B – Low voltage inter-ictal activity

heart beat returning at 10 minutes and spontaneous respiration established at 90 minutes. On day 8, the EEG was continuous and within normal limits. Over the subsequent 3 days, without a change in her clinical condition, the EEG became progressively more paroxysmal in nature (See Figure 3A) until on day 11, a continuous paroxysmal pattern was seen (See Figure 3B).

Neurologically throughout the period of the record, she had decerebrate posturing, and absent brainstem reflexes, except for spontaneous respiratory effort. She died aged 13 days.

2.   Baby boy W. born at 32 weeks gestation, wt. 1310 gms. The pregnancy was complicated by premature and prolonged rupture of the membranes and he was delivered by emergency LSCS for suspected foetal infection.   Infection screen soon after birth revealed E. coli meningitis, and at 12 hours of age, he was first noted to have seizures. Thse seizures were clinically very frequent, and treated with phenobarbitone and paraldehyde. Our record was started prior to the first dose of anti-convulsants and revealed almost continuous electrographic seizure activity (See Figure 4A). Interictal activity was bilaterally inactive, and as time progressed the interictal flat periods lengthened until finally prior to his death, he had several hours of inactive EEG (See Figure 4B). He died aged 72 hours.

These cases illustrate that two channels of EEG are sufficient to identify the three severely abnormal patterns reported in the literature, and did correctly predict the grave outcome of these two neonates. It is too soon to report on the clinical usefulness of this technique in less severe neurological insult.

The two major limitations encountered have been: firstly, difficulty in excluding respiratory artefact as a possible cause of EEG pattern abnormality and secondly lack of information of sleep-state making interpretation of the EEG more difficult.

To overcome these limitations, we are at present refining a method of recording respiratory pattern onto the channel previously used for time signal and event marker, and nursing staff are being asked to record behavioural observation regarding sleep-state as frequently (half-hourly or hourly) as their work load allows. With these two additional pieces of information, we may in future, have an indication of sleep-state throughout the recording.

Conclusions

The preliminary conclusions are:

1.   Prolonged EEG and ECG recording is possible in neonatal intensive care units.

2.   A respiratory pattern record is necessary to improve interpretation of the recordings.

3.   Prolonged two-channel EEG with ECG records are clinically more useful than the standard EEG in the differential diagnosis of abnormal behaviour.

4.   Two channels of EEG have been sufficiently to identify severely abnormal patterns in seriously ill neonates, correctly predicting the poor prognosis. More time and subjects are required to assess the clinical usefulness of this technique in assessing less severe neurological insults.

References

1. Harris R., Tizard T.P. (1960) J. Paediatr. **57**, 501-520.
2. Dreyfus-Brisac C., Monod N., Salama P. Ducas P., Mayer M. (1961) Verne Congres. Intern. Excerpta, Med.**37**, 228-230.
3. Dreyfus-Brisac C., Monod W. (1964) In: Neurological and Electroencephalogramic Correlative Studies in Infancy. Eds: P. Kellaway and L. Petersen. pp. 250-272. Gnine and Stratton, N.Y.
4. Schulte F.J. Hermann B. (1965) Monatsuhr Kindechedk. **113**, 457-465.
5. Monod N., Ducas P. (1968) In: Clinical Electroencephalography of Children. Eds: P. Kellaway and L. Petersen. pp.61-76. Gnine and Stratton, N.Y.
6. Monod N., Dreyfus-Brisac C., Sfuello Z. (1969). Arch. Fr. Pediatr. **26**, 1085-1102.
7. Monod N., Pajot N., Guidasu S. (1972) Electroencephalogr. Clin. Neurophysiol. **32**, 529-544.
8. Rose A.L. and Lombroso, C.T. (1970) Paediatrics. **45**, 404-425.
9. Engel R., (1975) Abnormal Electroencephalograms in the neonatal period. Charles C. Thomas. Springfield, Illinois.
10. Schulte F.J. (1960) Dev. Med. Child Neurol. **8**, 381-392.

Discussion

DR. SOUTHALL: The baby who had prolonged apnoea, and had EEG afterwards - why was that not picked up clinically or by the use of an apnoea monitor in the ward? Obviously, it lasted long enough to produce an EEG change, and therefore was probably harmful.

DR. EYRE: Apnoea was being detected clinically by an apnoea mattress and the baby was resuscitated if she did not restart breathing spontaneously. The EEG was not being displayed and the suppression was noted on review of the tape. The clinical problem was to exclude seizure as the cause for the recurrent profound apnoea.

DR. SOUTHALL: For how long did the apnoea go on before the EEG change became apparent?

DR. EYRE: We are unable to tell from the tape record because respiratory pattern was not recorded. Suppression of the EEG is seen during hypoxia. In our study, the EEG of some infants seemed to be suppressed soon after the onset of bradycardia, whereas in other infants, there was little change in the EEG pattern despite marked bradycardia.

DR. SOUTHALL: The bradycardia continued for a long time, did it not?

DR. EYRE: The infants are usually allowed to remain bradycardic for about 20 sec. to see if they will restart breathing again.

DR. SOUTHALL: Presumably, aminophylline would be given for the prolonged apnoea? Do these EEG recordings influence management of the prolonged apnoea?

DR. EYRE: If we thought that the apnoea was due to seizure activity, we would not give aminophylline as a therapy. In particular, this infant was ready for discharge home, and we needed to find out the cause for the apnoea.

DR. SOUTHALL: What was she treated with finally?

DR. EYRE: She was diagnosed to have an obstructive cause for the apnoea and had to remain in hospital until the episodes ceased.

EXPERIENCE WITH AMBULATORY MONITORING IN CHILDREN

D.M.B. HALL

St. George's Hospital & Medical School,
Tooting, London, SW17, UK.

Summmary

Ambulatory EEG records were made using the Oxford Medical System's Medical System's Medilog Recorder in 20 children. There were no major clinical problems. Recordings were successfully made even in young and handicapped children. Ambulatory EEG's were obtained in schools and at home. Eleven of the 20 records made a significant contribution to management. The indications for ambulatory records include uncertainty over the nature of episodic disturbances of consciousness, or behaviour and management problems in known epileptics

Introduction

This paper analyses clinical experience with ambulatory EEG monitoring in children and attemmpts to answer three questions:
1.   How practical and how useful is ambulatory monitoring in handicapped children?
2.   Is it practical and is it useful to carry out truly ambulatory recording with children?
3.   What are the main indications in paediatric practice for ambulatory EEG monitoring?

Patients and Methods

All recordings mentioned in this paper were made using the Oxford Medical Systems Medilog 4:24 EEG Recorder and were examined using the PMD-12 playback unit. The recorder was the standard instrument, except for one useful modification. A special connector was fitted which allows a choice betweeen ECG or accelerometer on channel 2. This option is particularly useful in paediatric practice where the distinction between cardiac and epileptic events is often less relevant than in adult practice.
    All electrodes were attached using the collodion technique. Parents and/or nursing staff checked them several times each day. With boisterous children it was found necessary to attach the preamplifiers with collodion as well as the electrodes and to tape the connections.
    A letter was sent beforehand. In particular, this emphasized that for comfort, the patient should wear a cardigan or shirt rather than jersey and T-shirt, so that they could readily remove their clothing.
    At night, the recorder and belt were removed from the patient's waist and either attached to the bed-head or placed under the pillow.

With very young or handicapped children night supervision may be
needed as there may be some risk of the child becoming entangled in
the wires and even strangled.

The parent, nurse or school-teacher responsible for the child
was provided with a record sheet, and asked to record all attacks,
funny turns, etc. and also to note the times of meals and teeth-
cleaning, since both cause confusing artefacts which may be mistaken
for spike and wave activity.

The present report is based on the 20 most recent recordings.
Most of the patients described here were drawn from seizure and
handicap clinics at a London teaching hospital, but 4 were referred
by other doctors specifically for monitoring. It is not possible to
assess from my results how many children in the population at large
might benefit from this method, because referral patterns in London
are very variable.

Results

Experience with handicapped children:
The sample of 20 children includes 3 with severe handicaps.
Successful recordings were made in all 3 without undue difficulty,
although supervision was needed. It has proved possible to complete
a recording in every handicapped child in whom it has been attempted.
Surprisingly, there was little attempt by children to remove the
electrodes after the first few minutes. The design of the pouch made
it difficult for the child to remove the recorder or to open it, and
to date there have been no problems with malicious damage. The
following two cases are given as examples.

Patient C.S. F - 18 months:
Mental retardation, ataxia, microcephaly; due to congenital
cytomegalovirus infection.
She was a very active child, but fell frequently, often striking
her head. It was not clear whether these falls were due to myoclonic
epilepsy. The recording was obtained without difficulty and confirmed that this was so; paroxysmal discharges were noted in association with each fall.

Patient L.M. F - 9 years:
Ataxic diplegia, mental retardation, aetiology unknown. Myoclonic epilepsy suspected; considerable patience was required to
obtain a recording, but this was accomplished. No abnormal events
occurred and it was, therefore, non-contributory.

Experience with monitoring outside the hospital:
Of the 20 patients cited, 11 were studied for all or part of the
recording while outside the hospital. Three (aged 8, 10 and 12 years
respectively) attended school; the remainder travelled home and returned once or twice daily as long as needed. Of the remaining cases,
3 were fully mobile within the hospital, including attendance at the
hospital school, and one recording was done in the Department of
Psychology. Only in the case of handicapped children was constant
supervision necessary. The following examples illustrate the versatility of this technique.

Patient P.H. M - 8 years:
    Sensori-neural deafness. His teacher reported "absence" epi-
sodes; the description was compatible with complex partial seizures.
These had never been noted outside school. Conventional EEG was
unhelpful. The ambulatory record was made in school. No change
occurred in the EEG during an absence. This added weight to the
previous suspicion that the attacks were in fact psychogenic.

Patient N.H. M - 10 years:
    He presented with photosensitive fits induced by television at
age 4. At age 6, he developed generalized tonic clonic seizures
without any precipitating factor. Both seizure types responded readily to medication. At age 9, he showed a compulsive fascination for
sun-light at certain angles and while staring at this, would go blank
for a few seconds. Self-induced epilepsy was considered but his
mother felt that the attacks were attention-seeking behaviour. The
recording was made out-of-doors and confirmed paroxysmal discharges
were associated with each episode. They improved considerably when
carbamazepine was discontinued.

Patient T.M. F - 8 years:
    Intellectual deterioration, cause not known. This girl was
known to have severe petit mal epilepsy which proved resistant to
therapy and was associated with deteriorating school performance. An
EEG performed just before the ambulatory record suggested a marked
improvement and showed very little spike and wave activity. For this
reason, it was suspected that she was faking many of her attacks.
The recording was carried out with the girl in hospital. While in
the hospital school, she had a prolonged run of almost continuous
spike wave activity lasting several hours. The attacks were obviously genuine and she was suffering from petit-mal status (1) or
spike wave encephalopathy (2). The previous EEG had been done in the
morning. The 24-hour record showed only a few bursts of spike wave
in the morning, not associated with clinical attacks, and the
prolonged attacks were all in the afternoon.

Patient G.T. F - 6 years:
    This girl displayed several seizure types but attacks of clas-
sical petit-mal absences were the predominant feature. School performance was very poor and it was not clear whether this could be
attributed to epilepsy, her medication or to non-medical factors.
The recording showed a few brief attacks very early in the morning,
but none during a long session with a psychologist, while her intel-
lectual problems were analysed. We concluded that her academic
difficulties were not directly related to inadequate control of
petit-mal.

Discussion

What are the indications for ambulatory EEG monitoring? Indications
for continuous monitoring in these 20 patients fell into two groups.

Group 1: In these cases, the child was experiencing episodic events

of disturbed consciousness or behaviour, of undertermined origin.
The conventional EEG either was normal, or showed an abnormality of
doubtful relevance to the clinical problem.

Patient D.P. F - 14 years:
    This girl was thought to have episodes of paroxysmal tachy-
cardia, but monitoring clearly demonstrated that the attacks were
epileptic and were of left-sided origin.

Patient J.G. M - 12 years:
    The history here suggested absence attacks, but the attacks were
infrequent. Repeated conventional EEG's were normal. The recording
confirmed the tentative diagnosis.

Group 2: This group contained children who had been confidently
diagnosed as having epilepsy. Ambulatory monitoring was used to
obtain furher information about the attacks. Some examples have
already been given (patients N.H., G.T., T.M., above).

Patient B.D. M - 8 years:
    The diagnosis of classical petit-mal type absences in this boy
presented no difficulty, but his mother was strongly opposed to
medication and claimed that the attacks were so infrequent that they
caused him little problem. The recording clearly demonstrated innum-
erable attacks over a 24-hour period and was helpful in obtaining
parental compliance.

Patient D.G. F - 12 years:
    In this girl also, the diagnosis of classical petit-mal was
straightforward, but she claimed to suffer a variety of different
attacks. It was not clear if this was genuine; she was a very
manipulative and demanding girl. The record combined with careful
ward observation showed only 3 per second spike wave episodes and
these reduced dramatically in her frequency as her medication was
given regularly in the hospital.

Conclusion

My experience shows that ambulatory monitoring is acceptable and well
tolerated even in young or handicapped children. It need not be
restricted to the hospital environment; indeed, in many cases the
full benefits are only realised if the child is returned to his usual
surroundings while the recording is made. In some cases, attacks
only occur in certain well-defined circumstances; also some children
with epilepsy seem to have fewer attacks in the hospital, presumably
because of regular medication and a predictable daily routine.
    School recording is practicable if the child is sensible, but
requires full co-operation from the teacher and careful explanation.
It is essential to give the teacher a contact telephone number and to
make oneself available throughout the period of recording in school,
if confidence is to be maintained.
    The age distribution of these cases is probably a fair reflec-
tion of the age at which problems occur. The small proportion of

children under 5 reflects the relative rarity of diagnostic difficulties in the age group rather than any intrinsic technical problem. When introducing any new diagnostic technique, one should
consider the extent to which management decisions are altered; in
other words, what would have been done had the technique not been
available. In the 20 cases which formed the basis of this report,
management was significantly influenced in eight. In two cases, a
diagnosis of epilepsy was unexpected; in two, the relevance of the
epilepsy to the observed behaviour pattern might have been substantially underestimated, and in another, the opposite error might have
been made. Among the remaining cases, useful confirmatory information was obtained in three, but management would probably have been
the same in the absence of monitoring. Thus nine of the twenty
records was non-contributory. This would be a good yield for any
investigation, but careful case selection is the main determinant of
yield. Because of limited technical assistance, my cases were very
carefully selected, and one would probably accept a lower proportion
of positive results when more recordings are made. On the other hand,
the equipment is expensive and should be used with care and discrimination. Outside major referral or research centres, the paediatric
workload alone would not justify the purchase of this system, but the
same equipment can be used without any modification for adult work.

On the basis of the cases reported here, I suggest the following
indications for ambulatory monitoring in children:
1. Undiagnosed episodes of disturbed behaviour or consciousness,
with:
    (i) Negative or equivocal standard investigation, and
    (ii) Occurring sufficiently frequently, perhaps once a week, to
have some hope of success.
Where events are much less frequent than once a week, the patient will need to be very disabled or frightened by the attacks to
persevere long enough with the recording.
Although cardiac rhythm disturbances are less commonly the cause
of odd attacks than is the case in adults, the possiblity should be
remembered and a simultaneous ECG record must be made.
My experience of recording breath-holding attacks has been dis-
appointing. Although there is usually no diagnostic difficulty,
occasional cases with an atypical story are worrying; however, the
recorder seems to have had an inhibitory effect on their occurrence.
Further study will be needed to determine the relevance of monitoring
in this problem and in the reflex anoxic seizures described by Stephenson (3).

2. Unequivocal epilepsy, with unanswered questions about:
    (i) Frequency of attacks
    (ii) Possible simulated attacks
    (iii) Relevance of epilepsy to learning or behavioural disorder
    (iv) Type of epilepsy.
In this group, recordings can often be of shorter duration; an
answer is often obtained in less than 24 hours. Simultaneous ECG is
of less importance and the accelerometer can be substituted; this
may be helpful in the interpretation of equivocal areas on the record.
Ambulatory monitoring using the Oxford Medilog is not necessar-

ily the best technique for elucidating the exact onset and propaga-
tion of an epileptic event, because of the limitation of channel
numbers. In these cases, telemetry with simultaneous video-recording
may be a more useful technique. It should be noted that several
cases referred for ambulatory recording had not had a sleep recording, in spite of the undoubted increase in yield of positive results
that this provides.

Further work will be needed to refine the indications for ambulatory monitoring and to determine the best way of making the technique widely available, at reasonable cost, within the National Health
Service.

Acknowledgement

I am grateful to Dr. Stores and Miss Talbot at the Park Hospital,
Oxford, to the Neurophysiology Department at the National Hospital,
Queen's Square, and to Dr. J. Foley at the Cheyne Spastic Centre, for
advice; also to those paediatricians who referred cases for study.

References

1.   Brett E.M. (1966) J. Neurol. Sci. **3**, 52-75.
2.   Chevrie J.J. and Aicardi J. (1972) Epilepsia (Amst) **13**, 259-271.
3.   Stephenson J.B.P. (1978) Arch. Dis. Ch. **53**, 193-197.

Discussion

DR. MILES: Dr. Hall mentioned the desirability of doing a sleep
recording to try to bring out the focus. Are children ever sleep-
deprived?

DR. HALL: No, that is not done as a normal routine. In fact, at the
unit that does our only EEG recordings we have considerable difficulty in getting any sleep recording. That is why I commented that it
surprises me that in many centres this is still not recognised as an
essential part of the routine. We have not sleep- deprived children.

DR. MILES: It is extremely difficult to get a pre-adolescent child
to sleep in the daytime. They have an extraordinary alertness. It
might have to be done just after their usual bedtime by keeping them
awake for a while longer than usual.

DR. HALL: We have found that sedation is quite often effective and a
number of records have been positive following heavy sedation, such
as Vallergan (trimeprazine). I know that this is not the optimal
technique, but it works in a number of cases.

AMBULATORY MONITORING AND CHILD PSYCHIATRY

G.C. FORREST AND C. CRAWFORD

EEG Department, Park Hospital for Children, Oxford, UK

Summary

The use of ambulatory monitoring in the assessment of attacks of
disturbed behaviour in 76 children referred to the Park Hospital EEG
Department is described. Recording provideds additional evidence of
psychiatric disorder in 18 cases, and confirmed the attacks as seizures in 20. In the remaining 38 cases, recordings were inconclusive.
Guidelines for the use of ambulatory monitoring in child psychiatry
are suggested.

Introduction

Children with seizure disorders are known to have a high incidence of
behaviour and emotional disorder (1) and so the clinician often finds
himself trying to distinguish between a change in type of seizures,
feigned seizures or psychological disturbance. Even in children with
no history of seizure disorder, it is sometimes difficult to make a
confident diagnosis when there are many causes of episodic behaviour
disturbance, including both physical and psychiatric conditions (2)
(Table 1).

Table 1

Differential Diagnosis

Physical Conditions	Non-Organic States
Complex partial seizures	Habit spasms
Absence seizures	Temper tantrums
Cardiac arrhythmias	Panic attacks
Migraine	Depersonalisation syndrome
Hypoglycaemia	Psychoses
Transient ischaemic attacks	Conversion hysteria

Although in many cases the psychiatrist will reach a diagnosis
based on the history of the attacks and clinical assessment of the
child's behaviour and mental state, in selected cases, a knowledge of
EEG or ECG changes accompanying the attacks will facilitate diagnosis. The Oxford Medilog system can provide such information by
means of a lightweight, unobtrusive cassette recorder, which allows
the child to continue in his normal routine at home and school.
Between October 1978 and March 1981, 76 children, aged between

four years six months and seventeen years six months, were monitored
with the Medilog system. Their intelligence ranged from severely
subnormal to above average. They were all referred with attacks of
disturbed behaviour, which included falls, lapses of concentration,
visual hallucinations, various abnormal movements, flushing and
sweat-ing attacks. 58 children had a history of seizure disorder,
the remaining 18 had no history of seizures.

106 recordings were taken, 3 of which were technically unsatisfactory. EEG alone was carried out in 99; EEG/ECG combined in 7.
86 recordings were made in the hospital (where the children are up
and dressed, attend school and take part in all sorts of activities)
20 were made at home. Most recordings lasted 24 hours, although 10
were continued for 2 days and 2 for 4 days.

The recordings can be divided into 3 groups:
1.   Children who had attacks during recording which were not
     accompanied by seizure activity (18 cases).
2.   Children who had attacks which were accompanied by seizure
     activity (20 cases).
3.   No attacks occurred during recording (38 cases)

Group 1: Attacks Without Accompanying Seizure Activity

Of the 18 children in this group, 7 had no history of seizure disorder and the recording provided confirmatory evidence of a diagnosis
of psychiatric disorder. For example, a 16-year old girl had a 10-
year history of daily visual hallucinations of a boy who had grown up
with her. During her attacks, which might last 20 minutes, she would
talk with him and then appear distant and unresponsive. A CT scan,
skull x-ray, and standard and sleep EEG had all been normal, but she
had been treated with anti-convulsant and anti-psychotic drugs. During 86 hours of continuous monitoring, she had two 'attacks' with no
evidence of organic pathology in the EEG. It was concluded that
these visual images were psychological phenomena, in a lonely,
isolated girl, who had produced an imaginary companion to meet her
needs.

Another case, a 9-year old girl had a 12-month history of daily
attacks of feeling unsteady, seeing things in miniature and a sense
of unreality, lasting up to a minute. Her normal EEG throughout
several attacks supported the diagnosis of Depersonalisation Syndrome (a neurotic disorder, where there is an unpleasant state of
disturbed perception, such as external objects being changed in
quality or size, or becoming unreal).

Table 2A summarizes the diagnoses of the attacks of the children
with no history of seizure disorder in this group.

The other 11 children in the group had a history of seizures.
Their attacks were diagnosed as listed in Table 2B.

Group 2: Attacks With Accompanying Seizure Activity

In this group, the recording confirmed the diagnosis of the attacks
as a seizure. Of the 20 children in the category, only one boy had
no previous history of seizures. He presented at age 12, with brief
outbursts of overactivity and verbal aggression. The attacks were
followed by headache and then sleep. He had had a brief febrile

Table 2

Oxford Child Psychiatry Series

A No History of Epilepsy	B History of Epilepsy
Imaginary companion..........1	Simulated seizures......5
Depersonalisation syndrome...1	Sleep disorder..........3
Habit spasm..................1	Anxiety state...........2
Anxiety state...............3	Stereotypies............1
Emotional disorder...........1	

convulsion at age 3. Standard and sleep EEG's were unhelpful but his EEG during an attack showed a predominantly right-sided slow wave disturbance with sharp wave components (Figure 1). These findings supported the diagnosis of psychomotor seizures.

Seven of the other 19 children in this group with a past history of seizures were causing concern because the form of their seizures had changed and there was doubt as to whether these new attacks were feigned. For example, an 8-year old severely sub-normal girl with cerebral palsy, had tonic-clonic seizures from age 12 . Six months

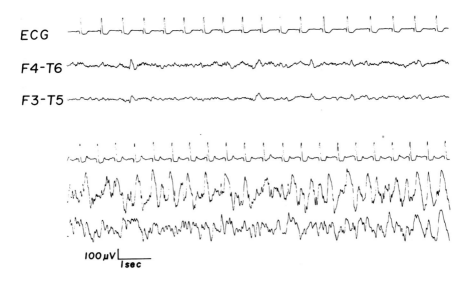

ECG

F4-T6

F3-T5

100 μV |
1 sec

Fig. 1   Example of seizure activity found in EEG of 12 year old boy.

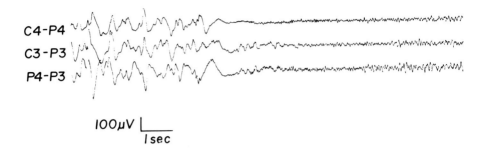

C4-P4

C3-P3

P4-P3

100μV |___
      1 sec

Fig. 2   Sample EEG during an attack in an 11 year old girl

ago, she began having attacks in school, where she would suddenly drop forward. Her teachers were convinced that these were feigned attacks to avoid certain situations. However, continuous monitoring during an attack showed desynchronisation of the EEG (Figure 2). Appropriate adjustment of her anti-convulsant medication has subsequently controlled these myoclonic seizures.

The other children in this group were being monitored so that their seizure activity could be quantified for objective assessment of seizure control, or to determine emotional or psychological precipitants. They will not be discussed further in this paper.

Group 3:   No Attacks During Recording

In this group of 38 children, the results were inconclusive. In some cases the attacks were occurring so infrequently that monitoring was inappropriate. In others, monitoring was clearly discontinued too soon (after 24 hours). 10 children had seizure activity at times on their recordings; 9 of these were known to have a seizure disorder, but one boy, who was having repeated brief attacks of impaired consciousness and no previous history of seizures, had spike and wave on his recording, suggesting that these attacks might well be absences.

Conclusions

A number of important points have emerged as our experience of this system has grown.

First, the attacks must be occurring frequently enough (once or twice a week) to make continuous monitoring practicable.

Second, monitoring can only be used properly if it is part of planned EEG studies. For instance, requests for monitoring to establish a localised disturbance are inappropriate as recording is unlikely to be helpful with the limited number of channels available in this system.

Third, having established the appropriateness of the recording, it is important to continue monitoring until an attack of the type in question occurs. It is important to note that in a child with a known seizure disorder, a   normal EEG during an attack will not confirm that all attacks are therefore 'feigned' seizures. Also, a normal EEG during an attack will not exclude epilepsy - merely provide additional evidence increasing the likelihood of psychological disturbance when taken in conjunction with a clinical assessment of the child's behaviour and mental state.

Lastly, it is essential to ensure that EEG/ECG combinations are used where necessary, particularly in those attacks where anxiety or cardiac arrhythmias are suspected as the cause.

In conclusion, from the point of view of a child psychiatrist, ambulatory monitoring offers diagnostic possibilities not available by other traditional means - provided that the guidelines are followed and adequate clinical detail is provided with the request for monitoring.

References

1.   Rutter M., Graham P.& Yule W.(1970) In: Clinics in Developmental
      Medicine No 35. Spastics International Press, Heinemann, London.
2.   Stores G. (1981) In: Advances in Epileptology, Ed.M. Dam et al.,
      Raven Press, New York.

Discussion

DR. SAYED: Dr. Forrest quoted a case in which a child was hallucinated and talking to a grown up. In this case, I would have thought that it would be a focal disturbance. Is Dr. Forrest sure that it was possible to exclude that on the limited channels? She mentioned in her guidelines that this sort of case should be excluded.

DR. FORREST: In this case, the monitoring was carried out as part of a planned series of studies, not as an investigation on its own, so we had already checked to make sure that on a sleep-recording there was no focal abnormality present.

DR. SOUTHALL: I am worried about the possiblity of one of the electrodes coming off during the recording. What sort of pattern would that produce? On a 24-hour ECG an artefact due to a loose electrode would be observed, but with EEG what pattern is produced if an electrode comes loose? Can it be distinguished from no activity on the EEG? That is very important when there are attacks, but no seizure activity.

(Dr. Forrest referred the question to Miss Talbot, a Member of the EEG Department, Park Hospital, Oxford.)

MISS TALBOT: If an electrode becomes loose, the problem mostly encounterd is 50 Hz interference or, if it is very bad, the channel is lost altogether.

DR. SOUTHALL: What about the spike?

MISS TALBOT: It would go flat. There is a whole new realm of artefacts when we start to look at continuous recording, and we soon learn what an electrode artefact looks like - in the same way as with any other EEG recording.

MR. IVES: Are the suspected temporal lobe patients investigated with sphenoidal electrodes?

MISS TALBOT: Not routinely.

THE VALUE OF PROLONGED EEG MONITORING TO THE CLINICIAN IN A PSYCHIATRIC LIAISON SERVICE

E.B.O. SMITH

Department of Psychiatry, John Radcliffe Hospital, Oxford

Summary

This paper describes the initial experiences gained in the selective application of ambulatory EEG recording during the first six months that it was available in a psychiatric liaison service. Examples of the advantages obtained by its use, in a variety of clinical situations, are given and suggestions are made for its application to a number of other problems commonly encountered by psychiatrists working in medical and surgical settings. Some of the practical problems, which emerged, are discussed briefly and preliminary conclusions are drawn on its effectiveness as an investigative technique.

Introduction

The psychiatrist, who practises in medical and surgical settings, encounters a high proportion of patients, who present difficult problems in clinical assessment and management. Invariably, they have been admitted to hospital as physically-ill people, do not perceive themselves as in need of psychiatric attention and are often reluctant to accept it. Severe emotional disorder and behavioural disturbances are commonplace. The reasons for psychiatric referral are often complex; in many cases, it is uncertainty and anxiety in the minds of the referring physician or surgeon, which lead to the psychiatrist becoming involved. The patient is not seen as being primarily in need of a neurological opinion, yet the assessment and clarification of impaired cognitive functioning, particularly of an episodic nature, is an everyday task within the broader brief of a comprehensive somatic and psycho-social appraisal of the patient. Working with inadequate information and in a setting, where decisions on psychiatric management have to be reached quickly, the clinician is grateful for any investigative tool, which may yield relevant and reliable information.

In traditional psychiatric practice, the contribution of electro-encephalography has proved to very limited, except when the psychiatrist has been functioning in the role of a neurologist seeking to confirm or exclude a diagnosis of epilepsy, or some other generalised or focal cerebral disorder. Even in neurological or general medical practice, reliance on relatively brief, "routine", EEG recordings, particularly at times, when the relevant clinical phenomena have been absent, has not only demonstrated its disadvantages as a routine diagnostic aid, but has led to the abuse and the devaluation of the technique. (1).

However, the development in recent years of ambulatory recording equipment with the capability of capturing electro-physiological data over long periods of time, in a wide range of environments and during intermittent or episodic clinical events, has provided new oportunities for the application of the EEG in psychiatric practice, particularly in the general hospital.

This paper describes the initial experience gained in the selective application of ambulatory EEG monitoring, during the first six months that it was available to patients referred to the Psychiatric Liaison-Consultation Service at the John Radcliffe Hospital, Oxford. The intention is not to review all the cases studied, but to indicate some of the advantages gained by its application and to suggest ways in which it offers new opportunities in the clinical evaluation, and tactical value in the management, of a number of problems commonly encountered in psychiatric practice in this setting. In association with colleagues in the EEG Department at the Park Hospital for Children, recordings were made with the Oxford Medilog System, employing a four-channel, 24-hour battery-operated cassette recorder with head-mounted pre-amplifiers and the data was reviewed with a PMD 12 page-made display unit. In every case, before ambulatory monitoring was commenced, a conventional 16-channel, EEG recording was made with the usual routine provocative measure of hyperventilation and photic stimulation. In most cases, it was also preceded by a natural sleep recording.

Evaluation of Episodic Clinical Events

(a) Previously Unidentified Seizures: The value of ambulatory EEG monitoring in the diagnosis of epilepsy has been well-established by several groups working in Montreal, (2, 3), Bethesda, (4), London (5) and Oxford (6, 7). Its usefulness in confirming the diagnosis, in detecting the laterality of foci, and in quantifying seizure activity have been demonstrated. Psychiatrists are rarely called upon to investigate patients with easily recognised seizures and in many cases, the referring physicians strongly suggest that the episodic disturbance is psychogenic. Such patients have usually been investigated neurologically, including routine EEG recordings, and in most cases, there is other evidence of psychiatric disorder, which may camouflage the fit-related activity.

> Case 1: A 66-year old man was referred with an 18 month history of severe depression and anxiety, which had been preceded by emergency admission after nocturnal restlessness, of a nonspecific type, was followed by his being unrouseable for an hour. At that time, he had been extensively investigated neurologically, including EEG recordings and a CT scan, without any abnormality being found. The emergence of a florid depression state, in an otherwise healthy man, with a history of a similar affective illness ten years earlier, led to prolonged treatment with anti-depressants, without any sustained response. Among the many psychiatric symptoms he decribed, were occasional brief episodes of loss of concentration and awareness of his environment. When his wife's attention was drawn to these attacks, she noticed that he looked dazed and made stereo-typed chewing movements. He was referred for ambulatory monitoring and an intermittent focal disturbance was found in the left fronto-

temporal area. A further CT scan showed no abnormality. Following the introduction of carbamazepine, the attacks ceased, there was a radical improvement in his self-esteem, and, despite the withdrawal of anti-depressants, the affective illness remitted and he returned to his former personality. Neurological vigilance is being maintained.

Although the diagnosis of complex partial seizures in such cases must inevitably be a clinical one, the use of prolonged ambulatory EEG recording increases greatly the chances of detecting confirmatory evidence.

(b) Recognition and Management of Simulated Seizures: The evaluation of questionable seizure activity is often a time-consuming and difficult undertaking, even when a psychogenic explanation seems likely on neurological or psychiatric grounds. The diagnostic advantages of ambulatory EEG monitoring, in such cases, has been demonstrated by Stores (7), with examples illustrating the unexpected outcome in some cases. An awareness that genuine seizure activity can occur without any detectable EEG disturbance, while concomitant electro-physiological abnormalities may be unrelated to the clinical events observed, only complicates the diagnostic task. For the neurologist, the establishment of the true nature of simulated attacks may conclude his clinical contribution; for the psychiatrist, however, it is a preliminary stage in the carrying out of a comprehensive social and biological assessment, forming a working relationship with the patient, and persuading him or her to face the under-lying emotional problems and find more appropriate ways of coping. In attitudes and behaviour, the patient is usually committed, with varying degrees of awareness, to resisting attempts to establish the psychogenic nature of such attacks, and is reluctant to engage in the frequently disturbing task of exploring feelings and problems. At this stage, ambulatory EEG monitoring can be of tactical value to the psychotherapist.

Case 2: A 21-year old undergraduate was admitted to hospital on several occasions, following attacks in which she suddenly fell to the ground, appeared to lose consciousness for some 15 minutes, and to display "post-ictal" weakness, lasting for many hours affecting her right face, arm and leg.

Following comprehensive medical assessment and observation of further attacks in the medical ward, a strong suspicion that these were of hysterical origin gained ground. An initial but comprehensive psychiatric assessment failed to expose any other problems. The patient denied that she had any other difficulties and resented referral to a psychiatrist. Her tutors declared that she was progressing satisfactorily with her studies and that she was a popular member of her College. Her mother gave an account of normal development, good health and a seemingly well-adjusted personality in childhood, adolescence, and early adult life, apart from a few fainting attacks when she was aged 14 years. In order to clarify the nature of the attacks, ambulatory EEG recording was arranged. After 56 hours of continuous recording, three attacks occurred, during which the EEG showed no significant abnormality. Faced with this evidence, the patient, for the first time, showed a willingness to examine her own emotional reactions and began to work on her problems. Subsequently, fears of academic failure, emancipatory problems in her relationship with her parents, and disturbances in psycho-sexual development emerged. No further attacks occurred and, after a period of severe anxiety and depression accompanied by self-injurious impulses, the patient settled down emotionally and returned to her studies.

(c) Hyperventilation Syndromes: The role of hyperventilation in the genesis of conscious awareness and a wide range of symptoms, affecting many systems, as been well-recognised, since the early accounts of White and Hahn (8) and Kerr et al (9). Although it is mentioned frequently in the differential diagnosis of many symptoms discussed in the ward rounds of a liaison psychiatric service, it is rarely possible to observe either acute episodic, or chronic habitual, hyperventilation in the hospital setting. Recently developed, non-invasive, techniques for prolonged ambulatory monitoring of both respiration and the EEG offer new opportunities to investigate such symptoms in the anxiety-provoking environments, where they occur.

Management of Patients Known to Have Epilepsy

(a) New Episodic Symptoms: patients, who have established epilepsy and who then develop brief, episodic disturbances of emotion or behaviour, are often referred to the Liaison Psychiatrist in the belief that their symptoms are neurotic in nature. The task of clarifying the nature of such episodes is not an easy one, especially as the presence of other neurotic features in the personality may be an independent concomitant feature. The patient often recognises that such attacks may well be psychogenic, yet fears that they represent a new form of seizure. The value of ambulatory EEG recordings, in such cases, cannot be over-emphasized.

Case 3: A 24-year old staff nurse had suffered from temporal lobe epilsepy since the age of 10. The original seizures were accompanied by a feeling of "being in two places at once", malaise, nausea, fear, a variable olfactory hallucinosis and subsequent partial amnesia. She had also suffered from occasional grand mal seizures. After many years of being free of attacks while on phenytoin, she began to experience very brief episodes of anxiety, akin to momentary fear, accompanied on occasions, by a subtle change in the quality of consciousness and sometimes by transient olfactory sensations, which were usually unpleasant. The patient realised that such episodes might be entirely psychogenic, particularly as she was experiencing lethargy, mild feelings of depression and intermittent insomnia. Her mental state was unremarkable and the neurological examination showed no abnormality. A routine 16-channel EEG recording showed only occasional left temporal slow waves and a natural recording revealed frequent sharp waves in that region, with a tendency to phase-reverse anteriorly. After 31 hours of continuous ambulatory recording, the patient experienced several of the new attacks, sometimes with olfactory experiences with durations ranging from a few seconds to 3 minutes. One olfactory experience was possibly associated with bilateral, irregular, slow activity but, in general, the patient's experiences were not associated with any convincing changes in the EEG. The patient was greatly relieved by these findings, lost her secondary anxiety, focused on a relationship with a boyfriend, who was inappropriately entertaining ideas of marriage, and was soon reporting far fewer episodes. She became symptom-free when her anti-convulsant medication was adjusted to a slightly higher dose.

In this case, as in many others, it was noticeable that the patient found the routine and sleep recordings, during neither of which she had an attack, as irritatingly irrelevant while the continuous ambulatory recording seemed an appropriate, sensible and effective investigation.

Case 4: The parents of a 32-year old, mentally-handicapped man, with severe epilepsy and a previous history of schizophreniform psychotic episodes, who had been under the care of the author for over 10 years, reported that he had developed an annoying habit of staring vacantly, grunting, turning his head to the right and pausing in mid-sentence when talking. In some ways, this appeared to be an attention-seeking device. The patient seemed unaware of, but embarrassed by, its occurrence. Ambulatory recording showed that 3 episodes were accompanied by bilateral synchronous spike and slow wave discharges lasting up to 30 seconds

(b) Fluctuations in Seizure Activity: From time to time, patients suffering from epilepsy report an unusually high frequency of seizures under certain conditions. Ambulatory recording techniques offer an effective means of obtaining confirmatory evidence of such fluctuations and may prove valuable in throwing more light on conditions, which facilitate the occurrence of fits.

Case 5: A 22-year old secretary had suffered from psychomotor seizures, since the age of 8, with good control of seizures by conventional anti-convulsant medication. Following the insertion of an intra-uterine contraceptive device, she experienced prolonged menstrual bleeding, lasting up to 14 days of each 28-day cycle. During the fortnight of menstrual flow, she reported a recurrence of fits on most days, but none during the remainder of the month. Ambulatory EEG recording for 24-hours was arranged under the two conditions. When menstruation was absent, occasional spike discharges were found in the right posterior temporal region only. During menstruation, spike discharges were recorded over the left posterior temporal area as well. Following removal of the coil, menstruation returned to normal with seizures becoming infrequent and confined to the time of menstrual flow.

Other Applications

One of the commonest problems faced by a Liaison Psychiatrist is the evaluation of a patient, who may be showing intermittently the psychiatric manifestions of an organic illness. Classical cases of delirium, with impairment of consciousness, disorientation, disturbances of memory, incoherence of thought and obvious perceptual disorders are seldom referred by the physician or surgeon, unless advice on management is required or the condition is believed to be superimposed on pre-existing psychopathology. Where disturbances of cognitive functioning are intermittent and less obvious, or lead to other irrational or behavioural abnormalities, particularly when no organic disease has been found, psychiatric opinion may be sought in the belief that neurotic or functional psychotic processes are responsible. In a busy general hospital ward, with frequent staff changes, continuous skilled observation of the mental state is not possible and crucial signs may be missed. The application of continuous EEG monitoring to detect evidence of intermittent global impairment of cerebral activity, as well as episodic focal abnormalities, could be invaluable in identifying sub-acute organic reactions due to metabolic disorders, drug intoxication, non-convulsive complex partial states and other similar disturbances in cerebral function.

Disturbances of sleep and wakefulness inevitably occupy the attentions of the Liaison Psychiatrist, from time to time, and in the investigation of morbid somnalence, insomnia and sleep-induced respiratory disorder, the technique of prolonged ambulatory recording is likely to yield relevant and valuable information in the patient's natural environment.

Practical Problems

The equipment at present available seems extremely reliable and robust, but its use in the face of severe restlessness and confusion may call for additional protection. The limited number of channels available present problems in deciding the placement of electrodes in some cases. For it to be of greatest value to the clinicians, it needs to be readily available and this implies the capability of initiating recordings at any time outside normal working hours. Since intermittent and episodic clinical events may be infrequent, the need for very prolonged recordings sometimes lasting several days, will often occur. The interpretation of the records can present difficulties at times, particularly in identifying artefacts, and the frequent use in medical and surgical units of drugs, which affect the EEG can set limits on the applicability of the technique, in some cases. For the Liaison Psychiatrist, however, probably the greatest problem concerns the conclusiveness of negative findings, especially when there is an urgent need to establish that symptoms probably have no organic basis.

Preliminary Conclusions

The initial experiences in the first six-months of applying ambulatory EEG monitoring, using the Oxford Medilog System in selected cases, referred to a psychiatric consultation-liaison service, suggest that it has considerable potential in clarifying the nature of atypical, intermittent or episodic clinical events. Quite apart from its role as a neurological investigative tool, it offers tactical advantages in the evaluation of symptoms as a prelude to psychotherapeutic intervention in cases of psychogenic disorder. It appears to many patient as a most appropriate and sensible investigation. It is a time-consuming technique, which needs to be used in a discriminating and flexible way and, in our view, should almost always be preceded by routine and natural sleep recordings. Although the clinician will occasionally be surprised by the findings on a prolonged recording, particularly during episodic disturbances, the diagnosis of epilepsy must remain a clinical one. As with the other expensive neurological investigations, there is a danger, that it could be abused by inappropriate and excessive demands for its use.

Acknowledgments

The author wishes to thank Dr. Gregory Stores and Miss Christina Crawford, of the Park Hospital for Children, Oxford, for their encouragement, advice and technical help in carrying out these studies. Thanks are also due to the Oxford Hospital Services Development Trust for a grant to purchase the recording equipment.

MR. IVES: In relation to Dr. Hall's inconclusive or negative findings during seizures, in over 100 temporal lobe patients, whom we investigated, of the patients, who just had their aura while their EEG was being recorded, only 10% showed an epileptic abnormality in surface and/or sphenoidal tracings. When the aura progressed to overt seizure, with head-turning and/or lip-smacking, 80% of the patients demonstrated epileptic activity in their EEG, but 20% still did not. How does Dr. Hall feel these negative findings in his EEG tracings should be dealt with?

DR. HALL: I cannot answer that - but perhaps Mr. Ives could comment. How much better does he do with the sphenoidal recordings than with surface recordings?

MR. IVES: Sphenoidal recordings will show interictal epileptic discharge in about 20% of the cases in which nothing is seen on the surface EEG.

DR. RAMSAY: Mr. Ives has asked a question which nobody can answer.

DR. SOUTHALL: I am new to long-term EEG recordings. I have been doing ECG for a long time and I am very worried about artefacts. Unless the contact between the electrodes and the skull or skin is monitored, there is no way by which we can be sure about what is being seen.

DR. RAMSAY: Having scanned several 100 patient recordings, it becomes very obvious that it is not possible to look at only one section. It is really unfair to many of the presenters (of today's papers) to do that because very frequently it is possible to tell what is happening only by the evolution of what happens in a channel. An epileptic event may not be spike wave, it may be a rhythmic buildup of slow activity. If an event is found to have occurred, and within a few minutes, the electrode obviously becomes filled with artefact, it has to be presumed that whatever was recorded earlier was artefact - or, at least, it should be disregarded. It is necessary to have the advantage of a long period of observation on the entire recording.

DR. SOUTHALL: Is there anything against the use of impedance technique to check the quality of the electrode contact?

DR. IVES: We have monitored impendance before and after recordings, and have found that until it becomes severely high, it generally does not relate to the amount of artefact. It is really related to the drying-out of the jelly or to the loosening of the electrode on the skin. If there is 5, 10 or 25 K impedance, it will not bother the cassette recording - it only does so when it is much higher than that.

DR. BINNIE: Mr. Ives' answer to the question about negative findings seems to have produced a rather resounding silence, but it is a very important issue, which needs to be considered further. The incidence of negative findings during established epileptic seizures is well-documented, particularly for simultaneous video-recording with

surface EEG and depth recordings. These are mostly series of
patients with partial epilepsy, who are being investigated for
possible surgical intervention. In some series the incidence of
complete lack of any change in the EEG - not only the absence of
spikes, but the absence too of any other changes - has been as high
as 40%. In one series by Weiser of what he called "psychic seizures"
the incidence of negative surface EEG was 100% - if there are people
here from Zurich, they may correct me on that. In relation to this,
it is important to realise that patients who present a problem of
differentiation between epileptic seizures and non-epileptic events,
are particularly those in whom, if the seizures are epileptic, they
are likely to be partial. Very few patients simulate tonic-clonic
convulsions - and, if they do, they are not very convincing. Usually,
the differential diagnosis is particularly with complex partial
seizures, many of which are electrographically negative. Also, we
have the same experience as Mr. Ives; in someone whose seizures
sometimes never go beyond some preliminary event and sometimes do,
EEG change is often seen only after he has been going about 30 secs.
- that is, in the longer seizures.

MR. IVES: I am not sure whether my epileptic population is different, but a large number of the patients I see, do simulate major
motor seizures - probably about half of those, which we decide in the
long-run are functional. Many of these are difficult to discern.
The most recent one, which was disturbing to me, was probably a true
epileptic seizure, not a psychogenic seizure, but there was an
absolutely normal EEG before, during a grand mal seizure and afterwards. I am still convinced that the patient has epilepsy, but I was
very disturbed to have recorded her EEG's by radiotelemetry - 16-
channel radiotelemetry, not only 4-channels - and still they were
normal. The concern is very proper. The other concern, obviously,
is that some seizures do not begin in the typical temporal lobe or
frontal lobe. The selection of electrodes is very important, if we
are to pick up the abnormal activity.

DR. BLUMHARDT: With regard to the importance of not reading too much
into the negative EEG at the time of an attack, not only is it
possible that the patient has deep discharge in the amygdala or
hippocampus and is actually just having an aura, but also it may be a
functional attack at that time. If we look only at the strips of
tape where there are attacks, quite marked seizure activity at other
periods may be missed. We have had cases with definite clinical
temporal lobe epilepsy, who have absolutely negative recordings at
the time of what seems otherwise to be a genuine attack. Yet, some
hours later, without any symptoms, there will be quite a lengthy
paroxysmal discharge (it does not have to be a short attack) from one
temporal lobe, which is clearly epileptic.

SIMULTANEOUS AMBULATORY MONITORING OF THE EEG AND ECG IN PATIENTS WITH UNEXPLAINED TRANSIENT DISTURBANCES OF CONSCIOUSNESS

L.D. BLUMHARDT AND R. OOZEER

University Department of Neurology , The Radcliffe Infirmary, Oxford, UK

Summary

Sixty-eight   patients with unexplained attacks of disturbed consciousness have had simultaneous EEG and ECG ambulatory monitoring to determine the clinical usefulness of the technique. Symptomatic episodes were captured on tape in 34% of cases, but were positively diagnostic in less than one-fifth of these patients. The majority had normal records during their attacks. In some paroxysmal episodes, artefact prevented a firm conclusion being reached. 'Silent' EEG and ECG abnormalities may also provide a guide to further investigation or treatment.   Epileptic discharges were associated   with characteristic ECG changes which may be of some value in differentiating epileptic from hysterical attacks.

Introduction

Despite thorough clinical investigation, the causes of transient disturbances of consciousness are often difficult to establish. Diagnosis may be confounded by the lack of a clear account of the course of events while symptoms may be non-specific for cardiac or cerebral dysrhythmias. The routine laboratory EEG and ECG are often unhelpful in this context. The introduction of techniques for ambulatory monitoring of cardiac (1) or cerebral activity (2, 3, 4, 5, 6, 7) has increased the chances of recording symptomatic events.

The usefulness of 24-hour ambulatory EEG recording in the investigation of patients with paroxysmal attacks of unknown aetiology has recently been reported (8). However, such patients also show a prevalance of cardiac arrhythmias on ambulatory ECG monitoring of between 10 and 64% (9, 10, 11, 12) and this remains a controversial area of clinical practice. Furthermore, seizures may follow cerebral anoxia from any cause while cardiac arrhythmias may occur as secondary autonomic accompaniments of epileptic fits (13, 14). For this reason, it is clearly important to establish the primary cause of unexplained attacks by monitoring heart and brain activity at the same time.

We report here some preliminary observations from a continuing study of simultaneous ambulatory monitoring of the ECG and EEG (SAMMEE) in patients with undiagnosed attacks of disturbed consciousness.

Patients and Methods

The criterion for entry to the study was repeated episodes of disturbed consciousness for which no diagnosis could be established by routine methods. Patients with a past history of epilepsy or cardiac arrhythmias were excluded. Migraine, ischaemic heart disease, syncopal attacks or other disorders were not considered grounds for exclusion if the attacks under investigation could not be attributed to these pre-exising conditions. The patients were seen soon after their initial presentation and the majority were not taking anti-convulsant or anti-arrhythmic medications. Patients were not selected on the basis of the frequency of their attacks. Sixty-eight patients with idopathic attacks have been recorded to date. Their mean age was 43.7 years (range 10-79 years). Thirty healthy controls and 20 epileptics, mostly with temporal lobe epilepsy, have also been recorded.

All recordings were made with Oxford 4-24 cassette recorders with two channels for EEG, one for ECG and one for a time-base with an event marker facility. Patients wore a digital watch synchronised with the recorder and completed a diary of activities and symptoms. The majority of recordings were made during normal daily activities, at home, school or work. A few patients were recorded during a hospital admission.

Recordings were made onto standard C120 cassettes using 9mm Ag/AgCl electrodes and preamplifiers (HDX-82) attached firmly to the scalp with collodion. Impedance was reduced below 5K by scarification. The EEG electrodes were placed on the 10-20 positions T3-T5 and T4-T6.

Each tape was visually screened independently by the two investigators using a fast playback device (Oxford Instruments PMD-12). Sections of record with features of interest were transcribed onto an 8-channel ink jet mingograph. Only unequivocal epileptic activity such as spikes or sharp waves, spike-and-wave-bursts or rhythmic epileptic slow wave discharges were accepted as abnormal in the EEG traces. Many records contained bursts of theta activity but these were not included in this analysis as the distribution and extent of such activity in the 24-hour records of healthy controls has not been established. For the same reason, single ventricular extrasystoles, although often very numerous in the patients' records, were not considered abnormal. The criteria used for 'significant' cardiac arrhythmias were those of Luxon et al (12).

Results

A total of 2376 hours of recordings, representing an average of 35 hours per patient (range 24-102 hours), have been screened. One or more symptomatic events were captured on tape in 23 of the 68 cases (34%) with unexplained attacks (see Table 1).

Eleven of these 23 patients (48%) considered their recorded attacks to be 'typical'. In seven of these cases the ECG and EEG were normal during the symptomatic episodes. Two patients had abnormalities during their attacks. One of these had undergone extensive cardiological investigations (Case 1). Her record showed several attacks each of which coincided with epileptic discharges.

TABLE: Dysrhythmias detected in patients with unexplained attacks (n = 68)

Symptomatic Event Captured	n	Associated Dysrhythmia*	Equivocal Record During Event	Normal Record During Event	Silent Abnormalities	Total Abnormal
Typical attack	11	2(1)	2(2)	7	2	4/11(36%)
Minor	12	1	1(1)	10	1	2/12(17%)
Nil	45	-	-	-	5(3)	5/45(11%)
Totals	68	3	3	17	8	11/68(16%)

* EEG and ECG abnormalities excluding cardiac arrhythmias occurring as an autonomic effect of seizure activity. Figures in parentheses represent number of EEG abnormalities in each category.

The recording of the other case, whose attacks had been attributed to possible temporal lobe epilepsy, showed a normal EEG trace and a cardiac arrhythmia which accounted for her distressing symptoms (Case 2). The other two patients with captured attacks had equivocal results. In one case, the EEG was obscured by muscle activity during a suspected epileptic seizure, and in the other irregular slow wave activity at the time of the attack was not significantly different from similar, asymptomatic activity recurring throughout the 'interictal' record (Case 3).

Twelve of the 23 patients (52%) experienced symptoms during the recordings which either were trivial or appeared to be unrelated to their presenting complaints. No abnormalities were seen in the records of ten of these twelve cases during their symptomatic episodes. In one patient in whom there was a suspicion that the attacks were not epileptic and possibly 'functional', trivial symptoms were associated with several dramatic events characterised by an excess of muscle activity and high voltage movement artefact in the EEG and a tachycardia in excess of 200/minute (Case 4, Fig. 1). Attacks with similar features were recorded in cases with mixed organic and psychiatric features who were included in our epileptic 'controls'. The remaining patient, who had presented with four attacks of loss of consciousness thought to be associated with an irregular cardiac rhythm, complained during the recording of palpitations and these were clearly associated with a supraventricular tachycardia.

Thus a positive diagnosis for the captured symptomatic events was established in 3/23 cases (13%) (Table 1). A further 3/23 (13%) had equivocal findings at the time of their attacks and an underlying EEG abnormality could not be excluded. The remaining 17/23 (74%) with symptoms during the recordings had normal ECG and EEG records at the indicated time of their symptoms. Three of these had 'clinically silent' (asymptomatic) cardiac arrhythmias at other times including episodes of ventricular tachycardia, salvoes of coupled ventricular extrasystoles and junctional tachycardias (Case 5, Fig. 2).

Most recorded attacks in the two patient groups, whether definite temporal lobe discharges or dubious episodes, were associated with alterations in the ECG rate or rhythm. Attacks which were considered to have a 'functional' basis or to be equivocal due to EEG artefact, were invariably associated with a sinus tachycardia. In most cases, this began well before the onset of the muscle or movement artefact associated with the symptomatic episode (e.g. Case 4, Fig. 1). Patients with clinically definite temporal lobe seizures, in which there was secondary generalisation in the EEG record, also showed a tachycardia, but its onset was often abrupt and closely correlated with the cerebral discharge. In addition, a short period of slowing of the cardiac rate sometimes preceded the seizure and marked irregularities including abrupt rate changes, sinus arrest and extrasystoles became prominent near the termination of the abnormal cerebral discharge (Fig.3).

Forty-five patients were asymptomatic during their recordings. In five the tapes revealed 'clinically silent' abnormalities. Three had epileptic activity during sleep, two with lateralised spikes and sharp waves during slow wave sleep while the third (Case 6, Fig. 4) had a temporal lobe seizure during light sleep. The two other cases had asymptomatic cardiac arrhythmias.

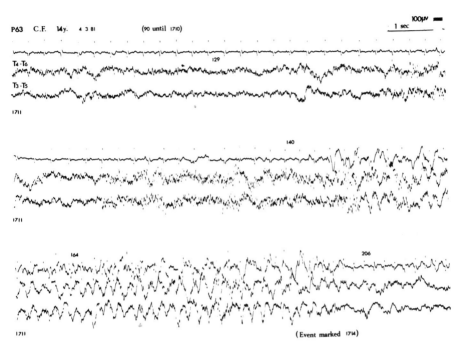

Fig. 1   Recorded attack at time of 'tiredness and weakness' in Case
          4. Note gradual increase in muscle activity over both
          sides of scalp obscuring the EEG traces which is followed
          by considerable movement artifact on ECG channel coinciding
          with rhythmic high amplitude 3-4 cps bilateral slow waves.
          Note steady increase of sinus tachycardia from 90 to
          206/minute.

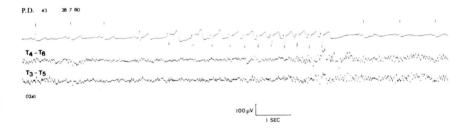

Fig. 2   Asymptomatic junctional tachycardia during light sleep
          (Case 5).

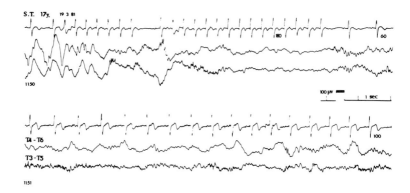

Fig. 3   Cardiac irregularities at end of temporal lobe seizure.
Generalised rhythmic epileptic slow activity ceases at left
hand end of top trace. Right-sided postictal slow activity
is seen in the lower trace. Note extra-systoles, irregularity of rhythm and the flattening of EEG which coincides
with tachycardia of 180/minute.

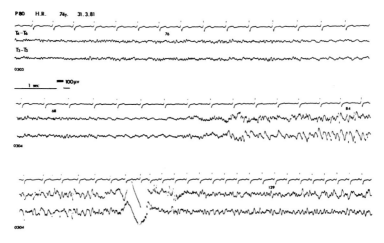

Fig. 4   Asymptomic noctural seizure. Note flattening of EEG and
slowing of cardiac rate at onset, the appearance of mixed
sharp and slow waves on the right and increase in heart
rate as the seizure activity develops and spreads to the
left. Despite the single myoclonic jerk the patient did
not rouse.

Case Histories

Case 1: Female, 22 years. Identical twin. 5-year history of stereo-typed episodes varying from 20/day to four months clear. A transient warning at onset consists of nausea with 'weak and clammy hands'. A choking sensation occurs in some attacks. Typically slumps forward gripping mother tightly but otherwise limp with eyes closed, rapid respiration, trembling and pallor. There is some awareness of surroundings throughout, but for three to four minutes she is unable to speak. Recovery is rapid but lethargy and malaise persist for a further ten minutes.

Twin sister has neurofibromatosis and similar 'dizzy turns and blackouts' diagnosed as cardiogenic and treated with a demand pacemaker.

Examination showed subcutaneous neurofibromata and cafe-au-lait spots. CAT scan, ECG and EEG all normal. Ambulatory ECG recordings and physiological studies of cardiac conducting tissue showed no abnormalities. SAMMEE (120 hours): several attacks captured in 'cluster', all of which were associated with focal right-sided seiz-ure activity with secondary generalisation and an accompanying sinus tachycardia.

Case 2: Female, 42 years. History of birth trauma. Diagnosis of temporal lobe epilepsy considered at 19 years following eclampsia and myoclonic jerks during pregnancy and episodes of fear, dysphoria and auditory hallucinations lasting up to one hour. B-blocker (Atenolol) commenced at 40 years for hypertension.

Presented with two-year history of episodes generally occurring on waking in the morning characterised by fear, sweating, blurred vision, bursting and thumping sensations in the chest, a reluctance to talk and a sensation of falling lasting up to two hours. Physical examination normal. ECG and CAT scan normal. EEG showed asymptomatic bursts of right-sided theta activity. SAMMEE (24 hours): two captured attacks coincided with long bursts of ventric-ular bigeminal rhythm and normal EEG. Attacks ceased after Atenolol was discontinued.

Case 3: Male 67 years, with recent left hemisphere infarction assoc-iated with occluded left carotid artery. Continuing episodes of amaurosis fugax. Presented with 18-month history of two to three 'blackouts' weekly. Transient warning consisting of hazy vision and giddiness followed by 'collapse' with loss of consciousness, limpness and pallor for up to 10 minutes. Thought (by paramedic) to be 'pulseless' in one attack. Sequelae of confusion for several min-utes. Past history of undiagnosed 'blackouts' at 35 years.

Examination revealed aphasia and residual right hemiparesis. EEG showed slow waves over left hemisphere lesion consistent with clinical and CAT scan findings. ECG normal. Diagnoses considered included Stokes-Adams attacks, intermittent cerebral flow problem ('cerebral steal') or epilepsy. SAMMEE (192 hours): one captured attack showed only a possibly increased amount of left-sided slow-wave activity but this was similar to the intermittent bursts of asymptomatic left-sided slow waves at other times in the 'interictal' record. The ECG was unchanged in the attack.

Case 4: Male, 14 years, with pre-existing migraine, behavioural disorder and obsessional neurosis; one sister with idiopathic grand mal epilepsy. Presented with six months' history of 'blank spells' varying from several attacks per day to one month clear. Warning of dizziness and 'closing-in' sensation for a few seconds followed by a transient 'blank' spell of several seconds. Sequelae of dizziness and nausea for up to one hour. No outward signs observed by his mother. Physical examination, ECG and EEG all normal. Features in history all suggestive of 'functional' attacks but temporal lobe epilepsy considered. SAMMEE (24 hours): multiple episodes of 'tiredness and weakness' coincided with movement artefact and marked tachycardia (Figure 1). Result equivocal.

Follow-up: further interrogation suggested attacks consisted of compulsive head-shaking. All symptoms have ceased.

Case 5: Female, 43 years with 15 months' history of attacks varying in frequency from 3/week to three months clear.. Transient warning, seconds, with 'curious feeling in stomach' and generalised sensation of warmth, followed by sudden collapse, with loss of consciousness, limpness and pallor for up to five seconds. Rapid recovery with no sequelae. Physical examination, ECG and EEG all normal. SAMMEE (24 hours): asymptomatic. Two 'clinically silent' episodes of junctional tachycardia during sleep (Figure 2).

Case 6: Male, 74 years with myocardial ischaemia. Twelve months' history of attacks with 1-2 second warning consisting of sensation that sounds are receding accompanied by momentary unsteadiness. This is followed by speech and activity arrest with unresponsiveness for five to six seconds. No loss of consciousness. Rapid recovery with 'scarlet flushing' of face in some attacks.

Examination revealed bilateral carotid bruits and ECG showed antero-lateral ischaemic changes. EEG normal. SAMMEE (24 hours): Asymptomatic nocturnal seizure with right-sided onset and postictal slowing (Figure 4).

Discussion

Although this study has just begun, our preliminary results confirm the value of recording ECG and EEG simultaneously in patients with unexplained attacks. If this technique is applied in the initial stages of the clinical work-up in patients with non-specific episodic symptoms, inappropriate investigations may be avoided. Nevertheless, it is clear that unequivocally positive diagnostic records will only be obtained in a minority of patients. Attacks occur with such widely varying frequencies that high capture rates cannot be expected, even if recordings are extended for periods up to a week in duration. In a few patients with predictable clustering of paroxysmal episodes a higher success rate may be achieved by repeated recordings at appropriate intervals. A 'baseline' 24-hour record is obtained in those cases where attacks are too infrequent to attempt to capture one. Our 'hit-rate' for typical attacks in our unselected series to date is 16%. The much higher capture rate of 46% in the only comparable series to date, of 26 cases with 'suspected epilepsy', is due to the selection of cases with frequent attacks (15).

Even where typical attacks were captured, we found the records were negative or equivocal in the majority (82%) of cases. Only two of 11 (18%) with characteristic episodes had a clear ECG or EEG abnormality accounting for their symptoms. This compares with four of 12 patients (33%) in Woods and Ives' (1977) report (15). Despite the technical advances which have made it possible to record high quality EEG from unrestricted patients, and even though scrupulous attention is paid to electrode technique, it is inevitable that such records will contain large quantities and varieties of artefact. While most of these can be identified and differentiated from abnormal activity, muscle potentials and movement artefact remain particularly troublesome during some paroxysmal attacks. In a few cases, we were unable to come to any firm decision due to obscuration of the EEG at the time of the symptomatic attack (e.g. Case 4, Figure 1), a problem also encountered by other workers in this field (15).

The clinical usefulness of ambulatory monitoring is not restricted to positive correlations during attacks although this information is most valuable diagnostically. Negative results, although more difficult to interpret, may also be of considerable value in narrowing the range of diagnostic possibilities (e.g. Case 3). The interpretation of minor symptoms in association with a normal record is complicated by the observation that the majority of auras in patients with temporal lobe eiplepsy do not result in alteration of the scalp-recorded EEG (16). Nevertheless, the absence of EEG changes during a major attack with loss of consciousness is strong evidence against an epileptic basis for that episode. However, while a negative finding may confirm that a particular attack is not a generalised seizure, it does not exclude a diagnosis of epilepsy, as the coexistence of functional and genuine seizures in some patients is well recognised in neurological practice. Our recordings from patients with established epilepsy have demonstrated the occurrence of 'non-epileptic' and epileptic events on the same tape. Thus negative results in our patients must be cautiously interpreted and the outcome established by long-term follow-up studies.

While previous reports of ambulatory EEG monitoring of patients with 'suspected epilepsy' have stressed the importance of capturing symptomatic events (8, 15), no mention has been made of the occurrence and significance of 'silent' abnormalities. Studies of ambulatory ECG monitoring in patients with transient neurological episodes have revealed a high prevalence of cardiac arrhythmias, albeit mostly asymptomatic (11, 12). While the detection of such silent arrhythmias does not establish a causal link with the patients' attacks, they may provide important clues for further appropriate investigations or treatment. The occurrence of asymptomatic focal sharp waves and spikes and a nocturnal seizure in three of our patients emphasises the value of the cassette recorder in obtaining a sleep record and provided strong circumstantial evidence of an epileptic basis for the symptomatic attacks in these patients. Although epilepsy remains primarily a clinical diagnosis and normative data for the 24-hour EEG recordings in ambulant subjects is not yet available, we believe that such findings taken in the overall clinical context of these cases provides a reasonable objective basis for a therapeutic trial of anti-convulsants. The relevance and importance for prognosis of such asymptomatic findings must be further explored by carefully controlled studies and by long-term follow-up.

Ambulatory monitoring of either ECG or EEG alone in the type of patient in this study is clearly inefficient and the results open to misinterpretation. All types of cardiac arrhythmias have been reported as autonomic concomitants of epileptic seizures (13, 14). The abrupt changes in cardiac rhythm, sinus arrest and extrasystoles we have recorded during temporal lobe seizures are similar to the arrhythmias reported by White and his colleagues (14) and may occur in such patients more commonly than is recognised. They have important implications for cardiologists who investigate patients with blackouts or dizziness by ambulatory ECG monitoring. The autonomic effects on the heart which can accompany quite non-specific attacks of temporal lobe epilepsy could well account for some of the puzzling cases whose episodes, recorded by ambulatory ECG monitoring, are associated only with an apparently insignificant sinus tachycardia. We are currently investigating the usefulness of the cardiac rhythm changes in distinguishiing epileptic from functional or hysterical episodes simulating seizures. Despite the high prevalence of cardiac arrhythmias reported in patients presenting with suspected epilepsy (11, 12), we have not so far encountered the situation where a cardiac arrhythmia has precipitated an epileptic seizure.

While the combined detection rate of 'abnormalities' in this study so far is only 16%, this figure does not take into account the usefulness of negative correlations in some patients. It must also be remembered that in the cases under investigation, a diagnosis has not been achieved by conventional methods. With further developments, in particular the provision of more EEG channels to improve the recognition of artefact, and with the acquisition of healthy control data, this technique should improve our diagnostic accuracy and our understanding of the mechanisms underlying transient unexplained disturbances of consciousness.

Acknowledgements

We should like to thank Dr. Roger Quy for valuable technical advice and the neurologists and cardiologists of the Oxford Region for referring their patients for recording..

This work was supported by a Medical Research Council Project Grant.

References

1.   Holter N.J. and Generelli J.A. (1949) Rocky Mountain Med. J., **46** 747-751.
2.   Ives J.R. and Woods J.F. (1975) Electroenceph. clin. Neurophysiol., **39**, 88-92.
3.   Ives J.R. (1976) Postgrad. Med. J. **52** (Suppl. 7), 86-91.
4.   Apple H.P and Burgess R.C. (1976) Postgrad. Med. J. **52** (Suppl.7), 79-85.
5.   Quy R.J. (1978) J. Physiol. **284**, 7P.
6.   Horwitz S.J., Burgess R.C. and Kijewski K.N. (1978) Am. J. EEG Technol. **18**, 133-139.
7.   Quy R.J., Willison R.G., Fitch P. and Gilliatt R.W. (1980) In: ISAM 1979: Proceedings of the Third International Symposium on Ambulatory Monitoring, ed. Stott F.D., Raftery E.B. and Goulding

L. Academic Press:London, 393-398.

8.   Ives J.R., Hausser C., Woods J.F. and Andermann F. (1981) In:
     Advances in Epileptology: XIIth Epilepsy International Sympo-
     sium, ed. Dam M., Gram L. and Penry J.K. Raven Press: New York,
     329-336.
9.   Walter P.F., Reid S.D. and Wenger S.K. (1970) Annals of Int.
     Med. **72**, 471-474.
10. Van Durme J.P. (1975) Am. H. Journal, **89**, 538-540.
11. Schott G.D., McLeod A.A. and Jewitt D.E. (1977) Br. Med. J. **1**
     1454-1457.
12. Luxon L.M., Crowther A., Harrison M.J.G. and Coltart D.J. (1980)
     J. Neurol. Neurosurg. Psychiat. **43**. 37-41.
13. Phizackerley P.J.R., Poole E.W. and Whitty C.W.M. (1954) Epi-
     lepsia, **3**, 89-96.
14. White P.T., Grant P.G., Mosier J. and Craig A. (1961) Neurology,
     11, 354-361.
15. Woods J.F. and Ives J.R. (1977) In: Epilepsy, 8th International
     Symposium, ed. Penry J.K. Raven Press: New York, 109-113.
16. Ives J.R. and Woods J.F. (1980) In: ISAM 1979: Proceedings of
     Third International Symposium on Ambulatory Monitoring, ed.
     Stott F.D., Raftery E.B. and Goulding L. Academic Press: Lon-
     don,. 383-392.

Discussion

DR. HALL: With regard to Dr. Blumhardt's cases with sudden increase
in heart rate and temporal lobe attacks, an alternative diagnosis in
that is panic reaction - which I am sure he has also seen a number
of times. We have monitored one young man who had a history suggestive of temporal lobe epilepsy, whose attacks always seemed to coincide with an event. The event we captured was associated with his
dropping a plate while he was washing up - this event was associated
with a sudden rapid rise in heart rate, a sinus tachycardia, but no
EEG change.
DR. BLUMHARDT: I think that the functional attacks nearly always
have tachycardias. What surprises me is the normal range of an
emotional sinus tachycardia - the cardiologists would not accept 210
or 220 beats/min (which is the sort of heart rate I observe) as being
within the normal range for a sinus tachycardia, even under severe
emotional stress. Nevertheless, it is common. In fact, every known
ECG arrhythmia has been recorded, usually towards the end, in temporal lobe discharges. There are numerous examples of cases who have
had umpteen ECG tapes - and the attacks have switched off with
Epanutin (Phenytoin) after they have been demonstrated to begin.
     The other point in this regard, is that the tachycardia may
appear to come before paroxysmal discharge or afterwards in the same
patient, who is otherwise having identical, stereotyped attacks.
DR. STORES: I was interested in Dr. Blumhardt's accounts of the
movement and muscle artefact, and I wonder whether he has experimented with placing the electrodes in different positions. I imagine
that there is most muscle interference when recording over the
temporalis. Does the problem remain if the electrodes are moved
elsewhere - probably not much would be forfeited diagnostically by
doing that?

Secondly, where does Dr. Blumhardt think that the movement artefact originated on the case he showed?

DR. BLUMHARDT: The movement artefact probably originates in the scalp. Obviously, it could be scalp movement - in some cases, there is tremendous bilateral slow wave, which looks quite rhythmic and beautifully sinusoidal, and which happens when a patient washes his face in the morning. In other cases, it is unilateral, when they scratch or just move an electrode. It is probably a combination of electrode, electrolyte, shearing, generating triobelectric potentials and also scalp movement. I do not have the time to show a library of artefacts, but it is worrying to know that spikes can be simulated by very simple movements of the heard, such as nodding, which are indistinguishable from the sort of spikes observed in some temporal lobe epileptics - so we do not know what they are up to during the 24 hours' recording. We have experimented with different positions, but if we are trying to diagnose "funny" turns, the differential diagnosis of temporal lobe epilepsy is already a possibility so the electrodes have to be placed somewhere over the temporal lobes.

It is not possible to simulate what a patient's activities are during 24 hours. A routine number of movements are done: eye movements, scalp movements, they brush their hair, the electrodes are wiggled, they chew, bite, close their eyes, look to left and right and so on, in order to exclude this sort of artefact. But that does not account for what that young boy was doing in those episodes not witnessed by his mother. It is difficult to simulate all those things that people may do. Perhaps there is a case here for video split-screen techniques - but not when the patient has an attack only once every four months.

PRECIPITATING FACTORS AND SEIZURE ACTIVITY

G. STORES AND R. LWIN

National Centre for Children with Epilepsy, Park Hospital
for Children and University Department of Psychiatry,
Oxford, UK

Introduction

Despite even careful use of anti-epileptic drugs, many people with
epilepsy continue to have seizures. Often these seizures do not occur
at random and close enquiry may well reveal that particular factors
or circumstances are consistently associated with their occurrence.
Among the many factors that have been recognised or suspected as
important precipitants of seizures are sleep loss, emotional stress,
boredom and monthly or diurnal cycles. At times, specific sensory
stimuli may trigger attacks. Occasionally, patients appear to be
able to abort attacks themselves by concentration, or their seizures
may be curtailed by arousing stimuli.

Most of this information about precipitating and inhibiting
factors is based on clinical impression or anecdotal case reports.
The classical studies in this area are those by Gowers (4) and
Symonds (13) as well as the extensive review by Gastaut and Tassinari
(2). Servit's (11) study was designed specifically to explore precipitating and inhibiting factors, but was of limited scope. In all
these studies, however, specific factors were said to be identified
in a high proportion of cases but in the main detailed EEG and
clinical correlations were not examined. Although few statistical
data are available on precipitating and inhibiting factors on adults,
there is even less information of this type on children with
seizures. This is so in spite of suggestions that such factors are
of particular importance in young patients, whose seizure frequency
may be affected by attentive factors (3,7), certain types of school
activities (5) and other types of mental and motor activity (9).

A disincentive to collecting information on such matters has
been the difficulty of obtaining objective, quantified information
about the occurrence of seizure discharge over long periods of time.
Attaining this is generally considered to be most difficult in the
case of non-convulsive seizures. Similarly, adequate reporting of
environmental and especially psychological factors is not easy to
achieve especially as such information is usually provided by parents, teachers or others without professional training in observational methods.

In the study by Sato et al (10), an eight-channel portable
cassette recorder was used to compile charts which showed the patterns of occurrence of seizure discharge in epileptic patients in
relation to their activities in hospital and at home. The results
confirm that emotional stress and boredom can act as precipitants of
seizures in some patients. The wider application of Sato's recording
method was hampered by the prominent nature of the equipment used for

long-term EEG recording. Patients had to carry equipment in a har-
ness with components held in pockets on the front and back of the
chest, and the transmitter was mounted on the top of the patient's
head. Fortunately, recent technical advances have made possible the
design of a system which allows satisfactory EEG and other physiological recordings to be made unobtrusively over long periods in real-
life situations (12). Although the system has been used mainly for
purposes of differential diagnosis in attacks of uncertain origin, it
lends itself to the collection of data about the occurrence of
seizures over long periods of time.
    The present study was concerned with the use of this system for
such long-term monitoring of EEG (and also EKG as an attempt object-
ively to monitor emotional state), for comparison with an account of
the child's activities over the same recording period.

Methods

From the EEG Department of the Park Hospital for Children in Oxford
and Lingfield School in Surrey, 28 children were identified who, in
spite of anti-epileptic medication, were still having absence seizures associated with generalized spike and wave activity in their
EEG. The age range of these children was 6-16 years and all were of
about average intelligence. Eighteen of the group were boys.
    After permission for inclusion in this study had been obtained
from the children's parents and their paediatricians, continuous 24-
hour ambulatory EEG/EKG recordings were carried out by means of the
Medilog system (12). Two channels of EEG were recorded from
positions C4 - P4 and C3 - P3 using standard electrodes. The third
channel was used for recording EKG, with electrodes placed on the
sternum and left side of the chest. The fourth available channel
recorded time and an event marker.
    Parents, teachers and nursing staff provided a record of the
child's behaviour throughout the recorded period by completing standardized sheets, which allowed an open-ended description of the
child's activities, but also required entries each 15 minutes on
specific aspects of behaviour, namely, whether the child appeared to
be excited, anxious, frustrated, inattentive, co-operative, bored,
sad, happy, talkative, or tired. The child was assumed to have slept
continuously during the night unless there was definite evidence to
the contrary. Each 24-hour tape was replayed on the PMD-12 visual
display system (12), which allowed artefacts to be excluded and the
duration of each burst of generalized seizure discharge to be
measured by hand. A bar chart was then compiled showing the total
duration of spike-and-wave activity in each 15-minute epoch over the
24-hour period. Heart rate was also counted for each 15-minute epoch.
The distribution of seizure activity and changes in heart rate were
considered in relation to the written account of the child's activities as illustrated in Figure 1.

Results

Individual differences in the distribution of seizure discharge over
the 24-hour periods were clearly seen. Some of these occurred in
relation to the sleep/wake cycle; in others, there appeared to be

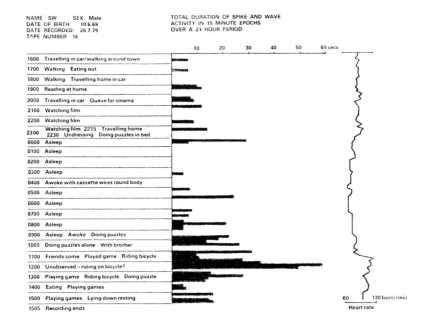

Fig. 1   Spike-wave activity related to occupation over a 23 hour period.

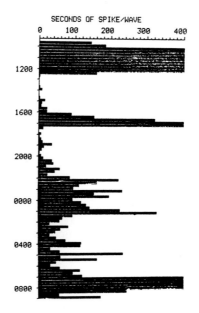

Fig. 2   Spike wave activity pattern over 24 hrs as found in the case of an 8 year old boy.

an association between peak occurrence of seizure discharge and more specific factors.

In 21 cases, seizure activity occurred predominantly in the awake state, but in two the reverse was seen. In the remaining five, seizure activity was equally distributed between the awake and sleeping hours.

In Figure 1, the uneven distribution of seizure discharge can be seen over the 24-hour recording period, not only between the awake and sleep periods, but especially during the time when the child was awake. Most activity is seen during the four hours after awakening and much of this was at the time when the child was riding a bicycle. The relationship in this case between seizure discharge and physical activity was confirmed by further observations.

Figure 2 illustrates the striking pattern of occurrence in seizure activity in another patient. This child was an eight-year old boy, with subtle absence seizures and prolonged periods of drowsiness or confusion, both associated with generalized irregular spike-and-wave activity. The print-out in Figure 2 (produced by an automated spike-and-wave analyser, discussed by Bailey,(p.204, this volume) and validated against manual analysis) shows intense seizure activity which is reduced dramatically within 15-30 minutes of each meal taken at mid-day, 16.00 hours and 08.15 hours the next day. The reduction of seizure activity, in this way, was associated with a transformation in the child's mental state from drowsiness and confusion to normal behaviour. These clinical and electrographic changes were reproducible and were not associated with any change in blood sugar levels.

In one of the children in this series, the peak occurrence of seizure activity seemed to be convincingly associated with his emotional distress. In another child, inactivity and complaints of boredom appeared to act as precipitants.

Conclusions

The results of this preliminary investigation suggest that ambulatory EEG monitoring by means of the Medilog system, combined with observational reports, can provide important information about patterns of occurrence of seizure discharge which might not be available by other means. This type of investigation of individual cases might demonstrate patterns of occurrence which had previously been unsuspected. This was the case, with most of the children, in the present series. The recording period was purposefully limited to a 24-hour period and for practical purposes it would be necessary to demonstrate consistency in these patterns of occurrence. If such consistency was demonstrated, there could be important implications concerning alterations in blood levels of anti-epileptic drug treatment in the case of the diurnal variations, or for non-pharmacological forms of intervention especially where psychological precipitants appear to be important.

Manual analysis of information from prolonged ambulatory monitoring is time-consuming and tedious. However, reliable results appear to be obtainable by automated means in most types of spike-wave discharge (Bailey, this volume). Improvements are still required in the means of obtaining a prolonged account of children's behaviour, which is of sufficient sensitivity, when used by parents or teachers as well as nursing staff unfamiliar with this type of assessment. As yet, there appears to be no way of monitoring the physiological aspects of emotional state in children in an unobtrusive and acceptable fashion. The attempt to achieve this in the present study by measuring heart rate was unproductive as heart rate is readily affected by physical exercise, whatever the child's emotional state at the time.

Finally, it might be objected that ambulatory EEG monitoring provides information only on seizure discharge contained in the EEG without regard to the presence, or otherwise, of clinical accompaniments. It is true that such clinical and EEG events are inconsistently related (8). In general, bursts of seizure activity of less than three seconds' duration are unlikely to be accompanied by clinical manifestations. Longer bursts may be associated with obvious absence seizures or by subtle effects on performance only detectable by special testing. In the present series, the vast majority of bursts of seizure activity was in excess of three seconds.

Acknowledgements

We are grateful to Dr. Nicol and his colleagues at Lingfield Hospital School for their help, and to the British Epilepsy Association for funding this project.

References

1. Bailey C. Proceedings of the 4th International Symposium on Ambulatory Monitoring, Gent. June, 1981 (in press).
2. Gastaut H., and Tassinari C.A. (1966) Epilepsia 7, 85-138.
3. Geier S. (1971) Epilepsia 12, 215-223.
4. Gowers W.R. Epilepsy and Other Chronic Convulsive Diseases;. Their Causes, Symptoms and Treatment. Churchill, London, 1881.
5. Guey J., Bureau M., Draver C. and Roger J. (1969) Epilepsia 10, 441-451.
6. Lee S.I., Sutherling W.W., Persing J.A. and Butler A.B. (1980) Arch Neurol. 37, 433-436.
7. Ounsted C. and Hutt S.J. (1964) Proc. Roy. Soc. Med. 5, 1178.
8. Penry J.K. In: Brazier M. (ed) Epilepsy Its Phenomena in Man. Academic Press, New York, 1973, 171-188.
9. Ricci G., Perti G. and Cherubini E. (1972) Epilepsia 13, 785-794.
10. Sato S., Penry J.K. and Dreifuss F.E. In: Kellaway P. and Petersen I. (eds) Quantitative Analytic Studies in Epilepsy. Raven Press, New York, 1976, 237-251.
11. Servit Z., Machek J., Stercova A., Dudas D., Kristof M., Cervenkova V. (1962) Epilepsia 3, 315-322.
12. Stores G. (1980) J. Int. Biomed. Info and Data, 1, 1-7.
13. Symonds C. (1959) Brain 82, 133-146.
14. Wilkins A.J. Zifkin B., Andermann F. and McGovern E. (unpubl.)

Discussion

DR. SAYED: Was the consistency of recurrence of sub-clinical discharges in response to precipitating factors measured by statistical analysis?

DR. STORES: No. It is important that the demonstration of a pattern, the way I have shown, over a particular 24-hour period needs to be shown to be a consistent finding in a child. I am not suggesting that that information by itself provides the basis for psychiatric intervention. I am simply using those cases to illustrate how insight might be gained into a situation which otherwise would be misinterpreted. That kind of finding needs to be followed up by further enquiry to see whether it is a consistent feature, or indeed to elaborate the details of the relationship.

DR. SOUTHALL: With regard to the children who show more activity during the night, it might be interesting to look at sleep apnoea in this group, and whether it could be related to epilepsy. Has Dr. Stores thought about trying to look at that?

DR. STORES: That has not been done yet. We are about to embark on some studies using the Medilog system for overnight sleep recording which would allow that sort of enquiry.

LONG-TERM EEG CASSETTE RECORDINGS
ADVANTAGES, LIMITATIONS AND FUTURE

J.R. IVES

Montreal Neurological Hospital and Institute,
Montreal, Quebec, Canada

Introduction

The major advantage of a 4-channel, 24-hour ambulatory cassette recording of a patient's EEG is the ability to obtain the record on a completely ambulatory out-patient over a significant period of time (1). However, this creates two major problems, 1) dealing efficiently with the vast amount of data collected, and 2) doing so in a reasonable amount of time. Traditionally, a conventional EEG is written out at a paper speed of 30 mm/sec. If this was also done for a 24-hour cassette recording, it would amount to 8,640 pages of EEG, or a length of 2.6 Km or 1.6 miles. It is also not very efficient to take 24 hours to replay the 24-hour tape, so replaying the tape at high speed is desirable, if one can deal with the increased data rate.

Analog Methods

The replay equipment will play back the 24-hour tape between 20x to 120x as fast as it was recorded (speed-up of at least 20x is required to recover low frequency signals) (2). The basic problem here is dealing with the higher bandwidth when the replay speed is increased, as shown in Table 1.

TABLE 1

Replay Speed	Bandwidth	Replay Time
x1	0.5 Hz to 35 Hz	24 hrs.
x10	5 Hz to 350 Hz	2.4 hrs.
x20	10 Hz to 700 Hz	72 mins.
x60	30 Hz to 2.1 KHz	24 mins.
x120	60 Hz to 4.2 KHz	12 mins.

Conventional EEG galvanometer pen-type chart recorders cannot resolve a bandwidth higher than 100 Hz (allowing only a speed up of x2). However, the use of ink-jet type recorders permits replay at x60 which resolves the significant information (1,3), while a replay at x20 is used to produce readable diagnostic EEG.

By taking advantage of the frequency shift due to increased replay speed, the EEG can be "heard" and this aids in reviewing the 24-hour for "interesting bursts of activity" (1).

Analog detection circuits, such as bandpass filters, 1st or 2nd derivative circuits, etc. are useful in highlighting specific events such as epileptic spikes or sharp waves, bursts of 3/sec spike-and-wave activity or rhythmical epileptic discharges (1, 3, 5).

As with all data analysis and data reduction techniques, it is very helpful to know beforehand what you are looking for. With epileptic patients, who have 3/sec spike-and-wave type discharges in their EEG, bandpass filters can be specifically tuned to the predominant discharge frequency as demonstrated in Figure 1.

By replaying the 24-hour cassette at x60 and writing out in a compressed form the signal that is derived from the bandpass filtered summation of the 4 original EEG channels, a one-page summary of the entire 24-hour EEG can be obtained in 24 minutes.

The first patient, illustrated in Figure 2a, is a 7-year-old male diagnosed with Lennox-Gastaut syndrome, who demonstrated atypical 2/sec spike-and-wave in his EEG. This compressed 24-hour recording indicates that the patient is more active during wakefulness than during sleep and that his bursts could be up to 10 min. in length.

The second patient (Figure 2b) is a 13-year-old female with a similar clinical diagnosis and atypical 2/sec spike-and-wave. In the compressed record it can be clearly seen that there is a marked difference in the morphology and time distribution of these discharges.

Analog methods are a very efficient means of reducing a 24-hour 4-channel record to a reasonable, meaningful quantitative result, particularly in specific areas as demonstrated above.

However, some events and desired results are more applicable to digital techniques.

Digital Methods

Digital computers in the form of mini and/or micro computer systems will become more and more prevalent in this field as technology advances in the areas of data acquisition, data analysis and large memory systems, combined with the trend of cost reduction.

Table 2 illustrates the main problem in the area of capacity since a 24-hour cassette contains about 70 M Bytes (or 560 M bits) of information. New disc systems (Winchester) have this capacity at a reasonable cost and could serve as a dumping area for the entire 24-hour cassette, as it is not practical to split up the 24-hour record onto separate discs, tapes, etc; besides losing continuity, too much time is spent changing medium.

TABLE 2

---

4 channels of EEG
200 samples per second per channel
8 bit resolution (1 Byte = 8 bits)
24 hours of recording
2.94 Bytes per hour
70.8 M Bytes per 24-hour recording.

Since the data contained on the 24-hour tape is analog, it has to be digitized before it can be analysed by a computer. In prac-

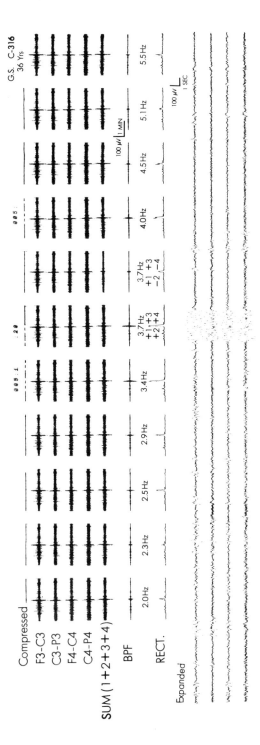

Fig. 1   Illustrates the tuning of the bandpass filter (BPF) and the addition and subtraction of channels to optimise the detection of a 3 per sec spike-and-wave discharge of a particular patient. The BPF is then used to represent the time distribution of discharges over the entire 24 hour recording period

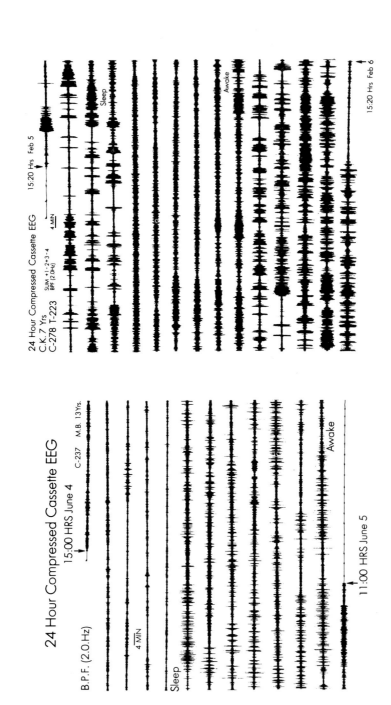

Fig. 2 (A and B) A 24 hour time distribution of slow 3 per sec spike-and-wave activity in two patients with Lennox-Gastaut syndrome

tice, this would be a 2 pass operation, the 1st to digitize and store the entire 24-hour EEG and the 2nd to analyse the record for specific or general events.

Another practical problem is to balance replay time and analysis time against playback speed and digitizing (or memory/tape/disc access time) throughput rate (Table 3). Computer time is so expensive that the faster the better; however, there are physical limitations that must be taken into consideration.

TABLE 3

4 channels of EEG
200 samples per second per channel
8 bit resolution

Playback Speed	Throughput rate (Bytes/sec)	Replay Time	
x 1	0.8 K	24	hrs.
x 2	1.6 K	12	hrs
x 4	3.2 K	6	hrs.
x 8	6.4 K	3	hrs.
x 16	12.8 K	1.5	hrs.
x 32	25.6 K	45	mins.
x 64	51.2 K	22.5	mins.
x128	102.4 K	11.25	mins.

At present using a PDP-11/60 mini computer system with software programmes, adapted from the 16-channel cable-telemetry data acquisition and analysis programmes (6, 7), a replay at x16 can be used to digitize about 8 hours of 4 channels of EEG onto digital tape. This tape can then be analysed for epileptic spikes and sharp waves and provide a time distribution of the spikes as affected by medication, seizures, sleep/awake states or stress conditions.

References

1. Ives J.R. and Woods, J.F. (1980). In Clinical Ambulatory Monitoring, Ed. by W.A. Littler, Chapman & Hall, London, 122-147.
2. Morris J.R.W. and Simpson A.F. (1980) In: Clinical Ambulatory Monitoring, Ed. by W.A. Littler, Chapman & Hall, London, 1-26.
3. Ives J.R. (1976) Postgrad. Med. J., **52**, (Suppl. 7), 86-91.
4. Stores G., Hennion T. and Quy, R.J. (1980) In: Advances in Epileptology: The Xth Epilepsy International Symposium. Ed. by J.A. Wada and J.K. Penry, Raven Press, New York, 89-93.
5. Quy R.J., Fitch P., Willison R.G. and Gilliatt R.W. (1980). In: Advances in Epileptology: Xth Epilepsy International Symposium, Ed J.A.Wada and J.K. Penry, Raven Press, New York, 69-72.
6. Ives J.R., Thompson C.J. and Gloor P. (1976) Electroenceph. Clin. Neurophysiol., **41**, 422-427.
7. Gotman J., Ives J.R. and Gloor P. (1979) Electroenceph. Clin. Neurophysiol., **46**, 510-520.

Discussion

MR. CROSBY: What were Mr. Ives' computer algorithms for the recognition of spikes?   Is this correlation match-filtering, or something like that?

Secondly, has he done any work on power spectral density displays of these data to aid data reduction?

MR. IVES: We have done no spectral analysis of these data, although the capability to do it is available.   We have used it only on patients with tumours several years ago.   It has not been found useful on temporal lobe patient groups, so it is not done.

With regard to the error rate of detection of spikes, it is probably best to refer to the several publications by Dr. Jean Gotman, in which this has been closely correlated with conventional traditional EEG's...

MR CROSBY: What algorithm is used? Is it match-filtering or something else?

MR. IVES: It is the detection of slope and duration.

THE ROLE OF PROLONGED AMBULATORY MONITORING IN THE DIAGNOSIS OF NON EPILEPTIC FITS IN A POPULATION OF PATIENTS WITH EPILEPSY

JOLYON OXLEY AND MARGARET ROBERTS

Chalfont Centre for Epilepsy, Chalfont St. Peter, Bucks, U.K.

Introduction

Some 120 people are admitted to the Chalfont Centre for Epilepsy each year for assessment. Over the last several years, about 10% of those admitted were considered to be displaying non-epileptic fits. Their fits were deemed to be non-epileptic on the evidence of direct clinical observation. The term "non-epileptic" is preferred instead of hysterical or simulated in order to avoid any pejorative overtones. The other causes of epileptiform fits (e.g. cardiac and metabolic) had been excluded.

The limitations of routine 20-minute EEG recordings in the differential diagnosis of paroxysmal attacks are well known. The advent of techniques for prolonged EEG monitoring should, therefore, significantly enhance clinical diagnostic accuracy. 8/16 channel EEG telemetry and video monitoring have been used successfully in this differential diagnosis (1 and 2). An alternative system for prolonged EEG monitoring has been described by Ives (3) and Stores (4) which permits ambulatory recording of four channels of EEG onto tape cassette and rapid data analysis. The system is less expensive than video telemetry, allows the subject complete freedom of movement and continuous recording for long periods is quite feasible.

The chief limitation of this technique in diagnosis would appear to be the restriction of the EEG signal to only four channels and the lack of simultaneous visual record of the attacks. Before employing four-channel EEG monitoring as a routine diagnostic aid to conventional clincal observation, it was considered essential to validate the EEG data produced by this technique in a controlled study. This entailed comparing the data obtained in a group of subjects who displayed clinically definite epileptic fits, with that obtained from a group, who were felt to display non epileptic fits.

Subjects and Methods

18 subjects have been assessed so far. All subjects had previously been diagnosed as suffering from epilepsy and were taking conventional anti-epileptic drugs, often in combination. All subjects, nevertheless, continued to have fits and they were admitted to the Chalfont Centre for Epilepsy for assessment.

Subjects were assigned to one of three clinical groups depending upon the assessment of their fits by members of the nursing staff at the Centre.

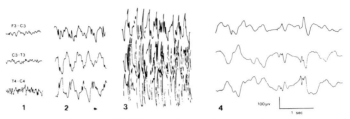

Fig. 1   Subject A (Group I) Three channel recorder used. 1. back-
          ground. 2. spike-and-wave. 3. EEG discharge and movement
          artefact characteristic of a tonic/clonic fit. 4. postictal
          slowing.

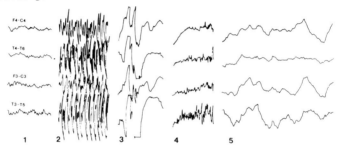

Fig. 2   Subject B (Group II) 1. background. 2. EEG discharge and
          movement artefact. 3. -5 post ictal changes.

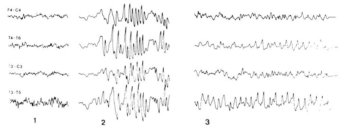

Fig. 3   Subject F (Group I) 1. background. 2. polyspike burst
          associated with clinical fit. 3. post ictal.

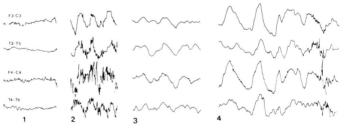

Fig. 4   Subject Q (Group I) 1. background. 2. artefact associated
          with tonic phase. 3. slow wave activity. 4. slow wave
          and movement artefact.

Group   I   Epileptic fits only (EP) 9 subjects - 5 male,
                   4 female
Group   II   Both epileptic and non-epileptic fits (MIXED)
                   2 subjects - 1 male, 1 female.
Group III   Non-epileptic fits only (NON EP) 7 subjects -
                   2 male, 5 female.

4-CHANNEL TAPED EEG - recordings were made for periods during which
subjects had at least one fit. The majority of subjects were recorded for 24 hours, but a few for much longer periods (up to 216
hours). The Oxford Medical Systems (OMS) Medilog-4 cassette recorder, standard C120 cassette tapes, silver electrodes and on-head preamplifiers (OMS HDX-82) (5) were used to record the EEG. A standardised electrode placement was used in most cases (F4-C4, T4-T6, F3-C3,
T3-T5). An event marker facility is provided by means of a button
attached to the recorder which produced a characteristic signal on
Channel 4 (Figure 5). The tapes were analysed visually on the Page
Mode Display, a speed of 20 x real time being found most satisfactory. Relevant sections were transcribed onto paper and the recordings coded for further analysis, which was made blind. Clinical
descriptions were noted for the recorded fits and their occurrence
noted on the tape using the event marker. Subjects remained at the
Centre for the duration of the recording, but their movements were
not restricted and they were thus not under continuous close observation. Only fits for which EEG data and clinical descriptions are
available have been used in the analysis.

Results

The results of all assessments are summarised in Table 1. Details of
the EEG findings and fit descriptions are given in Table 2.A total of
57 fits (23 EP and 34 NON-EP) have been recorded, at least one per
subject (Median 3, range 1-9).
    Some of the EEG findings in Group I are illustrated in Figures
1-4. These abnormalities were detected at the time of clinical fits.
7/9 subjects demonstrated fit-related epileptic activity. In 2 subjects (M & R) epileptic activity was seen throughout the record but
there was no significant change at the time of the fit. (Figures 5 &
6) and only one (Subject W) showed any epileptic activity which
occurred during sleep (Figure 7). The EEG findings in Group II
(MIXED) correspond exactly with the clinical assessment of the fits.

Discussion

Fit related epileptic activity was seen in 21/23 clinical EP fits
recorded. The EEG changes detected by the four channel recorder
were quite clear and largely free from obscuring artefact (See Figures 1-4). The apparent failure of two of the clinical EP fits
(subjects M & R) to produce fit-related epileptic activity may have
been due to inaccurate timing and marking of the fit with the event
marker, or the subjects may have been originally mis-diagnosed on
clinical grounds. However, it was notable that the recordings in
both subjects showed epileptic activity at other times which did not
produce clinical fits. These subjects require further study. Move-

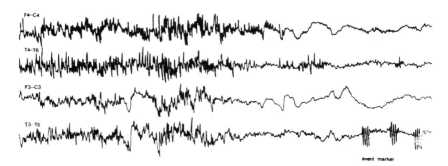

Fig. 5   Subject K (Group III) movement artefact (cf. Figs. 1 & 2)
            but no post ictal changes. Note three event market
            'blips' on Channel 4. These are produced by a non-
            standard attachment fitted to the recorder.

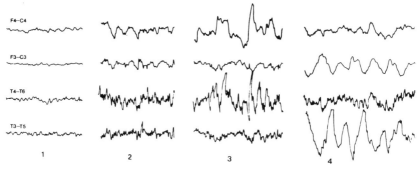

Fig. 6   Subject V (Group III) 1. background. 2.- 4. various forms
            of movement artefact. The 'slow waves in 4. are seen only
            in the left leads and are due to head moement.

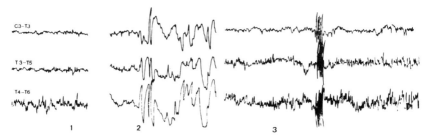

Fig. 7   Subject W (Group III) Three channel recorder used.
            1. background. 2. epileptic activity seen during sleep.
            3. no abnormality at time of clinical fit. The event
            marks were produced by an earlier marking system which
            superimposes a tone burst onto all data channels.

Table 1

Summary of Results of Assessments

Subject	Clinical Diagnosis	Fits Recorded	Taped EEG
Group I			
A	EP	3	F.R.E.A.
C	EP	2	F.R.E.A.
F	EP	3	F.R.E.A.
J	EP	1	F.R.E.A.
M	EP	1	E.A.
N	EP	1	F.R.E.A.
P	EP	3	F.R.E.A.
Q	EP	5	F.R.E.A.
R	EP	1	E.A.
Group II			
B	MIXED	* NON-EP 2	N.A.
		EP 2	F.R.E.A.
E	MIXED	NON-EP 3	N.A.
		NON-EP 2	E.A.
		EP I	F.R.E.A.
Group III			
D	NON-EP	2	N.A.
G	NON-EP	7	N.A.
K	NON-EP	1	N.A.
L	NON-EP	2	N.A.
S	NON-EP	3	N.A.
V	NON-EP	9	N.A.
W	NON-EP	3	E.A.

KEY: N.A. - no abnormality
         E.A. - epileptic activity
  F.R.E.A. - fit related epileptic activity
       * - based on clinical diagnosis.

bent and chewing artefact are relatively easy to recognise and if
doubt arises this can usually be resolved by reference to the clinical description. Thirty-one NON-EP fits have been recorded and none
of these produced significant changes in the recorded EEG.
    This technique may be of particular value in differentiating EP
from NON-EP fits in patients who display both types. In Group II,
the clinical diagnosis of the fits corresponded exactly with the EEG
findings.   Subject B (Group II) was considered to have a personality
disorder and his fits had previously been considered to be non-
epileptic on clinical grounds only. All anti-epileptic drugs had

Table 2

Fit Types and EEG Findings

Subject	Fit Description	Resting EEG	Taped EEG
Group I			
A	Tonic/clonic	s.w., s. & ps.	Movt.art.,p/i slow
C	Tonic, semi-purposive	s.w. & s.	Movt.art.,p/i slow
F	vacant, semi-purposive movements, confusion	s.w., sh. & s	Parox.s., ps.& s.w.
J	Tonic/clonic	s. & s.w.	Movt.art., p/i slow
M	Tonic/atonic	sh. & s.w.	Sh.& s.w.unrelated to fit
N	Wild semi-purposive movements with incontinence	s.w. & s.	Parox. s.w. & s.
P	Vacant semi-purposive movements	R slow focus	Parox. slow
Q	Tonic/atonic	bitemp. slow	Parox. slow
R	Cry, semi-purposive movements, may fall	gen. s.w.	S.w.unrelated to fit
Group II			
B	(i) Various often not witnessed	Bilat. slow	No abnormality
	(ii)Tonic/clonic	" "	Movt.art.,p/i slow
E	(i) Generalised shaking	Asymmetry	No abnormality/ sh. & s.w.*
	(ii) Tonic/clonic	"	Movt.art.,p/i slow
Group III			
D	Cry, stiffens with various movements	Occas. slow	No abnormality
G	Generalized shaking ± confusion	L temp. slow	No abnormality
K	Falls with mild movements	Occas. slow	No abnormality
L	Stiffens, various movements	Bitemp. slow	No abnormality
S	Jerking of limbs, falls	Occas. slow	No abnormality
V	Wild movements of limbs	L slow	No abnormality
W	Thrashing movements of limbs and trunk	Slow waves and spikes	s.w. & s. in sleep not related to fits

KEY: Movt.art. = movement artefact,
      s   = spike,
      sh.   = sharp,
      s.w.   = slow wave,
      p/i   = post ictal,
      p/s   = polyspike
      *   = 2 recordings on different days.

been withdrawn, which had no adverse effect on his fit frequency, and he was discharged from the Centre. However, after one year, readmission was sought because his fits were said to be more severe and of a different type. Prolonged EEG monitoring was undertaken (9 days) during which he had a number of his usual fits without abnormalities on the recorded EEG. On Day 9, he had a clinical tonic/clonic fit with appropriate EEG changes (Figure 2).

The absence of EEG changes in the clinical NON-EP group cannot be taken as being conclusive proof that this diagnosis is correct. Doubt has been expressed about such negative findings with only four channels of EEG data. Certainly localised EEG changes might well be missed, but it should be noted that all subjects in Group III were displaying fits which, if epileptic, would be of a generalized type and be expected to produce the kinds of changes seen in Group I. Other means of assessment, such as psychiatric evaluation and neuro-endocrine changes (6), should be used in conjunction with EEG and clinical findings to formulate a final diagnosis.

A further validation of this technique will derive from the clinical outcome in the patients with NON-EP fits. Preliminary results in 13 such patients (including the 7 reported above) suggest that AED can be safely withdrawn, and that striking improvements are sometimes seen not only in fit frequency but also in psychological well-being.

At this preliminary stage, 4-channel EEG taped monitoring would appear to give satisfactory results in the diagnosis of non-epileptic fits in the population of patients admitted to the Chalfont Centre.

It would appear advisable for a number of criteria to be satisfied:
1. The fits under study should be of a generalised kind.
2. The fits should be reasonably frequent - preferably several per week - although long recordings are quite possible.
3. Continuous expert observation is desirable, although probably not essential.
4. Various activities of the subjects should be noted during the recording: e.g. eating, sleeping, washing.
5. Other diagnostic criteria should be employed to achieve a final diagnosis.

Acknowledgement

We are indebted to Dr. Roger Quy of Oxford Medical Systems for expert technical assistance and to the Nursing Staff of the Chalfont Centre for their expert clinical observations.

References

1.   Bowden A.N., Fitch P., Gilliatt R.W.G., Willison R.G. (1975) The place of EEG telemetry and closed circuit television in the diagnosis and management of epileptic patients.
2.   Desai B.T., Porter R.J., Penry J.K. (1979) Neurology (Minneap.) 29, 602,
3.   Ives J.R. and Wood J.F. (1975) Clin. Neurophysiol. 39, 88-92.
4.   Stores G., Hennion T.S., Quy R.J. (1979) In: Proceedings of the 10th Epilepsy International Symposium. Ed: J.A. Wada and J.K. Penry. Raven Press. New York. 69-72.

5.   Quy R.J. (1978) J. Physiol (London) **284**, 23-24P.

6.   Oxley J., Roberts M., Dana-Haeri J., Trimble M. In: Advances
     in Epileptology. Ed: Dam M., Gram L. and Penry J.K.   Raven
     Press, New York (in press).

EVALUATION OF A SPIKE AND WAVE PROCESSOR FOR USE IN LONG-TERM AMBULATORY EEG MONITORING

C. BAILEY

Park Hospital for Children, Oxford, UK

Summary

This paper is an evaluation of a spike and wave processor developed by Oxford Medical Systems (O.M.S.) from a prototype system described by Quy (1).

The processor is designed to be used with Medilog system EEG recordings, replayed at 60 times real time. Its purpose is to detect the occurrence of spike and wave discharges in a selected EEG signal and quantify the total amount found in 15 minute epochs. A bar chart of the number of seconds of spike and wave activity per 15 minutes is produced.

The present paper is concerned with the reliability of the processor and sources of variability in the analysis procedure.

Method

Prior to performing each analysis, the processor was adjusted to suit each patient. This was carried out by varying the thresholds of operation of the spike detector and wave detector, both to suit he morphology of the spike and wave complexes of the patient, and to achieve the maximum discrimination against artefact.

A detector output is produced only when both the spike and wave components exceed their threshold levels.

Four 24-hour recordings of EEG made on the Medilog recorder were chosen, covering a wide range of types of spike and wave discharge.

Each of these four tapes was then, automatically, analysed by the O.M.S. processor on six different occasions.

After this each 24-hour record was written onto paper and a manual evaluation of the amount of spike and wave discharges present was carried out.

The results from these two operations were compared.

Results

Since each automatic analysis was repeated six times and re-adjustment of the processor was carried out each time, a range of results was obtained for each tape. Although each gave a very similar picture of the pattern of activity, the absolute amounts detected varied. In the following results, an average machine analysis was used.

The first tape analysed contained spike and wave activity, which could be described as 'classical' spike and wave. It was regular, well-organised, bilaterally synchronous and of approximately 3 Hz. Each burst had a well-defined start and finish. The comparison between manual and automatic analysis for this tape is shown in Figure

1. It can be seen that there is good agreement during the patient's waking hours, but an underestimation by the processor during sleep.

The second tape analysed contained bursts of spike and wave activity, which although still bilaterally synchronous, were less well-organised than in the previous case, of less well-defined onset and finish, and with some polyspikes.

As can be seen in Figure 2, the agreement between manual and automatic analysis is good during waking hours, but night-time activity is underestimated. As there is less overall activity, the underestimation is small.

In the third patient, the spike and wave activity was fragmented, poorly defined and not equally distributed on all channels. In this case (Figure 3), the analyser, while providing a reasonably representative picture of the overall pattern of activity, underestimates the amount of activity in both the sleep and awake states.

In the last patient, the spike and wave discharges are of low frequency, very irregular, poorly developed, fragmented and not easily distinguishable from background activity. As can be seen in Figure 4, the agreement between automatic and manual analysis is poor. Throughout the day, there is erroneous detection of spike and wave activity, although during sleep the correlation is good.

Discussion

The sources of variability in the results obtained appear to fall into the following groups:
    (1)   Adjustment of the analyser for each tape
    (2)   Sleep
    (3)   Artefact
    (4)   Low amplitude spike and wave activity, which merges with background.

1.   Analyser adjustments.

These analyses were all performed by one operator, and a range of results was obtained for each patient. When other operators with less experience were asked to set up and analyse a tape the range of results was even wider.

2   Sleep

Most variation between manual and automatic analysis occurred during sleep. Even in patients whose daytime spike and wave activity is of the 'classical' type, sleeping spike and wave activity is often slow, poorly defined, has polyspikes and is very fragmented, often into single spike and wave complexes. Where single spike and wave complexes occur, the design limits of the processor cause them to be undetected. If the spike and wave complexes are grouped together in an irregular burst, they are correctly detected.

The result of this is that many seconds of spike and wave activity are undetected by the processor during sleep, accounting for the difference between manual and automatic analysis already noted.

3.   Artefact

Here, a combination of waves of the appropriate frequency (2-4

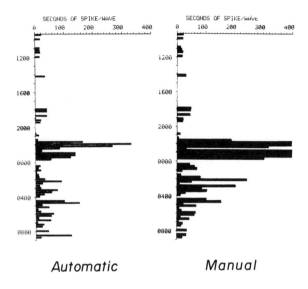

Fig. 1   Comparison of automatic with manual analysis — first tape.

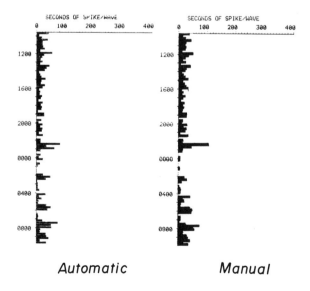

Fig. 2   Comparison of automatic with manual analysis — second tape.

BAILEY

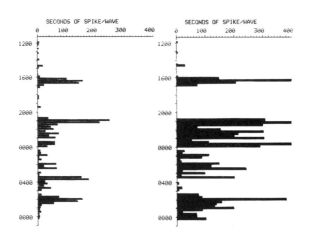

Automatic   *Manual*

Fig. 3   Comparison of automatic with manual analysis – third tape.

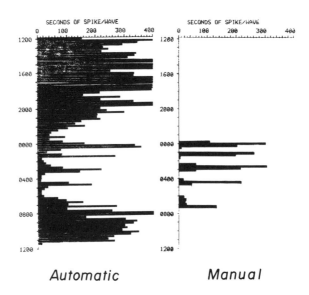

Automatic   *Manual*

Fig. 4   Comparison of automatic with manual analysis – fourth tape.

Hz) and superimposed spikes caused by muscle activity, for example chewing or scratching, cause a false detection of spike and wave activity by the processor. It was nearly always possible by appropriate adjustment of the processor to reduce this problem considerably. In practice, it only occurred when the setting up procedure had been performed carelessly, or had proved impossible to perform correctly, as in the case of the fourth problem area - low amplitude spike and wave activity, which merges with the background.

4. Low amplitude activity

In the fourth tape studied, the spike and wave activity, which only occurred during sleep, was of very low amplitude and difficult to distinguish from background activity. It did prove possible to detect this activity by appropriate adjustment of the processor, but in order to do so, the criteria for acceptance of waves and spikes became so wide that much normal EEG activity was recorded as spike and wave. This accounts for the large over-detection ofday-time activity in patient R.N.(Figure 4).

A comparable, though simpler, system to the one described here, has been evaluated by De Vries et al (2), with apparently good results, but it is important to note that in that study, patients were especially selected for the unequivocal nature of their spike-wave discharges, only portions of each patient's EEG recordings were used, mealtimes were specifically excluded from the study to minimise artefactual effects, and only 20% of the recordings were taken during sleep.

Conclusion

In spite of the problems outlined here, the Oxford Medical Systems processor produced an accurate account of the spike and wave activity occurring over a 24-hour period in tapes of the first three types discussed. Examination of records shows at least 60% of patients with generalized seizure activity at the Park Hospital EEG Department, Oxford, come into these categories, and for these patients, the processor can provide an objective account of the spike and wave activity occurring over a 24-hour period, which can be of considerable clinical value and which is not readily obtainable by any other means.

Acknowledgements

This work was supported by a grant from Ciba-Geigy Pharmaceuticals (UK) Ltd.

References

1.   Quy R.J., Fitch P. and Willison R.G. (1980) Electroenceph. & Cl. Neurophys. 49, 187-189.
2.   De Vries J., Wiseman T. and Binnie, C.D. (1981) Electroenceph. and Cl. Neurophys. 51, 328-330.

EVALUATION OF INTENSIVE EEG AND VIDEO MONITORING IN EPILEPSY

J.H.P.AARTS,* P.T.E.VAN BENTUM-DE BOER,* C.D. BINNIE,*
P.W.M. VAN DE GEEST,* A. KAMP,** F. LOPES DA SILVA,***
J. OVERWEG,* J.A.P.VAN PARYS,* A. VANWIERINGEN,*
A.J.WILKINS,****

*Instituut voor Epilepsiebestrijding Meer en Bosch, Heemstede,
** Medical Physics Institute TNO, Utrecht, ***Dierfysiologisch
Instituut, Universiteit Amsterdam, The Netherlands,
**** Medical Research Council Applied Psychology Unit,
Cambridge, UK

Summary

For those clinical problems most often requiring EEG monitoring of
patients with epilepsy, cable-telemetry appears the most appropriate
technology. A review of 178 consecutive monitoring studies showed
that some 80% of recordings yielded clinically useful information,
influencing treatment in approximately 2/3.

Introduction

Monitoring is increasingly used for the study of epilepsy, both for
research and for routine clinical purposes. Various technologies
have been employed. Valuable work has been done with conventional
hard-wired EEG machines (1); though the patient is severely
restricted in the range and nature of his activities, this appears to
be tolerable for up to 24 hours. Radio-telemetry gives good mobility
out-of-doors, but reception is often poor within hospital buildings,
bandwidth and channel capacity are limited to varying degrees by
telecommunication regulations of different countries (2) and the
apparatus is often so heavy as to restrict significantly the movement
of the patient. Cable-telemetry (3, 4, 5) is in our view the most
satisfactory solution for use in a hospital environment. In practice
the cable restricts mobility less than does the need for observation
or video-recording. The available bandwidth and channel capacity
are adequate even for depth electrode studies. Finally, miniaturized cassette recorders (6) allow great freedom of movement and
permit investigation of the patient in his natural environment and
during a wide range of activities. The price to be paid in terms of
limited bandwidth and channel capacity is, however, unacceptable for
many applications.
A technology looking for an application is unfortunately a
common phenomen in biomedical engineering and ideally the applications should determine the technology.

Applications of Monitoring in Epilepsy

The applications of EEG monitoring in epilepsy are summarized in
Table 1 which shows a breakdown of the clinical problems leading to

TABLE 1: Indications for monitoring and results: 161 consecutive patients June–December 1980.

PROBLEM	PATIENTS	REGISTRATIONS	QUESTION ANSWERED			CONSEQUENCE FOR TREATMENT		
			Yes	No	Additional Information	Yes	Minimal	No
Are Seizures Epileptic	67	73	39	34	24	34	1	38
Focus Localization	11	13	9	4	4	9	2	2
Seizure Incidence/ Evaluation Pharmacotherapy	43	48	46	2	21	40	4	4
Sensory-Precipitation/ Self Induction	35	39	38	1	5	38	0	1
Cognitive Impairment During Discharges?	7	7	6	1	2	1	3	3
Miscellaneous	11	11	11	0	3	3	1	3
	174	191	149 (78%)	42 (22%)	59 (30%)	131 (68%)	11 (6%)	49 (26%)

13 Patients & Registrations are common to 2 categories

Total Patients = 161

Total Registrations = 178

referral to our monitoring unit over a period of seven months.The pattern is similar to that found by others, notably Stalberg (7). The most common indication was differentiation between epileptic and non-epileptic attacks, a problem made the more difficult by the fact that psychogenic seizures arise most commonly in persons with epilepsy who may well have abnormal inter-ictal EEG's (8).

The attacks presenting diagnostic problems are, if epileptic, usually partial seizures. Ictal changes in the scalp EEG are often absent (9, 10, 11), or confined to a small region of the head. They may well be not recognizably epileptiform in nature, a reduction in amplitude or a change in frequency for instance (12, 13). From these considerations it follows that for this particular clinical application a high quality, multi-channel EEG is essential, preferably combined with reliable observation and video recording.. The supposition that the absence of spikes in a 3 or 4-channel recording during a seizure excludes an epileptic basis is demonstrably false and will probably result in over a third of complex partial seizures being misclassified as psychogenic.

The requirement for ictal registrations for purposes of locating a focus arises chiefly in patients being considered for neurosurgical intervention. For this application too, the maximum possible number of the recording channels is desirable and even a 16-channel system is arguably inadequate. The quantification of discharges in assessing the severity of epilepsy and responses to anti-epileptic drugs is self-explanatory, and is of course an application for which alternative systems particularly cassette recorders, may perhaps more conveniently be used.

As the main stress at this session is on monitoring EEG in a natural environment and during normal behaviour two applications in particular will be discussed.

The first is investigation of self-induced epileptic seizures. Until recently, these were regarded as very rare, typically found in photosensitive, mentally subnormal patients, who elicit attacks by gazing at the sun or at a bright light and waving one hand in front of the eyes (14). Attacks may also be induced by eye-closure. However, a direct consequence of our monitoring studies, was the discovery that this phenomenon is quite common and occurs in approximately a quarter of photosensitive epilepeptic patients, usually of normal intelligence, mostly by means of eye-closure (15). Self-induction may be suspected when a patient with photosensitive epilepsy exhibits repeated eye-closures of about one second's duration with forced upward deviation of the eyes, possibly associated with grimacing, smiling and touching or concealing the face. The movements are slower than blinks or the eyelid flutter of absence attacks. Overt seizures which may be induced are typically absences, occasionally a partial or tonic-clinic attack. The incidence of eye-closures increases under stress and in a well-lit environment and decreases in darkness. Self-induction will rarely be recognized under the conditions of a routine recording with the patient lying in bed with eyes shut or gazing at the ceiling. To establish the diagnosis one must monitor the EEG usually for several hours, with the patient engaged in normal activities in a well-lit room. If necessary the effects of mild stress (interview with doctor) and of darkening the environment may be tested. We now routinely monitor all new photosensitive

patients and find self-induction in a third. Self-induced epilepsy
is usually resistent to conventional therapy with anti-epileptic
drugs and effective treatment (16) requires that the condition first
be recognized.

Many investigations have shown that during generalized spike-
wave discharges, even in the absence of overt seizures, transitory
cognitive impairment (TCI) may often be demonstrated by appropriate
psychological tests (17, 18, 19; see Binnie (20) for review).

It is, therefore, of obvious importance for the management and
counselling of any person with "subclinical" spike-wave discharges to
determine whether or not these are accompanied by TCI. Unfortunately, the techniques employed for research studies are not generally
appropriate for such routine clinical investigations. Patients are
prepared to work at, for instance, continuous performance tasks for
only a few minutes and during this time, there may be insufficient
discharges to allow any adequate assessment, particularly if the
incidence of epileptiform activity is reduced by tension.

In view of these considerations, we were reluctant to undertake
monitoring studies for recognition of TCI. However, recently we have
developed tests which appear suitable. A task for detecting cognitive impairment in routine clinical EEG practice must meet the
following criteria:
1.   Epileptiform activity must not be suppressed by the test
itself. This is determined by arousal level, rate of data
transmission and intensity of the stimulus.
2.   The task must be acceptable even to poorly motivated patients,
for administration over a period of at least half-an-hour.
3.   Testing should be continuous as random stimuli may fall between
the discharges.
4.   Task difficulty must be adaptive to individual performance
levels.
5.   The task must have face validity demonstrating cognitive defic-
its of practical consequence.

Various tasks have been developed to meet these requirements;
all are presented in the form of video-games. The most successful so
far is a short-term memory task, essentially an automated version of
the Corsi blocks test. The patient is confronted with a TV display
of 7 blocks, which flash in a random sequence and he is then required
to reproduce the sequence by means of a light pen.

The length of the sequence is adaptive to the patient's level of
performance. Motivation and interest are enhanced by the use of
colour and sound effects; correct reproduction of the sequence causes
the apparatus to play a tune. Subjects from 7 years upwards whether
performing at a high or a low level will readily play the game for
half an hour or longer and are often reluctant to stop. An output to
the EEG machine is provided indicating the stimulus presentations and
correct or erroneous responses. The task suppresses epileptiform
activity little in most subjects and enhances it in a few. It has
demonstrated transitory cognitive impairment at a high level of stat-
stical significance in subjects where this was not suspected and conversely shown others to be unimpaired during generalized spike-wave
discharges of several seconds' duration. Our preliminary results
suggest that discharges during stimulus presentation are more disrup-
tive of performance than those occurring during the response.

Evaluation of Results

We first attempted to evaluate this clinical monitoring service by
the rather crude criterion of ability to answer the questions of the
referring physicians (21). Our overall success rate on 181 records
during 1978-1979 was 57% and on 178 in the last 7 months of 1980
(Table 1) was some 78% It is considerably higher where the nature of
the question (determination of seizure frequency for instance) is
such that an answer can almost always be provided. When the investigation requires the occurrence of particular clinical phenomena, as
in the case of seizure registrations, success depends largely on
perseverance, patient selection and recording under optimal conditions, for instance during a cluster of seizures in a patient whose
attacks occur in groups.

We are now carrying out a follow-up study in order to assess
this service by the more stringent criterion of its influence on
subsequent patient management. Our preliminary results suggest that
two-thirds of registrations materially influenced patient management, albeit sometimes in the negative sense that a proposed change
was shown to be unnecessary. At 2 months follow-up, clinical decisions based on monitoring appeared to have favourably influenced
patient care in 30%.

Acknowledgements

This work was supported by grants from the epilepsy research fund
"De Macht van het Kleine" and the Commissie Landelijk Epilepsie
Onderzoek.

References

1. Escueta A.V., Kunze U., Waddell G. and Boxley J. (1977) Neuro-
    logy (Minneap.) **27**, 144-155.
2. Manson G. (1974) Neurophysiol. **37**, 411-413.
3. Ives J.R., Thompson C.J. and Gloor P. (1976) Electroencephalogr.
    Clin. Neujrophysiol. **41**, 422-427.
4. Saint-Hilaire J.M., Bouvier G., Lymburner J., Picard R. and
    Mercier M. (1976) Union Med. Can. **105**, 1538-1541.
5. Binnie C.D., Overweg J. and Rowan A.J. (1980) In: Lechner H. and
    Aranibar A. (Eds) Proceedings of the Second European Congress of
    Electroencephalography and Clinical Neurophysiology. Exerpta
    Medica: Amsterdam. 83-88.
6. Ives J.R. and Woods J.F. (1975) Electroencephalogr. Clin. Neuro-
    physiol. **39**, 88-92.
7. Stalberg E. (1976) In: Kellaway P. and Petersen I. (Eds) Quan-
    titative analytic studies in epilepsy. Raven Press: New York.
    269-278.
8. Roya A. (1979) Arch. Neurol. **36**, 447.
9. Geier S. (1971) Electroencephalogr. Clin. Neurophysiol.
    31, 499-507.
10. Lieb J.P., Walsh G.O. and Babb T.L. (1976) Epilepsia, **17**, 137-
    160.
11. Wieser H.G. (1979) Z.EEG-EMG, **10**, 197-206.

12. Neundoerfer B. and Fuchs U. (1970) Dtsch. Z. Nervenheilkd. **197**, 133-148.
13. Dreyer R. and Wehmeyer W. (1978) Arch. Psychiatr. Nervenkr. **225**, 263-264.
14. Andermann K., Oaks G., Berman S. et al (1962) Arch. Neurol. **6**, 49-65.
15. Binnie C.D., Darby C.E., de Korte R. and Wilkins A.J. (1980) J. Neurol. Neurosurg. Psychiat. **43**, 386-389.
16. Orweg J. and Binnie C.D. (1980) Acta Neurol. Scand. Suppl. **79**, 98.
17. Mirsky A.F. and van Buren J.M. (1965) Electroencephalogr. Clin. Neurophysiol. **18**, 334-348.
18. Tizzard B. and Margerison J.H. (1963) Br. J. Soc. Clin. Psychol. **3**, 6-15.
19. Hutt S.J. (1972) Epilepsia, **13** 520-534.
20. Binnie C.D. (1980) In: Kulig B.M. Meinardi H. and Stores G. (Eds.) Epilepsy ahd Behaviour 1979. Swets and Zeitlinger: Lisse. 91-97.
21. Binnie C.D., Rowan A.J. Overweg J. et al (1980) Neurology (Minneap.), **31**, 298-303.

Discussion

DR. STORES: I was very interested in Dr. Arrts' television-type tests. Is it possible to alter the level of test difficulty by altering the rate at which the display flashes?

DR. AARTS: There is a sequence of flashing blots, and every time that the patient gives the correct response another one appears. The rate therefore depends on the patient's own short-term memory.

DR. STORES: So it is self-paced? (Dr. Aarts agreed). I asked the question - as I am sure Dr. Aarts will know - because people like Hyatt suggest that cognitive impairment is not an all-or-none effect, but that it varies with the level of task difficulty from one subject to another.

MR. IVES: How long was the average recording time in each patient in order to establish that efficiency rate of 78%?

DR. AARTS: The average recording time was 24 hours, depending on the sort of question to be answered in individual patients. If the referring physician asked for seizure diagnosis and the patient had five seizures within two hours, the recording was of course shorter. When there was a blot study, for instance, it is mostly done in 48 hours - because of the test/retest stability.

DR. BINNIE: Clearly we are seeing a different population of patients from a number of other speakers today. Both the most appropriate technology and the success rate may therefore well be different. This seems to be fairly typical of the experience of other specialist epilepsy centres, in terms of proportions of various kinds of clinical problems. We have enough trouble in the interpretation of 16-channel EEGs, and I wonder how people manage with only three channels.

DR. STORES: The test about which I asked earlier seems to lend itself to the study of possible adverse effects on behaviour - on cognitive function - of antiepileptic drugs. Is that something Dr. Aarts or Dr. Binnie has in mind to do?

DR. BINNIE: It is something that is already being done, but not with this particular test. If we look at the literature of psychological tests for detecting the effects of antiepileptic drugs, the answer is that there is not any clear evidence on which to base a selection of tests. We have been using a complex reaction time and the Wrighton trail-making test so far, but we are going to do a prospective study in normal subjects taking antiepileptic drugs to try out a whole battery of tests to see which are the most appropriate for detecting intoxication.

DR. STORES: Will these be patients taking a single drug?

DR. BINNIE: In the first case, the studies on all the subjects will be, but already, on a purely ad hoc basis, the trail test and reaction time are being used as part of the whole monitoring package. All patients who have serial blood level measurements also have the psychological testing. In fact, those who develop obviously toxic levels do show impairment on the Wrighton trail test. It is sometimes helpful for interpreting borderline blood levels; the phenytoin level may go up to 24, but does that matter for the particular patient? If the Wrighton trail test time also increases, it probably does matter.

PANEL DISCUSSION

MR. IVES: If Ms.Bailey could get three other volunteers also to read the records, that would demonstrate that the machine is probably not too bad - this is in reference to a paper by Penry, in which he reported various electro-encephalographers of varying experience reading the same records and having a variation of about $\pm$ 20%. Taking herself as the truth, there is quite a variation in the way in which electro-encephalographers even interpret spike-and-wave records, particularly in sleep.

MS. BAILEY: I tried to show that there is some disagreement, that there is a lot of room for manoeuvre, in fact, in deciding on the length of a burst.

DR. HALL: Mr. Ives raised the worrying problem about the negative record. I wonder how naive we are in assuming, as did the people from Chalfont, that we are looking for big changes. Is Mr. Ives' comment mainly applied to complex partial seizures, and does he think that it is valid to assume that in the other seizures being described in Chalfont, the absence of major EEG changes means that epilepsy can be ruled out as the problem?

MR. IVES: Most of our experience is with the temporal lobe patients - it is really a matter of providing the statistics to see how they fit with the other type of epileptic patient.

DR. STORES: I am glad that we have returned to the topic of negative findings - I very much wanted to say something about it earlier, but did not have the opportunity. It is, of course, undeniable that some patients will have seizures which are shown to be seizures by means of depth electrodes, including sphenoidals, with nothing very much happening in the surface electrode recordings. There is inevitably, therefore, an element of diagnostic uncertainty with negative findings. It would certainly be quite impracticable for a service such as ours, to do sphenoidal recordings. I would be interested to know about other people's experience of trying to do them on a large scale with children. We have been deterred from it, except in an extremely small number of cases, who seem to be very good candidates for temporal lobectomy - then that procedure forms part of the assessment. Beyond that, I would be very hesitant to embark on sphenoidal recordings on children to any large extent. That maintains the diagnostic uncertainty, therefore - but I do not think it matters all that much, because it would be foolish to expect any diagnostic procedure to provide diagnostic certainty one way or another, except when there is consistently unequivocal seizure discharge at the time of an attack. If there is nothing going on, however, at the time of an attack in a scalp-recorded EEG, it simply adds to the probability that this is not epilepsy; it does not mean that it is definitely not epilepsy, but makes it less likely that it is. For the clinician, that is very useful information on which to proceed. He will then proceed by treating the patient as having something other than epilepsy, in the light of the sum-total of clinical information.

DR. OXLEY: It is right to asssume that iof there is nothing on the tape, that may not be an epileptic manifestion - but it does not mean to say that the patient does not have epilepsy. That is a different proposition - as the silent abnormalities show.

If we really think that these people do not have epilepsy, they should be taken off their anti-convulsant drugs. The problem is that it should never have happened in the first place - many of these people have been labelled as having epilepsy quite unreasonably. I did not discuss the clinical outcome because the study is on-going, but of the 13 patients we have so far decided do not have epilepsy. using the criteria that I showed (it was not only the one criterion of the EEG) most of them have been successfully taken off their anti-convulsants. Some of them are put on psychotropic drugs for one reason or another - but that is a different issue.

DR. SOUTHALL: With regard to the high heart rates that Dr. Blumhardt observes, what happens to the clock track, or is a clock signal recorded to be sure that the high heart rate that is observed is not artefact?

DR. BLUMHARDT: Yes, there is a time base - there is the great conflict about giving up my time base, throwing it away and using another channel EEG. This is one of the problems with the Medilog Mark 1. After the first 100 cases, I have come to the conclusion that is what I must do. I do not see how these could be artefacts, unless it was a tape drive problem...

(DR. SOUTHALL: That is what I was thinking")...If someone is lying quietly in bed with a base pulse rate of 67 - which then shoots up to 130 and he remains asleep without any movement, why should that be the result of the recorder? These pulse changes are well-documented experimentally in dogs and also in humans with induced temporal lobe seizures.

.DR. SOUTHALL: I do not question that. However, I still make the point that unless the clock is actually being observed to make sure that the time is recorded accurately, it cannot be said with certainty that the high heart rate is true. It may be due to tape speed variability. Everybody is nodding their head, but from my experience in the ECG, using the synclock system on the Medilog, if it is switched off, there are changes in heart rate, which are due to be tape speed variability which look exactly like those described by Dr. Blumhardt.

DR. BLUMHARDT: If that is so, I give up.

DR.IVES: If there is a speed change on the tape recorder, this will also show up in the EEG - there should be a speed change there too.

DR. RAMSAY: I shall show some examples this afternoon, of heart rate changes that were the result of changes in tape playback. The difference can be observed, usually by looking at the EEG. I agree completely with Dr. Ives.

24-HOURS-EEG ANALYSIS: ULTRADIAN PERIODICITIES OF SPIKE-WAVE PATTERNS

W. BURR AND H. STEFAN

Universitatsnervenklinik - Epileptologie 43-Bonn 1 (FRG)

Summary

Spike-wave (s-w) activity is one of the most easily comprehensible EEG correlates parametrizing epileptic excitability, at least as far as generalized epilepsies are concerned. In this study, a method is proposed to analyse the existence and qualities of a hypothetical ultradian periodicity. In absence-patients ambulatory 24-hour EEG monitoring is repeatedly performed before and during anti-epileptic drug therapy. The records are scored by a computer programme in order to evaluate the time-profile of s-w activity. The resulting chronograms are subjected to different chronobiological analysis methods: harmonic analysis and complex demodulation (CD). Periodicities changing in the course of the day turned out to be better represented by the CD approach. Before and during anti-epileptic treatment, two main components of ultradian periodicity are found in the region of 8 and 2 hours respectively.

Introduction

For a great number of epileptic patients, the time course in the occurrence of their seizure attacks seems not to have a random structure. For instance, there are special forms of rhythmicity, such as morpheic or matutinal and the catamenial epilepsy. Expressed in chronobiological terms, the former may be said to have a circadian periodicity, the latter an infradian. In patients with frequent epileptic attacks within one 24-hour period, the density of epileptic patterns can show a time course that gives rise to the hypothesis that there exists an underlying, ultradian cyclic variation of epileptic excitability (5, 8).

The aim of this methodological study is to find out an appropriate analytical method for detecting and describing this kind of ultradian periodicity, as far as it is reflected by electro-encephalographic findings.

Material and Method

In patients suffering from frequent absence attacks, a 4-channel EEG is recorded during 24 hours. Using a portable mini-recording system (Oxford 4-24), this can be done without reasonably disturbing the patient's behaviour. The 24-hour records are automatically analysed by means of an individually adjustable computer programme (1) for pattern recognition. An algorithm, comparing the configuration of subsequent minima and maxima of the EEG curve with a pre-defined

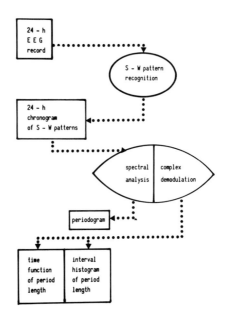

Fig. 1   Block diagram of chronobiological analysis.

parameter set, decides continuously about the occurrence of a spike-wave (S-W) pattern and causes the storage of a corresponding time code on magnetic disc. A subsequent computer runout of these disc-stored data, builds up a 24-hour chronogram of the density of S-W patterns with a sampling rate of 200s. According to previous studies (2, 3, 4), two different ways of chronobiological analysis were tested: The harmonic analysis (Fourier transformation, variance spectrum (6)), working in the frequency domain and the method of complex demodulation (CD) working in the time domain (7). In EEG analysis FFT has become rather well known, whereas the CD technique is less in use in spite of some of its advantages (9). (Figure 1). In the following section, the mechanism and some of the features of the CD approach are to be illustrated.

Complex demodulation

In Figure 2, the mathematical operations of CD are applied on a realistic S-W chronogram and the results are plotted stepwise: on the left hand, the functions in time, on the right hand - in order to have a better impression of the effect of the operations - the corresponding frequency representations. The original chronogram has been adapted to the FFT algorithm by trend removing, cosine tapering and adding zeros at the borders (A). Complex demodulation, strictly speaking means to multiply the (real) signal function by an unimodular complex function:

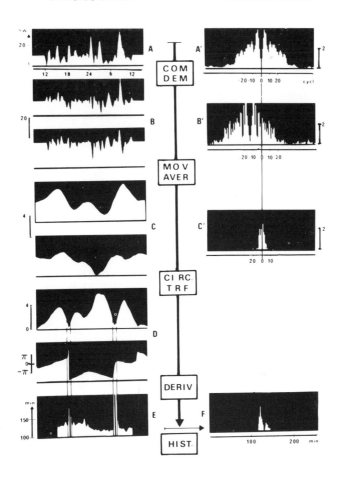

Fig. 2   Steps of analysis demonstrated in a realistic chronogram
            (left:time domain, right:frequency domain)
                CD frequency : $w_o = 14 * 2 \quad N$
                A - original chronogram
                B - chronogram after CD
                C - chronogram after CD + smoothing over.
                D - same as C expressed in circular co-ordinates
                    MO - modul,   PH = phase
                E - time course of period length
                F - histogram of period lengths (MO-weighted)

$$\bar{f}\,(t) = f\,(\,t\,) * \exp(-i\ \omega_o t) \qquad \text{(Com Dem)}$$

In the demodulated form, there is an easy way to perform a digital filtering: The moving average

$$\hat{f}\,(\,t_i\,) = \sum_{k=-n}^{k=n} \bar{f}\,(\,t_{i+k}) *g_k \qquad \text{(Mov Ave)}$$

(i.e. low pass filtering in demodulated form) is equivalent to band pass filtering in the original function (cf. spectral plots) with a centre frequency of ω_o . For the data shown in Figure 2, two successive iterations with a span of 60 data points were used. In order to allow a comparison between the original and the filtered signal the real part of the demodulated function is also plotted (Figure 3).

$$\bar{\hat{f}}\,(\,t\,) = \hat{f}\,(\,t\,) * \exp\,(=i\,\omega_o t)$$

As a next step in Figure 2, the complex function $\hat{f}$ (t) (C) is trans-formed into circular co-ordinates. Modul (MO) and phase angle (PH) reveal the amplitude and phase variation about the frequency ω_O. A constant slope in the phase plot is a direct measure for a rhythmicity inherent in the chronogram. An estimate of the time course of the corresponding period length is plotted in the lowest line of Figure 2. Obviously, this estimation is of less relevance at the signal borders (due to the averaging process) and in those re-gions where the modul gets too small. For compensation of this effect, the period-length histogram (F) is calculated by weighting each phase-slope value with the corresponding modul value.

Example of Application

Finally, to the previous example of Figure 2, the results of a later registration is to be added. For the same patient now, however, under anti-epileptic treatment (Carbamazepine), another 24-hour EEG was recorded and S-W paroxysms were automatically traced. In Figure 3, the results have been contrasted to the previous ones. In both cases, the periodogram reveals a lower and a higher frequency peak: 3-4 cycles (ca.8 hour) and 12-15 cycles (ca.115-140 min). In the later record (under drug application), S-W density seems to be atten-uated during the night. According to this phenomenon, the amount of lower frequency contribution gets more prominent compared to the higher component. In both cases, however, the CD technique reveals a change of the higher periodicity component in the middle of the night. To what extent these observations may contribute to the inves-tigation of epileptic mechanisms or the improvement of anti-epileptic treatment still remains a task for future studies.

25. 5.1979   1. 8.1979

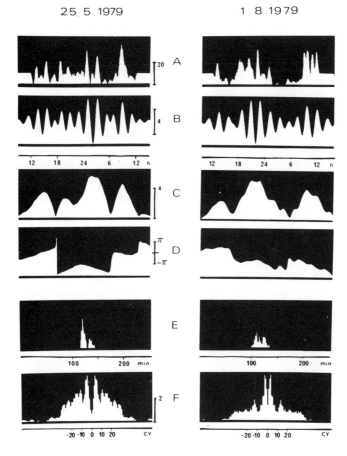

Fig. 3   S-W density function and chrono-analysis results for two
          registrations in the course of antiepileptic treatment
          (left: before tr. right: during tr.)
          A - original chronogram
          B - chronogram after remodulation
          C - modul
          D - phase
          E - histogram of period lengths
          F - periodogram

Conclusion

Comparing both approaches, we conclude as follows:
1. A rough idea which frequencies are involved is provided by the periodogram (FFT spectrum).
2. Some features, however, are not detectable in the spectrum, particularly those concerning phase relations. E.g.'an exact frequency in the data that undergoes a phase change of   radians midway through the record would contribute nothing to the frequency spectrum' (7).
3. In this example, by complex demodulation, this frequency would be easily detected, together with the phase change.
4. CD works with a higher resolution and results are a function of time. Actually this is an important aspect in our example, since it shows a dynamic structure of the ultradian periodicity in this case:
   In the middle of the night, a remarkable change in the slope of phase occurs which corresponds to a change of the period length from 135 minutes to 118 minutes.
5. As a restriction, however, it has to be pointed to the fact that the results of CD analysis depend rather sensitively on the choice of the filter parameters (centre frequency and bandwidth). Therefore, a combined use of both approaches seems favourable to us.

(Supported by Ministerium fur Wissenschaft und Forschung des Landes NordrheinWestfalen und Deutsche Forschungsgemeinschaft.)

References

1. Burr W. (1980). Z. EEG-EMG **11**, 135-141.
2. Burr W. and Lange H. (1977) Sleep Res. **6**, 141.
3. Burr W., Lange H. Penin H. and Vogt J. In: Sleep 1976 3rd Europe. Congr. Sleep Res., Eds: Koella W.P. and Levin P., Montpelier 1976. Karger, Baserl 1977, 474-478.
4. Burr W. Lange H., Platte M. and Strehmel D. In: Sleep 1978 4th Europ. Congr. Sleep Res. Eds: Asgian B. and Badiu B. Tirgu-Mures 1978 Karger, Basel 1980, 565-568.
5. Kripke D.F. (1974) In: Advances in Sleep Research. Ed: Weitzman E.D. Spectrum, New York, 305-325.
6. Kunkel H. (1969) Die Periodik der paroxysmalen Dysrhythmie im Elektro-enzephalogram. Thieme, Stuttgart, 1-80.
7. Orr W.C. and Hoffman H.J.K. (1974) IEEE Trans. Biomed Eng. BME **21**, 130-143.
8. Stevens J.R., Kodama HJ.,Lonsbury B. and Mills L. (1971) Electroenceph. clin. neurophysiol., **31**, 313-325.
9. Walter D.O. (1969) Electroenceph. clin. neurophysiol. Suppl. **27** 53-57.

Discussion

DR. BINNIE: Can Dr. Burr comment on the findings of Kellaway's group in the light of his own?   I think that Kellaway found a rather faster periodic process, with a period of 90 mins - but he also claimed two different periodic processes superimposed on each other.

DR. BURR: This is only one example, and it is a fact that periodicity is not found - or is not detectable - in by any means all patients.   I am sure that this cyclical variation is not directly dependent on sleep-waking.   I am not astonished therefore that there is a wide range of results.   I cannot make any further comment.

DR. CROSBY: Would Dr. Burr care to comment on the accuracy of determining the periodicity when there are only 12 or 15 cycles in one 24-hour period.

DR. BURR: I cannot give any level of significance of these results. It is similar to factor analysis of EEG frequency groups.   I could compare the results only with random data - and in random data the same level is not found, but no true level of significance can be given.   I think it is only a base on which to investigate whether with drug application, perhaps at a particular time of the day, there is any effect.

AMBULATORY MONITORING OF THE EEG IN THE ASSESSMENT OF ANTI-EPILEPTIC DRUGS

N. MILLIGAN* AND A. RICHENS**

*Institute of Neurology, Queen Square, London, WC1,
**Welsh National School of Medicine,
Heath Park, Cardiff, UK

Summary

Assessment of anti-epileptic drugs using prolonged ambulatory monitoring of the EEG is limited to patients with absences, where quantification of spike-wave activity provides a more objective index of seizure occurrence. However, long period of EEG registration create problems in data analysis and interpretation. The uses and limitations of this technique are discussed.

Introduction

Clinicians regard with suspicion changes in the EEG's of epileptic patients following medication as these often do not reflect an improvement in seizure control. Patients with absence seizures are a exception, however, as the frequency of absences closely parallels the amount of spike-wave (S-W) activity in the EEG. The EEG is potentially the most reliable tool for assessing response to medication although prolonged periods of EEG recording are necessary. Quantification of S-W activity provides a more objective assessment of seizure occurrence and serial recordings can be done to demonstrate an improvement with medication (1). Ambulatory monitoring of the EEG lends itself well to the assessment of patients with absences and enables long periods of EEG registration to be achieved with minimum patient restriction (2). Increasingly widespread use of this technique demands a critical appraisal of the information that is provided.

Data Collection Analysis and Interpretation

Prolonged recording of the EEG requires a system of automated analysis if the large quantities of EEG data are to be analysed rapidly. We have had experience with a technique for monitoring S-W activity using ambulatory taped EEG recordings and computerised analysis developed by Quy (3). The EEG is recorded using head-mounted preamplifiers and a four-channel cassette tape recorder (Oxford Medical Systems Medilog Recorder). The EEG recordings are replayed at sixty times real time with S-W activity being quantified by an analogue detection system. Arbitrary thresholds are pre-set for both spike and wave components independently so that the occurrence of a paroxysmal discharge will result in simultaneous opening of both spike and wave gates and detection by the computer. Spike and wave detector thresholds are set according to the individual morphology of the

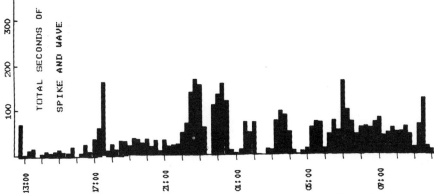

Fig. 1   Computer printout showing distribution of S–W activity   over
         a 24 hr period beginning at 12.45 in an epileptic   patient
         who showed frequent paroxysms of atypical S–W   activity in
         his EEG. Each bar represents the number of seconds of S–W
         activity in 15 mins. Total S–W = 4262   seconds in 24 hrs.
         Note the cyclical pattern of epileptic   discharges during
         sleep (22:00–06:00), each cycle lasting 1.25 hrs. This
         amounted to 40% of the total S–W activity   recorded. (Re-
         produced from (7) with permission).

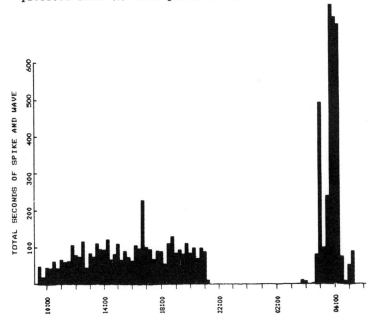

Fig. 2   Computer printout on a 24 hr EEG recording where nocturnal
         discharges (22:00–05:00) were phased out . Note the ex-
         cess of S–W activity after 05.00 hrs in relation to wake-
         fulness.   Total S–W = 5123 seconds in 24 hrs.

paroxysmal discharge relative to the amount and type of artefact. Bar charts of S-W activity over a 24-hour period are automatically plotted by micro-computer and dot matrix printer. The result is a histogram showing the amount and distribution of S-W activity in 15 min. epochs over 24-hours. (Figure 1). The site for electrode placement is determined from the resting EEG. Complete technical details are reported elsewhere (4).

The reliability of this system depends on the "cleanness" of the recordings. Movement artefact can be reduced by using head-mounted preamplifiers (5) but other types of artefact are more of a problem. The electromyographic artefact from chewing bears a superficial morphological resemblance to S-W activity having both spike and slow wave components (Figure 3). Detection of this artefact can be minimised only by siting electrodes away from the temporalis muscles. Whether or not this is feasible depends on how clearly defined the paroxysms are at other sites.

In addition to artefactual difficulties, automatic analysis of the 24-hour EEG introduces problems in data interpretation from physiological variations in epileptic activity. Many patients have

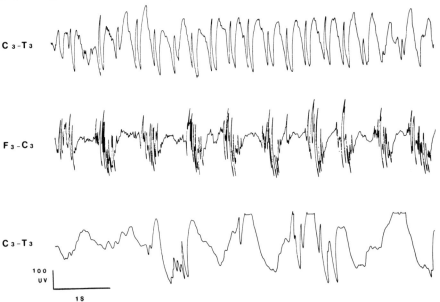

Fig. 3   EEG samples from a patient with frequent absences illustrating:
a)   well defined paroxysmal S-W activity
b)   high amplitude chewing artefact which hears a superficial resemblence to (a) having both spike and slow wave components.
c)   sleep record showing large amplitude slow waves with irregular high voltage spike potentials. These exhibit a periodicity throughout the night in relation to different stages of sleep, being suppressed during REM periods and enhanced during deep slow wave sleep.

an excess of S-W discharges during sleep. These bear little morphological resemblance to diurnal S-W activity (Figure 3) and are
closely related to slow wave sleep with relative suppression during
REM periods. Whether this activity should be included in the clinical
assessment of patients is debatable and raises a philosophical point
as it could be argued that patients do not have absences during
sleep. Moreover, Figure 1 clearly shows that nocturnal epileptic
discharges exhibit a cyclical pattern throughout the night, in this
case S-W activity between 10.0 p.m. and 6.0 a.m. amounting to 40% of
the total recorded. True ictal activity does not demonstrate such
periodicity. In other subjects, it is possible to "phase out" activity recording during sleep if the discharges are of low amplitude and
sufficiently non-rhythmic to pass undetected by the computer. Figure
2 shows the computer print-out of such a patient, who also exhibits
an increase in seizure incidence in relation to wakefulness, an
occurrence common to many patients with absence seizures (6). However, in view of the uncertain significance of nocturnal discharge,
S-W activity recording during sleep should be excluded from calculations when using this system in assessing a clinical response t
medication. This can easily be done by reference to the numerical
computer print out listing the number of seconds of S-W activity in
each 15 minute epoch. As it is not possible to judge the exact onset
of sleep from the computer print-out, however, calculations or
recordings should be made over a fixed number of hours of wakefulness. Ideally, this should include the early morning if excessive
S-W activity on waking is not to be overlooked and from a practical
viewpoint subjects should refrain from sleeping during the day.

Evaluation of the System

The results of the analysis of recordings from a thirteen-year old
girl, who demonstrated both a clinical and electro-encephalographic
response to sodium valproate are summarised in Table 1.
     48-hour ambulatory taped EEG recordings were made in the home
environment, each recording being analysed first automatically, and
then manually, by writing the tape out on paper and counting the S-W
paroxysms by eye. Calculations of S-W activity were made over 12
hours of wakefulness per 24-hours' recording. S-W activity was progressively reduced with successive increments in dosage, there being
little difference between a divided dosage and monodosage regime.
Overall, the performance of the automatic recognition system was
impressive. Correlation between the two methods of assessment was
high (r = 0.98) although the agreement between individual analyses
showed considerable variation. This may be acceptable, however, as
the value of a percentage difference is directly related to the total
amount of activity recorded, tapes containing very little S-W activity tending to indicate larger percentage errors even when the
actual difference (in seconds) between the two methods is slight.
     It sometimes proved exceedingly time-consuming analysing automa-
tically tapes containing a minimum of S-W activity. The time required to locate discharges, setting of detector thresholds and
checking and re-checking detection, or otherwise of artefact was
often very much greater than scanning the recordings once by eye and
playing parox-ysms out on paper as and when they arose. The use of

MILLIGAN AND RICHENS

Table 1

Total Amount of S-W Activity (in seconds) in the Period
(8.0 a.m.-8.0p.m.) as Assessed by Eye (E) and by Automatic
Analysis (A)

Treatment	Day 1	Day 2	Mean
None	(E) 369 (A) 333 (0.90)	(E) 221 (A) 227 (1.03)	(E) 295 (A) 280 (0.95)
SV 200 x 3	(E) 137 (A) 155 (1.13)	(E) 159 (A) 209 (1.31)	(E) 148 (A) 182 (1.23)
SV 500 x 2	(E) 24 (A) 34 (1.42)	(E) 55 (A) 36 (0.65)	(E) 40 (A) 35 (0.88)
SV 500 x 2 200 x 1	(E) 51 (A) 59 (1.16)	(E) 0 (A) 0 (1.0)	(E) 26 (A) 30 (1.15)
SV 500 x 3	(E) 3 (A) 1 (0.33)	(E) 1 (A) -	(E) 2 (A) -
SV 1500 x 1	(E) 11 (A) 3 (0.27)	(E) 12 (A) 10 (0.83)	(E) 12 (A) 7 (0.58)

Figures in ( ) = Agreement: $\underline{\text{No. A}}$
$\qquad\qquad\qquad\qquad\qquad$ No. E
SV = sodium valproate
- = no autommatic analysis. Total S-W <1sec (below threshold of
detection).

the event marker facility easily identified the evening limit (8.0
p.m.).

In addition to enhancing the accuracy of the results, manual
analysis provided information that could not be derived from the
automatic recognition system. Details of paroxysm frequency and
duration could be determined reflecting response to medication.
Table 2 shows that long duration paroxysms were shortened following
initial introduction of sodium valproate and this was succeeded by
progressive reduction of both frequency and duration of S-W
discharges, the optimum response occurring at 1500 mg./day in divided
dosage.

For patients with very frequent or prolonged paroxysms in their
EEG, manual analysis is a much less attractive proposition. Automatic analysis is ideal for these recordings as it is labour saving
and yet it is a paradox that such recordings are often least suited
to analysis using this system. Experience with institutionalised
epileptic patients shows that these subjects often have S-W activity
most clearly defined over the temporal regions with relatively poor
definition elsewhere. Whilst this may indicate a temporal origin to
the discharge, it also increases the degree of computer error due to

Table 2

Detailed Analysis of Spike-Wave Discharges

	No Treatment	SV 200x3	SV 500x2	SV 500x2	SV 500x3 200x1	SV 1500x1
No. paroxysms 1-3 sec.	7	1	3	0	1	6
No. paroxysms 4-10 sec.	6	14	4	3	0	1
No. paroxysms >10 sec.	18	1	0	0	0	0
Total No. paroxysms	31	16	7	3	1	7
Mean duration (secs)	9	9	5	7	2	2

Each taped EEG recording was played out onto paper and the S-W paroxysms were counted by eye.
Individual figures are the means from two consecutive 12-hour recordings. Fractions of paroxysms are taken as 0.
SV = sodium valoproate.

detection of chewing artefact.

Siting electrodes elsewhere may not be practical as this leads to under-estimation of S-W activity due to poor definition of complexes. Moreover, these patients exhibit changing morphology of S-W discharges even within the same paroxysm (Figure 4). Thresholds set to detect paroxysms with low amplitude spikes as in Figure 4 (c) - (d) result in continual opening of the spike gate, the S-W detector being triggered by any large amplitude slow wave. An automatic recognition system based on pre-set spike and wave detector thresholds is clearly not well-suited to this type of epileptic activity.

Reduction of S-W paroxysms following appropriate therapy is the best indicator of a therapeutic response in patients with absence seizures. However, changes in total S-W activity over isolated 12 or 24-hour periods may be misleading. Table 3 presents the results from two institutionalised patients with drug-resistant epilepsy recorded over six consecutive days. During the recordings, daily routines were unchanged and medication was constant throughout. Less control of the environment occurred at weekends however. The results indicate that S-W activity can show marked spontaneous fluctuations from day to day. Environmental influences may be of major import in the assessment of drug effects in these patients, though attempt at standardisation over long periods are difficult. In general, the accuracy of automatic detection in these patients is less due to a combination of factors previously mentioned. The daily variation in S-W activity complicates considerably the assessment of patients especially those that are relative non-responders. Unless the drug administered is highly effective in reducing S-W paroxysms, any partial beneficial effect could well be masked by the spontaneous

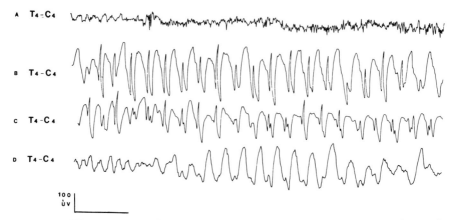

Fig. 4   EEG samples from the same patient and montage (T4-C4)
          illustrating (a) normal background activity, (b) well0
          defined paroxysm which stands out from the background
          making automatic detection easy, (c) irregular S-W dis-
          charge. During the paroxysm spikes are attenuated, at
          times becoming polyspikes. This leads to under-detection of
          S-W activity if thresholds are set to detect regular paro-
          xysms as in (b). (d) very irregular paroxysm. Only the
          slow waves are clearly defined, the spikes being barely
          recognisable.

daily fluctuations of S-W activity. Single 12-hour recordings may,
therefore, not be sufficient to demonstrate an improvement with
medication in these subjects.
     Inaccuracies from automated analysis of EEG recordings from
patients with irregular S-W paroxysms can only be resolved by manual

Table 3

Number of Seconds of S-W Activity per 12-hour EEG (7.0 am-7.0 pm)
Assessed by Eye in Two Patients with Severe Drug-resistant Epilepsy

Subject	Mon.	Tues.	Wed.	Thurs.	Fri.	Sat.	Sun.
1	2362 (0.76)	1275 (0.98)	561 (0.59)	347 (0.49)	311 (0.91)	375 (0.77)	
2	–	908 (0.77)	1226 (1.01)	1598 (0.76)	2027 (0.83)	3525 (0.99)	2349 (1.12)

During the recordings, medication was kept constant and daily
routines changed little except at the weekend.
Figuresin parenthesis = Agreement: <u>Automatic Analysis</u>
                                     Eye   Analysis

data analysis. Obviously, this increases considerably the workload
if long periods of EEG registration are made. However, modification
of trial design may help resolve this problem especially for drugs
given in an acute situation. A single subject prone to frequent
absence status has been studied by connecting him to the ambulatory
monitoring equipment whilst well and waiting for an absence status to
occur. EEG monitoring was then initiated and treatment given, in
this case, either diazepam, or a placebo administered rectally. Assessment was by counting S-W activity in 10 minutes of control EEG
and in seven 10 minute periods following treatment, each treatment
being repeated on six occasions. Automatic EEG analysis is not
required for such a short study as the tape can be written out on
paper and the S-W activity counted by eye. Figure 5 shows that
diazepam administered rectally is highly effective in terminating
recurrent absence status as judged by reduction of S-W activity in
the EEG. The difficulties in obtaining pharmacodynamic data during
clinical seizures are self-evident. The ambulatory monitor largely
resolved these problems and enabled data to be collected with little
inconvenience to the patient.

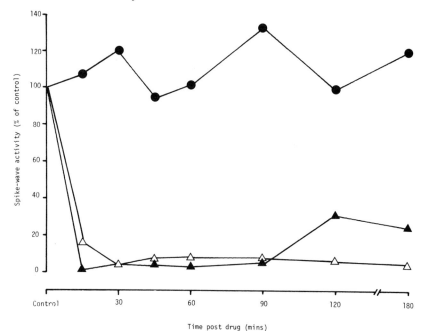

Fig. 5   Results (means of six treatments) of S-W analysis from a
          patient in recurrent absence status after rectal administra-
          tion of saline (●), diazepam solution 20mg (▲) and an   ex-
          perimental diazepam suppository 20mg (△) made at the John
          Radcliffe Hospital, Oxford. Assessment was by counting S-W
          activity in 10 minutes of control EEG and in   seven 10
          minute periods following treatment. Differences from saline
          (P<0.01) except at 120 minutes after diazepam   solution
          (P<0.05). Differences between diazepam solution   and diaze-
          pam suppository at 15 minutes and 180 minutes   (P<0.05).

Conclusions

Ambulatory monitoring of the EEG provides a means of obtaining long periods of EEG registration with minimum patient restriction and inconvnience. When used for assessment of a therapeutic response in patients with absence seizures, the foremost problem is accuracy of rapid data analysis. This is directly related to the individual morphological characteristics of the paroxysmal S-W discharge and to the amount and type of artefact. Consequently, the reliability of automated analysis is variable. Manual data analysis increases the accuracy of results at the expense of time and labour. Modification of study design for drugs given in an acute situation can minimise this, though the opportunities presenting for such studies are limited. In view of the uncertain significance of nocturnal epileptic discharges, response to medication using long-term monitoring should be determined from changes in the amount of diurnal S-W activity recorded during periods of wakefulness.

References

1. Penry J.K., Porter R.J. and Dreifuss F.E. (1971) Epilepsia **12**, 278-279.
2. Ives J.R. and Woods J.F. (1975) Electroencephalogr. Clin. Neuro-physiol. **39**, 88-92.
3. Quy R.J., Willison R.G., Fitch P. and Gilliatt (1980) In: ISAM 1979 Proc. of 3rd Int. Symp. on Amb. Mon. Eds. Stott F.D., Raftery E.B. and Goulding L. Academic Press, London 393-398.
4. Quy R.J., Fitch P. and Willison R.G. (1980) Electroencephalogr. Clin. Neurophysiol. **49**, 187-189.
5. Quy R.J. (1978) J. Physiol (Lond) **284**, 23-24.
6. Kellerway P., Frost J.D. Jr. and Crawley J.W. (1980) Ann. Neurol. 8, 491-500.
7. Milligan N. and Richens A. (1981) Br. J. Clin. Pharmac. **11**, 443-456.

Discussion

DR. HALL: Is there any fundamental reason why the automatic analysis should not improve as time goes on? Is it simply a problem of improving the technology and the programming?

DR. MILLIGAN: I think that Dr. Hall has really answered his own question. We hope that further improvements in technology will lead to improved automatic recognition systems, but I am not in a position to say how best to achieve this.

DR. IVES: Has Dr. Milligan gone back, say, two weeks later and read the records again, or given the records to somebody else to read?

DR. MILLIGAN: The results are from my own analysis, which was done only once. Manual data analysis can be a very time-consuming and laborious process.

DR. IVES: Secondly, when the same patient is re-done - in other words, off-medication and on-medication - are the levels of the analyser adjusted each time, or are the same parameters set for the same patient?

DR. MILLIGAN: Detector thresholds are set for each individual taped

EEG.

DR. IVES: With the girl whose medication was changed, were the settings of the automatic detector left the same?

DR. MILLIGAN: No.   As I mentioned, the detector thresholds are adjusted to suit the morphology of the spike-wave complexes in each tape. They can change from one recording to the next, even within the same patient.

CLINICAL USEFULNESS OF AMBULATORY EEG MONITORING OF THE NEUROLOGICAL PATIENT

R. E. RAMSAY, MD

Department of Neurology, Veterans Administration Hospital,
Miami, Florida, USA

Introduction

In 1975, Ives and Woods (1) reported on the technical feasibility of
long-term recording of EEG from an ambulatory patient. In 1979,
these authors reported the results of recording in 100 epileptic
patients and found that the ambulatory EEG was "also 3 to 4 times
more efficient than conventional EEG in documenting patients spontaneous seizure activity." (2) Several authors have suggested that the
extended four channel EEG recordings are beneficial in specific
instances (3, 4, 5). However, the utility of the procedure in a
general neurological population has not been adequately assessed.

Method

To evaluate the usefulness of 24-hour ambulatory EEG's, results from
two EEG laboratories were reviewed and combined. One was a
University-based EEG laboratory and the other was an active private
neurological service, with both an office and a hospital-based
laboratory. All laboratories served as referral facilities running
EEG's for physicians in the vicinity. When the tapes were recorded,
they were initially reviewed by the recording EEG technologist and
then reviewed again by the electroencephalographer. The results of
previous routine EEG's were obtained and when available the original
records were reviewed. In most cases, the patient's records were
available for review, and an assessment of the usefulness of the
findings on the 24-hour EEG could be made.
    The EEG's were obtained, using a four-channel Oxford Medilog
recorder. When four channels of EEG were recorded, the montage
consisted of F_3-F_7, T_3-T_5, F_4-F_8, and T_4-T_6. The montage consisted of
either F_3-F1, F_4-T_2, C_3-O_1, or T_5-T_3, T_1-T_2, T_4-T_6, when EKG was
recorded on the first channel. A few recordings were made using a
timing and event channel in which case, the montage consisted of EKG,
F_3-T_3 and F_4-T_4. Tapes were played back through an Oxford Page Mode
Rapid Scanner. Hard copies of segments of the recording were made
though a standard EEG instrument. In some patients, with primary
generalized seizure disorders, the frequency of discharges of various
durations were visually quantitated for the 24-hour period.

Results

Ambulatory EEG's were obtained in 465 patients and a total of 508 recordings were obtained. Patients ranged from 15 months to 90 years of age. In 449 of the patients a single 24-hour record was made. Longer recordings were obtained in 16 patients with a maxiumum being 96 hours. 21 of the tapes were felt to be technically inadequate and had to be repeated. The ambulatory EEG was obtained on most of the patients because of a history of undiagnosed episodes of loss of consciousness or unusual behaviour. Eight per cent of the patients had previously been diagnosed as epileptic. The records were obtained to correlate the electrographic with the clinical findings or to quantitate the number of significant electrographic discharges, which in some patients occur without their awareness.

The results of the routine EEG were either not available or the record could not be reviewed in 64 patients (Table 1). Of the remaining patients, 262 had normal routine EEG's. Five of these patients had ictal generalized convulsive episodes during which some portions of the EEG were not completely obscured by muscle and movement artefact and there was no apparent change in the recording.

TABLE 1

Comparison of findings from routine EEGs and from 24-hr ambulatory recordings

24-HourEEG	Normal	Abnormal	Unknown
Normal (Clinically useful)	209 (5)	48 (1)	54
Abnormal (Clinically useful)	53 (26)	91 (14)	10 (? 3)

Up to seven ictal events were recorded in these patients with no evidence of electrographic build up and no ictal or post-ictal changes. A generalized convulsive seizure was recorded in one further patient, which showed no changes in the record before or after the seizure. Although the ictal portion of the recording demonstrated prominent muscle activity, which limited visual analysis, the auditory play out was rather characteristic of a seizure discharge. Only two patients who were felt on clinical grounds to have epilepsy had normal routine and 24-hour EEG's in the interictal period. CT scan on these patients revealed a right frontal lobe AVM located near the cingulate gyrus and a right sphenoid wing meningioma. An interictal epileptiform pattern was present on each of the 24-hour tapes recorded on the remaining patients who were diagnosed as having epilepsy. In 53 of the patients with normal routine recordings, the 24-hour EEG was interpreted as abnormal. The abnormality was felt to be epileptiform and a diagnostic finding in 26 of the patients. The finding in the remaining 27 patientw were intermittent lateralized

theta or delta activity. Clinical and electrographic seizures were
recorded on the ambulatory monitor in 5 of the 53 patients, while no
seizures were recorded on the routine EEG.

Case Reports

1. The EEG of a 46-yeav old patient is shown in Figure 1. He had
two episodes of loss of consciousness, occurring early in the morning, while driving his truck to work. During the first episode, he
was involved in a two-car accident. As a result of the second episode, he awoke on the floor of his truck, which had gone off he road
and struck a tree. On both occasions, he was admitted to the hospital
and was extensively evaluated including several EEG's all of which
were normal. 24-hour ambulatory EEG revealed a right-sided spike
focus which became evident in the second cycle of sleep.

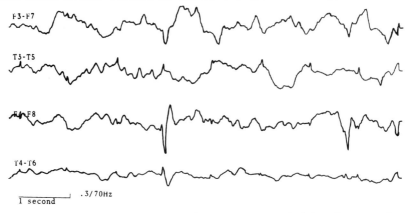

F3-F7

T3-T5

F4-F8

T4-T6

.3/70Hz

1 second

Fig. 1   **A right temporal spike focus was recorded in the second   and**
third cycle of sleep after two routine electro-encephalo-
grams were normal.

2. Patient RC was a 14-year old boy, who had a three-year history
of episodes of which were described by his parents as his becoming
"weak in the knees". He would slowly sink to the floor and apparently would be unresponsive to verbal commands for up to two minutes.
Over a three-year period, he had been evaluated by three different
neurologists and had several EEG's, all of which were either normal
or showed minor slowing of the background rhythms. He had also been
evaluated by a psychiatrist, who felt he had a functional disorder.
He had been treated with anti-convulsants at the onset of his symptoms, but he demonstrated no sustained improvement. At the time of
his 24-hour EEG recording, he had been without anti-convulsant medication for six months and he was having at least daily episodes.
Routine EEG the previous day showed only mild slowing of the background rhythms.
    Findings on the 24-hour EEG included a slow background frequency
and slow spike wave discharges up to 30 seconds in duration (Figure
2) suggesting a diagnosis of Lennox-Gastaut Syndrome. The discharges
occurred most promently late in the evening and again early the next

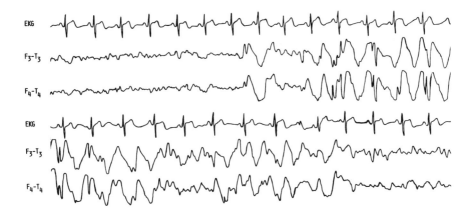

Fig. 2   Slow spike wave discharge was recorded from a 14 year old
boy who had episodes of his knees getting weak and being
unattentive to his parents.

morning, which is the reason routine EEG recordings failed to show
the abnormality.

Normal ambulatory EEG's were reported in 48 patients whose
routine tracings were felt to be abnormal. The abnormality in all
but 5 cases was slowing of the background rhythm, without lateralized
or paroxysmal activity. The electrode placement was limited to the
more anterior head regions, thus preventing the recording or interpretation of the more prominent occipital rhythms. In the other 5
patients, a questionable abnormal slow wave built up on a routine
recording in one patient and focal slowing (Temporal in 2 and frontal
in 2) in four patients. Several clincal events were recorded in one
patient in this group, during which there was no alteration in the
background EEG, supporting the clinical impression of pseudo epileptic seizures.

Abnormal routine EEG's as well as 24-hour ambulatory EEG's were
found in 91 of these patients. The findings in most patients consisted of slowed background rhythms or asymmetries, which were sub-
stantiated by the ambulatory recording. Although the abnormality was
clearly shown on the four-channel recorder, the results did not alter
the diagnosis or improve the care of the patient. Nine of these
patients had a clinical symptomatology during the recording without
evidence of changes in the EEG.

The significance of a negative finding in this instance was
difficult to assess. Recordings were obtained in five patients as
part of their work-up for lobectomy. Ictal events were recorded in
all patients and demonstrated the same lateralization as found on
routine and depth electrode recordings. In patient JN, the results
of the ambulatory EEG first suggested that her clinical symptomatology were indeed epileptic seizures. She had a long history of
seizures, which were significantly exacerbated after a very mild head
trauma a year and a half previously, and litigation was pending. She

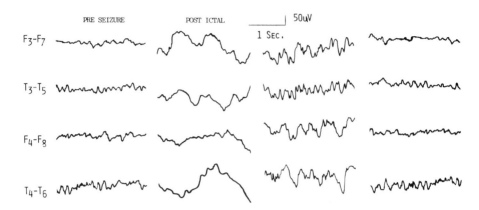

Fig. 3   31 year old patient with uncontrolled post-traumatic
          seizures. Ictal recording was obscured by muscle, but pro-
          minent slowing is noted in the post ictal period par-
          ticularly in the right hemispheric channels.

reported frequent seizures (1 to 2 per day), which by history were
simple partial with secondary generalization. During two hospital-
izations, she had only two seizures, which did not occur in the pres
ence of the hospital staff. Three ictal events were recorded on the
ambulatory EEG (Figure 3). There is no change in the record prior to
the event and the ictal period was obscured by muscle. Post-ictally
there was rather marked slowing most prominent over the right hemisphere, with return of normal background activity after ten minutes.
Depth electrode recording revealed a very active left mesial temporal
focus and the patient underwent a left temporal lobectomy, with the
pathology revealing a grade 1 glioma.
     The other utility of the ambulatory EEG has been to quantitate
patients' clinical seizures. TM is a 26-year old male, who was
reported to be having 20 to 30 petit mal seizures a day, while he was
taking high doses of Phenobarbital and Ethosuximide. 24-hour EEG at
the time revealed 67 spike wave discharges of 5 to 15 seconds in
duration and discharges of less than two seconds occurring continuously throughout the day-time. Medications were switched and
sevenmonths later, on a combination of Valproic Acid, Tridione and
Phenobarbital, only 21 discharges of 5 to 15 seconds were seen and
the frequency of the brief discharges had reduced to every 5 to 10
minutes. Although the patient realized he was having frequent seizures, he was unable to quantitate accurately the frequency or the
duration of the seizures. Quantitation of the number of discharges
aided in the objective assessment of his response to changes in his
medical regimen.

Technical

As experience was being gained with use of the system, 21 of the
tapes were inadequate due to technical difficulties. The accuracy of
the hook-up was assured by taping on each electrode in a specific

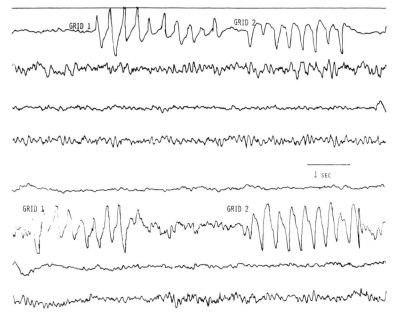

Fig. 4   Tapping on the individual electrodes produces a transient
          negative potential. At the start of a recording, the elec-
          trodes should be tapped in sequence to insure that the
          channel and grid attachment is correct.

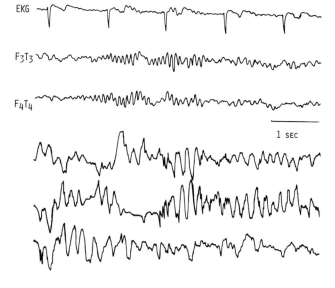

Fig. 5   High amplitude activity may spill over and be recorded on
          adjacent channels. During a period of movement, the EEG
          channel is obscured by activity from the second channel.

sequence at the start of the recording) channel 1- Grid 1 and Grid 2; then channel 2 - Grid 1 and Grid 2; etc). A distinctive artefact is produced as shown in Figure 4. Movement of the connection of the electrode to the preamplifiers was found to produce a very prominent artefact. At times this result in blocking of the channel, which could persist for the duration of the recording. High voltage activity occurring in one channel could also be reflected or cross-talk into other channels (Figure 5).

Recording in all channels will be lost if the ground wire becomes loose or breaks. A major portion of these artefacts were eliminated by attaching the preamplifiers and ground wire firmly to the scalp with collodion. Muscle, chewing and eye-movement artefacts are still prominent when the patient is awake and active. Generalized epileptiform discharges can easily be distinguished from chewing and movement both visually (Figure 6) and by listening to the auditory output. Seizures sound like a combination of a few pure tones, while chewing and muscle artefact is perceived as an irregular mixture of high frequency components. If the tape in the cassette sticks, the tape may be pulled across the head at an irregular speed producing an erratic recording. This was noted on two tapes and produces a fluctuation in the amplitude and frequency, which is evident in all channels synchronously. An example is shown in Figure 7, where there appears to be prominent arrhythmia. As the EKG complexes become closer together, the amplitude diminishes and an increase in the EEG frequencies is also prominently noted. The clue to potential sticking or irregular play-back is that as the frequency of the recorded activity increased, or in the case of the EKG, the complexes get closer together, the amplitude of the activity becomes much lower. This problem is eliminated by the use of timing marks on one channel as the sequencing of the play-out is defined by the distance between the time marks and any fluctuation in the recording speed would effect the timing marks - the same as it would the EEG/EKG channels.

Discussion

The majority of the recordings were done as out-patients. The frequency of recording difficulties and technically inadequate records diminished as experience with the system increased. When sequential 24-hour EEG's were recorded, the patients were requested to return to the EEG laboratory on a daily basis to have the integrity of the system checked. Using this technique up to 96 hours of continuous EEG has been recorded. Cassette recordings have proven to be a very efficient way of obtaining prolonged electrographic recordings. In a previously unselected population, we found this to be of definite help in 46 of 401 patients (11%) by either making a positive diagnosis or significantly aiding in the care of the patient. This was similar to what was reported by Green, et al (4) "an increase of 10% yield in electrophysiological abnormalities..." In the series reported here, only two patients felt to be epileptic failed to show any abnormal electrographic findings on the 24-hour recording.

Selection of the proper montage is imperative to maximize the chance of recording interictal epileptiform activity. Ebersol and Leroy (6) compared the montages used with the ambulatory recorder vs. standard 16 channel recordings. They found using montages that did

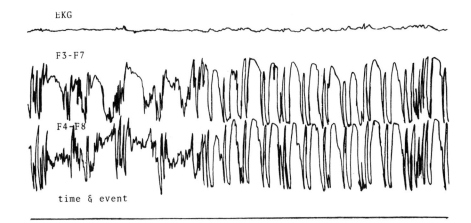

Fig. 6 Generalised spike wave discharges (right half record) can be distinguished from the artifact produced by chewing.

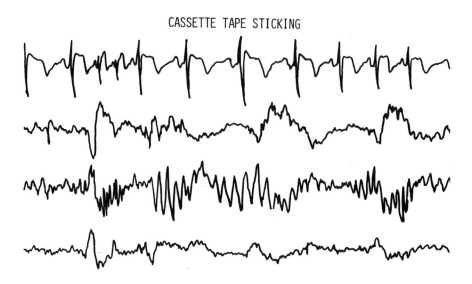

CASSETTE TAPE STICKING

Fig. 7 Sticking of the cassette tape during recording produces uneven recording. At playback, the frequency and amplitude of the activity will fluctuate simultaneously. The amplitude becomes lower as the frequency appears to increase.

not utilize common electrodes in two channels and that concentrated on the temporal leads (F^7, F^8, T^3, T^4, T^5, T^6), that 85% of the interictal epileptiform activity will be seen with the four-channel recorder. When recording from patients who have clinical seizures, which suggest a non-temporal focus, the montage   should be appropriately changed. We found normal ambulatory recordings in only 2 (4)% of known epileptic patients. The problem still remains in assessing the significance of abnormal 24-hour recording with focal seizures, as Ives and Woods (1) reported no EEG changes in 21% of the auras that they recorded. However, an abnormal interictal recording was found in all the patients. Recording of ictal events is significantly improved using an ambulatory recorder. Excluding patients evaluated for lobectomy, clinical and electrographic seizures were recorded in 16 patients on the ambulatory recorder and in another 15 patients, clinical events were recorded which were felt to be non-epileptic in origin. Only three seizures occurred while the patients were being recorded in the EEG laboratory.

Conclusion

With proper patient selection, the 24-hour ambulatory recordings adds a significant dimension to the evaluation and treatment of patients, who present with transient alteration in neurological function. Overall, a significant positive finding was found in 11.2% of the patients. Excluding patients with absence seizures, clinical 'seizures' were recorded in 31 patients (6.7%), with electrographic seizure activity found in 16 patients. In 15 patients (3.8%) the ambulatory EEG was normal during a clinical episodes resembling a convulsive seizure, supporting the diagnosis of pseudo-epileptic seizure. Only 4 seizures, three epileptic and one pseudo-epileptic, were recorded on routine EEG. The results must be evaluated considering the limitation of the methodology. These consist of :
1.   a limited number of scalp areas which can be recorded from,
2.   the prominent movement, muscle and chewing artefacts present particularly during the waking state, which may obscure some findings, and
3.   difficulty in timing EEG and clinical events when the timing channel is not used.
      The method has been found to be particularly useful in recording interictal and ictal seizures activity, which can be useful in supporting the diagnosis of epilepsy, lateralizing onset of seizure discharges, ad quantitating the number of clinical and electrographic seizures. Lastly, the possibility that a clinical symptom may be non-epileptic in nature can be suggested by the presence of normal EEG activity during the period of clinical symptomatology.

References

1. Ives J.R. and Woods J.F. Proc. of 3rd Int. Symp. on Ambul. Monitoring (1979) Ed: Stott F.D., Raftery E.B. and Goulding L., Academic Press, London, 383-92.
2. Ives J.R. (1976) Post Grad. Med. **52**, 86-91.
3. Horwitz S.J. Burgess R.C. and Kijewski K.N. (1978) Am. J. EEG Technol., **13**, 133-139.
4. Green J., Scales D., Nealis J., Scott G. and Driber T. (1980) Clin. EEG, **11**, 173-179.
5. Riley T.L., Peterson H., Mounaimue (1981) Abst. Am. EEG. Soc. Meeting.
6. Ebersole J.S. and Leroy R.F. (1981) Abst. Am. EEG.So. Meeting.

Discussion

DR. MONSTER: How long does it usually take to review these 24-hour tapes in this page mode that Dr. Ramsay uses?

DR. RAMSAY: In practice, I always have the technologist review it first, which usually takes her between 1 and 1.1/2 hours. Without knowledge of her printout or impression I review it, and this usually takes 20 or 30 mins. I then compare our results - according to the discrepancies in our interpretations, or at least between her printout and my impression, this may take no longer than that, or another 15 or 20 mins. I rarely take longer than 1 hour in total - I try not to, anyway.

MR. LOVELY: When the recordings are done on the tapes, are the tapes re-used for several recordings, by wiping them and re-recording on them?

DR. RAMSAY: No, I do not do that - I think it is imperative, partly for legal reasons and also because I like to go back to them - as, hopefully, I am able to get computer analysis designed for spike-wave detection. But it is more for legal reasons that I maintain all the tapes.

LONG-TERM RECORDING OF TELEMETERED EEG AND PROFESSIONAL VIDEO AS A BASIS FOR SYSTEMATIC SEIZURE ANALYSIS

M.J.O'KANE, F.S.O'KANE AND I.W. MOTHERSILL

Swiss Epilepsy Clinic, 8008 Zurich, Switzerland

Summary

An off-line split-screen technique combining 16 channel telemetered EEG and pre-recorded video-taped seizures has been utilized as an aid for seizure documentation. The implementation of quad split and slow motion replay has proven to give more detailed information on the electro-clinical correlation of seizures.
  Video-recordings of seizures are edited and archived on master-tapes which become part of an extensive video library, thus providing a valuable diagnostic and didactic seizure documentation system.

Introduction

The idea of displaying the EEG and patient was described by Schwab et al in 1938 (1). The method consisted of using two separate 16 mm film cameras; after developing, a third film was produced of the composite picture, synchronizing being achieved by specially marking each film. Hunter and Jasper in 1949 (2) developed the idea further, using one cine camera instead of two and synchronizing with the aid of an elaborate mirror system. In 1953, Schwab et al used a lens splitter for this purpose (3). Fifteen years later, split screen video technology was applied (4), resulting in the simultaneous recording of EEG and patient with the aid of two video cameras, special effects generator, monitor and video recorder. The equipment was readily available; but logistic problems created by the need for continuous EEG write-out and frequent videotape changes remained unsolved. Since the introduction of radio transmission of the EEG - by Breakell et al in 1949 (5) - long term monitoring of patients uninhibited in their movements had become possible.
  Various radio-telemetry systems were reviewed by Porter and colleagues in 1971 (6) and 1976 (7); Ives et al introduced a cable-telemetry-computer seizure monitoring system in 1974 (8). In 1976, Kaiser described an eight-channel multiplexed-EEG and simultaneous video recording system (9); the multiplexed EEG was recorded on the audio track of a video recorder, the eight EEG channels being reformatted by a video modem and displayed on a TV monitor.
  Recent advances in video technology, especially in 1" format played an important role in the designing of our system. We defined our priorities as follows:

1.   To obtain sixteen channels of EEG and/or other physiological parameters from uninhibited patients, both in the monitoring room and

within the clinic grounds.
2. To document simultaneously the EEG and clinical manifestations of seizures on one videotape.
3. To procure a hard copy of the EEG when required, without resorting to continuous write-out.
4. To edit and copy videotaped seizures, thus allowing the production and archiving of master tapes (videothek).

The EEG System

A radio-telemetry system was chosen because it gave patients freedom of movement and was less likely to interfere with the clinical course of seizures. Instrumentation tape storage, transmission of data and subsequent processing of signal information are best met with a digital system. The equipment, weighing 1.85 kilos, is located in three leather pockets on a belt which the patient wears round the waist. It consists of a power supply and 10 mW sender transmitting at 433.4 MHz, 16 EEG amplifiers and 16 4-pole butterworth filters, together with a 16-channel PCM encoder of 10-bit resolution.

Silver/silver chloride electrodes are applied following the 10-20 system of electrode placement (10) and the appropriate montage is selected via a hard-wired plug-in module (11).

The encoded EEG information is received and subtracted from the 433.4 MHz carrier. This is simultaneously recorded on a digital head of one of two video-recorders (12) - thus enabling EEG-video synchronization - and on an instrumentation tape with a 30-second delayed reproduction. Porter et al in 1976 (3) proposed the conversion of the analog EEG-signal to digital format and the displaying of the information directly on a video monitor in analog format. Unfortunately, these systems up until now have been limited in resolution. We are currently installing a 16-channel EEG TV-converter with a much improved resolution than the older system.

The EEG is demodulated and displayed on a 16-channel monitor; this monitor has a long decay P7 phosphore which in combination with a variable time base, allows ideal on-line viewing of the EEG. The 30-second delayed EEG is available on a 16-channel write-out, which is activated by a pushbutton, should a hard copy be required; channel 17 is used for pulsed BCD timing. The schematic of the complete on-line recording/monitoring system is shown in Figure 1

The Video System

The criteria established for our video recording system were as follows:
1. The video-recorders to be capable of delivering high quality reproduction of split EEG and patient to the extent of being able to read the EEG from the video monitor.
2. That stop and slow motion forwards and backwards be available so as to enable a precise correlation between EEG and seizure. Repeated viewing, allowing detailed protocols of taped seizures would be essential.
3. The system to have available integrated insert and assemble editing facilities.
4. Multi-generation of copies from master-tapes to be possible

without visual degradation of the video-display.
5.   The copies to be of such a standard that large-screen video-projection or transfer to film would be possible.

These criteria were met by the 1" BCN 50 and 40 (14) (Bosch Fernseh); the BCN format utilizes short track segmented field technique (SMPTE 1" type B Standard).   Direct contact with the manufacturer and service were of primary importance in the choice of this system.   Three audio-tracks are available of which the second is used as sound track, the third for recording hours, minutes, seconds and frames from a time-code generator. Since the first audio head could not handle the digitized PCM-EEG signal, it was replaced with a digital read/write head; the record and reproduce cards were easily fitted below the tape deck.   The digitized 16-channel EEG is thus recorded simultaneously with the video.

Because intensive monitoring sessions can last for hours and sometimes days, we provide the patients with a comfortable room, furnished with armchairs, desk, radio, television, washing facilities and a bed; children can choose from a large selection of toys, including computerized television games, useful also for performance tasks. A remote-controlled camera with motorized lens ad zoom is mounted on a vertically adjustable pan-and-tilt unit; this system has proven to give adequate video coverage.

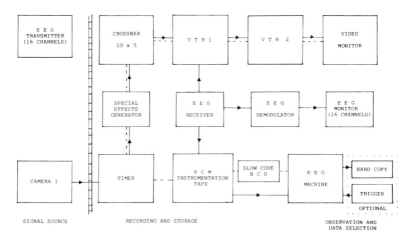

Fig. 1   On-Line System.

The video-recorders are used in series in case a seizure occurs during tape change-over, the average duration of a tape being 98 minutes. Should an attack be recorded, the tape is kept for later off-line editing while an immediate write-out is obtained. A video time-coder generator (11) blends timing information in days, hours, minutes and seconds on the video and pulses the time in BCD format onto the 17th channel of the EEG write-out; this is critical for on-line assessment of the seizure.

Off-line Editing

Video signal distribution is facilitated by means of a 10 x 5 video crossbar switching matrix presenting following sources for selection: electronically marked input and output of video-taped seizures from a slave recorder, video text patient information fade in and out, EEG signal replayed from audio track one of the slave recorder, demodulated and viewed by a plumbicon camera placed above the EEG machine. A preview status edit through a special effects generator displays the mixed EEG and patient video; final adjustments are made, these normally concerning lighting, EEG, video, amplitude, etc. Control is passed on to a master recorder with timing and frame count on the third audio track. An edit mode - assemble or insert - is selected and the edit simulated before a final edit is produced.

Master tapes are normally of 60-minute duration and contain an average of 18 edits; two copies of each master tape are produced routinely, the original being kept unplayed should further copies be required. The schematic of the off-line editing system is shown in Figure 2.

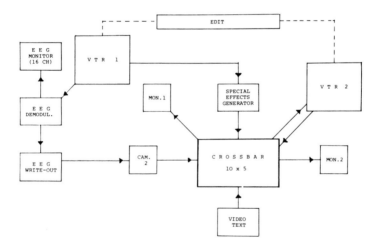

Fig. 2   Off-line editing system

The system was completed in May 1979 and since then 92 patients have been investigated over 964 hours of recording. 201 seizures have been documented and archived onto 16 60-minute master tapes in a video library.

Systematic replay and analysis of master tapes serve as an aid to diagnosis and classification of seizures. The material archived has also shown to be an invaluable tool in teaching programmes for medical and allied personnel.

References

1. Hunter J. and Jasper H.H. (1949) Electroenceph. Clin.Neurophysiol. **1**, 113-114.
2. Hunter J. and Jasper H.H. (1949) Ibid.
3. Schwab R.S., Schwab M.W., Withee D. and Chock Y.C. (1954) Electroenceph. Clin. Neurophysiol **6**, 684-686.
4. Köhler and Penin H. (1970) EEG-EMG **1**, 102-106.
5. Breakell C.C., Parker C.S. and Christopherson F. (1949) Electroenceph. Clin. Neurophysiol. **1**, 243-244.
6. Porter R.J. Wolf A.A. and Penry J.K. (1971) Am. J. Techn.**11**, 145-159.
7. Porter R.J., Penry J.K. and Wollf A.A. (1976) In: Quantitative Analytic Studies in Epilepsy, P.Kellaway and I. Petersen, eds. Raven Press, New York. pp 253-68.
8. Ives R.J., Thompson C.J., Gloor P., Olivier A. and Woods J.F. (1974) In: Biotelemetry II, P.A. Neukomm ed., Karger, Basel, 216-218.
9. Kaiser E. (1976) In: Quantitative Analytic Studies in Epilepsy, P. Kellaway and I. Petersen, eds. Raven Pres, New York, 279-288.
10. Jasper H.H. (1958) Electroenceph. Clin. Neurophysiol. **10**,371-375.
11. O'Kane M.J. and Sauter R. (1977) In: Epilepsy, the 8th International Symposium, J.K, Penry, ed.,Raven Press, New York.
12. O'Kane M.J., O'Kane F.S. and Mothersill I.W. (1980) In: 12th Epilepsy International Symposium, Copenhagen, Denmark.
13. Porter R.J., Penry J.K. and Wolf A.A. (1976) Ibid.
14. Zahn H.L. (1979) SMPTE Journal, Vol. 88,**12**, 823-831.

LONG TERM MONITORING OF MULTIPLE PHYSIOLOGICAL PARAMETERS USING A PROGRAMMABLE PORTABLE MICROCOMPUTER

L.E. MILES AND R.B. RULE

Stanford Sleep Disorders Clinic and Sleep Research Centre,
Stanford, California and Vitalog Corporation, Palo Alto,
California, USA

Summary

The Vitalog physiological monitoring system (PMS-8) is a portable,
general purpose microcomputer, designed for continuous analysis of
information from up to eight physiological sensors for up to weeks at
a time. At present, the PMS-8 provides sensor interfaces for ECG,
respirations, physical movement and body temperature; and the user
can programme the monitor to function in many different ways. The
PMS-8, and an earlier model, the TherMolog, have been used for several years by the Stanford Sleep Research Centre and Sleep Disorders
Clinic for studying circadian dyschronosis, sleep apnoea and the
distinction between sleep and wakefulness. The Vitalog PMS-8 has
allowed reliable, cost-effective and labour-saving studies in the
patients' own environment throughout the entire 24 hours.

Introduction

The Stanford Sleep Disorders and Sleep Research Centre, in collaboration with Vitalog Corporation of Palo Alto, has developed and applied
an intelligent, all-solid-state, portable physiological monitoring
system. The data is stored in solid-state memory for subsequent
rapid recovery, display and secondary analysis by a Data Manager,
which includes floppy diskette storage and hard copy graphics. (See
Figure 1).

Specifications of the PMS-8 Portable Monitor

The PMS-8 monitor (see Figure 2) has physical dimensions of 6.0 x 3.4
x 1.3 inches and weighs 12 oz (including batteries). Power consumption averages 1.5 mA from a 500 mAmp/hr rechargeable NiCad battery
pack. 36,864
bits of random access memory (RAM) are available for data storage,
with an expanded memory option of 102,400 bits. A recessed button
and LED display allow functional verification and event marking and
an optional output can indicate a pre-selected heart rate zone.
     We have developed and are using sensors, sensor interfaces and
software for monitoring ECG, respirations, physical movement and body
temperature. These signals enter through an eight channel A/D converter with the ECG also being processed by an analog R-wave
detector. Other sensor interfaces are in active development.

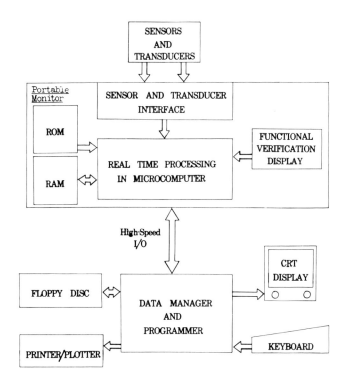

Fig. 1   Block diagram of Vitalog Portable Physiological Monitoring
          System (PMS-8) with Data Manager.

Specification of Data Manager

The data manager system consists of an Apple II computer (Apple
Computer Corporation of Santa Clara, Calif.) Data can be stored
permanently on five-inch floppy diskettes; can be numerically or
graphically displayed on a Sanyo video monitor or as hard-copy using
an Axiom or Florida Data Corporation printer/plotter and can even be
transmitted to another computer.   Vitalog provides a hi-speed Apple
/PMS-8 interface plus custom software.   Many standard software packages are commercially available.
     The data manager serves to:
     -    initialize the PMS-8, at which time it can define any

variables and even insert new programmes,
-        read and verify the complete contents of the PMS-8 memory,
in less than 15 seconds,
-        permit development of software for further analysis of the
data: e.g. statistical analysis,
-        allow users to develop their own software for the PMS-8,
-        provide for extensive PMS-8 hardware testing in the field.

Some Special Features of the System

Intelligence : Real-time Processing, Data Compression, Power-Down.

The portable microcomputer allows intelligent processing of
sensor information in real time. Depending on its instructions, the
monitor may store the converted analog signal directly in memory, or
use the information from one or more data points (or several different inputs) to calculate some mathematical or logical derivative.
Sensor input can be sampled at any time interval and the signal can
be screened to identify artefact or specific events. Only the most
pertinent information need be stored.

E. C. G.   MONITOR   RESPIRATION
SENSOR   SENSOR

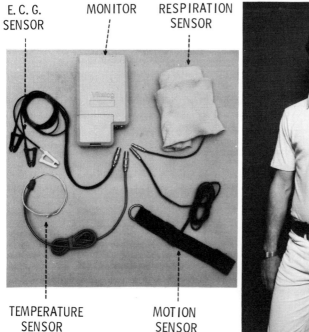
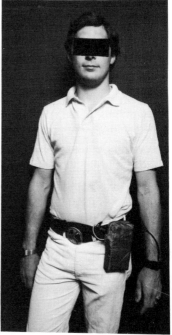

TEMPERATURE   MOTION
SENSOR   SENSOR

Fig. 2   Photograph of subject wearing the Vitalog Portable Physio-
          logical Monitor (PMS-8) with sensors for measuring tempera-
          ture, physical activity, and ECG. The inset shows the PMS-
          8 with its usual sensors.

Data compression techniques contribute to the efficient utilization of solid-state memory. Encoding of the data is often employed. In many applications, data compression can also be achieved by storing little or no data when the signal is "invalid" (outside some prescribed limits), " normal" (conforming to some specified criteria), or unchanging (such as when the sensors are unplugged). A "power-down" mechanism under software control allows the processor drastically to reduce power consumption whenever it is "idle".

This intelligent real-time "pre-processing" not only increases the duration of the recording by more efficient use of the memory and batteries, it also minimizes the amount of subsequent "off-line" data processing. The information finally recovered from the monitor can range from long trains of time series data points to a simple yes/no response.

Programmability

An unique feature of the PMS-8 system is that the portable monitor is externally programmable from the data manager. Programmes controlling the monitor can reside in the Read-Only-Memory (EPROM), in the Random Access Memory (RAM), or in a combination of both. Even when the monitor runs under the control of the programme in EPROM, certain variables (e.g. sampling rates, number and types of sensor inputs, definition of data encoding schemes) can be redefined by using the data manager to load values into Random-Access-Memory (RAM) at the time the monitor is initialized. Furthermore, the programme in EPROM can be augmented, modified, or even completely replaced by software loaded into RAM. A single instrument can, therefore, be reprogrammed for diverse applications.

The Apple II data manager has been provided with a Programme Development System with documentation to allow the user to write, assemble, debug, load and operate his own software for the PMS-8. The user is thereby able to develop sensor interfaces, create custom software and monitor a great variety of physiological signals through the eight-channel A/D converter

Both the external programming and the specification of variables are implemented through the data manager and transmitted to the PMS-8 via a high-speed bi-directional I/O channel. Hardware self-test, hardware debugging and custom monitoring programmes, supplied by Vitalog Corporation, all operate in this manner.

Functional Verification and Self Test

The user is given the ability to test the PMS-8 hardware in the field before each recording session and to verify the function of the monitor during actual operation. The data manager has programmes for testing all major aspects of the hardware (including the sensors), and can load software into the PMS-8 so that the monitor can test itself. Furthermore, the data manager can simulate a sensor input signal to allow "closed loop" testing. The LED display is used to verify the function during an actual recording, and the switch can be used as an event marker. These features provide for simple field maintenance and increase the confidence of the user.

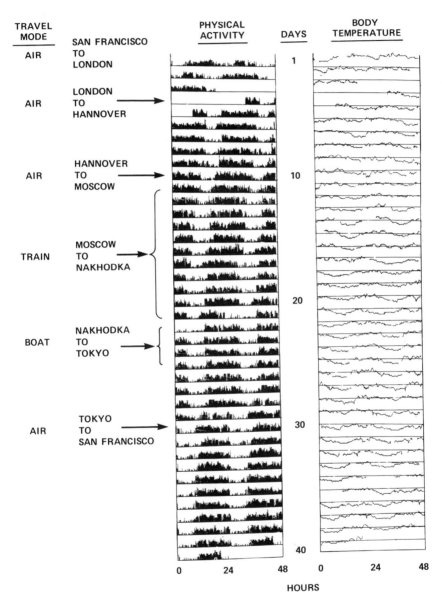

TRAVEL MODE		PHYSICAL ACTIVITY	DAYS	BODY TEMPERATURE

AIR — SAN FRANCISCO TO LONDON

AIR — LONDON TO HANNOVER

AIR — HANNOVER TO MOSCOW

TRAIN — MOSCOW TO NAKHODKA

BOAT — NAKHODKA TO TOKYO

AIR — TOKYO TO SAN FRANCISCO

HOURS

Fig. 3   Recording of Body Temperature and Physical Activity :   48-hr. double-plot of deep body temperature   and physical activity recorded by a Vitalog monitor from   a 44 year old male subject during a trip around the world.

Applications

The PMS-8 and an earlier model, the TherMolog, have been used for
several years by the Stanford Sleep Research Centre and Sleep Disorders Clinic for studying circadian dyschronosis, sleep apnoea and
the distinction between sleep and wakefulness (1, 2). Collaborators
and other investigators have found these devices useful for studying
such problems as stress, jet lag, shift work, insomnia, infection,
allergy, nutrition, exercise physiology, executive fitness, cardiac
rehabilitation, certain psychiatric disorders, infant behaviour and
the effects of certain medications.
     Figure 3 shows a typical 48-hour double plot of deep body temp-
erature and physical activity data. In this instance, the plot uses
data recovered from a TherMolog monitor carried by a 44-year old male
during a trip around the world. The subject travelled across time-
zones at different rates and in a variety of conveyances. Changes in
the amplitude and phase of his circadian rhythms are readily perceived.
     Figure 4 shows a plot of the fastest and slowest steady-state
heart rates occurring in successive five-second intervals, in a woman
complaining of excessive day-time sleepiness. The monitor was applied to the patient at mid-afternoon during an out-patient clinic.
At that time, a special programme was loaded into the monitor, the
function of the monitor on the patient checked and the monitor pow-
ered down by unplugging the electrodes. Late that night, in her own
home, the patient plugged the electrodes into the monitor which then
automatically began to process and store physiological data. The
record shows that about one hour after sleep onset (0130 hours) the
patient began to show the first of several episodes of the typical
bradytachycardia of sleep apnoea.
     Figure 5 shows a plot which indicates the amplitude and frequ-
ency of successive inspirations and expirations during the early part
of a nocturnal sleep period of an apparently normal 37-year old male.
The respiration sensor was the Respiratory Inductive Plethysmograph
(Respitrace. TM, Ambulatory Monitoring Incorporated, Ardesley, New
York).

Conclusion

The PMS-8 belongs to a new generation of "intelligent" instruments
and offers unique capabilities. In contrast to analog recorders,
this instrument has no moving parts, requires much less power and is
not subject to mechanical failure. It is capable of monitoring
multiple physiological parameters and recording variously derived
data points over periods of up to several weeks.
     The Vitalog PMS-8 enables physicians to carry out diagnostic
screening and to assess the outcome of treatment throughout 24 hours
and in the patients' own environment. The use of reliable, all-
solid-state intelligent portable monitors allows labour-intensive,
technically difficult and expensive in-patient investigations to be
reserved for those patients in whom the effort, expense and
restricted environment is unequivocally justified.

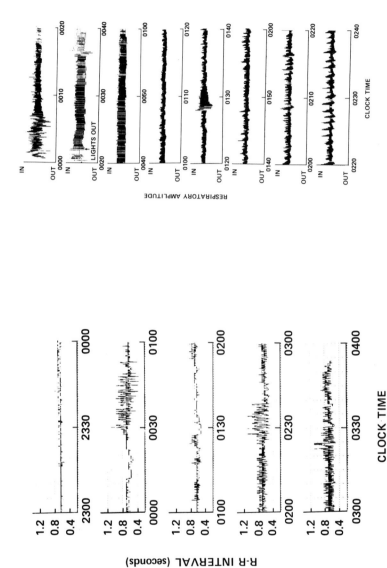

CLOCK TIME

R-R INTERVAL (seconds)

RESPIRATORY AMPLITUDE

CLOCK TIME

Fig. 4 (left)   Recording of ECG : Plot of the fastest and slowest steady-state heart rates in successive five second intervals, in a 35 year old female who complained of excessive daytime sleepiness.

Fig. 5 (right)   Recording of Respirations : Amplitude and frequency of respirations monitored, analysed, and recorded by a Vitalog PMS-8 during the early part of a nocturnal sleep period.

References

1.   Miles L., Cutler R., Drake K., Rule B., Dement W. (1978)
     Sleep Res., **7**, 293.
2.   Miles L., Flagg W., Rule B., Redington D., Dement W. (1979)
     Chronobiologia, **6**, 133.

Discussion

DR. SACKNER: What is the digitising rate on the ADC to the microprocessor for the various signals about which Dr. Miles was talking?   Was the digitising done at 20 points/sec, 30 points/sec - or what?

DR. MILES: at 16 points/sec.

DR. SACKNER: Do you think it will be possible to handle three channels of information for the respiratories, rib cage, and sum?

DR. MILES: Yes, that can be done in terms of what the microprocessor has to do.   The question is what will be stored away in memory.   At this point we really need to look at a lot of algorithms to see what can be appointed fairly confidently in order to have general agreement about what is truly normal respiration - and then we just have to believe the processor.   With some people who are having abnormal respirations all night, obviously we will soon run out of memory.   It is possible to drive a digital micro-cassette with this monitor if necessary and, as I said, for the respiration device (because we will probably want to have at least the R-wave detector, and perhaps even another respiration sensor) we will certainly go up to the larger memory option with the 160,000 bits of information. Even with that, we will want to be able to discard things that the processor and the physician reviewing it will confidently believe as being normal.   Of course, we want to use this as a screening device and not for characterising severe apnoeics.   If they have a problem, Society can afford to spend the $700 to treat these patients.

MR. EVANS: What type of transducer is used by Dr. Miles to record rest activity states?

DR. MILES: We use more than one sort of transducer.   Almost all of these data have been obtained using an array of 360° tilt switches - 6 of them orientated on the surfaces of a cube, so that there is approximately equal activity in all directions.   It is approximately quantitative, as can be seen from the data when patients are being calibrated on the treadmill test.   There is some debate about the best place to put sensors; in fact, the cardiac rehabilitation people seem to prefer to put the sensors on the leg, but most of our studies have been done with the sensors on the non-dominant wrist.   The group at San Diego (and also other people) have mostly used analog motion sensors, accelerometers or piezoelectric devices.   The one with the eye movements is a little sliver of a device made by Siemens.

DIPL.ING. RASCHKE: Is there any relationship between the sleep apnoea syndromes and the long-term recordings over several days?   Can any relationship be seen between the sleep apnoea syndromes and complaints observed on the recordings over several days?

DR. MILES: It depends what is being measured.   Certainly, the activitity in somebody with sleep apnoea is very abnormal in the daytime; in fact, some of these patients have a reversed rest-activity cycle. They are so incapacitated and restless at night that they often find it easier to sleep in naps in the daytime when they are sitting up in a chair.

DR. SACKNER: What about the sleep-staging with the microprocessor? Many more points per second will have to be digitised. Spectral analysis has to be done, or some other way of sleep-staging them. How can that be handled?

DR. MILES: That type of sleep-staging was not using the EEG. There is an effort to get away from using the EEG or, if it is used, perhaps to use on the alpha-power. There is a project at Stanford trying to get away from the classic methods of sleep-staging, and to look at the transition between sleep and wakefulness by doing a statistical evaluation of many different factors - up to 30 factors. We know that with a motion sensor it is possible to get very close to the sleep period, maybe even to the times that the eyes are shut, so perhaps even with a motion sensor and alpha-power itself we are getting into the right ballpark. That is a very promising area to investigate, not the area mimicking classic sleep-staging criteria of Rechtschaffen and Kales. Many of the most useful sleep parameters, such as the relative arousal and brief 10-second arousal, are not even in the Rechtschaffen and Kales' manual. The daytime consequences both of noise-aroused sleep and of disturbed sleep in the elderly appear not to relate very well to classic wake-after-sleep onset but far more to these brief arousals.

AMBULATORY MONITORING OF OESOPHAGEAL REFLUX USING A PORTABLE RADIOTELEMETRY SYSTEM

D.F. EVANS, F.J. BRANICKI, A.L. OGLIVIE, M. ATKINSON, J.D. HARDCASTLE

University Department of Surgery and University Hospital, Queen's Medical Centre, Nottingham, UK

Summary

Gastro-oesophageal reflux has been assessed in 10 patients at work and in the home using a newly developed pH sensitive radiotelemetry capsule (rtc) (1) and a portable receiving system (2). Oesophageal pH was continuously monitored by the tethered rtc and recorded with a portable receiver and a Medilog 24-hour cassette tape recorder worn on a waistbelt, allowing the patient complete freedom of movement. Outpatient studies were undertaken during activities of patients fully ambulant at work in factories, offices or shopping centres.

The mean number and duration of reflux episodes during a 24-hour study period was significantly greater during the day than at night, both for ambulatory outpatients and patients in hospital, and greater during outpatient studies than in hospital. Ambulatory outpatient oesophageal pH monitoring is useful in the management of patients with atypical symptoms and may demonstrate significant reflux when inpatient investigations and endoscopy findings show minimal abnormality.

Introduction

Oesophagitis, caused by reflux of gastric contents into the oesophagus, is a common problem in hospital practice. There are a number of objective measurements available to assess the severity of the complaint but there has been considerable debate as to their diagnostic accuracy and it is apparent that the diagnosis of symptomatic reflux is a significant problem (3).

Patients rejected for surgical treatment of gastro-oesophageal reflux because of negative endoscopy and biopsy findings, but often complaining of severe symptoms, sometimes return to hospital at a later date with an oesophageal stricture or advanced oesophagitis. A widely used method for the study of acid reflux is the measurement of oesophageal pH (4). Short term recordings during the day are less reliable than overnight measurements in the detection of pathological reflux and differentiation from reflux after meals (5).

Many patients claim that symptoms are most troublesome during activities at work which involve bending or stooping or any manoeuvres which involve an increase in intra-abdominal pressure.

Twenty four hour oesophageal pH monitoring may allow identification of high risk patients (6). Hitherto it has been impossible to monitor oesophageal pH in ambulatory patients at work or in the home; the flexible pH electrode technique involves continuous intubation, is unpleasant for the patient, and cannot be used (7) during activities at work. Radiotelemetry devices provide an attractive alternative. Early capsules suffered from electrical and temperature drift and proved unsuitable in clinical practice (8), but the development of an improved capsule (Model 7006 Rigel Research) and a portable receiving system have made the present study possible.

Patients and Methods

Patients

Oesophageal pH was monitored for 24 hours in 10 patients with a mean age of 45.5 years (SD $\pm$ 12.02). Symptoms were graded and oesophagitis graded at endoscopy and biopsy according to the criteria defined by Reid and Davis (9). Each patient was provided with a diet sheet detailing food and drinks with a pH value of < pH 5 to be avoided during ambulatory studies. Relevant medication for oesophageal reflux was witheld for the period of the test.

Procedure

The pH sensitive rtc measured 28mm x 6.6mm and utilised a coloured glass electrode and a self-contained reference cell to measure pH in the range pH 1 to pH 9, a small mercury battery, a transducer and a transmitter. The activated reference cap functions for up to 10 days from the time of initial activation and the battery life is approximately 40 days, sufficient for a number of studies. Overall drift is sufficiently low ($\pm$ 0.5 pH unit for 24 hours) to enable longterm continuous recording of pH within the body. The rtc was sterilised in a solution of 0.1% Cetrimide for 3-4 hours and calibrated in buffer solutions at pH 4.5, 9.0 and 7.0. The rtc was swallowed without difficulty and tethered in the oesophagus by a small bore polyvinyl tube (OD 0.54mm) which was attached to a thin silastic sleeve fitting tightly around the capsule. It was positioned 5cm proximal to the lower oesophageal sphincter high proximal zone, previously determined by oesophageal manometry. A 5cm length of clinifeed tubing was guided over the polyvinyl tube and positioned at the angle of the mouth to minimise discomfort. Graduation marks are visible through the clinifeed tubing, and following fixation of the polyvinyl tube to a metal t-piece this was taped in position to the cheek. The rtc was re-calibrated at the conclusion of each study to determine the degree of drift during the test, the recordings being considered acceptable if drift was less than one pH unit per 24 hour period of recording.

Outpatient Studies

Outpatient studies were performed using a portable receiving and recording system. This consists of a battery operated FM receiver and combined switching unit which recorded on to a Medilog 4-channel cassette recorder (Oxford Medical Systems Ltd). The portable receiver, previously described by us, and the Medilog recorder weigh only 1 Kg and are comfortably worn by the patient during normal activities at work and in the home. At night, the patient continues to wear the chest aerial belt, the waistbelt containing receiver and

recorder being placed at the bedside allowing the patient to turn
freely during sleep. Signals recorded on tape were replayed on
standard Oxford highspeed replay equipment and periods of gastro-
oesophagel reflux analysed.

Recognition of Artefact

Artefactual changes in records of oesophageal pH monitoring occur as
the result of signal loss. A simultaneous recording of signal
strength on a separate channel of the Medilog recorder enabled
periods of signal loss on ambulatory recording to be easily
identified (Fig. 1).

Inpatient Studies

Inpatient studies were also undertaken on the same group of 10

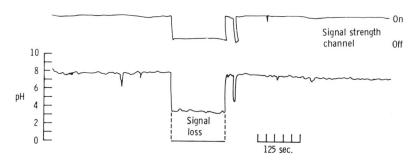

Fig. 1   Temporary signal losses in the pH recording indicated by
the addition of a signal strength channel.

patients using the same rtc. Signals were detected by a standard
receiver (Model 7040 Rigel Research, Sutton) and aerial switching
unit (Model 7043 Rigel Research, Sutton), permitting the frequency
changes which result from pH variation to be measured. A continuous
recording was achieved using a conventional pen recorder (Grass
Polygraph, Quincy, Mass, U.S.A.).

Handling the data

Reflux episodes have been defined as a sharp fall in pH of at least 2
pH units followed by a slow return to the baseline, the duration of
each reflux episode being dependent upon clearance of the oesophagus
by swallowing. (Fig.2) Subject to the condition that there was a
fall in pH of > 2 pH units, the following calculations were made for
each 24 hour outpatient and inpatient recording:

Number and duration of reflux episodes with a fall in pH to $< $ pH 5.

Number and duration of reflux episodes with a fall in pH to $< $ pH 4.

Twenty four hour recordings were analysed as day and night records

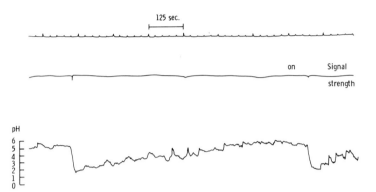

125 sec.

on   Signal

strength

pH
6
5
4
3
2
1
0

Fig. 2   pH recording during an ambulatory reflex episode of
18 minutes duration.

for a 16 hour day (6.30 am to 10.30 pm) and an 8 hour night (10.30 pm
to 6.30 am).   All the data was analysed using the X^2 test for
individual patient's records and the student unpaired t test for
group results.

Results

Number of reflux episodes

The mean number of reflux episodes with a fall in pH to < pH 5 was
significantly greater during the day and night for outpatients when
compared to hospitalised patients (t = 3.73, p<0.01, t = 2.12, p<0.05
respectively (Fig. 3), and greater during the day than at night for
both ambulatory outpatient and inpatient investigations (t = 3.39, p
< 0.01, t + 3.33, p < 0.01 respectively) (Table 1).

Duration of reflux episodes

The mean duration per hour of acid reflux episodes with a fall in pH
to less than pH 5 was significantly greater during the day for
outpatients than for inpatient studies (t = 2.22, p < 0.05) (Fig.4),
and greater during the day than at night for outpatient studies (t =
2.40, p < 0.05) (Table 2).

Relationship of symptoms, endoscopy and acid perfusion tests to acid reflux episodes

Four patients with mild (grade 1 to 2) symptoms had significantly
more episodes with a fall in pH to less than pH 5 during two hours of
recording when studied as ambulatory outpatients than as inpatients

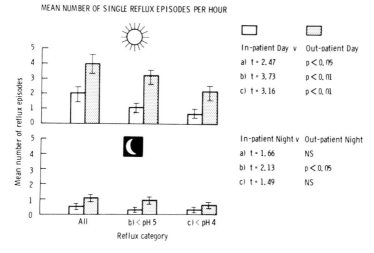

MEAN NUMBER OF SINGLE REFLUX EPISODES PER HOUR

In-patient Day v Out-patient Day
a) t = 2.47   p < 0.05
b) t = 3.73   p < 0.01
c) t = 3.16   p < 0.01

In-patient Night v Out-patient Night
a) t = 1.66   NS
b) t = 2.13   p < 0.05
c) t = 1.49   NS

Fig. 3   A comparison of the frequency of reflux episodes during
          ambulatory and inpatient recordings.

Table I.

MEAN NUMBER OF SINGLE REFLUX EPISODES PER HOUR ($\pm$ S.E.M.)

	In-Patient				Out-Patient		
	All	Fall to pH < 5	Fall to pH < 4		All	Fall to pH < 5	Fall to pH < 4
Day	2.10 ($\pm$ 0.36)	1.06 ($\pm$ 0.20)	0.64 ($\pm$ 0.16)	Day	3.98 ($\pm$ 0.67)	3.19 ($\pm$ 0.54)	2.08 ($\pm$ 0.43)
Night	0.49 ($\pm$ 0.27)	0.23 ($\pm$ 0.16)	0.22 ($\pm$ 0.14)	Night	1.10 ($\pm$ 0.30)	1.03 ($\pm$ 0.34)	0.70 ($\pm$ 0.29)
Total per 2 hours	2.59 ($\pm$ 0.57)	1.28 ($\pm$ 0.31)	0.85 ($\pm$ 0.26)	Total	4.98 ($\pm$ 0.80)	4.22 ($\pm$ 0.72)	2.78 ($\pm$ 0.57)

Number of reflux episodes during the day and night for
ambulatory and inpatient studies.

Table II.

MEAN DURATION (MINUTES) PER HOUR OF ACID REFLUX EPISODES (± S.E.M.)

	In-Patient				Out-Patient		
	All	Fall to pH < 5	Fall to pH < 4		All	Fall to pH < 5	Fall to pH < 4
Day	14.0 (± 3.4)	6.5 (± 2.0)	2.7 (± 1.1)	Day	22.8 (± 3.2)	17.2 (± 3.5)	7.8 (± 2.6)
Night	3.2 (± 1.2)	1.8 (± 1.2)	0.6 (± 0.5)	Night	8.6 (± 3.0)	6.2 (± 2.9)	4.3 (± 2.8)
Total per 2 hours	17.1 (± 4.4)	8.3 (± 2.9)	3.3 (± 1.5)	Total per 2 hours	31.3 (± 5.6)	23.5 (± 6.1)	12.1 (± 5.2)

Duration of reflux episodes during the day and night for ambulatory and inpatient studies.

(t = 6.08, p < 0.001) (Table 3). Similarly five patients with mild (grade 1 to 2) endoscopy findings had significantly more and longer episodes with a fall in pH to < pH 5 per two hours of recording time as ambulatory outpatients than as inpatients (t = 4.05, p < 0.01, t = 2.40, p < 0.05 consecutively) Table 3). Six patients underwent an acid perfusion test and all demonstrated a positive result. Again they had more frequent and longer episodes with a fall in pH to < pH 5 for two hours of recording time as ambulatory outpatients than as

Table III.

Patient Initial	Symptom Grade	Endoscopy Grade	Acid Perfusion Test	No. of Reflux Episodes		Duration of Reflux Episodes	
				In-pt	Out-pt	In-pt	Out-pt
P. H.	2	3	+	1.08	7.06	0.6	9.58
J. H.	4	1	+	0.89	5.45	4.51	29.67
D. H.	2	3	+	0	4.01	0	46.18
F. C.	3	1	+	1.35	1.5	4.19	14.06
B. E.	1	1	+	1.76	6.03	16.16	12.45
P. K.	3	4		3.47	6.78	27.46	66.01
B. W.	3	4		1.79	0.79	9.63	0.48
P. B.	4	1		1.13	4.25	17.56	21.59
G. G.	2	1		0.13	4.91	0.07	20.67
R. L	3	2	+	1.23	1.41	3.17	13.9

Comparison of symptoms and endoscopy grades to number and duration (mins) of acid reflux episodes with a fall in pH < 5 per two hours of recording for both ambulatory and inpatient studies.

inpatients (t = 3.19, p < 0.01, t = 2.58, p < 0.05 respectively (Table 3). Only one patient, BW, with severe symptoms and marked endoscopy findings (Table 3) was found to have had more and longer episodes as an inpatient than as an outpatient; we believe that in this case, as symptoms were severe, antacids may have been taken during the study, contrary to express instructions.

Discussion

We have found the tethered pH sensitive radio telemetry capsule in conjunction with a portable receiver and recorder to be a reliable, accurate and acceptable means of monitoring oesophageal reflux in the ambulatory subject. Signal loss and drift are sufficiently low to enable long term 24 hour monitoring of oesophageal pH in patients carrying out everyday activities, including in some cases heavy manual work. The capsule was well tolerated by our subjects who were able to eat and sleep without difficulty; indeed 30% of our patients had repeat tests which might have been refused with more conventional methods using an indwelling pH probe.

Using this method we have demonstrated that contrary to popular belief, there is a greater incidence of oesophageal reflux during the day than at night, especially for the ambulatory studies. More importantly, we have shown that the mean number and duration of reflux episodes with a fall to below pH 5 are significantly greater for an ambulatory outpatient than for the same person as an inpatient. The differences are less at night (Fig. 3) not surprisingly since the night activities for both in and outpatients may be presumed to be very similar.

The daytime difference is important because it indicates that patients with severe symptoms, but little evidence of either endoscopic or histological oesophagitis, may well be classified as normal during a hospital test despite severe reflux at home, thus delaying diagnosis, appropriate management, and the prevention of more serious complications.

We would thus recommend ambulatory assessment as described, as being more sensitive than conventional methods and giving a more realistic assessment of the problem in the patient's everyday environment. It can show, for example whether food or physical activity is the primary factor initiating the onset of acid reflux.

It may also assist in predicting those patients who are most likely to benefit from surgical correction.

References

1.   Colson R.H., Watson B.W., (1979) 209-212, Ed. Amlaner Jnr, C.J., MacDonald D.W. Pergamon Press, Oxford, New York.
2.   Evans D.F., Foster G., Hardcastle J.D., Slater E. Proceedings of IIIrd International Ambulatory Monitoring Symposium 1979, Ed. Stott, Academic Press, London & New York, 415-421.
3.   Lipschutz W.H.,in: Recent Advances in Gastroenterology (1976) 3, 1-26, Ed. Bouchier I.A.D. Churchill-Livingstone (Edinburgh, London, New York).
4.   Irvin T.T., Perez-Avila C., (1977) Scan.J.Gastroenterol. 12 (6),

715-720.
5.   Atkinson M., Van Gelder A., Amer.J.Dig.Dis. (1977) 22, 365-370.
6.   Demeester T.R., Johnson L.F., Joseph G.J., Toschano M.S., Hall
     A.W., Skinner D.B. Ann. Surg. (1976) 184-459.
7.   Wallin L., Marsden T., Boesby S., Sorensen O., Scan.J. Gastro-
     enterol. (1979) 14 (4), 481-487.
8.   Baron J.H., Clinical Tests of Gastric Secretion, Histology,
     Methodology, Interpretation (1978), Macmillan Press Ltd. (Lon-
     don, Basingstoke).
9.   Reed P.I., Davies W.A., Am.J.Dig.Dis (1978) 23   No.2, 161-165.

Discussion

DR. PHILLIPSON: I think that paper was fascinating. Mr. Evans said
that most people feel that reflux happens more at night. My
impression in talking to patients has been that on history numerous
symptoms during the day can be elicited which usually fail to show up
at night - just as demonstrated with the oesophageal overnight pH
monitoring.
MR. EVANS: We were rather surprised at this finding. The study is
obviously being continued. It was felt that it might be an erroneous
finding with such a small number of patients, but there is exactly
the same finding as the numbers of patients increase.
DR. PHILLIPSON: Where is it being positioned? Mr. Evans said that
it is previously determined by manometry. Is it lower or middle-
third?
MR. EVANS: It is positioned 5 cm above the high pressure zone of the
lower oesophageal sphincter.
DR. PHILLIPSON: Secondly, how is the capsule calibrated in terms of
its pH?
MR. EVANS: It is calibrated in three buffer solutions, at pH 4, 7
and 9, in a 37° water bath. They are temperature sensitive, of
course, so it is important to calibrate at the temperature at which
they are used.
DR. PHILLIPSON: Is the calibration reasonably stable?
MR. EVANS: Previous pH-sensitive radiotelemetry capsules have
suffered from drift problems to such a marked degree that they have
been little used in the clinical situation. This particular capsule
has drift characteristics of typically less than one-half of a pH
unit for a whole 24 hour period. In fact, calibration is repeated at
the end of a study, and if the calibration is greater than one pH
unit of drift that study is discarded. However, that has not
happened very often.
DR. MILES: I, too, am fascinated by this paper; I suspect that the
motivations of Dr. Phillipson and myself are very similar, working as
we do in a sleep disorders clinic. Of course in many patients who
are referred to our clinic with nocturnal arousals, choking or
regurgitation, and even with peculiar nocturnal choking attacks, it
enters strongly into the differential diagnosis of sleep apnoea when
they seem genuinely to have attacks of laryngeal spasm. It is a big
problem in our clinical practice because it requires a physician to
go in to put the tube down. I suppose that this capsule could be put
down during the day and still be there in the evening when the

recording is occurring. It is a beautiful technique. Many other centres also put a lot of reliance on acid-clearing tests. Has Mr. Evans used those tests during the night, or during these procedures?

MR. EVANS: Half (6) of the patients had the Berstein test, an acid perfusion test, and 5 of them were positive. Acid clearance is not done with this particular system, we find that the patients provide enough acid of their own. The duration of reflux is measured as well as the number of episodes of reflux, which provides an 'index' of oesophageal clearance.

MR. WOLFF: Perhaps I misinterpreted it, but I had the impression from the Table (the third from the last) that the correlation betwen time of reflux and either symptoms or endoscopy scale was almost non-existent. Measurements were made - people who were refluxing, for instance, 64% of the time seemed to have a scale which was 2 in one case and 1 in another, whereas people with much smaller degrees of reflux had much higher ratings. Has Mr. Evans any sort of feeling about whether these things are related at all?

MR. EVANS: Indeed, we have. This is the great problem of oesophageal function tests that there is no correlation between either symptoms and endoscopy or symptoms and actual acid reflux. There is great controversy in oesophageal circles, about whether any meaningful information is to be gained from oesophageal function tests. Some workers say that there is a good correlation between endoscopy and the degree of oesophagitis and the degree of reflux, whereas other workers find no correlation - which is what we find.

MR. WOLFF: So when this is said to be of benefit to the patient, it is not in fact any benefit?

MR. EVANS: We are hoping that with an ambulatory study we may have a more meaningful measure of acid reflux than the studies that are performed in hospital. Eight out of the 10 patients using a scoring system devised by Demester in the States fell into this category, yet they had proven oesophagitis. However, all but one of those 8 in the outpatient studies had positive scores. We are therefore saying that this is a better test than the hospital test.

DR. SACKNER: One of the other commonly held beliefs is that nocturnal asthma may be precipitated by reflux. First, has Mr. Evans looked at distance reflux by pulling back the pH electrodes so that it is possible to see how far the reflux goes - not 5 cm above, but perhaps higher?

   Secondly, has he considered studying patients who are awakened at night with asthmatic episodes to see whether this reflux might be occuring?

MR. EVANS: In answer to the first question, no we have not - the only studies that have been performed are at the 5 cm position. It would be interesting to do what Dr. Sackner suggests.

   Secondly, we have not even thought about looking at asthmatics at night. There is a clinician in Salford, Bancowitz, who is investigating this. His hypothesis is that it is the acid reflux oesophagitis that is causing the awakening, and possibly causing the asthmatic attacks.

DR. PHILLIPSON: With regard to the correlations, Mr. Evans does not need me to come to his defence, but the fact that there was poor correlation between various patients in terms of their symptoms and the degree of reflux is not the critical aspect. It is the fact that reflux can be demonstrated in the individual patient. Very often the clinical problem is the patient who has symptoms - chest pain, chest discomfort - day or night, and it is not sure whether it is due to reflux, angina or indeed some other disturbance. The demonstration of reflux in such a patient where it is suspected clinically provides confirmatory evidence. The fact that another patient with the same degree of reflux has no symptoms is fine; but another patient may have the same degree of coronary artery narrowing and still have no angina. My feeling is that this is useful in the individual patient, rather than simply trying to make correlations among various patients.

MR. EVANS: This system was used initially with proven refluxes to prove the efficacy of the system. There was one patient (whom I showed) with severe chest pain who had little proven reflux. Since the test was performed he has had his hiatal hernia repaired - we hope that that is our first successful case.

CALIBRATION TECHNIQUES FOR THE RESPIRATORY INDUCTIVE PLETHYSMOGRAPH

H. WATSON, A. SCHNEIDER, S. BIRCH, T. CHADHA, W.M. ABRAHAM
M.A. COHN AND M.A. SACKNER

Division of Pulmonary Disease, Department of Medicine,
Mt. Sinai Medical Centre, Miami Beach, Florida 33140, USA

Summary

The purpose of this study was to review existing calibration techniques and introduce a new calibration technique for the Respiratory
Inductive Plethysmograph. Existing calibration techniques discussed
include:
(a)   The isovolume angle manoeuvre (1)
(b)   The Stagg, Goldman, Davis method (3), and
(c)   The simultaneous equation method (2, 4).
A new two body position calibration technique is described and its
extension to a single position method is also described. These
calibration procedures were compared to spirometry with changes in
body posture, to each other, and to isovolume angle determinations.
We conclude that:
(a)   The accuracy of the new calibration technique is greater,
      or equal to the other methods, when body position is
      altered, and,
(b)   That isovolume angle calibration in a single position pro-
      vides the most accurate calibration of rib cage to abdom-
      inal contribution, but only in the position calibrated.

Introduction

In 1967, Kono and Mead described a method of measuring respiration
using magnetometery and devised a single position method for calibrating the device (1). In 1977, Cohn et al described repiratory
inductive plethysmograph (RIP) and another method of calibration
using data from two positions (2). The first technique required a
trained subject and maintained volume accuracy only in the position
used for calibration, while the second technique used natural breathing and maintained volume accuracy in all positions, but it was
subject to mathematical distortions, when calculating compartmental
gains.
    Ideally, a calibration technique should:
1.   Be done in a single position
2.   Require no patient co-operation
3.   Minimize the time spent breathing on a spirometer
4.   Provide simple calculation of compartmental gains, and
5.   Remain valid in all positions for long periods of time.
We have devised a new method of calibrating the RIP that is not

ideal, but it combines some properties of the previous techniques, is simpler to calculate, and generally produces more accurate results. The purpose of this study is to review the methods for the calibrfation of the RIP and review previous studies comparing these methods for volume and compartmental distribution accuracy.

Methods

A common calibration feature considered is the rib cage (RC) and abdominal (AB) channels can be scaled against an internal reference, so the gains of each channel can be increased or decreased a known percentage against that reference. All calibration procedures begin with the gains of the two compartments equal and set to a value of 1.00. The electrical sum of the two scaled signals is generated internally and available as the sum output. A spirometer (SP) is used for the measurement of known volumes. Generally, there are two ways to compute the sum. One is to determine correctly the proportion of the rib cage and abdomen, sum them, and scale this output to match spirometry. The second way is to proportion and scale, correctly, the rib cage and abdominal signals and finally sum them for output. The second way is preferred because it provides correct volumes for all three signals of the rib cage, abdomen and the sum.

Isovolume angle manoeuvre (ISV)
      This method has been described previously (1). Figure 1a shows a typical trace obtained from an isovolume angle calibration. A graphic display is used where the rib cage signal is shown on the

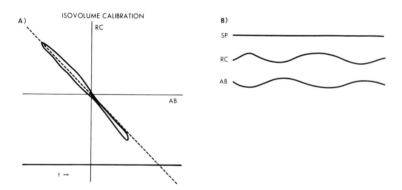

Fig. 1   Isovolume angle calibration technique. A: X-Y plot of
            isovolume manoeuvre (RC vs AB). B: Scalar plot of
            isovolume manoeuvre (SP, RC, AB vs time).

ordinate and the abdominal signal is shown on abscissa. The graphic display scaling is such that identical inputs will produce a trace of 45° for the line of identity. Figure 1b shows a time trace of the two compartments illustrating the movement of volumes from one compartment to the other.

The spirometer trace does not vary indicating that there is no movement of air in and out of the lungs during the manoeuvre. Actually, the tubing to the spirometer is closed off during the manoeuvre and the subject is asked to move as much volume as possible, back and forth, between the rib cage and abdomen with a standard continuous monitor of mouth presssure to assure there is no compression of the thoracic gas volume. Typically, mouth pressures should be less than $\pm$ 20 cmH$_2$0 during the manoeuvre. The gain of one of the two compartments is then raised or lowered to adjust the trace on the graphic display so that it reaches the 45 degree line. The sum output is then recorded against spirometry and the final proportional difference between the sum and the spirometer is established. Having done this, the individual gains of the rib cage and abdominal compartments are equally adjusted to compensate for the sum's proportion against spirometry.

Stagg, Goldman, David Method (SGD)

This method has been previously described and the calculations detailed (3). It makes the assumption that implicit in spontaneous breathing is enough variability both within and between breaths to determine the proportionality of the rib cage and abdominal compartments as well as the sum's proportionality to spirometry. This variability is attributed to a curvi-linear relationship of the rib cage and abdominal movement during natural breathing and the normal breath-to-breath variability. This approach is in effect a computerized way of calculating a miniature isovolume distribution during spontaneous breathing. We have placed two practical constraints on this technique. The first is that we limit data collection to a fixed time of 20 seconds, because the subject is re-breathing on a spirometer, and secondly, we assume the calculated values are stable at the end of the 20-second period. The technique uses only one posture (usually supine) and data are collected at 20 points per second for the rib cage, abdomen and spirometer signals. Delta values are calculated for each new sampled point as the difference between the new point and its previous mean. Means and standard deviations are accumulated on a point-by-point basis, using these deltas. Running correlation coefficients are computed for the rib cage against the abdomen, the rib cage against the spirometer, and the abdomen against the spirometer. Two parameters are derived from all these measured values, which are the correlation of the computed sum against spirometry and the ratio of the abdominal to rib cage gains. Finally, the rib cage and abdominal gains are computed. All these calculations are done 20 times a second and a time weighed window average is used to derive the final values at the end of 20 seconds. This window average (OLD = 0.8(OLD) + 0.2 (NEW)) is exponentially shaped with time and has a time constant of approximately 6 samples or 0.3 seconds.

Simultaneous Equation Method (SEQ)

This method is one that uses two postures and has been previously described (2). Figure 2 summarizes the method, which uses data recorded usually in the supine and standing postures. Delta volumes ($V_{max}-V_{min}$) are calculated for the spirometer, rib cage and abdominal signals in each of the two postures. These measured delta

values are then substituted in the equations shown and the rib cage
and abdominal gains are solved. In practice, we collect 20 seconds
of data at 20 points per second and measure the maximum and minimum
of each breath during that period. The maximum and minimum points
are determined from the spirometer and the corresponding time point
values are measured for the rib cage and abdomen traces. Deltas are
arbitrarily paired from the supine and standing data collections and

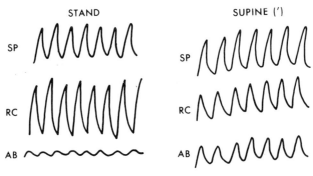

$$K(RC) + L(AB) = SP$$

SOLVE

$$K = \frac{(AB')(SP) - (AB)(SP')}{(RC)(AB') - (RC')(AB)}$$

$$L = -\frac{(RC')(SP) - (RC)(SP')}{(RC)(AB') - (RC')(AB)}$$

Fig. 2   Simultaneous equation technique – raw data from the
standing and supine positions used for calibration and the
algebraic solution for RC and AB gains.

the gains are computed for each available pair and then averaged,
yielding a mean, standard deviation and standard error for each gain.
The included statistics give an indication of the scatter of the data
and the reproducibility of the means. Scatter can be reduced by
using only the middle-half or third of a breath as a delta, which
tends to eliminate reactive phase irregularities at the beginnings of
inspiration and expiration.

In application, the solution of the gains is sensitive to the
denominator either being zero, or close to zero, resulting in the
calculations being either infinity, or at least skewed, so as not to
reflect accurately the true gains. This was evidenced as a need to
calculate a separation factor (4) as an indicator of the proximity of
this unwanted condition.

Least Squares Method (LSQ)
This method is a new method that combines qualities of the
previous methods to yield one that has increased accuracy and ease of
application (5). considering the following equations

$$RC + AB = 0 \qquad (1)$$
$$RC + AB = SP \qquad (2)$$
$$RC/SP + AB/SP = 1 \qquad (3)$$

Equation 1 is the equation of the model used for the ISV and SGD methods; equation 2 is used for the SEQ method, and equation 3 is the relationship used for the new least squares approach. Equation 3 reflects the proportionality of the sum of two compartments equalling a constant value as in the ISV method and being calculated with the spirometer as a reference as in the SEQ method. Figure 3 shows the graph of equation 3 as the solid line. This solid line has the same

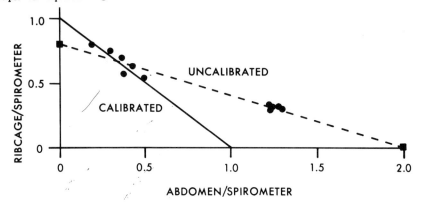

Fig. 3   Least squares method for calculation of RC and AB gains. Calibrated line (solid line), uncalibrated ratios (dots), least squares regression line (dotted line), X and Y intercepts (squares). See text for details.

slope as the isovolume line and its X and Y intercepts are 1.0 compared to the isovolume line intercepts of zero. Considering the calibrated line, if all the air from a breath goes into the rib cage, then the RC/SP ratio is 1.0. Conversely, if all the air from a breath goes into the abdominal compartment, the AB/SP ratio is 1.0. For all other distributions of ventilation then, the points would lie somewhere on the solid line if the respiratory inductive plethysmograph was correctly calibrated. In practice, data are collected for the spirometer, rib cage and abdomen in two positions, in the same manner, as the SEQ method. Delta values for the three signals are measured for each breath as $(V_{max} - V_{min})$ for each of the two postures and then the RC/SP and AB/SP ratios are calculated. The deltas for each breath can then be plotted as co-ordinate pairs with the RC/SP as the Y values and the AB/SP as the X values as in Figure 3. The solid line in Figure 3 is the graph of the calibrated line given by equation 3. The points denoted by (0) are the co-ordinate pairs measured from a data collection run, such as shown in Figure 2. The points in the upper left of Figure 3 correspond to the standing position run, and the points in the lower eft correspond to the supine run. A line (represented by the dotted line) can then be drawn through the uncalibrated points described by the raw data co-ordinate pairs. The minimum error line through these points can be derived with a least squares fit through all the raw data co-ordinate pairs. The X and Y intercepts for the uncalibrated line can then be derived. Multiplying the dotted line by the reciprocals of its X and Y intercepts rotates the dotted line back to the calibrated line,

since the calibrated line's intercepts are 1.0 and multiplication of
a value by its reciprocal yields a result of 1.0. Thus, the LSQ
calibration technique can be summarized as follows:

1. Collect the raw data in each of two positions and measure
    the RC, AB and SP deltas.
2. Compute the ratios RC/SP and AB/SP for each breath in the
    two positions.
3. Compute a least squares fit through all of the data where
    each breath's RC/SP value is used as the Y value, and the
    AB/SP value is used as the X value. Both positions data
    are fed into the same fit calculation.
4. Compute the X and Y intercepts. The RC calibration factor
    is the reciprocal of the Y intercept, and the AB calibra-
    tion factor is the reciprocal of the X intercept.

Figure 4 shows the resulting differences in the distribution of
ventilation in seven positions and how the differences shift up and
down on the calibration line. Also listed in Figure 4 are the percent
differences from spirometry for each of the seven postures.

It can be seen from Figure 3, that the changes in distribution
need not be as large as the ones occurring between the standing and
supine positions. In fact, only a slight difference in distribution
is required and any suitable method can be employed to accomplish
this.

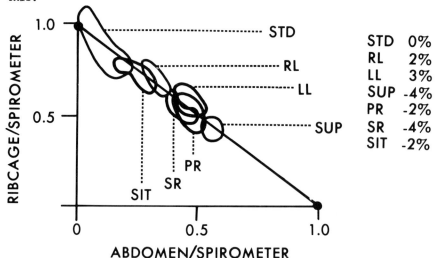

Fig. 4   Distributions of ventilation in the standing, right and
          left lateral, supine, prone, semi-recumbent and sitting
          positions with loops outlining the clustered areas
          obtained for each position. Also shown are the percent
          differences from spirometry in each position.

Extended Least Squares Method (XLSQ)
     This method is an extension of the LSQ method with the same
assumptions as the SGD technique, i.e. the method assumes there is
enough change within the distribution of ventilation during normal
breathing to allow the graphic calculation of the rib cage and abdo-

minal gains, using the method of the LSQ technique. Since the LSQ technique uses the ratios RC/SP and AB/SP, it is necessary to have finitely large values to prevent division by zero or skewing of the gains by near division by zero. Therefore, an extended sampling technique was devised to allow the LSQ calculation to be used with data collected at 20 point a second and still have large values for the rib cage, abdomen and spirometer, thereby preventing distortion of the calculations.

Figure 5 illustrates the transformation done on the data to get 20 samples a second, with the equivalent of a whole breath volume. If it is assumed that respiration is a sinusoidal shape, and that sinusoid is integrated for half of its period, the resulting integral is the amplitude of the sinusoid (Figure 5a). If the sinusoid is then fullwave rectified, the integration can be started at any point in the sinusoid and the same result will be obtained. Full wave rectification here is defined as making every part of the waveform positive with respect to the first point used as a reference. This is illustrated in Figure 5b.

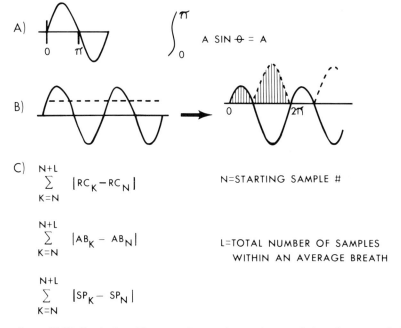

A) $\int_0^\pi A \, SIN \, \theta = A$

B)

C) $\sum_{K=N}^{N+L} |RC_K - RC_N|$ N=STARTING SAMPLE #

$\sum_{K=N}^{N+L} |AB_K - AB_N|$ L=TOTAL NUMBER OF SAMPLES
WITHIN AN AVERAGE BREATH

$\sum_{K=N}^{N+L} |SP_K - SP_N|$

Fig. 5   XLSQ Method: The sampling algorithm used in the extended least squares calculation. (A) Basic observations. (B) Illustration of applied transform. (C) Actual transform used.

If this same integration is done on the whole period of the full wave rectified sinusoid, then the final value would be twice the amplitude of the sinusoid. This type of transform integrated over the whole period of a waveform will always give a positive finite value for any type of a period waveform. Since the LSQ calculation uses

the RC/SP and AB/SP ratios, the exact scaling of the integration of
the above transform is not required when the same transform is applied to all three signals. Figure 5c shows the exact transform used
on the signals and represents the digital implementation of the
integration and full wave rectification, that is accomplished by
summing up the absolute values of the differences between the present
samples and the first reference sample point. These summations are
computed over an amount of time equal to the duration of an average
breath. That average breath is determined by computing the average
time of all breaths sampled within the 20 second sample of data.

Review of Previous Studies

Validation
        Our validation procedure is one that measures the sum signal of
the respiratory inductive plethysmograph and the spirometer simultaneously for 20 second at 20 points per second during natural breathing. The maximum and minimum of each breath are identified on the
spirometer signal and the corresponding time points are identified on
the respiratory inductive plethysmograph sum. The volume of each
breath as measured by both devices is then the maximum less the
minimum for each breath. The difference of the respiratory inductive
plethysmograph less the spirometer is then expressed as a percent of
the spirometer volume for each breath. Means and standard deviations
of these percents are calculated for the whole sampling period and
these means are what we refer to as the percent difference from
spirometry obtained from our validation procedure. Validations are
done routinely after calibrations, and in all studies, calibrations
are accepted only if the corresponding validation is within $\pm$ 10%,
of spirometry. If the validation results are greater than $\pm$ 10%,
the calibration process is repeated. If the validation is still
unsatisfactory, the position of either the rib cage or abdominal
bands, or both, are shifted by a few centimetres. The majority of
our subjects have been calibrated satisfactorily with one or two
trials. Once calibrated, validations can be done any time, to monitor, continually, the accuracy of the respiratory inductive plethysmograph.
        Isovolume angles can be used to assess the proportional accuracy
with which the rib cage and abdominal components have been calibrated. At angles of 46 and 47°, abdominal displacement relative to
rib cage displacement would be under-estimated by 3.4% and 6.7%; at
angles of 44 and 43° abdominal displacement would be over-estimated
by 3.6% and 7.2% relative to rib cage displacement (6). Since we
accept validations of $\pm$ 10% of spirometry, corresponding isovolume
angles of 45° $\pm$ 3° are also acceptable.

Simultaneous Equation Method (SEQ)
        Fifteen healthy non-smokers (9 males and 6 females) whose ages
ranged from 17 to 28 years, and eighteen asymptomatic smokers (8
males and 10 females) whose ages ranged from 19 to 42 years, were
volunteers in this experiment (7). Calibrations were done using SEQ.
Seven of the smokers (3 males and 4 females) had evidence of small
airway disease as judged by testing in our laboratory. Thus, there
were 11 smokers without small airway disease (smokers NSAD) and 7

smokers (smokers SAD) with small airway disease.   Each subject was validated in each of the following positions: sitting on a chair, standing, supine, semi-recumbent at 45°, prone and right and left lateral decubiti in a standard hospital bed. No special procedure was employed for positioning the bands in relation to position and shoulder girdle. Figure 6 shows the validation results between the spirometer and respiratory inductive plethysmograph determinations of mean tidal volume for each subject in the seven positions. The average maximum and minimum of the percent differences for all sub- jects ranged from -7% to 9%, For all positions, the accuracy of the respiratory inductive plethysmograph was not significantly different among the non-smoker and smokers except for the right and left lat- eral decubitus positions. In these positions, there was a slightly greater accuracy in the smokers than the non-smokers. Considering all positions, 88% of all observations were within ± 10% of spiro- metry in all positions.

Least Squares Fit (LSQ)
        Seven sheep were prepared for the measurement of respiratory mechanics by restraining them in a cart, intubating them through one nostril and placing a balloon catheter into the lower oesophagus for estimation of pleural pressure (8).   Respiratory inductive plethysmo- graph bands were placed around the rib cage and abdomen. The LSQ method of calibration was used and the distribution of ventilation was changed one of three ways. The first two ways were by cinching either the rib cage, or the abdomen, and the third way allowed the sheep to re-breathe on the spirometer, so that as the carbon dioxide increased within the spirometer, the accompanying increase in tidal volume was sufficient to alter the distributions.
        Following calibration, the respiratory inductive plethysmograph was validated and baseline mean pulmonary resistance was measured. Subsequently, increasing doses of carbachol aerosol were administered to the animals. When sufficient broncho-spasm was achieved, the validation of the respiratory inductive plethysmograph was repeated. Figure 7 shows all had tidal volumes as measured by the respiratory inductive plethysmograph within ± 6% of spirometry on validation. Carbachol aerosol challenge resulted in mean pulmonary resistance going from a baseline of 1.5 to 8.8 $cmH_2O/1/sec$, which is an increase of 487%. Validations after challenge showed five of the sheep re- maining with ± 6% of their initial validation values, while in two others, the validation percent changed by ± 11%. These errors were most likely a result of a change in the placement of the coils during the study. The animal that had the highest absolute resistance value and largest increase in resistance, i.e. from 0.6 to 14.7 $cmH_2O/1/sec$ only, had a change of only 1% from the spirometric values from begin- ning to end of the experiment.
        Five sheep were then prepared by placing them in a cart and intubating them so validation procedures could be done (8). Once they were calibrated in the supported position, they were lifted out of their carts and allowed to stand while a second validation mea- surement was obtained. The LSQ method of calibration was used in the same manner as the broncho-provocation study. The supported valid- ation showed differences within ± 10% of spirometry, and changes less than or equal to 5% of the original validation value in four of

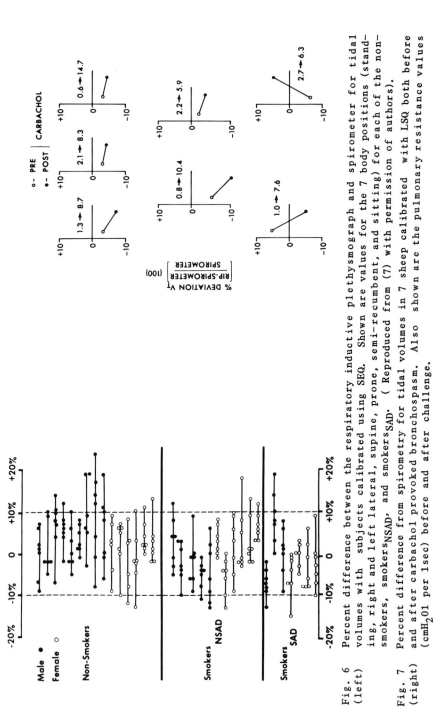

Fig. 6 (left) — Percent difference between the respiratory inductive plethysmograph and spirometer for tidal volumes with subjects calibrated using SEQ. Shown are values for the 7 body positions (standing, right and left lateral, supine, prone, semi-recumbent, and sitting) for each of the non-smokers, smokers NSAD, and smokers SAD. (Reproduced from (7) with permission of authors).

Fig. 7 (right) — Percent difference from spirometry for tidal volumes in 7 sheep calibrated with LSQ both before and after carbachol provoked bronchospasm. Also shown are the pulmonary resistance values (cmH₂0l per 1sec) before and after challenge.

the five animals after position change. The largest difference observed was 8% in one animal, but all changes were still within ± 10% of spirometry.

Validation Versus Isovolume Angle

Eight subjects were calibrated using LSQ and then validated in the prone, left and right lateral, supine, standing, sitting and semi-recumbent positions. Isovolume angles were also determined at functional residual capacity, near total lung capacity, and near residual volume for each subject in all positions (7). The functional residual capacity angles compared against the percent differences in tidal volume validations showed that 50% of 56 observations fell within ± 3⁰ of the 45⁰. This compares to the accuracy of the validations where 86% of the values fell within ± 10% of spirometry. In 16 instances, the isovolume angle was ≥ 50⁰ or ≤ 40⁰ and yet the deviation of the validations was less than ± 5% of spirometry. In six instances, the isovolume angle was within ± 3⁰ of 45⁰, the validation results ranged from -10% to -20% and from 10% to 20%.

Figure 8 shows the isovolume angles for all three lung volumes for each subject in all positions. In 45% of all observations, the isovolume angles at the 3 lung volumes were parallel (within ± 2⁰ of 45⁰). In others, wide variation of the isovolume slopes as a function of lung volume were observed, but the data did not correlate with the magnitudes of volume differences between respiratory inductive plethysmography and spirometry.

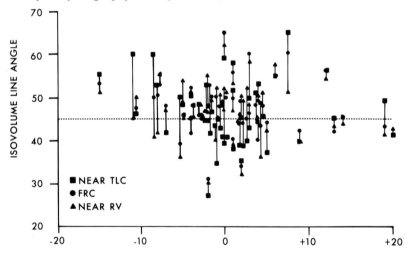

% DIFFERENCE BETWEEN
RESPIRATORY INDUCTIVE PLETHYSMOGRAPHY AND SPIROMETRY

Fig. 8   Plot of isovolume angle (degrees) versus percent difference from spirometry for eight subjects in seven different body positions while breathing quietly at functional residual capacity (FRC), mean total lung capacity (TLC), and mean residual volume (RV). (Reproduced from (7) with permission of authors)

New Studies of Calibration Procedures

Comparison Among Methods
   In this study, raw data were recalled from the computer that
were collected on 10 normals in the position validation study (7).
As pointed out, the calibration runs were selected for the lowest
validation error using the SEQ technique. The standing and supine
positions were recalled and the LSQ calibration done as a comparative
two-position calibration. Additionally, the SGD and XLSQ calibrations were done on the data from the supine position only. Validation runs were then done on the exact same data from the prone, left
and right lateral, supine, standing, sitting and semi-recumbent positions using each set of calibration factors (5). Figure 9 shows the
histograms of the absolute values of the validation results expressed
as percent occurrences. Taking the absolute value of the validation
results makes all the differences positive thereby increasing the
resolution of the histograms. As can be seen, the LSQ has the tight-
est distribution with 61% of all values having validation results
within ± 5%$ of spirometry. both LSQ abd SEQ had 89% and 90% of all
validations with ± 10% of spirometry. The single position calibration techniques were too noisy to give dependable calibration results.

LSQ Versus ISV
   Ten subjects were calibrated with the LSQ method, and isovolume
in the standing (ISV (stand)) and supine (ISV (supine)) positions
(9). Validations and isovolume angle determinations were then done
in the standing and supine positions after each calibration. Table 1
shows the validation results. With LSQ, there is no systematic
difference between the standing and supine positions and the data are
centred about zero per cent.

Table 1

Calibration	Position	Validation Mean ± SD		
LSQ	Stand	1.1%	±	5.1%
	Supine	−1.0%	±	5.6%
ISV (Supine)	Stand	5.0%	±	8.5%
	Supine	−0.9%	±	6.9%
ISC (Stand)	Stand	−0.7%	±	6.7%
	Supine	10.8%	±	14.5%

ISV (supine) position reflects the same degree of accurcy as LSQ, but
both positions show increased variability over LSQ. ISV (stand)
standing position reflects the same degree of accuracy as LSQ, but
the mean of the supine position is outside of the acceptable error
range of 10% and both positions again reflect increased variability
over the LSQ method.

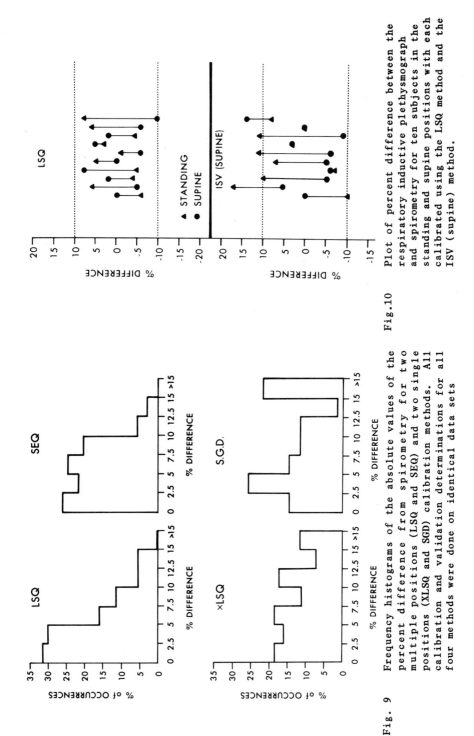

Fig. 9   Frequency histograms of the absolute values of the
percent difference from spirometry for two
multiple positions (LSQ and SEQ) and two single
positions (XLSQ and SGD) calibration methods. All
calibration and validation determinations for all
four methods were done on identical data sets

Fig. 10   Plot of percent difference between the
respiratory inductive plethysmograph
and spirometry for ten subjects in the
standing and supine positions with each
calibrated using the LSQ method and the
ISV (supine) method.

Figure 10 shows the LSQ and ISV (supine) data for all 10 subjects. All observations were within $\pm$ 10% with the LSQ method, 80% for ISV (supine) and only 65% for the ISV (standing) which is not shown. As Table 1 indicates, the LSQ validation data are centred randomly about 0%. The ISV (supine) data show that the technique gives very tight calibration 30% of the time and a much looser calibration 70% of the time.

Table 2 shows the isovolume angle results. LSQ standing, ISV (supine) supine, and ISV (stand) standing all show mean angles essentially parallel to the 45° line. ISV (supine) supine and ISV (stand) standing show little variability. Figure 11 shows the isovolume angle determinations for all three methods. As in Table 1, the figure shows the tightness of the ISV (supine) supine and the ISV (stand) standing positions. The LSQ plot illustrates the tendency of the method to split the difference between the angles and centre them about zero, with the exception of two subjects. Even though the angles on those two were both low, the validations were within $\pm$ 6% and -5% for both positions in the two subjects.

Table 2

Calibration	Position	Isovolume Angle Mean $\pm$ S.D.	
LSQ	Stand	46°	$\pm$ 5.2°
	Supine	40.2°	$\pm$ 6.1°
ISV (Supine)	Stand	50.7°	$\pm$ 6.4°
	Supine	46.1°	$\pm$ 1.7°
ISV (Stand)	Stand	46.4°	$\pm$ 1.6°
	Supine	42.4°	$\pm$ 7.2°

Conclusions

Both SEQ and LSQ methods are accurate within $\pm$ 10 of spirometry volmes in 90% of instances, no matter which body posture is assumed. The LSQ method has a higher probability (61%) of giving a validation within $\pm$ 5% of spirometry. Since the precision is still only within $\pm$ 10%, we believe that respiratory inductive plethysmography should be considered a stable, semi-quantitative method in terms of volume equivalency to spirometry. Errors tend to be random and although any single instance may appear to have a high or low error, the accuracy of the device increases with the sample size. The power of this device is its ability to monitor non-invasively the pattern of breathing for extended periods.

LSQ appears to give as good a volume calibration in a single position as an isovolume manoeuvre but the isovolume manoeuvre still provides the best compartmental proportion accuracy for a single position. The LSQ method centres the differences between its two calibration positions as can be seen in Figure 11 probably account-

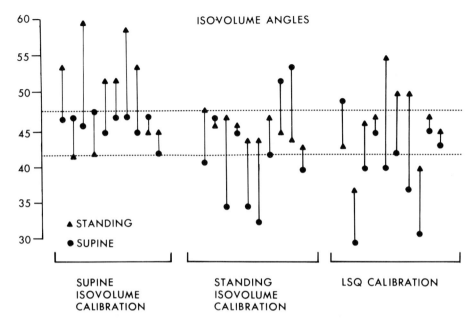

Fig.11   Plot of the isovolume angles for ten subjects in the
standing and supine positions with each calibrated using
the ISV (supine), and ISV (stand), and LSQ methods.

ing for its decreased accuracy in isovolume angles.As previously
noted, the rib cage can be 12% high and the abdomen 10% low and the
volume accuracy would still be roughly 2% (4). Going to another
position might make this proportion swing in the opposite direction,
still maintaining a tight volume accuracy. Nevertheless, there still
appears to be a loose relationship between the isovolume angle and
volume accuracy and the physiologic basis requires more investigation.

The XLSQ method can obviously be used in one or more positions,
and in fact, gives the same result as LSQ with two positions. When
applying either XLSQ or SGD in a single position, they are correct (
± 10%) about 65% of the time. This is not reliable enough for
routine calibration, but the supposition that a miniature isovolume
distribution can be calculated during spontaneous breathing is an
attractive idea. Both of the present methods could be used in conjunction with spirometry to determine these angles, but the question
of noise in the method appears to interfere with reproducibility.
Additional work in these areas might provide more accurate calibration and distribution determination methods.

Finally, in sheep we found we were not able to obtain accurate
calibrations with SEQ. The LSQ method eliminated that problem and
its increased reliability was due to the fact that only small differences in the distribution of ventilation are needed for LSQ because
of its graphic solution. The respiratory inductive plethysmograph
provided satisfactory data, both with position change and after
induced broncho-constriction.

References

1. Konno K and Mead J. (1967) J. Appl. Physiol. **22**, 407-422.
2. Cohn M.A., Watson H., Weisshaut R., Stott F. and Sackner M.A. In: ISAM 1977: Proceedings of the Second International Symposium on Ambulatory Monitoring, Eds: F.D. Stott, E.B. Raftery, P. Sleight, L. Goulding, London, Academic Press, 1978, pp. 119-128.
3. Stagg D., Goldman M. and Davis J.N. (1978) J. Appl. Physiol. **44**, 623-633.
4. Watson H. In: ISAM 1979: Proceedings of the Third International Symposium on Ambulatory Monitoring, Eds: F.D. Stott, B. Raftery L. Goulding, London, Academic Press, 1980, pp. 537-558.
5. Watson H.L., Birch S.J., Gruen W.G., Cohn M.A., Schneider A.W. and Sackner M.A. (1981) Am. Rev. Respir. Dis. **123**, 181 (Abstract).
6. Sharp J.T., Goldberg N.B., Druz W.S. and Danon J.(1976) J. Appl. Physiol. **39**, 608-618.
7. Cohn M.A., Rao A.S.V., Broudy M., Birch S., Watson H., Atkins N., Davis B., Stott F.D. and Sackner M.A. (Submitted for publication).
8. Abraham W.M., Watson H., Schneider A., King M., Yerger L. and Sackner M.A. (1981) J. Appl. Physiol. (Accepted for publication).
9. Chadha T., Birch S., Jenouri G., Schneider A., Watson H., Cohn M. and Sackner M.A. American Physiological Society (Abstract in press)

Discussion

DR. E. PHILLIPSON: Is it correct to assume that for routine clinical use, it is best to calibrate, using the least-squares in the supine posture, for a sleep study?

MR. WATSON: Two postures were used for the least-squares approach. The extended approach was trying to do it in a single posture, but I found that a single posture was too noisy. We have found that the most reliable calibrations are obtained using the two-posture least-squares approach.

MR. CROSBY: Have drift characteristics of the calibration over 24 hours, with movement of the bands been examined?

MR. WATSON: Movement of the coils will cause a change in the calibration factor. The sensitivity of the coils to movement depends on the shape of the individual on which they are placed. The gain of the coil itself is a function of the volume that it is enclosing; if it shifts up and down and the compartmental volume changes, its sensitivity will also change. As long as the coils do not move, there should be no change in the calibration characteristics.

NON-INVASIVE MEASUREMENT OF RESPIRATORY MECHANICS IN LAMBS

J.C. WOLLNER, J.E. FEWELL, P. JOHNSON

Nuffield Institute for Medical Research,
University of Oxford, UK

Introduction

The larynx is an important component of the respiratory system. Apart from its obvious protective role against aspiration, it plays an important part in ensuring an adequate lung volume and respiratory rhythm in sleep during early post-natal development in lambs (1, 2). During quiet sleep and quiet wakefulness, there is a reciprocal relationship between contraction of the diaphragm during inspiration and contraction of the thyroarytenoid (the major laryngeal adductor in sheep) during expiration. This increased expiratory resistance to gas flow provided by the larynx helps to ensure an adequate lung volume. In contrast, during rapid-eye-movement sleep, the thyroarytenoid ceases to adduct and post-inspiratory activity of the diaphragm helps to maintain lung volume; up to 45% of total diaphragmatic activity may fulfil an expiratory function. Thus, it is obvious that lung volume is protected during expiration by different mechanisms which depend upon behavioural state. These mechanisms are particularly important in young animals because they have very compliant chest walls and their breathing frequency decreases during development.

Since adduction of the larynx during expiration affects the expiratory gas flow pattern, we reasoned that this could be detected by a continuous measurement of chest and abdominal dimensions. The aim of this study was to see if a non-invasive system, suitable for use in human infants, could detect these changes in the mechanics of breathing in lambs.

Methods

Studies were done on lambs (5 to 45 days of age), several days after electrodes for the following measurements were implanted:

    Electrocorticogram, electro-oculogram, electrocardiogram and
    thyroarytenoid and diaphragm electromyograms.

These electro-physiological signals were used to assess behavioural state and also allowed us to correlate electromyographic data with non-invasive measurements using respiratory inductive plethysmoraphy.

The system used for the non-invasive measurements was the Respitrace (Ambulatory Monitoring, Inc., Ardsley, NY). This device utilizes two elastic bands, one worn around the chest and one worn around the abdomen. Into each band is sewn a coil of wire wound in such a manner so as to cause a variation in the inductance of the coil with a change on area which occurs during each respiratory excursion. The coils are fed independently by high frequency oscillators whose frequencies change in relation to the area bounded by the bands. This frequency change is converted into an analogue signal; thus three signals arise - thoracic excursion, abdominal excursion and a third signal, which if appropriately calibrated, gives a measure of tidal volume. Since we were mainly interested in the wave-form of the chest and abdominal signals, the Respitrace was set up such that their gains were equal. All signals were recorded on to a pen recorder (Beckman R411 8-channel dynograph).

Results

The effect of thyroarytenoid activity on the Respitrace waveform is shown in Figure 1.

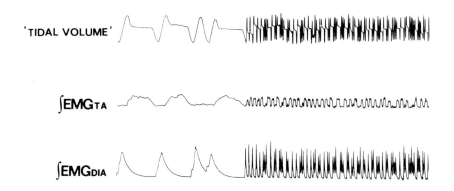

Fig. 1 Effect of thyroarytenoid activity on Respitrace waveform. $\int EMG_{TA}$ = integrated thyroarytenoid electromyogram $\int EMG_{DIA}$ = integrated diaphragm electromyogram.

Thyroarytenoid activity produces a characteristic "shoulder" on the waveform indicative of the effectiveness of the larynx in maintaining lung volume during expiration. Note that the thyroarytenoid is not active during every respiratory cycle and that the waveforms of these breaths are more symmetrical in shape.

In order to provide additional evidence that these waveform changes during expiration were related to activity of the upper airway, we made recordings from animals after tracheotomy and insertion of a fenestrated tracheostomy tube (Figure 2). When the tracheostomy was closed and the upper airway intact, thyroarytenoid activity produced a subglottic pressure of 3 to 4mmHg and the characteristic "shoulder" on the Respitrace waveform. However, when the tracheostomy was open and the upper airway bypassed, thyroarytenoid activity did not produce a positive subglottic pressure or a "shoulder" on the Respitrace waveform.

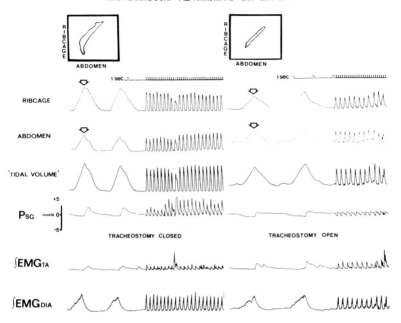

Fig. 2 Effect of tracheostomy on Respitrace waveform. P_{SG} = subglottic pressure $\int EMG_{TA}$ = integrated thyroarytenoid electromyogram $\int EMG_{DIA}$ = integrated diaphragm electromyogram.

Figure 3 shows a recording taken from a lamb as it changed sleep states (quiet sleep to rapid-eye-movement sleep to quiet sleep). as the lamb enters rapid-eye-movement sleep, rib-cage excursions decrease and the ventilation becomes almost entirely diaphragmatic. In rapid-eye-movement sleep, thyroarytenoid activity ceases and the "shoulders" on the Respitrace waveform disappear. During this time, we also plotted abdominal excursions against rib-cage excursions on an oscilloscope. Polaroid pictures of these X-Y plots were taken approximately every tenth breath (Figure 4). As the animal cycled into rapid-eye-movement sleep, the slope of the plots changed, indicating the predominant role of the diaphragm during this sleep state. It is also possible to detect changes in the initial portion of the expiratory plot, which are related to the thyroarytenoid activity; this is evident on frames 3, 4, 33, 35 and 36.

Conclusion

This study demonstrates that important changes in the mechanics of breathing can be detected non-invasively by respiratory inductive plethysmography (Respitrace). These findings, in addition to the evidence recently provided by Duffty et al (3), suggest that tidal volume can be accurately measured with this system in neonates, and that respiratory inductive plethysmography can be a powerful tool for other respiratory investigations in newborns. In particular, this system provides a viable alternative to measurement of respired

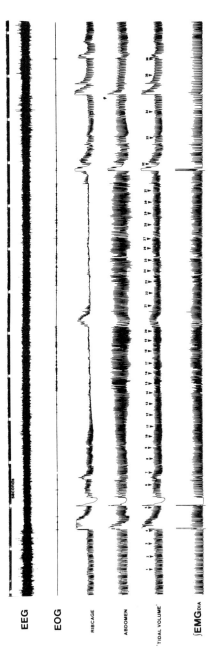

Fig. 3   Typical recording from lamb during quiet sleep and rapid-
eye-movement sleep. EEG = electrocorticogram   EOG = elec-
tro-oculogram ∫EMG$_{DIA}$ = integrated diaphragm electromyogram.

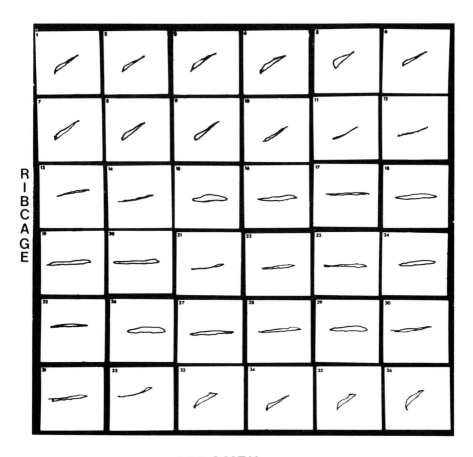

ABDOMEN

Fig. 4   X-Y plots of ribcage excursion against abdominal excursion
during quiet sleep and rapid-eye-movement sleep. Numbers
indicate respective breaths on Fig. 3.

airflow with a face mask and pneumotachometer. This is important because mask application alone alters the pettern of breathing and increases minute ventilation (4). Since it is now becoming apparent that abnormalities of ventilation other than apnoea (e.g. central hypoventilation, chronic lung disease) underly respiratory failure in early postnatal life, respiratory inductive plethysmography, which is relatively easy to use, may be well-suited for incorporation into monitoring systems.

Acknowledgements

Supported by Wellcome Trust 9594-1.5, The Foundation for the Study of Infant Death, and National Institutes of Health Pulmonary Faculty Training Grant HL07159.

References

1.   Johnson P. Comparative aspects of the control of breathing during development. In: Central Nervous Control Mechanisms in Breath-ing, Pergamon Press, Oxford, 1979, 337-353.
2.   Harding R., Johnson P., McClelland M.E., The expiratory role of the larynx during development and the influence of behavioural state. In: Central Nervous Control Mechanisms in Breathing, Pergamon Press, Oxford, 1979, 353-359.
3.   Duffty P., Spriet L., Bryan M.H., Bryan A.C. (1981) Am. Rev. Respir Dis..**123**, 542-546.
4.   Avery M.E., Chernick V., Dutton R.E. Permutt S. (1963) J. Appl. Physiol. **18**, 895-903.

Discussion

DR. PHILLIPSON: Mr. Wollner is probably aware that the paediatric group at the Hospital for Sick Children, Toronto, have done similar measurements in terms of the abdominal rib-cage contributions to ventilation and intercostal and diaphragmatic EMG's in healthy adolescents. They found exactly the same as in the lambs - that is, in REM sleep, the diaphragmatic EMG and the abdominal contribution both increase. They also noted that going from wakefulness to non-REM sleep, there was an increase in the rib-cage contribution. Has that been observed in the lambs?
MR. WOLLNER: We have not studies wakwfulness in detail.
DR. PHILLIPSON: Is there any idea physiologically why the thyro-arytenoid is not firing on every breath?
MR. WOLLNER: The thyro-arytenoid controls respiratory frequency by the regulation of expiratory time. Thus, depending on the frequency the animal needs to maintain adequate lung volume, the thyro-arytenoid is active whenever necessary.
DR. PHILLIPSON: So you look upon it more as a mechanism for maintaining FRC or adequate lung volume?
MR. WOLLNER: Yes, essentially - and respiratory rhythm by the generation of positive expiratory pressure, which we believe acts on pulmonary stretch receptors.

ANALYSIS OF BREATHING PATTERN DURING PROVOKED BRONCHOCONSTRICTION UTILIZING RESPIRATORY INDUCTIVE PLEYTHYSMOGRAPHY

M.A. SACKNER, T.S. CHADHA, A.W. SCHNEIDER & S. BIRCH

Div. Pulmonary Disease, Dept.Medicine, Mount Sinai Medical
Centre, Miami Beach, Florida 33140, USA.

Summary

Utilizing respiratory inductive plethysmography, the monitoring of breathing pattern was carried out in normal and asthmatic subjects. They were given either aerosolized saline or methacholine aerosol in a double-blind cross-over trial. We wanted to ascertain whether a characteristic alteration of breathing pattern occurred with minor degrees of bronchoconstriction insufficient to produce clinical symptoms. A consistent increase of mean inspiratory flow (V_T/T_I) was found with bronchospasm in both the normal and asthmatic subjects. All other components of the breathing pattern, i.e., tidal volume, minute ventilation, frequency, inspiratory time, and fractional inspiratory time, showed variable inconsistent changes. We conclude that analysis of the breathing pattern obtained by non-invasive respiratory monitoring may be helpful in detecting disease processes.

A major purpose of non-invasive respiratory monitoring, i.e. measurement of breathing pattern while the subject is breathing naturally without the encumbrances of a mouthpiece and nose clip or face mask, is to utilize changes in the volume, time and flow components of the breath for detection of disease processes. With the exception of monitoring for central and obstructive apneas during clinical polysomnographhy, there has been little attention directed towards continuous monitoring in respiratory disease.

Bronchomotor tone is ordinarily assessed from discrete rather than continuous measurements on a long-term basis. Such   tests which include measurements of forced expiratory volumes and flows, and resistance of the airways, lung and chest-lung system, depend to a greater or lesser extent upon special breathing manoeuvres, breathing through a mouthpiece while the nose is occluded, placement within a whole body plethysmograph and insertion of an oesophageal balloon catheter. Recently, it has been shown that acute bronchoconstriction produces an increase in inspiratory muscle activity as measured directly from surface electromyography (1). Inspiratory muscle activity may be assessed indirectly by an increase of pressure developed during the first 0.1 sec of inspiration against an occluded airway ($P_{0.1}$). Although this measure is not satisfactory for long-term respiratory monitoring because it requires breathing from a mouthpiece, changes in the pressure magnitude directly correlate with one of the flow components of the breathing pattern, mean inspiratory flow (V_T/T_I) (2, 3). The purpose of this study was to investigate whether changes in this parameter (which might be expected to increase with bronchoconstriction) or other components of the breathing pattern (measured by respiratory inductive plethysmography) would be altered by minor degrees of bronchial provocation.

Materials and Methods

We studied four men and two women normal non-smokers, with a mean age of 27 years (range 21 to 35 years) and three men and three women with bronchial asthma with a mean age of 29 years (range 25-31 years). The asthmatics were in a stable clinical and functional state and had not been taking maintenance oral bronchodilators and corticosteroids. They had not utilized aerosolized bronchodilators for at least 48 hours prior to the study.

Baseline pulmonary function evaluation consisted of spirometry, measurements of airway resistance and functional residual capacity by body plethysmography and distribution of ventilation by the single breath nitrogen test.

On a previous day, all subjects underwent standard bronchial inhalation challenge with methacholine aerosol delivered through a dosimeter system (4). Specific airway conductance was calculated in order to generate a standardized dose response curve for each subject. The initial dose which lowered the specific airway conductance by 35% was designated provocation dose 35% (PD 35) and this dose was subsequently used for challenge on later days. With this dose, none of the subjects experienced the sensation of bronchospasm and none had wheezing audible with the stethoscope.

Detailed descriptions of the AC coupled respiratory inductive plethysmograph and calibration methods have been published previously (5, 6). Briefly the device consists of two coils of insulated wire about the rib cage and abdomen which are excited by an oscillator circuit. The change in self inductance of these coils with movement of the rib cage and abdominal compartments during breathing is proportional to change in thoracic volume which can be made equivalent to tidal volume measured at the mouthpiece with spirometry (SP). In the present study, we employed a new calibration technique which is described by Watson elsewhere in this volume. This method depends upon changing rib cage (RC) and abdominal (AB) contributions to the tidal volume by assuming two body positions, utilizing the equation $RC/SP + AB/SP = 1$, and employing a least squares fit for its graphic solution. The gain factors on the RC and AB components of the respiratory inductive plethysmograph are then set through the calibration circuit. In all subjects, the difference of respiratory inductive plethysmography volumes from spirometry was less than 5%, both in the standing and supine positions; the mean difference was 3.1%, S.D.0.9%.

The investigation was designed as a randomized double blind cross-over. After validation of the respiratory inductive plethysmograph, $FEV_{1.0}$ was obtained by spirometry. At the end of the observation period, $FEV_{1.0}$ was repeated. The subject rested semi-recumbant on a bed in a quiet room for 15 minutes and data were collected from the respiratory inductive plethysmograph over the next 15 minutes by means of a microprocessor system. The subjects were given either the aerosolized buffered saline as a control or the PD 35 dose of methacholine at the bedside while in the semi-recumbant position and data were collected for another 15 minutes. On day 2, the procedure was repeated with the aerosol which had not been given on day 1.

The microprocessor system digitized the analog signals at 20 points per second, measured the amplitude, inspiratory and expiratory times for each breath of the rib cage and abdominal excursions and their sum. It calculated and plotted in a variable compressed time-scale the following parameters: minute ventilation, tidal volume, frequency, inspiratory time, fractional inspiratory time and mean inspiratory flow (V_T/T_I) (8) (Fig.1). It also calculated the mean and standard deviations and plotted the frequency histograms of each parameter for the whole recording period. A paired t-test was used to test for differences between treatments with $p<.05$ taken as significant.

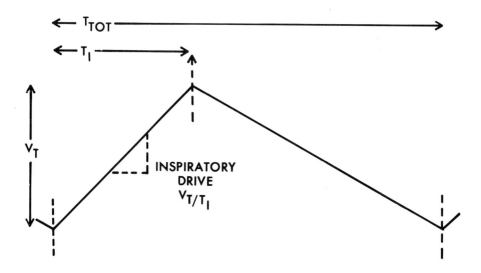

Fig. 1   The timing, volume and flow components of a breath which are used to analyse the breathing pattern

Results

There were no differences on the two study days between the normals or asthmatics for the baseline, minute ventilation, tidal volume, frequency, inspiratory time, fractional inspiratory time, mean inspiratory flow, $FEV_{1.0}$ and specific airway conductance. Furthermore, with the exception of mean inspiratory flow and minute ventilation, no consistent changes were seen in the group means of the components of the breathing pattern, although variability from subject to subject occurred. All normal and asthmatic subjects showed an increase of mean inspiratory flow (V_T/T_I) after methacholine aerosol compared to the baseline period. Normal subjects showed an increase in

(V_T/T_I) of 56 ml/sec (S.D. 12) above the baseline after methacholine administration. This was significantly higher than the figure of 6 ml/sec, (S.D. 12) after buffered saline (p<.01). Corresponding values in asthmatics were 71 ml/sec (S.D.12) and 31 ml per sec (S.D.8) (p<.01).

The frequency histogram demonstrating this change shifted uniformly for all breaths (Fig. 2).

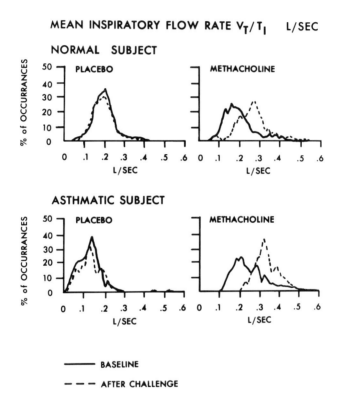

MEAN INSPIRATORY FLOW RATE V_T/T_I L/SEC

Fig. 2   Frequency histograms of mean inspiratory flow in a normal and asthmatic subject. A uniform shift to the right is seen after methacholine administration with no change after saline control

In normals minute ventilation increased from 5.30 L/min to 6.3 L/min after methacholine (p<.05) but not with normal saline. The frequency histogram demonstrating this change showed a uniform shift.

Mean FEV $_{1.0}$ change from baseline to 15 minutes after aerosolized saline was 2% and 5% after aerosolized methacholine in normal subjects and 6% and 9% in asthmatic patients, respectively (p</05).

Discussion

Analysis of breathing pattern during airways obstruction is complicated by such variables as lung and airway mechanics, change in chest wall properties, abnormal gas exchange and cortical conditioning (9, 10, 11). Most data are based upon assessment of ventilatory response to hypercapnia, which may not simulate the underlying disease process. Mann et al (12) assessed the breathing pattern of normal adults who breathed on the mouthpiece with the nose occluded after bronchoconstriction was provoked with aerosolized methacholine. These authors produced a greater drop of specific airway conductance (75%) than we did and their subjects wheezed. They found no consistent changes in minute ventilation, tidal volume, inspiratory time and mean inspiratory flow but both frequency and fractional inspiratory time increased. Furthermore, in all subjects P_{100} increased together with increase in functional residual capacity of 920 ml. This failure to observe an increase in mean inspiratory flow is inconsistent since both $P_{0.1}$ and V_T/T_I reflect respiratory centre output. In part, this inconsistency might have been due to cortical influences provoked by mouthpiece breathing.

In the present study, we found that the most consistent change with bronchoconstriction was an increase in mean inspiratory flow. That this can be taken as an increase in inspiratory muscle drive is consistent with other clinical observations. Thus, patients with acute bronchospasm generally increase their alveolar ventilation beyond the level to maintain after saline control. the normal alveolar carbon dioxide tension. Asthmatic patients during spontaneously occurring acute bronchospasm of variable severity show a pattern of rapid breathing with high mean inspiratory flow rates and normal tidal volumes (13).

Changes in FRC can alter the response to resistivee loaded breathing. An increase in functional residual capacity produces a decrease in the length of the inspiratory muscles and by depressing the diaphragm will alter the force-tension relationship of this muscle, placing it at a mechanical disadvantage. Hyperinflation depresses mouth occlusion pressure ($P_{0.1}$) and thereby one would expect a decrease of mean inspiratory flow. In our study, the level of FRC was not measured, but would either remain normal or increase following methacholine administration. The increase in mean inspiratory flow, therefore, is over and beyond that necessary to overcome the potential mechanical disadvantage of the inspiratory muscles and reflects the high inspiratory muscle activity as related to respiratory centre output. This increase in inspiratory muscle activity has also been observed in bronchoconstriction induced by aerosolized histamine administration as indicated by carry-over of inspiratory muscle tone (measured by surface electro-myography) to the expiratory phase and accounts for the hyperinflation found in association with bronchospasm (1).

The mechanism of the increased drive to breathe with bronchospasm is unclear. We have shown in other experiments that metha-

choline does not produce stimulation of irritant receptors so that it
is directly related to bronchoconstriction. Thus, the minor degree
of bronchoconstriction in some way sets up a neurally mediated reflex
to increase respiratory centre output.
    This study demonstrates the potential application of non-inva-
sive respiratory monitoring to detect alteration of clinical state.
Bronchoconstriction should be suspected as a non-specific sign if
mean inspiratory flow increases over an observation period. If the
end-expiratory level rose as well as a result of hyperinflation, then
this diagnosis would be strengthened. The DC coupled respiratory
inductive plethysmograph should be capable of monitoring such a
change and this is presently under study.
    From clinical observations, one might further speculate that
mean inspiratory flow would increase in pulmonary oedema. In this
situation, one might observe a decrease in end-expiratory level along
with a shallow rapid breathing pattern. Our future intent is to
develop algorithms using the analysis of breathing patterns to indicate various groups of respiratory diagnoses. In addition, monitoring
of hemodynamics would be an extremely helpful adjunct under a variety
of circumstances. For example, non-invasive monitoring of systolic
time intervals to indicatge a decrease in myocardial contractility
would strengthen the diagnosis of early pulmonary oedema in the
example just cited, given the change in breathing pattern.

References

1. Muller N., Bryan A.C., Zamel N. (1980) J. Appl. Physiol. **49**,
    869-974.
2. Clark F.J., von Euler C. (1972) J. Physiol. **222**, 267-95.
3. Milic-Emili J., Grunstein M.M. (1976) Chest (Suppl.) **70**, 131-
    133.
4. Chai H., Far R.S., Froehlich L.A. et al (1976) J. Allergy Clin.
    Immunol. **56**, 323-27.
5. Sackner J.D., Nixon A.J., Davis B., Atkins N. and Sackner
    M.A.,(1980) Am. Rev. Respir. Dis. **122**, 867-71.
6. Watson H.L., Birch S.J., Gruen W.G., Cohn M.A., Schneider A.W.,
    Sackner M.A., (1981) Am. Rev. Respir. Dis. **123**, 182. (Abstract).
7. Watson H., Schneider A., Birch S., Chadha T., Abraham W.M., Cohn
    M. and Sackner M. (1981) ISAM Proceedings of the Internatinal
    Symposium on Ambulatory Monitoring.
8. Newsom D., Stagg D. (1975) J. Physiol. **245**, 481-98.
9. Sorli J., Grassino A., Lorange G., Milic-Emili J., (1978) Clin.
    Sci. Molec. Med. **54**, 295-304.
10. Bechbache R.R., Chow H.H.K., Duffin J., Orsini E.C. (1979) J.
    Physiol. **293**, 285-300.
11. Garrard C.S., Lane D.J. (1979) Clin. Sci. **56**, 215.
12. Mann J., Bradley C.A., Anthonisen N.R. (1978) Resp. Physiol. **33**,
    339-47.
13. Guz A. (1977) In: Asthma - Physiology, Immunopharmacology and
    Treatment, Ed. L.M. Lichtenstein K. Frank Austen, Academic
    Press, New York, (1977) 211-22.

Discussion

DR. PHILLIPSON: It seemed to me that in the normals 5% of the breaths had a tidal volume of less than 200ml. Were those breaths and, if not, what were they?

DR. SACKNER: Yes, they are breaths. It turns out that our concept of what is a normal tidal volume has changed considerably as a result of non-invasive monitoring. Healthy people are frequently seen with mean tidal volumes of 250 to 275ml, breathing at 25 times a minute if they are lying semi-recumbent in a quiet room with nobody disturbing them. If someone goes into the room the tidal volume may increase and the respiratory rate slow down. The normal tidal volume of 500 or 600 ml is related to mouthpiece breathing with a nose-clip, and it has a lot of cortical influence. I believe that the respiratory rate in most of our studies is closer to 20 to 24 breaths/min with much lower tidal volumes.

DR. PHILLIPSON: Secondly, a more clinical physiological question: it seemed to me that Dr. Sackner said very briefly that the dose of methacholine was the same in the asthmatics and in the normals. Is that right?

DR. SACKNER: No, I did not mean that. Each individual subject was calibrated for PD_{35}. The doses were all different, but for each subject a PD_{35} dose was determined. If I said what you suggest, that was wrong.

DIPL.ING. RASCHKE: In the first slide showing histograms of tidal volume Dr. Sackner demonstrated that there was a bimodal distribution. In the histograms following methacholine intake there was a trimodal distribution. Can it be said whether this polymodal distribution is due to higher periods of tidal volume change in the individual, or is it an effect of interindividual change?

DR. SACKNER: First, those frequency histograms were group data, although I must admit that if individual data points are looked at there are also irregularities. There are certainly lots of variations in tidal volumes while people are just lying quietly which may again be related to cortical influences - thinking of what is going to happen to them, for instance. In terms of sorting out the frequency histograms over this relatiely brief period of 15 mins, I would not be prepared to say whether we are looking at something that is real. A much longer period of time would need to be studied for us to be able to say that. We have looked at 8-hour data for tidal volume during sleep, and those data look quite Gaussian.

DR. RICHTER: First, has Dr. Sackner found any hints about any correlation between the real pulmonary resistance and his index of resistance, for example, with the forced oscillation technique?

DR. SACKNER: That is under study and will be done. So far, all we have is the FEV_1 before and after, and in fact the FEV_1 changes did not distinguish the saline from the methacholine group.

DR. RICHTER: Secondly, sometimes the expiratory resistance was increased in asthmatics, and I was very interested in the resistance loops and the pressure flow curves. Have the expiratory flow changes also been studied?

DR. SACKNER: Mean expiratory flow has been studied in these subjects, but no difference was found. The only parameter that was statistically significant - at least in this type of analysis - was mean expiratory flow.

MR. WATSON: The other point, certainly with the methacholine over a
short period of time, is that they would tend every now and then to
take a large breath which temporarily reverses the
bronchconstriction. According to the dose of methacholine that
remains, the bronchoconstriction will reappear over a period of
minutes, which may induce another deep breath and relieve the
bronchoconstriction.

DR. MONSTER: To achieve a more detailed interpretation of the
breathing patterns observed, we will be forced to make other types of
recordings simultaneously with the breathing patterns. Has Dr.
Sackner some thoughts about this?

DR. SACKNER: That was alluded to by Dr. Richter who mentioned the
possibility of doing oscillatory resistances. We shall do that.
With regard to the long-term continuous measurement of resistance,
Dr. Cohn will discuss that later. An oesophageal balloon can be
dropped in to look at it, but we did not wish to drop an oesophageal
balloon in this series of experiments because it was felt that this
would again give cortical influences that might knock out what we are
looking at. The breathing pattern itself is a non-specific
expression of an insult, or a stimulus. This is what we have found,
and that finding was consistent. A bronchoconstriction agent was
given which was known definitely to produce bronchoconstriction. The
intention of non-invasive monitoring should be early detection, then
proceeding to a definitive test - whatever that definitive test may
be. Airways resistance is the gold standard, and that would have to
be measured.

LONG-TERM MICROPROCESSOR MONITORING
OF BREATHING PATTERN

H. WATSON, A. SCHNEIDER, M. COHN AND M.A. SACKNER

The Samuel J. Kraver Scientific Data Processing Centre
and The Jane and Edward Shapiro Pulmonary Suite,
Department of Medicine, Mt. Sinai Medical Centre,
Miami Beach, Florida, USA

Summary

A Z-80 microprocessor-based computer system was developed for the
long-term non-invasive monitoring of the breathing pattern. Assembly
language computer programmes were written for calibrating, monitoring
and analysing the signals from the respiratory inductive plethysmograph (1).
     The calibration programme uses the method of Least Squares to
solve for the gain factors of the rib cage and abdominal signals of
respiratory inductive plethysmography (2). The data collection programme monitors the signals, breath by breath, and stores the information in a versatile data base on floppy discs. One off-line analysis programme displays the scalar plot of the following parameters
in a variably compressed time-scale: tidal volume minute ventilation, rate, inspiratory time, fractional inspiratory time and mean
inspiratory flow. The other analysis programme calculates the frequency histograms of the same parameters. The system has been used
to monitor breathing patterns during sleep and after broncho-provoca-
tion.

System Design

We have developed a microprocessor/software system for continuous
long-term monitoring of breathing patterns. This has potential diagnostic importance for critical care, sleep disorders and ambulatory
monitoring. Conventional methods of monitoring breathing require a
physical connection to the airways either with an endo-tracheal tube,
a mouthpiece, or a face-mask, connected to a pneumotachograph or
spirometer. These methods produce patient discomfort, enhance cortical stimulation and cannot be used for long periods of time. Further, the pattern of breathing is altered while breathing on a mouthpiece, with a nose clip compared to breathing naturally (3). The
respiratory inductive plethysmograph (RIP) (Respitrace, Ambulatory
Monitoring) allows continuous unobtrusive monitoring of respiration
without physical connection to the airways. Traditional methods of
respiratory analysis become ineffective, when considered over tens,
hundreds, or thousands of breaths. The ability to monitor respiration continuously, necessitates an automated system of analysis.
Therefore, we devised a microprocessor and software system to monitor
each and every breath, while identifying important points within each
breath and saving these data in an indefinite data base, which can

later be accessed and analysed with time series or histogram analysis.

The microprocessor system is a Z-80 based system with 48 Bytes
of memory, dual 8-inch floppy disc drives, a 12-bit precision analog-
/digital converter, a real-time clock, a CRT-terminal for programme
interaction, a video-monitor for graphics' data and status, and a
thermal printer for hard copy of text and graphics. The system runs
under the CP/M operating system supplied by Digital Research, Inc.
The applications programmes are written in Z-80 assembly language and
are enchanced by structured programming macros, floating point arithmetic macros and function library, and a plotting and graphics library. All programmes are written in a modular fashion and are combined using a linking loader providing the final executable form.

A system that is used in this fashion requires software that is
able to perform initial calibration and subsequent validation of the
RIP against a spirometer. Additionally, long-term analysis requires
a series of programmes both for data collection and analysis. We
developed a general purpose data collection programme that measures
important points on each breath and condenses all those points into a
data base, stored on a floppy diskette. This data collection programme can be run for very short times such as for 5, 15, or 30
minutes, or it can be run continuously for approximately 12 hours,
with a single density diskette, or up to 48 hours with a double
density, double-sided diskette. Once the data have been collected
and stored in the data-base, they can be analysed with respect to
time, including the ability to calculate means and standard deviations and to identify certain characteristic events, times or patterns, and also by time independent methods, such as histogramming.
This analysis yields probablility distributions and patterns associated with respiratory parameters in different time-blocks, and also
permits statistical analysis to test for significant differences
between sets of histograms.

The most important component of both the calibration programmes
and the long-term data collection programme is the detection of
individual breaths. It is important that only the fluctuations in
the signal due to respiration are detected and other small fluctuations in the signal due to movement are not detected as breaths.
These programmes use a technique, that defines a minimum acceptable
volume change to define a breath, rejecting any volume change less
than this amount. The default value is set at 100 ml., but this may
be changed at any time by the user. Breath detection is accomplished
by the critical point analysis routine. This routine identifies the
proper points for the minimum and maximum for each breath based on
the sum, the corresponding rib-cage and abdominal values, and determines the time since the last critical point. Timing and amplitude
measurements are also made for looping parameters when considering
the rib-cage versus the abdomen signals.

System Validation

This analysis was validated by monitoring 5 normal volunteers for a
4-hour period, comparing computer analysis with hand measurements
(4). Initial and hourly measurements were made at respiratory rates
of 10, 20, 40 and 60 breaths per minute and while breathing on a

fixed volume bag in both the sitting and supine positions. Hand measurements were made from a Grass Polygraph recording system and plotted against the computer measurements of tidal volume and frequency for over 500 points. These results fell within 10% of identity for all measurements, with a standard deviation of 4% and no systematic differences.

Applications programmes for the system are divided into two groups. The first group deals with the initial calibration and validation of the RIP and the second group consists of the long-term data collection and analysis of the RIP signals.

Respiratory Inductive Plethysmograph Calibration

There are two calibraton and validation programmes: NEWCAL and BAGCAL. Both of these programmes solve the Least Squares method of calculation for calibration factors. NEWCAL uses the spirometer input as a volume signal, and BAGCAL uses the Spirobag for fixed volume breaths. Both of these programmes have the capacity to begin collecting breaths in one posture and then halt collection and continue in another posture. A maximum of 100 breaths can be collected, so more than two postures can be used for the solution of the calibration factors if desired. After calibration has been done, the programmes have the capacity to validate the volume accuracy of the RIP sum against the volume standard and express the difference as a percent (100(RIP Vman - RIP Vmin/SP Vmax - SP Vmin)). The mean, standard deviation, and standard error are also calculated for the percent differences of each breath in the validation run.

Long-Term Monitoring

In the second group of programmes, there are a data collection programme, DKVEST. DKVEST collects the rib-cage, abdomen and sum signals continuously and measures the critical points on each breath, while saving that data in a data base on the diskette: it also provides a display of the incoming real-time data on the graphics monitor and has a limited capability to give an on-line indication of some of the analysis parameters included in the time-series analysis programmes.

Additionally, DKVEST has (1) an event marker so that a single breath can be marked with an event (2) a continuous display of the elapsed time to provide notations, if desired in a log, and (3) a collecton routine for O_2 saturation values at 5 second intervals.

Different combinations of the data collection programme are used for different types of protocols. Typically, a sleep study involves data collection of breathing pattern along with O_2 saturation over an 8-hour period. A study of exercise might run with 5 minutes of pre-exercise control, 5 minutes of exercise and 5 minutes of post-exercise recovery. Another protocol design might involve the identification of specific breaths within a long data-collection time, and use the event-marker capability.

The analysis programmes access the data base, which was built by DKVEST and perform their specific types of analysis. These are READ3, PLTHIST, and EVENT. Table 1 shows a menu from READ3. This programme is used for time-series analysis of data and plotting of

TABLE 1

Read3 Programme Menu Options

---

1 - Open Input File
2 - Random Access to Disc
3 - Exit Programme
4 - O_2 Saturation Values
5 - MV
6 - TV
7 - Rate
8 - TI
9 - T_I/T
A - T_V/T_I
B - Phase Angle
C - Variable Options
D - FRC Level
E - Mean Expiratory Flow
F - Plot O_2 Saturation
G - T-Total
H - Effort
I - % Rib Cage Contribution

---

all of the parameters listed in the menu against time, where the time
scaling can be expanded or compressed with the variable options.
Option 1 allows READ3 to open a data base file for analysis, and
option 2 allows random access to any specific time within the data
base. In this way, data within the computer can be correlated with
hard copies or with elapsed times that were logged during the data
collection run. Other parameters that are routinely calculated on a
breath-by-breath basis are minute volume, tidal volume, respiratory
rate, inspiratory time, inspiratory time as a percent of the total
breath-time, mean inspiratory flow, which is the tidal volume divided
by the inspiratory time, phase angle, which is a looping parameter,
FRC level or the absolute voltage value obtained from the sum signal,
mean expiratory flow, which is the tidal volume divided by the expiratory time, total breath-time, the percent rib cage or the percent of
the sum volume that went into the rib cage, and the tidal volume
combined with the effort, which is another looping parameter.

Variable options give the user the ability to expand or contract
either X or Y scaling, print the means and standard deviations of a
parameter ar regular time intervals, switching hard copy on or off,
and access to the next event recorded in the data base independent of
time.

Time Series Analysis

Figure 1 shows a schematic representation of an analog recording of
RIP signals and the corresponding computer display. The sum (V_T),
the rib cage (V_{RC}), and the abdomen (V_{ABD}) traces are shown. Three
specific ties are indicated. Time T1 is a relatively normal respiratory cycle, with some degree of paradoxic motion present in the rib

ANALOG RECORDING

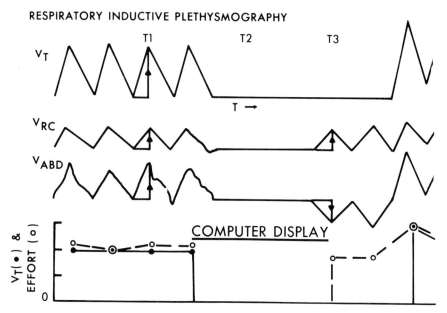

Fig. 1   Schematic representation of measurements made by the
          computer. (See text).

cage and abdominal compartments. Time T2 is a central apnoea period,
and time T3 represents an obstructive apnoea time. The computer,
when computing the effort trace measures the delta value (Vmax-Vmin)
for both the rib cage and abdominal components as well as the sum.
This is shown schematically at times T1 and T3. Effort is then
calculated by adding the absolute values of the two compartmental
values. Effort is either equal to the tidal volume when both compartments are in phase, or greater than the sum when the rib cage and
abdominal components are out of phase. The computer display is
represented in the bottom of Figure 1 as the opposite trace of the
tidal volume and effort. The dotted line represents the effort
signal and the solid line represents the tidal volume signal.

At time T1, the effort trace is higher than the tidal volume
trace indicating some paradoxic motion is present in the rib cage and
abdominal compartments. Time T2 shows what the computer algorithm
does with a central apnoea. If the time between breaths exceeds 10
seconds, the algorithm classifies this as a central apnoea and drops
the effort and tidal volume traces to the zero volume value. Time T3
represents an obstructed apnoea and here, the rib cage and abdominal
components are exactly 180 degrees out of phase. The scalar sum of
the two components as represented by the tidal volume trace is zero,
although the sum of the absolute values of the deltas obtained from
the individual compartments represents a large effort. This is shown
in the computer display as the tidal volume trace staying at zero

while the dotted trace representing the effort value rises from zero
to the summed value of the individual components. This way, the
READ3 programme allows the distinction between central, obstructive
and complex apnoeas. Additionally, the effort trace gives an indication of paradoxic motion even during periods of respiration. This
paradoxic indication is supplemented by the phase angle parameter
consisting of the measurement of the phase angle of a loop transcribed from each breath, with the rib cage against the abdominal
signals.

Histogramming Analysis

PLTHIST is a histogramming programme for the analysis of the same
parameters as contained in READ 3, but it allows time-iondependent
analysis and comparison of data. Any random time block of data can
be histogrammed with this programme. The data are accessed and the
length of time for the histogram is specified and analysis is performed by the computer. Trend analysis is computed on the raw data
to assure stationarity of the data throughout the period under consideration. PLTHIST has the ability to save the current histogram
data on the diskette, read it back from the diskette, or to combine
multiple histograms into a single one for display and analysis.
PLTHIST can compare two distinct histograms to determine whether or
not there is a statistically significant difference between them.
These statistics allow comparison of the general shape, as well as
tests on the medians and variabilities of the histograms.
    This analysis allows any individual component of the breathing
pattern to be used as a control after a stimulus. Measurements can
be made at one point in time and compared to another point in time on
the same individual and a determination can then be made using the
histograms as to whether or not a change has occurred within any of
the analysis parameters. Short, or long, time blocks can be considered against each other for analysis. Other uses could involve the
comparison of the effects of drugs by the measurement of a before and
after histogram.

Event Analysis

A third analysis programme is called EVENT. This programme again has
all the parameter options contained within READ3; however, it
searches the data base and it only deals with the breaths that are
marked with the event marker. When it encounters a breath that is
marked with an event, it prints out the preceding breath, the event
breath, and the breath following the event for the parameter selected. It also prints the elapsed time of the run in terms of
minutes. Breaths that are marked with an event are also indicated in
the analysis of the READ3 programme. A vertical tick mark is added
to the data as it is displayed on the graphics screen.

Time Series Data

The following figures show some of the typical data analysis obtained
with each of the programmes:

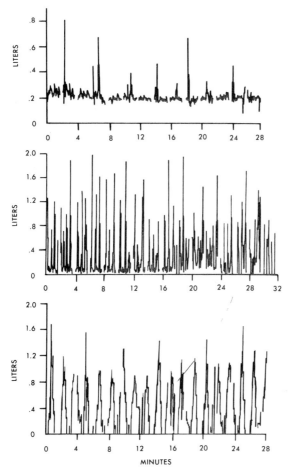

Fig. 2   A: (Top) Tidal volume during quiet sleep in a normal
              individual.
         B: (Middle) Tidal volume with sleep apnea.
         C: (Bottom) Tidal volume with Cheyne-Stokes Respiration
              during sleep.

Figure 2 shows tidal volume data obtained from three individuals
during a night. All of the traces show data highly compressed with 4
minutes per division on the time axis and volume scaling from 0 to 2
litres. Figure 2A shows a normal individual during quiet sleep, with
tidal volume shown ranging around 200 to 300 ml. One four-minute
block can show approximately 80 breaths, so that the data is highly
condensed and is used to show time-patterns. The high volume breaths
indicated, in Figure 2A, correspond to sighs occurring during the
sleep. Figure 2B is shown with the same scaling. The highly irregular tidal volume trace is produced by an individual that has both
central and obstructive apnoeas. The tidal volume trace is dropped
to the zero value during the apnoeic periods and the erratic nature

of the trace is very apparent. Figure 2C shows an individual with
the Cheyne-Stokes respiration. The characteristic cyclic nature of
the tidal volume is indicated in this time-volume trace. The volumes
shown dropping to the zero value indicate breaths that were below 100
ml in volume, even though the individual had a sustained effort.

Figure 3 shows the record of a patient with sleep apnoea syn-
drome.The scaling is 20 seconds per division on the time scale and
200 ml per division on the volume axis. At time T1, the tidal volume
trace drops to the zero value indicating a lack of volume in the sum
signal, but the effort signal continues on as indicated by the dotted
line. After the break of the obstruction, there is one breath, where
the rib cage and abdomen are in phase, and then the resumption of
breathing, where the effort is higher than the tidal volume indicating that the rib cage and abdomen are out of phase. Time T2 is
another apnoea, with a central onset because of a lack of effort
during that time, and then the effort starting in the middle of the
apnoea with no corresponding volume trace, indicating a complex
apnoea with a central onset. At time T3, there is a total cessation

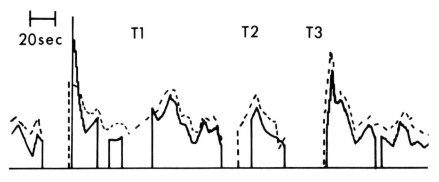

Fig. 3   Real sleep data of todal volume and effort during apneas.
          (See text).

of effort and volume at the same time and duration, indicating a
central apnoea. Again, at the end of the apnoeic period, a deep
breath followed by more breathing with the effort being higher than
the tidal volume. This type of trace represents the ability of the
computer system to distinguish between the three types of apnoeas.

Histogramming Data

Figure 4 illustrates the power of the histogramming analysis approach
and its ability to compress data into an easily recognizable format.
The minute ventilation is plotted on the X-axis with 10 litres/minute
per division and the percent of occurrences on the Y-axis with 10%
per division. Both histograms in Figure 4 were done for an entire
night's sleeps study. Figure 4A was done on a normal individual and
Figure 4B was done an individual with sleep apnoea syndrome. The
dramatic differences in shape and value are apparent. In the apnoea
display (Figure 4B) there is a Y-intercept of approximately 13% at
zero volume, this would indicate that approximately 13% of the night

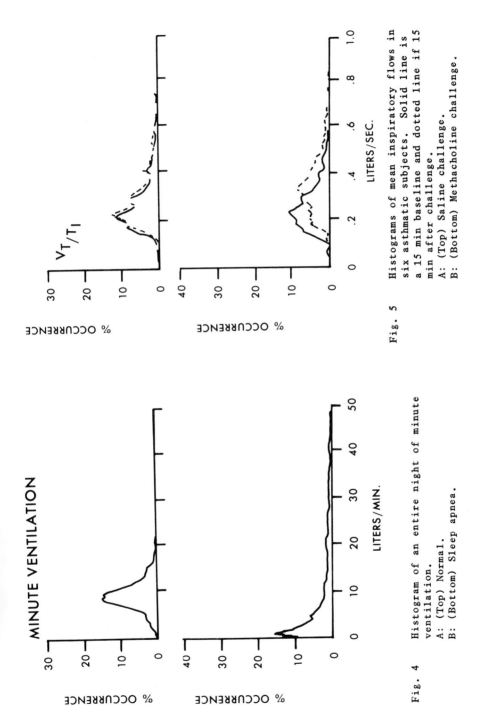

Fig. 5 Histograms of mean inspiratory flows in six asthmatic subjects. Solid line is a 15 min baseline and dotted line if 15 min after challenge.
A: (Top) Saline challenge.
B: (Bottom) Methacholine challenge.

Fig. 4 Histogram of an entire night of minute ventilation.
A: (Top) Normal.
B: (Bottom) Sleep apnea.

was spent with zero ventilation, as defined as breaths with volumes, less than 100 ml.

Figure 5 shows the results of histogram analysis in 6 asthmatic individuals. Data from all six subjects were combined into one histogram. Figure 5A shows the results from a saline challenge to these subjects. The protocol was such that data were collected for 15 minutes before the challenge for a control and then for 15 minutes again the challenge. The solid line represents the results of the control run and the dotted line represents the post-challenge data. Figure 5A shows no change in the mean inspiratory flow with the saline challenge and also illustrates the reproducability of the control run both in terms of shape and distribution of the histograms. Figure 5B shows the same 6 individuals, only this time they were challenged with a methacholine dose that reduced specific airway conductance by 35%. Again, the solid line is the control and the dotted line is the post-challenge data. A dramatic shift occurs in the mean inspiratory flow of these individuals. Upon examination of the individual components of tidal volume and inspiratory time, there was no statistically significant difference in the means, but there was a significant difference in the mean inspiratory flows. This parameter reflects respiratory centre drive and the experiment indicates heightening of drive with minimal degrees of bronchoconstriction.

References

1. Schneider A.W. (1981) Long-term monitoring of respiration. Masters Thesis, University of Miami.
2   Abraham W.M., Watson H., Schneider A., King M., Yerger L. and Sackner M.A. (1981) J. Appl. Physiol. (in press).
3. Sackner J.D., Nixon A.J., Davis B., Atkins N. and Sackner M.A. (1980) Am. Rev. Respir. Dis. **122**, 867-871.
4. Watson H., Schneider A., Frieden A. and Sackner M.A. (1980) Am. Rev. Respir. Dis. **121**(4), 203, (Abstract).

Discussion

DR. MILES: Have there been problems with artefact? What happens with artefact when the subjects wake up, or when the recording is continued for a whole night?

MR. WATSON: Movement times, shifts in position, can cause a movement artefact. However, the movement times, compared to the total recording time, are minimal, even though they may show up as artefacts in the trace. If we are looking at histograms, or means and standard deviations, everything should average out.

DR. MILES: There are some apnoeics, who for hours, never have a "normal" breath, are there not?

MR. WATSON: The algorithm that determines the breath is fairly noise-immune - that is the noise immunity, which is typed in as the minimum breath volumes, so any noise or short spikes on a breath less than 100 cc are ignored. With the physiologic filters, those can be turned on or off. The data can, therefore, be looked at while they are being analysed to see what artefacts are there; it is then possible to go back and analyse the data again with the physiologic filters to see what is being excluded. All those physiologic filters are under programe control, so reasonable values can be put in - that is, values which are thought to be reasonable for the data being analysed.

DR. COHN: Movement artefacts generally send the signal right off the screen. Therefore, if the assumption is made that even the largest breath is nominally 2 litres, every one of those movement artefacts will be excluded. Mr. Watson is really saying that data will be lost because the subject may be breathing when he is also moving, but that, even in the most restless subjects, there are still 20 breaths/min (1200 points/hr or 9600 in an 8-hour recording), so we are talking about thousands of data points and quite a lot of information can still be obtained even excluding the movement artefacts. If the movement artefacts were within the range of the tidal volume, however, that would cause a lot of trouble because it would not be known what was movement and what was tidal volume. Fortunately, however, it does not work out that way - the movement artefacts are tremendous and send the signal right off the screen.

DR. SOUTHALL: I note that this is used in babies. Have babies in the supine position been compared with babies in the prone position, or even adults compared in the supine and prone positions?

MR. WATSON: The prone and the supine were two of the postures that were used in the 7-position studies. The greatest error occurred in the right and left lateral decubitus positions, which is probably due to change in the shape of the abdominal compartment.

DR. SOUTHALL: I am interested in baby monitoring. Babies' positions can vary considerably.

MR. WATSON: We have no data on babies at all - perhaps Dr. Phillipson has some data?

DR. PHILLIPSON: I do not have personal data, but the paediatric group at the hospital for Sick Children has. These data have just been published in the 'American Review'. They have found that the use of the respitrace system is very reliable in infants, and that it is quite independent of posture. I cannot quote the exact figures, but the details are available.

THE MEASUREMENT OF RESPIRATORY FLOW BY INDUCTANCE PNEUMOGRAPHY

S.L. HILL, J.P. BLACKBURN, T.R. WILLIAMS.

Department of Clinical Measurement, Westminster Hospital,
London, UK

Summary

The use of Inductance Pneumography for measuring volume and flow was investigated in fit volunteers.

The apparatus was easy to use and good correlations were obtained for both volume and flow when compared with conventional spirometry.

The technique is suitable for the non-invasive measurement of volume from which flow may be derived.

Introduction

A non-invasive method for measuring respiratory flow was required for the assessment of various types of oxygen mask.

The equipment had to be stable, accurate and unaffected by changes in gas composition. It could not be connected to the airway directly as this would affect the performance of the oxygen therapy device.

A number of methods have been reviewed by Sackner (1979). Inductance pneumography was selected as a technique suitable for detailed investigation. Previous reports showed good correlation when used for measurement of volume, but detailed studies of flow measurement by this method had not been carried out.

The apparatus has been described by Milledge and Stott (1977). It consists of two single turn coils attached in a zig-zag fashion to elasticated belts. These belts encircle the chest and abdomen at the level of the 4th costal cartilage and umbilicus respectively.

Movement associated with respiration alters the cross sectional areas of the two coils and thereby changes their inductances. These changes of inductance are detected as changes in the frequency of oscillators connected to the coils. The output from each oscillator is demodulated, filtered and summed to produce a signal proportional to volume. This is then differentiated to obtain respiratory flow rate. The two signals are displayed on a multi-channel recorder (Watson, 1979) (Fig.1).

Method

The belts are placed over the chest and abdomen of the subject. The subject then performs a series of iso-volume respiratory movements with an open glottis, shifting air within the lungs by alternate contractions of the intercostal muscles and the diaphragm. The gains on the thoracic and abdominal channels are adjusted so that this

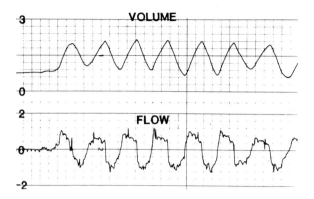

Fig. 1   Simultaneous volume and flow by Inductance Pneumography.

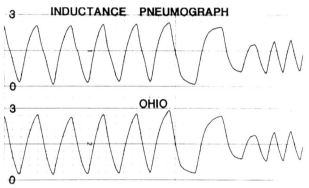

Fig. 2   Volume recorded by Ohio SLpirometer and Inductance
          Pneumograph.

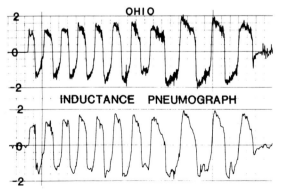

Fig. 3   Flow recorded by Ohio Spirometer and Inductance
          Pneumograph.

manoeuvre produces minimal deflection of the trace. This equalises the outputs of the two belts so that the thoracic and abdominal contributions to respiration are recorded correctly.

The patient then takes a series of breaths of different tidal volumes whilst simultaneously breathing into an Ohio dry spirometer. The output of the inductance pneumograph is matched to the output of the spirometer. The flow channel is calibrated electrically as the derivative of the volume channel. The volume and flow traces from the inductance pneumograph and Ohio spirometer are displayed on a four-channel recorder (Figs. 2 and 3).

The volunteers remained supine during measurements and breathed at rates up to 5 litres per second and volumes to 2.5 litres. A preliminary study showed that the calibration was not significantly affected by changes in position of the subjects.

At the end of the run, the calibration of the equipment was checked and baseline drift measured.

The flow and volume traces obtained from the inductance pneumograph were compared with the corresponding traces from the spirometer.

Results

The flow traces are of good quality and easily interpreted except at high flow rates combined with large tidal volumes when the pneumograph trace shows an exaggerated peak. This may be due to pressure changes within the alveoli at high flows, or to contraction of the auxiliary muscles of respiration under the belts.

Table 1

Results of Linear Regression of Paired Observations of Inductance Pneumograph and Ohio Spirometer (Figures 4 and 5)

	Volume	Flow
Slope	.972	.929
Intercept	.057	.075
Correlation coefficient	.991	.992

The scatter diagram shows that the discrepancy in flow recorded by inductance pneumography and the Ohio spirometer increased at fast flow rates and that correlation was much better at the more physiological level of up to 3 litres/sec.

The calibration of the volume channel did not alter significantly during the average run (about an hour), but some baseline drift occurred. The flow channel remained stable in all respects.

Discussion

The device is easy to use and relatively simple to calibrate. It is comfortable to wear and not particularly restrictive. Body movements produce quite large artefacts on the flow trace but in normal use the

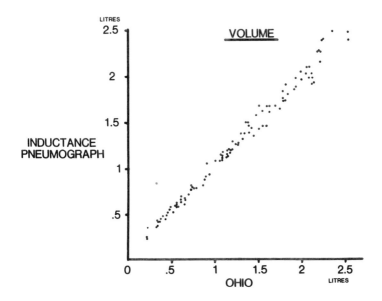

Fig. 4   Scatter diagram of Volume, Ohio Spirometer against
           Inductance Pneumograph.

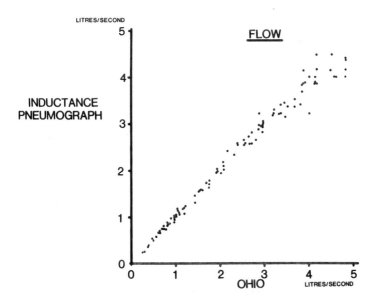

Fig. 5   Scatter diagram of Flow, Ohio Spirometer against
           Inductance Pneumograph.

trace is stable and easily read.

The cardiac impulse produces a clear output on the flow channel but this does not interfere significantly with the measurement of respiratory flow.

Some inaccuracy occurred at high flow rates but this was towards the limit of the physical capabilities of fit volunteers. This discrepancy may be due to the fact that inductance pneumography measures chest wall movement, whilst the spirometer measures gas flow and may be affected by the resistance of the apparatus.

Conclusion

Inductance Pneumography is a relatively simple and accurate method of measuring respiratory flow rate and volume where interference with the airway is to be avoided.

The inaccuracies occurring at high flow rates limit the useful range of this apparatus to about 3 litres per second.

Acknowledgements

We wish to thank Dr. Milledge and Dr. Stott for providing the body belts and oscillators used in this study and for their encouragement and advice.

References

1.   Sackner M.A. In: ISAM 1979: Proceedings of the Third International Symposium on Ambulatory Monitoring, ed. Stott F.D., Raftery E.B. and Goulding L., Academic Press: London.
2.   Milledge J.S. and Stott, F.D. (1977) J. Physiol. 264, 4P.
3.   Watson H. In: ISAM 1979: Proceedings of the Third International Symposium on Ambulatory Monitoring, ed. Stott F.D., Raftery E.B. and Goulding L., Academic Press: London.

MONITORING OF BREATHING DURING SPEECH IN EXERCISING SUBJECTS

J.M. PATRICK, M. ELIZABETH JACKS AND J.H. DOUST

Department of Physiology and Pharmacology,
University Medical School, Nottingham, UK

Summary

A respiratory inductance plethysmograph has been developed for ambulatory monitoring of ventilation. In a laboratory study, the hypothesis that speech imposes an extra requirement for ventilation in exercise has been examined. 15 male subjects performed steady-state exercise on a treadmill at three different work-intensities. While reading aloud a 100-word paragraph either once or six times without a break, there was a marked reduction in ventilation of around 40%. Afterwards, there was a small overshoot and a quick return to control levels of ventilation. It is concluded that any respiratory embarrassment associated with speech during exercise is not due to hyperventilation.

Introduction

The possibility of using indirect methods (i.e. those without physical connection to the airway) to record ventilation in ambulant subjects was reviewed at ISAM 1979 by Sackner (1) and by Patrick et al (2). Although inductance plethysmography was shown to provide adequate ventilatory records in subjects exercising on the treadmill or bicycle ergometer, this method does not seem to have been applied yet to the monitoring of subjects away from a recorder in the laboratory.

Ambulatory monitoring methods for ventilation are likely to be of most value when used to assess the ventilatory cost of activity, particularly in patients with impaired ventilatory capacity, in whom exercise tolerance is reduced. In a recent review, Cotes (3) estimated that coping with the activities of normal daily living requires the ability to sustain a ventilation of about 50 l/min, and he surmised that an additional 20 l/min would be required if speech were undertaken concurrently. This implies that a material fraction of the ventilatory capacity becomes monopolised during speech, leaving less available for the gas exchange requirements of exercise, and thus limiting the exercise to submaximal levels. Speech during exercise would be particularly difficult for patients with pulmonary disease, and the hypothesis above is indeed a basis for the clinical grading of breathlessness using the questionnaire of Cotes (4). The hypothesis is also the basis for one suggested method for setting safe limits to endurance-training activities (such as jogging) in normal subjects: that is, to keep the jogging speed below that which prevents simultaneous conversation (the 'talk-test' (5)).

Surprisingly, there are no detailed reports of measurements of the ventilatory cost of speech in exercise. A respiratory inductance plethysmograph has been used here to investigate the effect on ventilation of a short period of speech in normal subjects exercising on a treadmill. A preliminary report of some of these findings has already been published (6).

Methods

Exercise and Speech Protocol

Subjects walked or ran on a level treadmill at three different speeds, designed to give steady-state heart rates close to 85, 120 and 150 beats/min. Recordings of ventilation were made during a 30- or 60 sec. control period after at least five minutes of exercise had elapsed, and then during and after a period of speech. In Series I, the subjects read aloud a standard paragraph of 100 words. In Series II, the same paragraph was read six times without a break. The subjects then continued to exercise while ventilatory recordings were made for periods of 45 sec (Series I) or 3 min (Series II). No talking was permitted during this period. Calibration procedures were performed at the beginning and end of each exercise run.

Subjects

15 healthy adult males volunteered to be subjects: none had any knowledge of the expected outcome. Their mean age was 21.7 years, their weight was 70.7 kg. and their height 1.80 m. They were made familiar with the experimental procedure, and practised reading the paragraph. Six subjects took part in Series I and the other nine in Series II.

Ventilation Monitoring

A modification (2) of the single-coil inductance plethysmograph of Milledge and Stott (7) has been used. For calibration of the plethysmograph several breaths were recorded at each exercise intensity during re-breathing from an oxygen-filled spirometer. This provides tidal volumes (V_T) covering the range found in the experiment, and allowed V_T to be estimated with a precision of 5 to 20% from the relation between plethysmograph and spirometer excursions. An additional calibration check was obtained by collecting expired air in a Douglas bag during the fourth minute of the exercise period. The sum of the calibrated tidal volumes on the plethysmograph trace was compared with the actual volume collected. The average error was 1.7% and the standard error of the estimate was 5 litres/min.

Analysis

The plethysmograph signal was recorded on paper at 2.5 mm/sec. and the peaks and troughs of the record were later digitised manually to provide breath-by-breath values for V_T. Ventilation was calculated from the sum of the expired tidal volumes over the appropriate sections of the record, using the spirometer calibration described above.

Results

Table 1 gives the mean results for the two series of experiments and shows that expired ventilation at each intensity of exercise is substantially reduced during the period of speech. In Series II, when the ventilation is measured over three minutes rather than 30 seconds of speech, the depression is somewhat less marked.

Table 1

Average Ventilation (1/min; ± SEM) Before and During a Period of Speech at Three Intensities of Exercise

Exercise Intensity	Series I (n=6)		Series II (n=9)	
	Control	30-sec. Speech	Control	3 min. Speech
1	26.9 1.8	17.9 1.3	19.7 0.8	15.7 0.8
2	45.0 6.2	25.4 2.5	35.2 3.6	24.4 1.8
3	69.2 7.2	36.4 4.0	56.7 2.6	36.0 1.8

Figure 1 shows the data for individual comparions between the speech and control periods. Again, the depression is seen to be smaller during the longer speech period. The higher the initial ventilation, the larger the reduction during speech (both in relative and absolute terms) and the greater the ventilatory deficit. At the highest intensity of exercise, speech reduces ventilation by about 40%.

Table 2 (which is a continuation of Table 1) shows the ventilation immediately after speech in both series. After 30 seconds of speech (Series I), ventilation rises above the control level for about 15 seconds, while after 3 minutes of talking (Series II), the overshoot lasts about 2 minutes. The time course of the overshoot and the recovery can be seen in Figure 2, which gives the mean values for ventilation throughout the whole experiment for the nine subjects in Series II at the highest work intensity. The absolute size of the overshoot, expressed either as peak excess ventilation (10 1/min.) or as excess ventilatory volume (5 to 6 litres), is about the same at each intensity, and is, therefore, proportionally greater at the lowest exercise level.

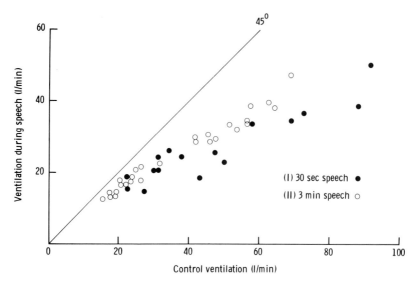

Fig. 1   The relation between ventilation during speech and ventilation during the control period beforehand, in 15   subjects
exercising at 3 different intensities on the treadmill.
The period of speech lasted 30 sec or 3 min. The line of
equality is shown.

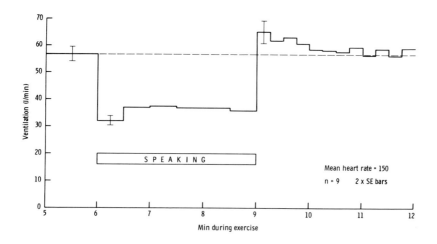

Fig. 2   Mean ventilation (+2 x SEM) before, during and after a 3 min
speech period in nine subjects running on a treadmill   with
steady-state heart-rates of about 150 beats/min.

Table 2

Average Ventilation (1/min; ± SEM) in Consecutive 15-second Periods
Following a Period of Speech Lasting about 30-seconds in Series I and
about 3 minutes in Series II, at Three Different Exercise Intensities

Exercise Intensity		1	2	3
Series 1 (n=6)	1	28.2 ± 3.5	56.7 ± 7.4	66.9 ± 10.5
	2	26.5 ± 3.1	45.1 ± 8.0	61.4 ± 9.9
	3	23.8 ± 3.6	44.3 ± 7.2	62.5 ± 12.1
Series II (n=9)	1	26.7 ± 1.6	46.4 ± 4.7	65.4 ± 4.2
	2	23.5 ± 1.7	40.5 ± 3.4	61.9 ± 3.5
	3	22.2 ± 1.5	38.0 ± 3.5	63.1 ± 4.3
	4	21.1 ± 1.6	38.4 ± 3.7	60.7 ± 2.8
	5	22.2 ± 2.1	38.9 ± 3.6	58.6 ± 3.7
	6	22.3 ± 1.7	37.8 ± 3.3	58.2 ± 2.9
	7	20.1 ± 1.1	39.1 ± 3.4	57.6 ± 3.2
	8	20.0 ± 1.5	36.7 ± 3.4	59.6 ± 3.6
	9	20.4 ± 1.6	37.1 ± 3.9	56.4 ± 3.4
	10	19.2 ± 0.9	36.6 ± 4.0	58.6 ± 3.3
	11	20.3 ± 1.3	36.4 ± 3.9	56.2 ± 3.5
	12	19.7 ± 1.5	36.9 ± 3.7	59.0 ± 3.2

Conclusions

The main finding of this study is that ventilation in exercising
subjects is markedly reduced during continuous periods of speech, and
has a modest brief overshoot afterwards.   There is a suggestion that
some recovery may take place even while speech is continuing, as the
deficit is less when averaged over 3 minutes of speech than it is
when averaged over the first 30 seconds only.
    Indirect methods like the inductance plethysmograph cannot meas-
ure ventilation with the precision of conventional methods, but there
can be no doubt about the direction and size of the ventilatory
 hange imposed here by speech during exercise.   Movement artefacts,
having predominantly the frequency of the footfall, do not obscure
the respiratory waveform or prevent the measurement of tidal volume.
    The limitation of ventilation during speech is presumably due to
the voluntary reduction of expiratory airflow down to the low values
required for phonation.   This aspect of the study is dealt with fully
elsewhere (8).   But although the period of speech makes particular
flow demands on the ventilatory system, there is no extra requirement
for ventilation per se.   Indeed there is a reduction.   After talking,
however, there is a small extra requirement which peaks at about 10
1/min. and last for about half the time of the speech period itself:
it involves the movement of about 5 extra litres of air.   This could

tax a very limited ventilatory capacity at modest workloads, but
cannot account for the difficulty in talking during hard but still
sub-maximal exercise. The contribution of speech to breathlessness
and to the limitation of exercise must be related to the altered
pattern of breathing rather than to an extra demand for ventilation:
that is, any respiratory embarrassment in exercise during speech is
NOT due to hyperventilation.

Acknowledgements

Mr. John Hillier developed the inductance plethysmograph with the
help of Miss Beverley Smith. M. Elizabeth Jacks was an undergraduate
medical student in the Department.   J. H.Doust is supported by a
grant from the Sports Council.

References

1.   Sackner M.A. (1980) In:ISAM 1979 Proc. of 3rd Int. Symp. on
      Amb. Mon. Eds: Stott F.D., Raftery E.B., Goulding L. Academic
      Press, London,   299-319.
2.   Patrick J.M., Ross A.M. and Hanley S.B. (1980) In: ISAM 1979
      Proc. of 3rd Int. Symp. on Amb. Mon. Eds: Stott F.D., Raftery
      E.B., Goulding L. Academic Press, London, 321-328.
3.   Cotes J.E. (1975) Br.J. Ind. Med. **32**, 220-223.
4.   Cotes J.E. (1979) Lung Function. Blackwell Scientific Publica-
      tions, 399.
5.   Fentem P.H. (1978) New Scientist 256-259.
6.   Doust J.H. and Patrick J.M. (1981a) J. Physiol. **312**, 57 P
7.   Milledge J.S. and Stott F.D. (1977) J. Physiol. **267**, 4-5 P.
8.   Doust J.H. and Patrick J.M. (1981b) Respiration Physiology **46**,
      134-47.

Discussion

DR. JAWAHIRI: The level of exercise was constant throughout, so I
conclude that the CO_2 production remained unchanged during exercise.
Therefore, it must be concluded that during the time that the people
were talking there was a rise in arterial PCO_2... (Dr. Patrick
agreed). The interesting point is that during ordinary exercise
$PaCO_2$ should remain unchanged. Therefore, when Dr. Patrick's subjects stopped talking, it would be expected that the same control
mechanisms come into effect and that their $PaCO_2$ should now return
again to normal. The overshoot should exactly equal the undershoot
that they had while they were talking.
DR. PATRICK: That is right, but in fact the overshoot is never as
much as the undershoot. I have tried to measure end-tidal PCO_2 and
PO_2 values during experiments like this. I did not want to show
these measurements today, because I am trying to get away from making
measurements at the mouth. The end-tidal PCO_2 rises very substantially during speech and then falls back again rather quickly at the
end of speech. Indeed, if CO_2 response lines are drawn, the overshoot will not be expected to be anything like as great as the undershoot originally. We can discuss the control aspects of this later,
outside this discussion. My results are very similar to those of Dr.

Phillipson during CO_2 breathing.

DR. PHILLIPSON: This is a very elegant study. It shows, as ours did, the interaction between the behavioural respiratory control system, of which speech is the best examle, and the automatic or the metabolic system. Dr. Patrick drove the metabolic system with exercise; we drove it with hypercapnia, but in both instances, it was over-ridden by the demands for a behavioural hyperventilatory activity, namely, speech. I suspect that the over-ride is within limits. I do not yet know of anyone who has killed himself by speaking, by getting hypercapnic and hypoxic.

     All our subjects spontaneously volunteered, that while speaking, even during the hypercapnic run, they were much less short of breath than during the quiet hypercapnic run - and, of course, they were breathing much less. Did any of you subjects comment that they were much less aware of the breathing while they were speaking?

DR. PATRICK: Yes, several said that.

DR. CASHMAN: What was the average age of the subjects? Secondly, what was the workload on the treadmill?

DR. PATRICK: They were all young male adults, 20 to 35-years-old. The workload was varied according to their heart rate response: 150 beats/min was the target heart rate for the highest exercise intensity during which they were running on the treadmill.

DIPL. ING. RASCHKE: Does Dr. Patrick think that his subjects compensate for their loss in O_2 by anaerobic mechanisms - or is that not possible? When there is a heart rate of 150 or 160 beats/min, that is surely above the endurance limit?

DR. PATRICK: Yes, they will be compensating in that way and it should be possible to detect any anaerobic metabolism by the size of the overshoot afterwards. The curious finding on my penultimate slide was that the overshoot was about the same at the highest intensity of exercise as it was at the lowest, so I cannot think that anaerobiosis during the speech period contributes very much to that recovery ventilation.

MEASUREMENT OF PULMONARY MECHANICS DURING QUIET BREATHING IN NORMALS AND ASTHMATICS USING A RESPIRATORY INDUCTIVE PLETHYSMOGRAPH

M. COHN, B. DAVIS, H. WATSON, M. BROUDY, S. BIRCH
AND M. SACKNER

Samuel J. Kraver Scientific Data Processing Centre and
the Jane and Edward Shapiro Pulmonary Suite, Division of
Pulmonary Disease, Department of Medicine, Mount Sinai Medical
Centre, Miami Beach, Florida, USA

Summary

Using a respiratory inductive plethysmograph and oesophageal and nasal catheters, we continuously monitored respiratory timing, nasal and pulmonary resistance and pulmonary compliance in six normals and six asthmatics, while lying quietly for four hours breathing air via a face mask. No significant differences between the groups for the time components of respiration were found. The mean pulmonary resistance of 5.1 $cmH_2O/L/sec$ and mean compliance of 0.12 L/cmH_2O in the asthmatics differed significantly from 2.8 $cmH_2O/L/sec$ and 0.21 L/cmH_2O, respectively, in the normals. Mean nasal resistance of 0.4 $cmH_2O/L/sec$ was similar in both groups. No significant differences in timing of respiration were observed when five subjects were restudied without the mask and catheters. Therefore, such systems are acceptable for long-term monitoring of the effects of exposure to aerosols, gases and pollutants.

Introduction

Usual methods for monitoring respiration require a mouthpiece, which alters the pattern of breathing and prevents long-term continuous monitoring. Magnetometers accurately measure tidal volume without need of a mouthpiece, but cannot be used to monitor respiration for long time periods, because of changes in calibration after postural changes (1). We have previously described the respiratory inductive plethysmograph, which is capable of accurately measuring tidal volume (2) and, when combined with an oesophageal balloon, pulmonary mechancis without physical connection to the airway (3). In this study, we expand our preliminary observations of breathing pattern in normals and asthmatic subjects during four hours of continuous monitoring (4) and include measurement of pulmonary resistance and compliance. In addition, we measured the effect, of the pulmonary apparatus (face mask, oesophageal catheter) on the breathing pattern.

Methods

Six healthy male subjects, ages 18 to 30 years, and six asthmatics (4 males, 2 females), ages 18 to 40 years, volunteered for the study and gave informed consent. All were asymptomatic, on no medication and had normal routine pulmonary function tests at the time of the study.

Calibration of the Respiratory Inductive Plethysmograph

Just prior to the study period, an AC-coupled respiratory inductive plethysmograph (Respitrace[R], Ambulatory Monitoring, Inc; Ardsley, NY) with an electrical frequency response that is flat fom 0.05 to 15 hertz and consisting of rib cage and abdominal coils, whose inductance changes during breathing are proportional to the volume displacements of each compartment was placed on the subject. For calibration, the subject breathed quietly into a dry rolling-seal spirometer for 30 seconds (Ohio 800, Ohio Medical Products, Houston, Texas) first, while standing and then, supine - a method previously described (2). In each position, the electrical signals from the spirometer and respiratory inductive plethysmograph were fed into a Harris computer system (Harris S110, Harris Corp., Ft. Lauderdale, FL) for calculation of rib cage and abdominal signals from the respiratory inductive plethysmograph and generated their sum. If ideally calibrated, this summation signal would be identical to the spirometer signal when the previous signals are generated, re-analysed and compared. For our study, if the mean amplitude of the calibrated summation signal of the respiratory inductive plethysmograph in the supine position was greater than $\pm$ 10% of the spirometer signal, the calibration procedure was repeated.

Placement of Oesophageal and Nasal Catheters

After calibration of the respiratory inductive plethysmograph, each patient inhaled into both nostrils, two puffs of a 0.05% solution of oxy-metazoline hydrochloride, a long-acting nasal decongestant. Then, each subject, while seated swallowed a 10 cm balloon tipped catheter, connected to a calibrated pressure transducer. The alloon was positioned in the lower third of the oesophagus by withdrawing it slowly from the stomach (determined by observing a positive pressure signal on inspiration) until 5 cm above the gastro-oesophageal junction (the position where the positive pressure signal changes to a negative signal on inspiration), filled with 0.5 ml air, and then securely taped in position. A second, smaller (3 cm) balloon tipped catheter connected to another pressure transducer, was passed nasally into the pharynx, gradually withdrawn until the deflection on the transducer produced by the subject's tongue during swallowing disappeared, and then taped into position. The oesophageal catheter was connected to both pressure transducers, using a Y-connector. One transducer was referenced to the mouth (face mask, mouthpiece of the spirometer, or room) to reflect total trans-pulmonary pressure (P_{TP}), the other referenced to the pharyngeal catheter in order to subtract the pressure component resulting from nasal flow resistance (P_{TP-N}). The pressure signals were digitally filtered by the computer (cut-off above 15 Hz) to reduce cardiac oscillations (5).

Computer Data Analysis

After the calibrated signals for volume and pressure were fed into the computer, tidal volume (V_T), breathing frequency (f), breath duration period (T), duration of inspiration (T_I), fractional inspir-

atory time (T_I/T), "mean" inspiratory flow (V_T/T_I), and minute ventilation (V_E) were measured and calculated for each breath from either
the spirometer volume signal or the summation signal derived from the
respiratory inductive plethysmograph. A digital derivative of the
volume signal, i.e. flow, was generated by the computer and along
with one of the transducer pressure signals was used for calculation
of pulmonary resistance and compliance for each breath (Figure 1).

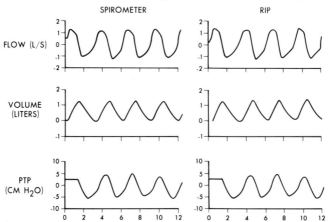

Fig. 1   Example of computer plot of tidal volume, pressure (PTP),
          and derived flow signals from the spirometer and respira-
          tory inductive plethysmograph used for calculation of air-
          flow resistance and compliance. Since the pressure signal
          is digitally filtered at frequences above 15 Hz, cardiac
          oscillations are not seen.

The transducer signal measuring P_{TP} was used to measure total pulmonary resistance (R_L) and the one measuring P_{TP-N} was used for total
pulmonary resistance less nasal flow resistance. Nasal flow resistance (R_N) was calculated by subtracting the latter from the former.
In two subjects, this value was compared to that obtained following
the study, using posterior rhinometry (6). Mean resistance was
calculated by computer determination of the inspiratory mid-volume
point and expiratory equal volume point on the volume signal (7). At
these exact time points, the pressure signal change was divided by
the corresponding flow signal change to calculate resistance. Dynamic lung compliance (C_L) was calculated by the computer by dividing
the inspiratory volume change (points of zero flow) by the corresponding change in pressure.

Validation of the Respiratory Inductive Plethysmograph
        Immediately before and after the four-hour monitoring period,
the volume signals from the spirometer and respiratory inductive
plethysmograph along with the total transpulmonary pressure (P_{TP})
signals were fed into the computer for analysis while the subject
breathed quietly for 25 seconds into the spirometer while standing.
This was repeated while supine. The mean and standard deviation of
each parameter were determined for all the breaths collected. The
mean values determined from the respiratory inductive plethysmograph

signals were compared to those from the spirometer signal and expressed as percent differences:

[(respiratory inductive plethysmograph value minus spirometer value)/spirometer value] x 100.

Long-Term Monitoring

After calibration and validation, the respiratory inductive plethysmograph and total transpulmonary pressure (P_{TP}) signals were fed into the computer for on-line analysis while each subject breathed air through a soft face mask (air flowing by the orifice at 30 litres/min) for four hours lying either supine or semi-recumbent. All signals were recorded on a Honeywell tape recorder for off-line analysis to determine pulmonary less nasal resistance using the transpulmonary minus nasal pressure signal (P_{TP-N}). For both analyses, forty-eight consecutive five-minute averages of all parameters were calculated and stored in the computer for final print-out and statistical analysis. The mean and S.D. of these 48 consecutive averages were determined for each subject. Following the study, nasal resistance was also measured in two subjects, using posterior rhinometry (6) and the values from the two methods were compared.

Effect of Catheter and Face Mask on Pattern of Breathing

To determine the effect of the catheters and face mask on the time components of the breathing pattern, three normal and two asthmatic subjects repeated the four-hour study twice; first, with only the face mask. and second, with neither the catheters nor face mask. The mean and S.L. of the 48 consecutive five-minute averages of the time components of respiration from these two studies were compared to the values from the long-term monitoring when the subjects wore the face mask and catheters.

Results

Validation of the Respiratory Inductive Plethysmograph

87% of mean tidal volumes measured by respiratory inductive plethsymography in the supine and standing positions before the study and 90% after the study, fell within ± 20% of those measured by spirometry. Similar accuracies were found for mean inspiratory flow and minute ventilation.

Table 1

Percentages of Pulmonary Resistance and Compliance Measurements by Respiratory Inductive Plethysmography Deviating from Spirometry

Cumulative % Deviation From Spirometry	± 10%	± 15%	± 20%	± 30%	± 40%
Resistance PreStudy	48	65	78	100	100
PostStudy	42	47	74	89	100
Compliance PreStudy	77	91	91	100	100
PostStudy	74	89	89	95	100

Table 1 shows the pre- and post-study percentages of measurements by respiratory inductive plethysmography deviating from spirometry for pulmonary resistance and compliance, regardless of body
position.

100% of mean pulmonary resistance values measured by respiratory
inductive plethysmograph before the study and 89% after the study,
fell within $\pm$ 30% of those measured by spirometry.

100% of dynamic pulmonary compliance values measured by respiratory inductive plethysmography before the study and 95% after the
study fell within $\pm$ 30% of those measured by spirometry.

All values of the remaining parameters (V_T, f T, T_I, and T_I/T)
measured by respiratory inductive plethysmography fell within $\pm$ 5% of
those measured by spirometry before and after the study.

Long-Term Monitoring

Figure 2 shows a plot of the five minute averages of
pulmonary resistance in the normals and asthmatics. A greater
variability as seen in the asthmatics compared to the normals.

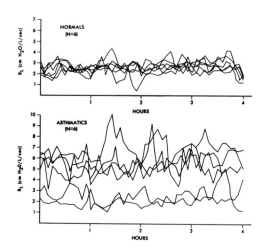

**Fig. 2   Plot of five minute averages of pulmonary resistance in the
normals and asthmatics. Note the greater variability in
the asthmatics than the normals.**

Table 2 shows the mean and S.D. of the 48 consecutive averages
for each parameter during the four hours of monitoring in the normals
and asthmatics. No significant differences for the time components
of respiration (V_T, f, T, T_I, $T_I T$, V_T/T_I, and V^E) were found between
the normals and asthmatics. The mean (S.D.) total pulmonary
resistance (R^L) of 2.8 (0.5) $cmH_2O/L/sec$ in the normals was significantly less (p<.05) than 5.1 (1.9) $cmH_2O/L/sec$ in the asthmatics.
However, nasal resistance was similar in both groups. The mean
resistance measurements using two different methods in two subjects
were within 15% of each other.

The mean (S.S.) dynamic pulmonary compliance (C^L) of 0.21 (0.07)

L/cmH$_2$O in normals was significantly greater (p<.05) than 0.12 (0.01 (0.01) L/cmH$_2$O in the asthmatics.

The time constant of the respiratory system (R^L x C^L) was similar in both groups.

Effect of Face Mask and Catheters on Patterns of Breathing

Table 3 shows the mean (S.D.) of the 48 consecutive fiveminute averages during the four hours of monitoring in the three normals and two asthmatics:

    (a) with the face mask and catheters

    (b) with mask only; and

    (c) with neither mask nor catheter.

Although a small but significant, (p<.05), decrease in mean (S.D.) T from 3.40 (0.28) sec without mask or catheter to 3.13 (0.22) sec with both mask and catheter and a small but significant, (p<.01), increase in mean (S.D.) T^I/T from 0.37 (0.02) without mask or catheter to 0.40 (0.01) with mask only was observed, no significant differences in V^T, f, T^I, V^T/T^I and V^E were found. The physiologic significance of the differences in T and T^I/T is uncertain.

TABLE 3

EFFECT OF FACE MASK AND CATHETERS ON BREATHING PATTERN IN THREE NORMALS AND TWO ASTHMATICS

	V_T (L)	f (breaths/ min)	T (sec)	T_I (sec)	T_I/T	V_T/T_I (L/sec)	V_E (L/min)
Mask and Catheters	0.34 (0.10)	21.2 (1.7)	3.13* (0.22)	1.28 (0.14)	0.42 (0.05)	0.27 (0.06)	6.60 (1.65)
Mask only	0.32 (0.08)	19.4 (2.3)	3.28 (0.40)	1.29 (0.15)	0.40** (0.01)	0.25 (0.05)	5.84 (1.25)
No Mask or Catheter	0.32 (0.08)	18.9 (1.5)	3.40* (0.28)	1.24 (0.09)	0.37** (0.02)	0.27 (0.07)	5.83 (1.79)

Mean and standard deviation (parentheses) shown.
* p<.05, paired t-test.
** p<.01, paired t-test.

Table 2   Mean and S.D. of 48 consecutive averages shown in Fig. 2.

	VT (L)	f (breaths/	T (sec)	TI (sec)	TI/T	VT/TI (L/sec)	VE (L/min)	RL (cmH2O/L)	RN (cmH2O/L)	CL (L/cmH2O)	RLxCL (sec)
Normals (N=6) Mean	0.40	21.6	3.07	1.28	0.43	0.32	7.79	2.84*	0.38	0.21*	0.60
(S.D)	(0.09)	(1.5)	(0.18)	(0.11)	(0.03)	(0.06)	(1.40)	(0.52)	(0.57)	(0.07)	(0.21)
Asthmatics (N=6) Mean	0.33	26.3	2.80	1.17	0.44	0.27	7.01	5.12*	0.37	0.12*	0.63
(S.D)	(0.13)	(9.4)	(0.72)	(0.24)	(0.03)	(0.11)	(2.40)	(1.90)	(1.10)	(0.01)	(0.23)

Mean and stand deviation in parentheses.
*$p < .05$, unpaired t-test.

Conclusion

The evaluation of therapeutic aerosols, gases, and environmental pollutants on the breathing pattern is facilitated by their administration with a flowthrough face mask since exposures in environmental chambers are quite costly. The experiments here reported were designed in part to assess the influence of such apparatus on respiration. We previously described the breathing pattern during four hours of continuously monitoring normals and asymptomatic asthmatics while lying quietly in bed using a respiratory inductive plethysmograph (4). Table 2 shows that no significant differences in V^T, f, t, T_I T_I/T, V_T/T_I, or V^E were observed between the normals and asthmatics. In this study, we add the measurement of pulmonary resistance, nasal resistance and dynamic lung compliance during the four hours of continuous monitoring. Since use of a nose clip and mouthpiece has previously been shown to alter breathing pattern (8, 9), we also restudied the breathing pattern of 5 subjects wearing the face mask only (to assess any effect of the catheters) and without face mask or catheters (to assess any effect of the face mask). .

Measurements of volume pressure and flow-pressure relationships of human lungs to determine pulmonary compliance and resistance are based on indirect determination of pleural pressure from oesophageal pressure (10). Agreement between the two is maximized by positioning the balloon tipped catheter in the lower third of the oesophagus and inflating it with 0.5 cc air. In the supine and, to a lesser extent, the semi-recumbent position, cardiac oscillations are enlarged, interfering with computer determination of pressure changes for calculation of resistance and compliance. In this study, we employed a digital filter with an upper frequency cut-off at 15 Hz, which suppresses cardiac oscillations, without amplitude loss of the lower frequency respiratory related pressure changes. The supine position may also result in a positive shift in baseline oesophageal pressure presumably from the weight of the mediastinum on the balloon and causes an increase in pressure amplitudes (11). However, in our study, pulmonary compliance values measured in the supine and standing positions were comparable. Because of the low flow rates encountered during quiet breathing, a method for calculation of average pulmonary resistance was used (7).

All measurements of resistance and compliance using respiratory nductive plethysmography fell within $\pm$ 30% of simultaneous spirometry, an acceptable level of accuracy. The mean pulmonary resistance of 2.8 cmH$_2$0/L/sec in our supine or semi-recumbent normals is higher than the value of 1.0 cmH$_2$0/L/sec measured by Ferris et al in normals while sitting (11). This difference might be related to the different postures and may explain why nasal resistance contributed only 13% to total resistance in our normals but over 50% in Ferris' group. Another factor may be the pre-treatment with a nasal decongestant in our groups.

The asthmatic group had a significantly higher pulmonary resistance and lower compliance than the normals. The product of resistance and compliance (R^L x C^L) represents the time constant of the respiratory system and may determine respiratory frequency (13). The similar value of R^L x C^L in the two groups may explain why no significant differences in the timing of respiration were observed.

The use of the face mask and catheters did not produce any significant changes in the time components of respiration, especially mean inspiratory flow (V^T/T^I). The latter is considered an index of respiratory drive (14) and a sensitive indicator of mild degrees of provoked broncho-constriction (15). However, no difference in mean inspiratory flow between our normals and asthmatics was observed despite a higher pulmonary resistance in the latter. This may be related to the steady state achieved during long-term monitoring in this study in contrast to acute changes in pulmonary resistance during provocation with inhaled broncho-constrictors, such as methacholine.

Thus, this system for long-term monitoring of respiratory timing and mechanics using the respiratory inductive plethysmograph, face mask and balloon tipped catheters, is an acceptable semi-quantitaive method for evaluating the long-term pulmonary response to exposure to aerosols, gases and pollutants within defined limits of accuracy.

References

1. Ashutosh K., Gilbert R., Auchincloss J.H., Erlebacher J. and Peppi D., (1974) J. Appl. Physiol. **37**, 964966
2. Cohn M.A., Watson H., Weisshaut R., Stott F. and Sackner M.A. In: ISAM 1977: Proceeedings of the Second International Symposium on Ambulatory Monitoring, Ed: F.D. Stott, E.B. Raftery, P. Sleight and L. Goulding, London, Academic Press, 1978, 119128.
3. Cohn M.A., Lehrer L., Watson H., Davis B., Zarzecki S., Stott F. and Sackner M.A. (1978) Am. Rev. Respir. Dis. **117**, 322 (abstract).
4. Cohn M.A., Rao B.V.A., Davis B., Watson H., Broudy M.J., Sackner J.D. and Sackner M.A. In ISAM 1979: Proceedings of the Third International Symposium on Ambulatory Monitoring. Ed: F.D. Stott, E.B. Raftery and L. Goulding, London, Academic Press, 1980, 355365.
5. Laxminarayan S., Spoelstra A.J.G., Sipkema P. and Westerhof N. (1978) Med. & Biol. Eng. & Comput. **16**, 397407.
6. Taylor G., Shivalkar P.R. (1971) Clin. Allergy **1**, 63.
7. Cook C.D., Sutherland J.M., Segal S., Cherry R.B., Mead J., McIbroy M.B. and Smith C.A. (1959) J. Clin. Invest. **36** 440448.
8. Askanazi J., Silverberg P.A., Foster R.J., Hyman A.I., MilicEmili J. and Kinney J.M. (1980) J. Appl. Physiol. **48**, 577580.
9. Sackner J.D., Nixon J., Davis B., Atkins N. and Sackner M.A. (1980) Am. Rev. Respir. Dis. **122**, 933940.
10. MilicEmili J., Mead J., Turner J.M. and Glauser E.M. (1964) J. Appl. Physiol. **19**, 207211.
11. Mead J. and Gaensler E.A. (1959) **14** 8183.
12. Ferris B.G., Jr., Mead J. and Opie L.H. (1964) J. Appl. Physiol. **19**, 653658.
13. Mead J. (1960) J. Appl. Physiol. **15**, 325336.
14. MilicEmili J., Siafakas N.M., Gautier H. (1979) Bull. Europ. Physiopath. Resp. **15**, 1726.
15. Chadha T.S., et al. (1981) Am. Rev. Respir. Dis. **123**, 205 (abstract)

Discussion

DR. SOUTHALL: In which order were those last three tested out?   Did
Dr. Cohn start with the patient with the mask and oesophageal cath-
eters, going down, or start with nothing and move up?
DR. COHN: The initial study was with all the patients having the face
mask and catheters.   The subsequent two studies were in no particular
order.
DR. SOUTHALL: So they could have got used to the mask and catheters?
(Dr. Cohn agreed that they could have).
DR. SACKNER: What was the interval between studies?
DR. COHN: The interval was several months at least. We later asked
the question about the effect of the system and the timing of respiration,so the last two repeat studies were many months six months
or perhaps one year later. They were not together in time. However, the other two were done about one week apart: that is, the
mask only and without a mask studies.
DR. PHILLIPSON: That there were no differences was a surprising
finding. Did that happen because it was longterm monitoring?   Certainly,in the short term, over a matter of minutes, we have noticed
quite considerable differences when the subject is relieved of all
the encumbrances round the mouth and the face, using only the respitrace. The pattern of breathing is then usually quite different. Is
it because this is fourhours' data that something is being lost or
gained, according to the point of view?
DR. COHN: Yes, I believe that is probably true. There are marked
variations from minute to minute, perhaps depending upon the patient's comfort, distracts, pain at one point or another and so on.
We are simply looking at an overall level. The use of the frequency
histogram and other techniques for looking at large amounts of data
points may be helpful in gathering more information from such a
system, but in terms of the longterm effects over four hours, this is
the way in which we initially looked for the data anaylsis.   Nevertheless, it leaves much to be desired. Looking at fiveminute averages means that many small changes are lost although perhaps appropriately so.
DR. PHILLIPSON: Since the six asthmatics clearly had elevated resistances, why are they different from Dr. Sackner's six asthmatics
in that their mean inspiratory flow rate was lower than the normals,
whereas his were higher?
DR. COHN: In terms of the actual base line mean inspiratory flow
rates, they were lower in our study. This may be connected to the
duration of the study and relaxation after four hours. Two of our
asthmatics fell within our normal range of pulmonary resistance and
the others fell outside it. Of course, these measurements were made
semi-recumbent. Prior to the study and again afterwards, pulmonary
resistance was measured using body plethysmography, and they were
really within normal limits.
DR. PHILLIPSON: That increased pulmonary resistance presumably was
mostly airway resistance.
DR. COHN: But they were normal in the supine position in body plethysmography, which might suggest that the supine position further
increased the resistance, at least at the flow rates in which we
measured, which were quite low. I might comment that this average

pulmonary resistance measurement is used because of the low inspiratory and expiratory flow rates encountered during quiet breathing. This allowed us to measure resistance with less variability than measuring resistance at a fixed flow rate in all the subjects.

DR. SACKNER: In terms of this particular system, there is no valving. The subject is wearing a mask, and the air is flowing by at 30 litre/min, so he is taking in air from a stream going past the mask, so this is not precisely the same as a face mask with valving. That is one explanation for the slight differences. This system is set up to deliver pollutant mixtures - which is what we are really interested in doing, just flowing the air past the subject.

In terms of the resistance measurements, as Dr. Cohn mentioned, an attempt was made to use a standard Mead-Wittenberger technique, subtracting off compliance. It was completely unsuccessful because that method really depends upon panting to close a loop - and that cannot be done. There are definite problems with the measurement of resistance using this sort of approach. Dr. Cohn alluded to that in terms of the fact that the flow rates are very low and the variability is quite large - 30%. Therefore, it is very approximate, and should be considered only as a semi-quantitative approach rather than an absolute one.

COMPARISON OF FORCED VITAL CAPACITY AND FLOW VOLUME CURVES IN SMOKERS AND NON-SMOKERS UTILIZING SIMULTANEOUS SPIROMETRY, RESPIRATORY INDUCTIVE PLETHYSMOGRAPHY AND BODY PLETHYSMOGRAPHY

M.A. SACKNER, A.S.V. RAO, S. BIRCH, N. ATKINS AND B. DAVIS

The Samuel J. Kraver Scientific Data Processing Centre
and The Jane and Edward Shapiro Pulmonary Suite,
Dept. Medicine, Mount Sinai Medical Centre, Miami Beach,
Florida, USA

Summary

Respiratory inductive plethysmography can be utilized to measure the time-volume and flow-volume components of the forced expiratory vital capacity manoeuvre. It is not as precise as spirometry and body plethysmography and produces a pattern midway between the tracings obtained from these two devices. It provides acceptable semi-quantitative tracings during the breathing of air and the less dense helium-oxygen or more dense sulphur hexafluoride-oxygen mixtures.

Introduction

Respiratory inductive plethysmography serves as a semi-quantitative, non-invasive monitor of resting ventilation in non-smoking normal subjects and smokers with minimal respiratory disease. The device is calibrated to volume measured with simultaneous spirometry during tidal breathing. Its calibration is maintained over a wide range of body postures and during exercise on a treadmill and bicycle ergometer (1, 2). In contrast to spirometry, respiratory inductive plethysmography reflects changes in thoracic volume. During forced expiratory vital capacity manoeuvres, discrepancies may take place between spirometric volumes measured at the mouth and changes of thoracic volume. First, measurements by magnetometers indicate that inhomogeneity of rib cage and abdominal movements occur during the forced expiratory vital capacity manoeuvre, although the calibration of this device assumes that the rib cage and abdomen each move with one degree of freedom (3, 4, 5). Secondly, thoracic volume may be increased by compression of alveolar gas (6) and decreased by shifts of blood from the rib cage and abdominal compartments into the neck and extremities. Finally, displacement of abdominal viscera from the abdomen to the rib cage compartment may alter the scaling factors of the rib cage and the abdomen (1).

Neither inhomogeneity of rib cage and abdominal movements, nor shifts of blood and viscera, need to be considered when measuring changes in thoracic gas volume by body plethysmography with the subject breathing to the outside of the chamber. The purposes of this study included determination of:

1.   The relationship among spirometry, respiratory inductive pleth-

ysmography and body plethysmography in estimation of forced vital
capacity;
2.   The effects of breathing gases of differing density such as
helium and sulphur hexafluoride on the forced vital capacity and flow
volume curves, and
3.   Which devices and measures of the preceding distinguish smokers
from non-smokers.

Materials and Methods

Subjects: Nine non-smokers, ages 17 to 28 and twelve smokers, ages 21
to 39 were enrolled in the study. Baseline pulmonary function tests
included spirometry, body plethysmography, single breath nitrogen
test and measurement of closing volume. On the basis of these tests,
six of the 12 smokers were considered to be normal and six had small
airway disease.

Experimental Design
     The subject was seated within a whole body plethysmograph
modified such that an 8 inch inner diameter by 11 inch length port
was connected to a dry rolling seal spirometer for measurement of
volume changes within the body plethysmograph (Figure 1).

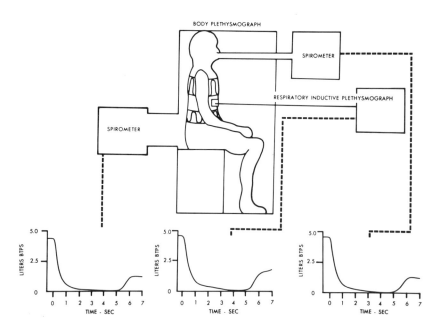

Fig. 1   Schematic diagram of the subject enclosed within a constant
           pressure variable volume body-plethysmograph.   Three
           tracings of forced vital capacity produced by the   subject
           are depicted: body plethysmography, respiratory   inductive
           plethysmography, and spirometry.

The subject breathed through a mouthpiece connected to 1.24 inch
tubing leading to a dry rolling seal spirometer located immediately
outside the chamber. The subject wore a respiratory inductive plethysmograph, which had been previously calibrated to spirometry during
tidal breathing (1). The frequency amplitude response of the body
plethysmograph was flat to within ± 5% to 8Hz and then fell off
rapidly. The frequency amplitude response of the dry rolling seal
spirometer located outside the chamber was flat to within ± 5% to
15Hz. The frequency amplitude response of the respiratory inductive
plethysmograph tested electrically was flat to 15Hz and rolled off
thereafter because of electronic filtering. The respiratory inductive plethysmograph when placed upon a subject was tested up to 5Hz
and found to have flat amplitude response within ± 10% up to this
frequency; it has not been tested at higher frequencies owing to the
characteristics of the sinusoidal pump utilized to generate these
data.

The subjects performed three to five forced expiratory vital
capacity manoeuvres. Simultaneous recordings of volume changes from
spirometry, respiratory inductive plethysmography and body plethysmography were obtained by inputting the analog signals from these
devices into a digital computer. The computer digitized the analog
signal at a rate of 60 points per second, displayed the raw data,
scaled and displayed the curves, calculated the various parameters
from the forced expiratory vital capacity curve, calculated the
derivitive from the volume tracing and displayed the flow volume
curve (for spirometry) or derivative of volume (dV/dt) volume curve
(for respiratory inductive and body plethysmography). The forced
vital capacity tracing selected for analysis was the one which had
the highest value of vital capacity measured by spirometry.

The subject repeated this forced vital capacity manoeuvre after
three vital capacity breaths from a reservoir bag containing a mixture of either 20% oxygen and 80% helium or 20% oxygen and 80%
sulphur hexafluoride. The curves selected for analysis from these
different density gas mixtures were the ones that had the highest
value of vital capacity as measured by spirometry.

Results

Figure 1 depicts a display of the forced expiratory volume tracing in
a smoker breathing air as obtained by the various devices. The basic
configuration of the curves are similar among the devices although
there are slight distortions late in the respiratory inductive plethysmography tracing. Inspection of the forced expiratory volume curves
and the flow-volume or derivative of volume - volume (for inductive
and body plethysmography) curves indicated that peak flows are generally greater with both plethysmographic methods. The pattern of the
respiratory inductive plethysmographic tracings generally fell between those of spirometry and body plethysmography.

Table 1 lists the representative values for the forced expiratory vital capacity and the differences among devices and between
smokers and non-smokers. Forced vital capacity and $FEV_{1.0}$ on both
helium and air breathing were greater in non-smokers for the body
plethysmographic compared to the spirometric data. There were no

TABLE I

REPRESENTATIVE VALUES FOR ANALYSIS OF FORCED EXPIRATORY VITAL CAPACITY CURVE[+]

	NONSMOKERS				SMOKERS			
	FVC LBTPS	FEV$_{1.0}$ LBTPS	Peak Flow or dV/dt LBTPS/Sec	Flow or dV/dt at 25% VC LBTPS/Sec	FVC LBTPS	FEV$_{1.0}$ LBTPS	Peak Flow or dV/dt LBTPS/Sec	Flow or dV/dt at 25% VC LBTPS/SEC
AIR								
Spirometry	4.31 ± 1.27	3.78 ± .92	8.0 ± 2.6	2.5* ± .3	3.92 ± .77	3.33 ± .57	7.5 ± 1.6	1.8* ± .6
Respiratory Inductive Plethysmography	4.36 ± 1.53	3.78 ± 1.10	9.5 ± 4.0	2.5 ± .2	4.27 ± 1.10	3.51 ± .91	9.1 ± 3.3	1.9 ± .9
Body Plethysmography	4.42 ± 1.30	3.93 ± 1.00	10.3 ± 4.5	2.4 ± .4	3.98 ± 1.00	3.46 ± .62	8.8 ± 3.1	2.0 ± .7
He 80% = O$_2$ 20%								
Spirometry	4.25 ± 1.25	3.89 ± 1.03	10.1 ± 3.8	3.1* ± .4	3.91 ± 1.03	3.46 ± .64	9.7 ± 2.8	2.1* ± .7
Respiratory Inductive Plethysmography	4.17 ± 1.52	3.87 ± 1.36	10.3 ± 5.1	3.3* ± .9	4.22 ± 1.36	3.63 ± .85	10.4 ± 2.1	2.2* ± 1.2
Body Plethysmography	4.33 ± 1.29	4.05 ± 1.10	11.7 ± 4.9	3.4* ± .9	3.94 ± 1.10	3.58 ± .65	11.0 ± 3.4	2.6* ± .6
SF$_6$ 80% = O$_2$ 20%								
Spirometry	4.18 ± 1.16	2.92 ± .76	4.7 ± 1.5	1.4 ± .2	3.84 ± .76	2.74 ± .49	5.2 ± 1.3	1.1 ± .3
Respiratory Inductive Plethysmography	4.40 ± 1.59	3.06 ± 1.12	7.7 ± 5.5	1.5 ± .3	4.23 ± 1.12	2.97 ± .82	8.0 ± 2.9	1.4 ± .3
Body Plethysmography	4.17 ± 1.11	3.07 ± .76	7.2 ± 3.8	1.5 ± .3	3.84 ± .76	2.89 ± .55	7.4 ± 2.5	1.4 ± .3

+ VALUES ARE MEAN ± S.D.
* SIGNIFICANT DIFFERENCES BETWEEN SMOKERS AND NONSMOKERS
  SIGNIFICANT DIFFERENCES BETWEEN DEVICES

differences between respiratory inductive plethysmography and spirometry. This trend in $FEV_{1.0}$ held for smokers, but there was little
variation among the forced vital capacity volume as measured by the
various devices and when utilizing different density gases.   In both
non-smokers and smokers, peak flows or peak dV/dt were greater with
body plethysmography than spirometry for all gases;   respective values for respiratory inductive plethysmography generlly fell between
those measured with the other two devices.   In both groups, the
variability of respiratory inductive plethysmography was much greater
than spirometry or body plethysmography.

The flow or dV/dt at 25% of vital capacity during breathing of
helium best differentiated non-smokers from smokers.   This was found
for all the devices and was therefore more sensitive than the single
breath nitrogen test and closing volume since only half the smokers
were diagnosed as having small airway disease by these criteria.   In
addition, the flow from spirometry breathing air at 25% vital capacity also differentiated smokers from non-smokers.

The forced expiratory vital capacity tracings derived from
respiratory inductive plethysmography and body plethysmography were
plotted against spirometry (Figure 2).

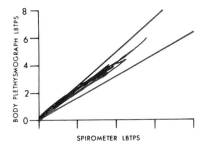 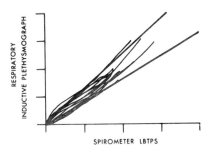

Fig. 2   Body-plethysmographic and respiratory inductive   plethysmographic determined forced vital capacity plotted against
simultaneous spirometry together with lines   indicating ±
20% deviation from identity. For body-plethysmographic
tracings, the curves for the most part   are deflected upward
in the early part of the vital   capacity whereas for the
respiratory inductive   plethysmographic there is a great
deal of scatter of the data.

In both non-smokers and smokers, the plots of the volume from
body plethysmography against spirometry for all the gas mixtures were
similar.   There was a tendency for greater volumes from body plethysmography than spirometry during the first half of the manoeuvre and
an approach to a line of identity during the second half of the
manoeuvre.   There did not appear to be any consistent difference in
this pattern between non-smokers and smokers. The plots of respiratory inductive plethysmography versus spirometry did not show a
consistent pattern;   in some tracings, there were greater values and
in others, lesser values than spirometry during the first half of the
forced vital capacity manoeuvre.

Conclusion

This study indicates that respiratory inductive plethysmography is an acceptable method for semi-quantitative assessment of dynamic events during the forced expiratory vital capacity manoeuvre. For all volume and flow parameters analysed, it showed more variablity than spirometry and body plethysmography. The analog tracings showed a pattern between spirometry and body plethysmography.

Theoretically, compression of thoracic gas by high alveolar pressure in the early part of the vital capacity manoeuvre should be detected by plethysmographic estimation of thoracic gas volume (6). This was a fairly consistent finding for the body plethysmographic measurements, but not for the respiratory inductive plethysmo-graph. The discrepancy is accounted for by the factors noted in the introduction of this paper, although it should be pointed out that the inconsistencies were minor. Further, the relationship between the three devices was similar among the different density gas mixtures.

The best test for discriminating non-smokers from smokers was the flow or derivative of volume at 25% vital capacity above residual volume during breathing of the helium-oxygen gas mixture. All three devices revealed such differences between the smokers and non-smokers.

The currently available respiratory inductive plethysmograph cannot be used as an accurate substitute for body plethysmography in the measurement of changes of thoracic gas volume during the forced vital capacity manoeuvre. Moreover, both spirometry and body plethsmography provide more precise measurements than this device. However, respiratory inductive plethysmography is a viable alternative for measuring serial changes of the time-volume and derivative of volume-volume components of forced vital capacity in subjects outside the pulmonary laboratory, such as in the bed-confined and ambulatory subject.

References

1. Cohn M.A. Rao A.S.V., Broudy M., Birch S., Watson H., Atkins N., Davis B., Stott F.D. and Sackner M.A. J. Appl. Physiol. submitted
2. Sackner J.D., Nixon A.J. Davis B. Atkins N. and Sackner M.A. (1980) Am. Rev. Respir. Dis. 122, 867-871.
3. Konno K. and Mead J. (1967) J. Appl. Physiol. 22 407-422.
4. Siafakas N.M. Morris A.J.R. and Green M. (1979) J. Appl. Physiol. 47 38-42.
5. Melissinos C.G., Goldman M., Bruce E., Elliott E. and Mead J. (1981) J. Appl. Physiol. 50, 84-93.
6. Ingram R.H. and Schilder D.P. (1966) Am. Rev. Respir. Dis. 94, 56-63.

Discussion

DR. PHILLIPSON: In view of the obvious measured and theoretical difference between the body plethysmograph and the inductive plethysmograph - one measuring thoracic gas volume, the other measuring thoracic volume - as Dr. Sackner said, it can be lost into the neck or elsewhere. At the moment, the respiratory inductive plethysmograph treats the system as a two-compartment model. If it was treated as a three-, four- or greater compartment model, by having an increasing number of coils, would that improve the situation? Theoretically, if the subject was wrapped, it should then become a plethysmograph.

DR. SACKNER: There is no question from the magnetometry data that, looking at the lower portion of the rib cage, the signal goes up rather than down. I carried out an interesting experiment on myself in which we looked at the CAT scan at RV (residual volume) position. It turns out that some of that distortion at RV position is related to change in thickness of muscle mass and not change in lung volume. The CAT scanner was used to measure soft tissue around the rib cage. We are not only measuring thoracic volume, but also muscle mass underneath the transducer, and if muscle mass changes in volume it is detected by respiratory inductive plethysmography.   I do not believe that we shall get much further in terms of accuracy by putting more bands around the chest. The major problem is really in the changes of neck volume. What we need to do now (and some experiments have been started) is to measure changes of neck volume by means of the inductive plethysmograph coil around the neck. There may not be much of a problem, since the neck can be approximated to a cylinder; it moves with one degree of freedom. Perhaps we can add this signal to the volume obtained with respiratory induction plethysmography.

THE EFFECT OF NITROUS OXIDE AND RESISTIVE LOADING ON BREATHING PATTERNS

D. ROYSTON, C. JORDAN AND J.G. JONES

Division of Anaesthesia,
Clinical Research Centre, Watford Road, Harrow, Middlesex, UK

Summary

We have studied the effect of sub-anaesthetic concentrations of nitrous oxide on the ventilatory response to an inspiratory resistive load in eight normal volunteers. A respiratory inductance plethysmograph was used to measure both tidal volume and the relative contributions of the rib-cage and abdomen/diaphragm to tidal breathing. When breathing an inspired concentration of 40% nitrous oxide, 20% oxygen with the balance nitrogen, there was a reduction in the rib-cage contribution to tidal breathing in both the unloaded and loaded conditions. There was also a decrease in the rib-cage contribution for the first loaded breath and an increase in asynchrony of the rib-cage and abdominal components both for the first breath on load and for the steady state on load, compared with the response breathing air.

Introduction

Nitrous oxide is used in dental surgeries in the technique of relative analgesia, and from premixed cylinders containing 50% nitrous oxide and 50% oxygen (Entonox) for analgesia in obstetrics and in ambulances. It is also used to provide analgesia in the post-operative period, particularly in patients with a limited respiratory reserve, because it is considered to have no deleterious effects on ventilation and is, therefore, safer than the conventional opiate type analgesic drugs, although this has not been unequivocably established.
     The effects of a drug on ventilation may be studied in a number of ways. One approach is to examine the response to a load. A commonly used test is the ventilatory response to an added chemical load such as the addition of carbon dioxide to the inspired gas. A less well-studied technique is the ventilatory response to an inspiratory mechanical load such as an added resistance, compliance, or a threshold load. There are very few studies on the effect of analgesic drugs on the response to mechanical loading in humans. It is likely that such tests may provide new and valuable information as there may be a dissociation in response to chemical and mechanical loads (1,2). The ventilatory response to added carbon dioxide is reported not to be depressed by nitrous oxide even in anaesthetic concentrations (3). In this study, we have examined the ventilatory response to a mechanical load, an added inspiratory resistance while breathing nitrous oxide in concentrations commonly used to provide analgesia.

Methods

Eight male volunteers (mean age 29 years) took part in the study, which was approved by the Northwick Park Hospital Ethical Committee. The subjects breathed through a mouthpiece attached to a heated pneumotachograph which, in turn, was attached to a non-rebreathing valve, the inspiratory limb of which had two parallel paths, one containing a laminar flow resistance, the other being capable of complete occlusion by the balloon of a Foley catheter. The pressure drop across the resistance line was linearly related to flow up to a flow of 0.5 litre.sec^{-1}. The inspiratory resistance of the system was 0.25 kPa l^{-1}. sec^{-1} with the balloon catheter deflated and 3.88 kPa l^{-1}.sec^{-1} with the balloon inflated.

Tidal volume and the rib-cage and abdomen/diaphragm components of tidal volume were measured using an inductance plethysmograph. The inductance plethysmograph was calibrated for each subject, using an isovolume manoeuvre followed by a period of breathing on an Ohio 840 electrical spirometer.

To obtain rib-cage and abdomen/diaphragm contributions of the volume change, the inductance plethysmograph was calibrated in accordance with the following equation, which describes total volume change (Vsum) in terms of the separate volume changes of abdomen (AB) and rib-cage (RC), with their respective scaling factors X and Y :

$$Vsum = X.AB + Y.RC$$

The ratio of X and Y was obtained by the subject performing an isovolume manoeuvre and adjusting the ratio to provide a zero sum signal. The absolute scaling factors X and Y were then determined following a period of quiet breathing on a spirometer enabling the rib-cage, abdomen and sum signals to be correctly calibrated in terms of volume change.

All subjects followed the same protocol. They were studied supine and breathed air through a physiological mouthpiece with a nose clip applied, via the unloaded system for 15 minutes. They then breathed for a further 10 minutes after the load was applied by inflating the balloon on the catheter. The inspired gas mixture was then changed to 20% nitrous oxide, 20% oxygen, the balance nitrogen. The subjects breathed this mixture for 20 minutes to allow equilibration with the inspired gas in the absence of the inspiratory load. The gas mixture was then changed to one containing 40% nitrous oxide and 20% oxygen and the procedure repeated as for the 20% nitrous oxide mixture. The load was always applied during an expiration, silently and without the subject's knowledge. Care was taken to ensure that the subjects were awake at all times. They were asked to keep their eyes open and could always respond purposefully to a vocal command. All subjects followed this protocol on a day preceding the full study to allow familiarisation with the equipment and its calibration.

Results

Only the tidal volume data and the contributions of rib-cage and abdomen are presented here, the results of other variables are presented elsewhere (4).

The mean value for each variable of a representative two-minute period of breathing prior to application of the load was taken as the control value for each subject. The "First Breath on Load" represented values for that breath and was used as an indicator of the response mediated via nervous pathways as there can be no change in chemical drive for that breath. The "Steady State on Load" was the mean value for each variable for each subject of a representative two-minute period toward the end of the time on load. All volumes are at B.T.P.S. To compare the effect of the drug on the response to the load, the difference between the non-load and load values of each variable while breathing air (the control responses) were compared with the difference while breathing each of the nitrous oxide mixtures, using the paired 't' test.

The effect of nitrous oxide on the tidal volume response is shown in the Table 1. There was a significant depression of the response for the first breath on load with 40% N_2O but no significant difference for the steady-state response. There was no significant change in the non-loaded (control) tidal volumes while breathing either of the N_2O mixtures (Table 1, Column 1), but there was a progressive reduction in the rib-cage contribution of the volume change with increased N_2O concentration (Table 1, Column 4). The rib-cage contribution when breathing the 40% N_2O mixture was significantly less (p = .04) than that breathing air.

The effects of loading on the rib-cage contribution of tidal volume are shown in Table 1, Columns 5 and 6). These data show that there is a highly significant reduction in the rib-cage component of the immediate response to he load while breathing 40% N_2O with a return to normal compensation during the steady-state period.

There was usually a degree of asynchrony between the abdomen/diaphragm and rib-cage components of the volume change, and the amount of asynchronous movement was invariably increased when breathing with an increased airway resistance, as shown in Figure 1. This figure shows the relative rib-cage and abdomen/diaphragm changes for one subject, expressed as X-Y plots.

The index used to assess the amount of asynchrony is shown in Figure 2, with a subject breathing 40% nitrous oxide in a steady state on load. We used the ratio of the length of the line representing abdomen/diaphragm and rib-cage movement during inspiration (A→B) to that during expiration (B→A). In the absence of obstruction, the expiratory movement is roughly equivalent to the Konno and Mead relaxation line (5). The end of the inspiration, represented by the break in the loop, occurred when there was zero flow at the mouth. A ratio of unity for:

$$\frac{A \rightarrow B}{B \rightarrow A}$$

would represent the same degree of movement of the abdomen and rib-cage for inspiration and expiration, whereas increasing values would represent a relatively greater degree of asynchrony during inspiration. This follows from the fact that expiration tends to follow a roughly straight 'relaxation line'.

The group results for this ratio in Table 1, Columns 8 and 9 indicate an increase in the amount of asynchrony of the abdomen/-diaphragm and rib-cage components with the first breath on load for

TABLE I

Inspire Gas	Tidal Volume(litre)			Rib Cage Volume / Tidal Volume			Inspiratory / Expiratory movement		
	Unloaded	First Breath on load	Steady State on load	Unloaded	First Breath on load	Steady State on load	Unloaded	First Breath on load	Steady State on load
Air	0.69 (0.07)	0.3 (.02)	0.04 (0.05)	0.39 (0.03)	0.01 (0.03)	0.006 (0.03)	1.08 ((0.03))	0.04 (0.04)	0.13 (0.03)
20%	0.67 (0.06)	-0.06 (0.13)	0.02 (0.08)	0.34 (0.03)	0.09 (0.04)	0.01 (0.03)	1.03 ((0.02))	0.23* (.0.08)	0.12 (0.18)
40%	0.68 (0.06)	-0.08* (0.17)	-0.06 0.05	0.33* (0.03)	0.09* (0.03)	0.03 (0.04)	1.08 (0.02)	0.43+ (0.11)	0.22* (0.09)

Results (mean and s.e.m.) for tidal volume, rib cage volume change as a ratio of the tidal volume change and the ratio of the inspiratory to expiratory rib cage and abdomen/diaphragm movement, for unloaded breathing and the response to the load (i.e. load minus unloaded) for the first breath on load and steady state on load. Values are compared with the air value at the head of the column using a paired 't' test.

* p< .05   + p = 0.02

* p< .05

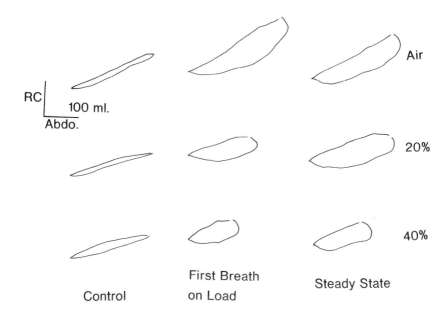

RC
100 ml.
Abdo.

Air

20%

40%

Control   First Breath   Steady State
               on Load

Fig. 1   Rib-cage and abdomen/diaphragm movement of representative
            breaths for each gas mixture and load condition.   Subject
            3.

each nitrous oxide concentration compared to the increase breathing
air. There was also an increase in the amount of asynchrony in the
steady-state with 40% nitrous oxide.

Conclusion

The aim of this study was to examine the effect of nitrous oxide,
given in sub-anaesthetic concentrations, on the ventilatory response
to an added inspiratory resistance. Our aim was to use a respiratory
inductance plethysmograph to separate this response into its rib-cage
and abdomen/diaphragm components, and analyse any difference in response for each component of the volume. We also developed an index
of asynchrony and paradoxical movement of the two components of
ventilation. An increase in this index would mean that gas in the
respiratory system would be moved from one region to another, thus
increasing the amount of dead space ventilation, and also increasing
the effort used to produce a comparable volume change at the mouth.
Using this approach, we have shown that 40% nitrous oxide produced a
reduction in the rib-cage contribution to tidal breathing in the non-
loaded state. There was also a decrease in the rib-cage component
from the first breath on load and an increase in paradox and asyn-

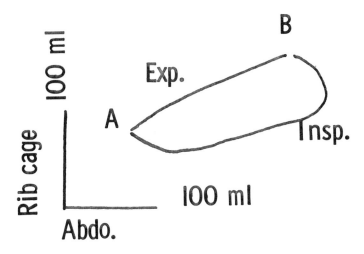

Fig. 2   Rib-cage and abdomen/diaphragm movement during inspiration
and expiration. This loop is the steady state on load
breathing 40% nitrous oxide shown in Fig. 1.

chrony of the rib-cage and abdomen components both for the first
breath and steady-state on load responses compared with the response
breathing air.   This implies that for a given load there is a con-
tinuum of alteration in response of the rib-cage movement with increasing analgesia and anaesthesia.

The index of paradoxical or asynchronous movement used in this
study would be of little value for any study where there was an
increase in expiratory resistance because the line B--A would no
longer follow the line of relaxation.

In conclusion, we have shown that when normal subjects breathed
sub-anaesthetic concentrations of nitrous oxide, there was a reduced
immediate compensation to inspiratory resistive loading, especially
of the rib-cage component of ventilation, and further, that there was
increased asynchrony between rib-cage and abdomen/diaphragm during
the steady-state period of resistive loading.

References

1.   Jordan C. et al (1979) Br. J. Anaesth. **51**, 497–502.
2.   Jordan C., Lehane J.R. and Jones J.G. (1980). Anaesthesiology,
     53, 293–298.
3.   Eckenhoff J.E. and Helrich M. (1958) Anaesthesiology, **19** 240–
     253.
4.   Royston D. Jordan C. and Jones J.G. (1981) Br. J. Anaesth. **53**,
     667–668P
5.   Konno K. and Mead J. (1967) J. Appl. Physiol. **22**,407–422.
6.   Jones J.G. et al (1979) Br. J. Anaesth. **51**, 399–407.

Discussion

DR. SACKNER: Dr. Royston has tackled a problem of great interest to us; an index of out-of-phasedness. Has the idea expressed in the last slide been compared to any other parameter, perhaps the area of the loop?

Secondly, is there any mathematical basis for what was done?

DR. ROYSTON: No, only on the physiological basis that if it is assumed that the expiratory portion is non-loaded that will represent a relaxation line and the two components will fall together. The difference between the two must represent a degree of wasted ventilation. The inspiratory loop must have more wasted ventilation because it is not relaxed but is active.

DR. SACKNER: Has this method of analysis been looked at during sleep? That is the other problem. During snoring, there may be paradoxing too - partial paradoxing. It would be helpful to know that as well, in order to put an index on it.

DR. ROYSTON: At the moment, a sleep study is running post-operatively. In subjects who have morphine by continuous intravenous infusion exactly the same thing is demonstrated. However, if a local anaesthetic technique is used to provide total analgesia, people do not paradox. As with alcohol, or many other depressant drugs, respiratory depression is allowed to develop.

DR. SACKNER: Is it the intercostals that get depressed first, while the diaphragm is still holding up?

DR. ROYSTON: I believe that myself. I know that Macklem and many other people do not, but I believe that in post-operative analgesia and in anaesthesia, it is the rib-cage which is totally depressed. Freis and many others have demonstrated this. In chronic obstructive airways disease patients, it might possibly be the abdominal component, but for post-operative respiratory depression, it is almost certainly the rib-cage.

DR. PHILLIPSON: On that very point, can it be said that because the first breath responses to the load were much more severely affected than the steady-state responses - that the effect of the drug is acting more on the spindle than on the muscle itself? Are there tests of other muscle function, say, knee-jerk or some other independent test that would demonstrate the mechanism, by which the drug acts?

DR. ROYSTON: This is being actively studied.

AUTOMATIC PATTERN RECOGNITION OF THE ONSET OF RESPIRATORY PHASES USING THERMISTOR TECHNIQUES

F. RASCHKE

Institut für Arbeitsphysiologie und
Rehabilitationsforschung der Universitat Marburg,
Ketzerbach 21 1/2, D-3550 Marburg, W. Germany

Summary

We developed an automatic procedure for exact and artefact-less determination (error < 3% as compared to the visual method) of the onset of spontaneous respiratory phases during sleep, wakefulness and strain. For this purpose, we used thermal recording of respiration in order to be independent from body movements, especially during sleep and physical work and we determined the onset points with very short latency ($\hat{t}$ = 10 msec) by means of pattern recognition. The procedure is described in detail and the results concerning phase co-ordination (entrainment) between the cardiac cycle and the onset of respiratory phases showed a marked coupling between cardiovascular and respiratory systems during sleep. 8 high-performance athletes (compared with 8 untrained subjects) showed a preference for a dia-stolic onset of inspiration and a systolic onset of expiration.

Introduction

The research into the factors determining inspiratory or expiratory time and the period length of the respiratory cycle has mainly been concerned with input variables such as pO_2, pCO_2, pH and lungstretch receptors. Little attention, however, has been paid to events within the cardiovascular system.

The determination of the exact onset of respiratory phases from a respiration curve shows that the inspiratory phase especially does not start at random but at distinct phases of the cardiac cycle. That means that cardiovascular events and the onset of respiratory phases are phase-coupled, or phase-co-ordinated. This phenomenon was first observed by Schoenlein in 1895 (1) in fish and in man by Galli in 1924 (2). Later on it was extensively followed up in different crustacens, fishes and mammals. Up till now, there have been about 70 papers which describe this phenomenon in different species (for ref. cf. 3).

The phase-co-ordination in man has so far been studied in detail after measured doses of physical work (4), during night-work with an inversion of the circadian rhythm (5), during anaesthesia in children and adults (6), in patients with an implanted pace-maker (7), after caffeine intake (8) and during night sleep (9).

All the investigations in man have shown that marked coupling

between the onset of respiratory phases and the cardiac cycle predominantly occurs during the resting and recuperative phases of the
organism. On the other hand, this coupling is very easily disturbed
even by low levels of strain. Therefore, it appears to be a
particular sensitive measure for recuperative processes.

Methods

All methods of respiratory recording have different disadvantages.
For our purpose, breathing by a mouthpiece or face mask would alter
the spontaneous breathing pattern and is not acceptable for sleep
research. Mechanical recording by cardiopneumogram, or plethysmography on the other hand, is susceptible to trouble from body movements.
       Because we are mainly interested in the exact determination of
the duration of respiratory phases, we used a thermoelectric method
which, however, gives no information about tidal volume or flow
velocity.   For this purpose, we developed a special nasal transducer
with great sensitivity for changes in air flow. The carrier is made
from aluminium, easily adaptable to the individual bridge of the
nose. The two thermistors are in series, in order to be independent
from lateral effects of airflow through the nostrils. The thermistors are protected against mechanical damage by means of an aluminium
funnel. The conical orifice concentrates the inspiratory airflow
onto the thermistors. We used this amplification of the instream
because several investigations in man have shown that the inspiratory
onset is more closely co-ordinated with the cardiac cycle than the
onset of expiration.
       The thermistors have the disadvantage of cooling down during
apnoeic phases, upon displacement and during flat inspiration curves,
thus making a sharp determination of the onset of inspiration impossible. We, therefore, heated them to a temperature of 28° leading to
a temperature change (even after breath-holding or apnea) for both
inspiratory and expiratory airflow.
       The diameter of the bead thermistor (Siemens K 19) is 0.4mm;
the time constant is given to 0.4 sec. For our purpose, however, the
cut-off frequency as calculated from the time constant is less
important, because we need a differential signal in the time domain.
       We therefore determined the actual time delay by means of an
apparatus for estimating the transfer function between a sinusoidal
airflow of 0.5 l amplitude through a mechanically driven pump and the
response of the transducer. This determination yielded a latency of
10 msec at a frequency of 15/min, which is regarded to be short
enough for exact quantification of the onset points. However, it
must be pointed out that this accuracy could only be obtained with
the aid of a pattern recognition system which is described as follows:
       Respiration curve and ECG are stored on magnetic tape (Tandberg
TIR 115), and replayed via a multiple ADC to a laboratory computer
(Plurimat-S from Intertechnique). The sampling rate of the AD-
converter was set to 436.37 Hz (tape speed 16 times the original
value), which gives sequences of 5 min. (32 blocks), 10 min, (64
blocks), or more in connection with the block size of 512 data
points.

The analysis of phase-coupling was done off-line in two steps. We stored the data sequences continuously on a magnetic disc and analysed the respiration and ECG curves from successive epochs of 18.75 sec. throughout the total sleep time. (Figure 1) shows the procedure we use for pattern recognition of the onset points from such a sequence.

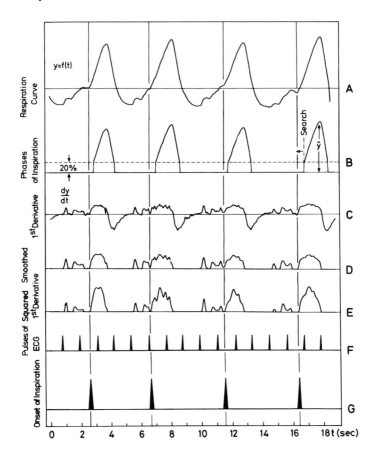

Fig. 1   Procedure for pattern recognition of the exact onset of inspiration: respiration curve (A), rectified and its level reduced (20% of **y**:B), differentiated (C), rectified and smoothed without altering the phase (D), and exponentially amplified (E), R wave trigger pulses (F), inspiration onsets defined by the computer (G).

The respiration curve at the top of the figure is taken from a light sleep phase of a healthy male subject. The thermoelectric recording guarantees artefactless records in respect of body movements, but it has the serious disadvantage of producing cardiac-tracheal artefacts, the so-called cardiopneumatic waves (10) which can be seen in curve A, especially during the endexpiratory pause. We, therefore, took great care to eliminate these artefacts because they would have produced an automatic coupling between cardiac events and respiration.

Furthermore, it is well known that apnoeic breathing patterns appear during sleep, even in healthy subjects, during the REM or inter-REM phases. These also have to be eliminated.

Thirdly, the procedure of pattern recognition should be independent of displacement of the transducer during the night, and of individual and inter-individual differences in the shape of the respiration curve. The procedure we follow from top to bottom takes account of all these points.

The criteria for automatic determination of the inspiratory onset are:
1.   That a steep positive increase can be taken to signify the onset point, and
2.   That this differential change occurs at the beginning of a clearly defined inspiratory phase.

In order to fulfil the second criterion, it is essential to know the future course of the curve comparable to the visual method. These phases, clearly identifiable as inspiration, are shown in B. B. only contains the crests which exceed 20% of the maximum value ($\hat{t}$) of the sequence length used, thus providing indepence from the amplitude and eliminating rudimentary and apnoeic respiratory phases.

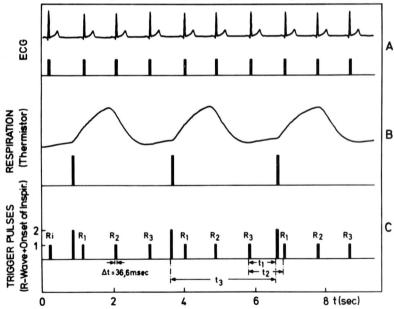

Fig. 2   ECG with R wave trigger pulses (A), respiration curve with inspiration onsets as defined by the automatic pattern recognition system (B), and interval lengths t1, t2, t3, and Ri calculated for each respiratory cycle (C).

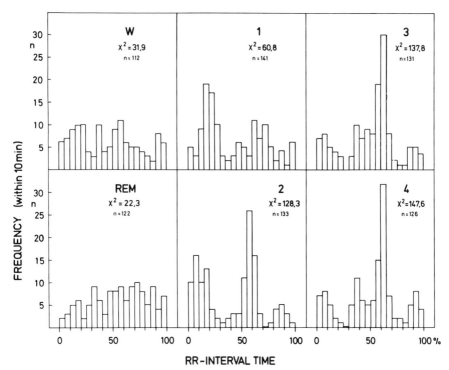

Fig.3   Frequency distribution of the onset of inspiration during
         cardiac cycle (normalized to 100%, divided into 20 ranges of
         5%   each).   Different sleep stages WAKE, REM, Stages 1-4
         Histograms of 10 min. records for each stage of a healthy
         male subject. Chi 2 values indicate deviation from an even
         distribution.

The first derivative of A is developed in C in order to obtain
the exact onset point. C is then digitally low-pass filtered without
altering the phase using the coefficients 1/4, 1/2, 1/4 and in D only
the positive changes are considered. An exponential amplification
and a reduction of the level, to exclude values under 2% of the
maximum, results in E, in which the cardiopneumatic movements are
either diminished or totally erased.

The logical connection between the two criteria can now be
followed up in B with a clearly defined inspiration. Starting at the
search mark, the computer picks up the nearest preceding point at
which curve E reaches zero. And now the inspiration onset is identified in G. The vertical lines which are drawn after the run of the
whole procedure indicate an accurate phase positioning. The pattern
recognition as described functions with a high level of accuracy,
with less than 3% error as compared to the visual method.

The interval times between cardiac and respiratory activity are
calculated as follows (Figure 2): t_1 = interval length between R
peak and the subsequent inspiration onset; t_2 = interval length

betweeen two R peaks; t_3 = interval length of the respiratory cycle and additionally, the number of R peaks during each respiratory cycle was computed. These four variables are considered continuously throughout the total sleep time.

Results

Figure 3 shows the result of a single male subject with 10-min. records during the different sleep stages. The 6 histograms represent a typical example of the phase co-ordination of inspiration onset time as a percentage of the cardiac cycle length (t_1/t_2 x 100), in order to be independent of the absolute values. The y-axis is the frequency of inspiration onsets counted for 10 min. in each sleep stage. During wakefulness, there is little deviation from an even distribution and during the REM-stage, inspiration onset really starts at random within the cardiac cycle. But during the light sleep (stage 1), an early peak emerges leading to a bimodal phase-coupling during stage 2, which changes to a conspicuous monophasic coupling during deep sleep in stages 3 and 4. These histograms indicate that there exist both a varying degree of co-ordination, represented by the height of the peaks and a preference for a certain temporal order.

Figure 4 confirms these results in a group of 10 healthy male subjects, whose R wave triggered histograms of inspiration onset are compiled for the total sleep time according to the actual depth of sleep of one undisturbed night. As already seen in Figure 3, the bimodal histogram again appears during light sleep and a monophasi structure can be seen in stage 4, whereas during REM-sleep and just after awakening, an even distribution indicates less or no phase-coupling.

From the histogram with standardized RR intervals, we calculated the X^2 values from 100 inspiration onsets each divided into 20 ranges. In Figure 5, the different stages of sleep, the relaxed supine and sitting position and increasing physical work on a bicycle ergometer are computed. This diagram now comprises the total range of different levels of consciousness and strain.

It reveals that the phase-coupling can only be observed during repose. The remarkable breakdown at 30 W proves that the slightest stress causes the two functions to respond with their own specific demand of regulation and thus the co-ordination, or in other words, the entrainment, is broken up.

If one takes into consideration, the mechanisms which are responsible for the coupling of respiratory phases to the heart beat, intensive studies on rabbits by Bucher and his colleagues (11) have shown that cardiovascular events are capable of triggering the respiratory phases, because cutting the left vagal nerve and cooling the right atrium diminished the coupling mechanism. On the other hand, he did experiments with artificial pressure pulses in the carotis sinus (12) which produced entrainment between the cardiovascular and the respiratory systems.

Because of the difficulty in applying these results to man and because there is a need for proof of functional meaning of the phenomena, we tried the following approach.

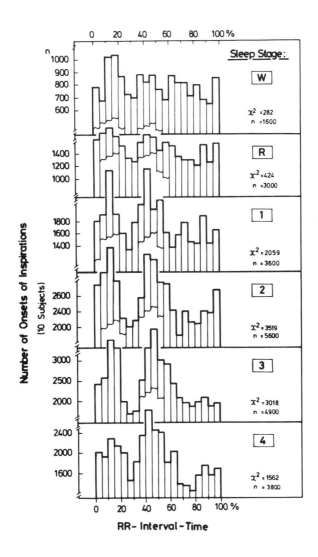

Fig.4   Histograms of the onset of inspiration during cardiac cycle
summed up for the total sleep time of 10 healthy male subjects. Events counted in sequences of 100 successive inspiration onsets for each sleep stage (n = 16 sequences
(Wake), n = 30 (REM), n = 36 (Stage 1), n = 56 (Stage 2), n =
49 (Stage 3), n = 38 (Stage 4).

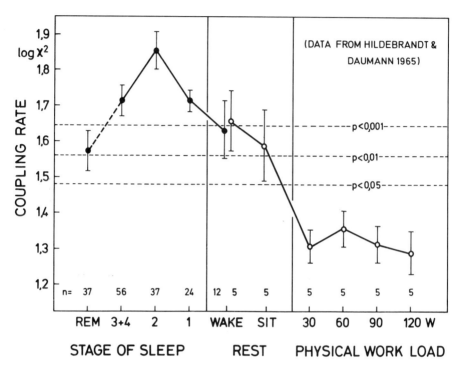

Fig. 5   Mean of logarithmic chi 2 values (coupling rate), separated
into different stages of sleep (n = 10 healthy male subjects). Lowered coupling rate during rest (supine and seated
position) and absent co-ordination during physical work
(ergometer) on the right (n = 5 healthy male subjects).
Bracketsindicatestandard error.Data on right from (4).

We compared the coupling mechanisms from 8 untrained subjects
with 8 high-performance athletes.
    As already seen in the histograms, there are usually two differ-
ent peaks: the one positioned early in the cardiac cycle, the other
positioned late. We therefore called them systolic and diastolic
peaks and computed the mean height of these peaks in Figure 6.   On
the x-axis, the 16 subjects are placed in order according to the
actual ratio of their pulse/respiration frequency during deep sleep.
Therefore, the sportsmen are clustered on the left, the untrained
subjects are clustered on the right.   The y-axis gives the mean
height of the systolic (above) and the diastolic peaks (below).   The

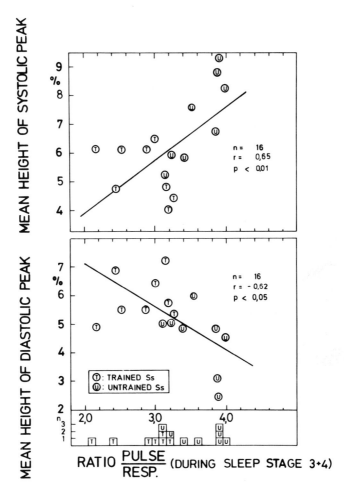

Fig. 6   Mean relative height of the two peaks (from the histograms)
with systolic (above) and (diastolic (below) inspiration
onset in 8 untrained and 8 trained subjects.. They are
ordered on the x-axis according to their instantaneous ratio
of respiratory to cardiac cycle length during deep sleep
(stages 3 + 4). Frequency distribution of the subjects
below shows accumulations at integer ratios.

sportsmen's behaviour indicates that they start inspiration more
often during a diastolic than during a systolic phase. We, furthermore, investigated the behaviour of the expiratory onset, which is
not shown here, but it gave clear results for the sportsmen. They
have their expiratory onset coupled to the systolic phase. The
untrained subjects have no coupling for expiration.

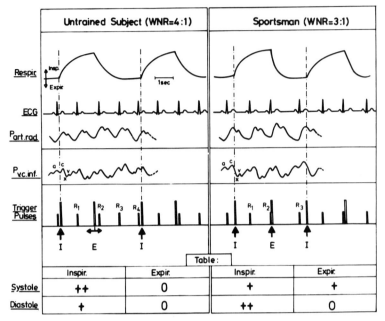

Fig. 7   Positions of inspiratory and expiratory onset within
         cardiac cycle during the stable entrainment state (co-ordina-
         tion).   Untrained subject on the left, high-performance
         athlete on the right.Pressure pulse curves from arteria rad.
         and vena cava inf. for haemodynamic phase comparison.   Table
         indicates the preferred positions for different subjects.

These results are summarized in Figure 7. On the left, there is
the untrained subject. In the stable entrainment state, he has a
whole-number relationship between heart beat and respiration of 4:1.
The inspiratory onset predominantly occurs in the systolic phase, the
expiratory onset is variable. The sportsman on the right has his
inspiratory onset predominantly at the beginning of the diastolic
phase and additionally couples the expiratory onset to R_2, the second
heart beat of the respiratory cycle.

Conclusions

The results have shown that the coherent state, which is an overt
biological principle for optimizing the organism's efficiency, is
realized between the cardiovascular and respiratory systems only
under resting conditions. The method of measuring phase-coupling
depends very sensitively on sleep stages and strain components.
     The pattern recognition process is easily programmed on a micro-
processor. Future studies can be done on line, thus providing an
instrument for measuring the autonomic state which is not disturbing
the subject.

As far as the functional meaning of our findings is concerned, we can only suggest from the sportsmen's results that the onset occurring during diastole supports and optimizes venous return and hence the pre-load and filling mechanism of the heart.

Further studies in connection with impedance cardiography, e.g. the determination of stroke volume and cardiac output and the determination of the abdominal part played by respiration in driving the venous return at the optimal moment, will show if this suggestion is right.

Acknowledgement

The respiratory transducer was developed by Mr. Richard Schneider, and Mrs. Margot Kampa drew the figures. Thanks for their skilled technical assistance.

References

1. Schoenlein K. (1885) Z. Biol. **32**, 511-547.
2. Galli G. (1924) Arch. Mal. Coeur. **17**, 208-221
3. Raschke F. (1981) Die Kopplung zwischen Herzschlag und Atmung beim Menschen - Untersuchungen zur Frequenz- und Phasenkoordination mit neuen Verfahren der automatischen Analyse. Inaug.-Diss. Univ.Marburg.
4. Hildebrandt G. an Daumann F.J. (1965) Int. Z. angew. Physiol. **21**, 27-48.
5. Engel P., Hildebrandt L., Pollman (1971) Arbeitsmed., Sozialmed., Arbeitshygiene, **38**, 95-104.
6. Engel P., Jaeger A., Hildebrandt G. (1972) Arzneim.-Forsch. (Drug Res.) **22**, 1460-1468.
7. Hinderling P. (1967) Helv. Physiol. Acta. **25**, 24-31.
8. Engel P. and Hildebrandt G. (1973) Psychol. Beitrage, **15**, 77-86.
9. Storch J. (1967) Methodische Grundlagen zur Bestimmung der Puls-Atem-Kopplung beim Menschen und ihr Verhalten im Nachtschlaf. Med. Inaug.-Diss. Marburg.
10. Meltzer S.J. (1898) Am. J. Physiol.**1**, 117-127.
11. Bucher K., Ebneter-Schwitter H., Bucher K.E. (1973) Res. Exp. Med. **162**, 1-6.
12. Bucher K. and Bucher K.E. (1977) Res. Exp. Med. **171**,101108.

Discussion

DR. PHILLIPSON: How is it possible to be certain that it is the
cardiac that is triggering the inspiration, for example, rather than
the other way round?   Sinus arrhythmia is a well-recognised
phenomenon.
DR. RASCHKE: (Slide) I have investigated that, and can rule out that
the reverse mechanism is responsible. This is a respiratory arrhythmia. In an experiment on breathing to a given beat, I investigated
what happened in this phase. When breathing to a given beat the
inspiratory onset does not change that heart beat after the point of
onset. The results of this investigation rule out an effect that
produces the onset of the next heart beat from the inspiration. Of
course, these modulating effects are dominant, but what happens here
in the microdomain is most important for our studies - and it is not
involved if the complete respiratory arrhythmia is considered.
DR. PHILLIPSON: If these were plotted out as a cross-correlogram...
DR. RASCHKE: I have plotted this for a cross-correlogram because
there are two modulated curves, so cross-correlation techniques can
be carried out. But this cannot be done with trigger pulses. There
are some statistical methods for binary cross-correlation, but they
only cause trouble, I think. Because this phase-coupling is only a
statistical event, it is called "relative co-ordination" in von
Holtz' definition - that means that the coupling mechanism is not
stable, it is present for some inspirations and absent in the following few respiratory cycles. Therefore, methods which require continuous registration would not be valid.
DR. PHILLIPSON: Do you think that the link is with sleep state per
se or with heart rate?   The strongest linkage was in stages 2, 3 and
4 when heart rate is slowest and the next strongest linkage was
awake and in REM sleep when the heart rate is the next fastest. The
linkage was the weakest during exercise (when heart rate is the
fastest). It could be argued that it was simply a function of basic
heart rate rather than sleep state as such.
DR. RASCHKE: As was said yesterday, in stages 1 and 2, in light
sleep stages, there are the greatest modulating effects. That is
exactly what I have seen in heart rate modulation. I have done many
studies on heart rate modulation during different stages of sleep and
it is highest in light sleep. That would suggest that the modulating
effects also produce the highest coupling bcause, as was shown in the
bimodal histogram, there is an early peak and then a second peak in
the light sleep stage.

RESPIRATION WORKSHOP

In the Chair Dr. E.A. PHILLIPSON

Discussion

DR. SACKNER: I should like to bring up the subject of a patient of Dr. Phillipson's who had obstructive lung disease, whose oxygen saturation fell during sleep with little change in tidal volume or respiratory frequency. There are modifications that could be made to the instrument to make it more useful. I think Dr. Phillipson was alluding to the fact that there was probably airway closure, perhaps due to retention of secretions. Thus, PCO_2 did not increase and oxygen saturation decreased, yet tidal volume remained stable -
DR. PHILLIPSON: - suggesting a drop in FRC, leading to arterial desaturation.
DR. SACKNER: Exactly. I think that if we are looking for advances in non-invasive monitoring with respitrace, we need the capability of measuring FRC levels. If the FRC level also dropped, that would make it almost crystal clear... (Dr. Phillipson agreed) The problem with measuring FRC level is that it needs DC coupling, which means that any changes in body position (since there can be visceral shifts) may send it off scale. Mr. Watson has been thinking about this in terms of future modifications, and perhaps he could discuss the techniques.
MR. WATSON: We have been doing some developmental work of advanced concepts for dealing with DC coupling and analysis techniques using the respitrace, leading to the design of what we call the digital calibration box. Within it there is a microprocessor system, so it can make certain measurements on respiration without the need for a large computing system and provide some data reduction.

We have the problem that if there is a change in body position there will be a large shift in baseline - and how can that be recorded during the night? Another situation that arises if one wants to look only at the apnoeic periods and thus wants a large gain during those apnoeic periods but does not want the pens blocking the rest of the time. In order to accomplish that, we have added what is essentially an auto-zero type of window. With the digital box there is the capacity to specify how large we want the trace to be. If it exceeds the maximum limit placed into the box, it automatically repositions the pen to the middle. Thus, it is possible to keep track of a large volume shift by counting the number of re-centrings and still maintain a fairly large sensitivity over a limited range, also keeping track of the DC level changes.

Frank Stott can give us insight too involving a redesign of the whole system because we need temperature stability in the oscillator, and temperature stability in the demodulator. The analysis features will be an added benefit.
DR. STOTT: The stability of transducer systems of this kind is important; the question is how stable and how important? If we want to measure FRC, the engineer needs to know the accuracy and sensitivity needed for this purpose. Obviously they will not be the same for a baby as for a large adult. Both these have to be known.

What should we do about the shift in baseline with body movement? If there is an artefactual shift with change in posture,

that cannot be distinguished with this sort of device alone from an
actual change in FRC due to change in posture.
     For, say, an adult and an child, what is the stability
requirement? What is the smallest change in FRC which would be
considered significant?
DR. PHILLIPSON: If it is a research study, we want to know whether
FRC is changing and we must decide what limits of change we wish to
detect. For a research study, a change of 50 or 100 ml in an adult
may be a very important change, depending on the particular question
that is being asked.
DR. STOTT: 50-100 ml for an adult, and scaled down proportionately
for a baby, is that it?
DR. PHILLIPSON: That is reasonable.
DR. STOTT: There may be much larger changes than that if there are
any major changes in posture. What do you propose to do about that?
Is all that will be asked of the respiration measurement device that
it should be accurate as long as the patient does not change his
posture?
DR. SACKNER: A large shift of the FRC level will take place if
someone rolls over.
DR. STOTT: Are you talking about a real shift of FRC, or an artefact
that looks like a shift in FRC?
DR. SACKNER: Something has moved – viscera have moved. Looking at
the DC recordings that we have obtained so far with the present
systems, if somebody moves suddenly the entire trace goes off,
whereas, for example, in our few bronchoprovocation studies, there is
a gradual increase in the FRC level.
     Returning to the 50 ml as the right figure in adults, if we look
at spirometric traces in somebody breathing with a mouthpiece,
changes in level of that magnitude are frequently seen, probably
resulting from a cortical influence, whereas looking at respitrace DC
over 15 minutes it is usually fairly stable – because again, changes
in thoracic volume are being measured, so that there are no RQ
problems. I like that figure of 50 ml – but I have to say that I can
visualise it only in the short-term. I cannot really give a number
over an hour.
DR. PHILLIPSON: Going back to the pre-respitrace era – if we can
remember back that far – when magnetometers were being used, say, for
a research study, we would accept data only if on direct visual
observation the subject did not move (because changing posture threw
out the calibration). Also, it was only over a short period of time.
Therefore, the studies, for example, in which the subjects suddenly
went from non-REM to REM sleep, and the magnetometers indicated a
fall in FRC, were felt to be reasonably reliable. I do not know how
we will get around the problem of the change in posture.   Part of it
is artefact, but part of it is a true change in FRC.
DR. STOTT: The only way we will find that out is to rehearse the
specific individual, is it not, and to carry out a simultaneous
respitrace and spirometer recording, getting the individual to roll
over in bed and to lie prone, supine, right and left lateral to see
how much change there is on the spirometer and on the respitrace
system.
DR. COHN: I might add that that has been done – at least on myself –
to see how quantitative one might be changing from sitting to supine

or standing posture while remaining continuously on the mouthpiece. This was done with a spirometer - it had to be done quickly because oxygen runs out. Indeed, during some of the posture changes, there were much greater effects observed of the respitrace FRC using the DC system compared to the spirometer. There is no doubt that one is adding and subtracting things other than gas to the compartments. I am not sure that doing that manoeuvre ahead of time will allow interpretations to be made of the respiratory inductive plethysmograph at a later time.

DR. STOTT: I was thinking of the manoeuvre more as a method of delimiting what information can and cannot be trusted. Dr. Cohn is talking about something more akin to the ambulatory problem rather than to the research investigation, where he is not dealing only with rolling over but actual changes such as sitting, standing, lying - which will be bigger changes than those resulting from simply rolling over from one lateral position to another, for instance.

DR. COHN: For everyone's information, I might add that we have looked at the DC system with a few of our obstructive apnoeic patients to obtain some idea of what happens to the resting lung volume. Indeed, during the apnoeas the resting levels of rib cage, abdomen and sum gradually fall. With resumption of breathing, the FRC level is markedly increased, perhaps several hundred cc in magnitude on the summation channel, with a gradual fall during the subsequent five or six breaths until the next apnoea begins. This would be an example of the order of magnitude of the changes in that clinical example. But they are quick changes; we are talking about 30-second changes and then restoration over a few seconds, in contrast to the other long-term FRC changes that may occur in chronic lung disease, for example.

DR. STOTT: It might therefore take a long time to find out whether it is possible to separate out genuine FRC changes in the presence of that sort of background noise by using statistical trend analysis methods. We would need to know whether if someone changes position and then returns to the original position there is a return to the starting point, or whether there is any sort of hysteresis effect. I think that estimates can be made of the limit of instrumental stability that is achievable. Roughly speaking, I would put that limit in the region of 0.1% of vital capacity provided that at least the microclimate in which the transducer system is contained did not change by perhaps more than 2 or $3^{\circ}C$. That is a not unreasonable requirement, and in fact is probably generally met in a sleep laboratory.

DR. PHILLIPSON: If we have solved the FRC problem, perhaps we could move on to some other points.

DR. ROYSTON: We are interested in the automatic quantitation of asynchrony or paradox for our postoperative studies. They are mainly drug and sleep studies. The questions that we are trying to answer are whether narcotic analgesics cause respiratory depression and, if so, how. A number of our patients who are given narcotic drugs - and even non-narcotic drugs, as I showed earlier today - develop asynchrony of the rib cage-abdominal signal loops.

DR. PHILLIPSON: In quiet breathing in the normal individual, as Dr. Royston showed, one tends to move up and down around the relaxation line, and the more that it leaves the relaxation line, in one direction or another, the more is either the abdominal or rib cage contribution. As Dr Royston showed, the problem is that in certain situations the patients had some paradox - that is, they were partially out of phase - so that the loop was moving down initially (that is, the rib cage was moving in as the abdomen was moving out) and then moving around and coming back down a relaxation line. He measured the length of that line, as opposed to that line to get some index of the degree of paradox. The problem that was discussed following his paper is that the length of the line, although certainly appealing at first glance, could also be misleading in that if you were totally obstructed you would be moving up and down the isovolume line and the lengths of the lines would be the same. It seems to me that we need something that combines both the width of the minor axis and the angle which that line forms; in other words, the width of the minor axis will tell us the size of the loop, and the angle will tell us how far out it is from the relaxation time.

DR. SACKNER: I do not think the minor axis will help because there can also be figure-of-eight loops.

DR. STOTT: With a computer we could get a best-fit ellipse to the curve that is actually found. It is then possible to specify with the appropriate number of coefficients exactly what is its eccentricity and its angle. If there is a figure-of-eight type loop, the computer will almost certainly say "no fit available" - and that might simply have to be accepted.

DR. PHILLIPSON: Something which only measures ellipse area will not be sufficient, as I see it, somehow the angle has to be brought into this.

DR. STOTT: Yes, we would need both the lengths of the major and minor axes, and their angles of inclination, or something equivalent to that, but it would be quite complicated to compute, and for most purposes I think something much more simple is required. One method which I am considering is what we might call an efficiency index. This is done by computing in the normal way from the two excursions, the rib cage and the abdomen (with the phasing taken into account) the volume that is obtained. It is in fact a simple summing, so that when they are in antiphase and there is an obstructive apnoea the volume is nil. Then we add the two components' magnitudes, disregarding the phase difference. As long as we can be satisfied that we have them for the same breath, their magnitude can be measured separately and added together as though they were perfectly in-phase. The volume actually found is then expressed as a percentage of the volume that would have been obtained if they were in phase.

When breathing at 100% efficiency, with everything absolutely in phase, there is a coefficient of 100 - that is, 100% efficiency. If it obstructs, it goes right down to zero, and there is zero efficiency. If it is partially out of phase, there is a figure somewhere in between.

DR. PHILLIPSON: So you are comparing the sum channel basically to the absolute sum of the other two...? (Dr. Stott agreed).

DR. SACKNER: Dr. Stott has a reasonable approach; we need some kind of single point, or two points on a moving trace. As you pointed out having all those plots is not satisfactory, and would be impossible to deal with, for a whole night's data. It is impossible to deal with several indices such as the area of ellipse and the angle - I do not know how that could be plotted. Dr. Stott's approach, in which an efficiency index could be developed, is perfect.

DR. STOTT: That would be good because it could then be done using a moving-window average to smooth out the irregularities. That would provide a very good trend indication.

I think, though, that Mr. Watson has an alternative approach to propose.

MR. WATSON: This suggestion arises as a result of discussion with Dr. Stott and is a simple approach which is easy to implement with a simple processing system.

For example, the rib cage flow might be essentially negative initially and then becomes positive to the peak value, the reverse for expiration, and if there is any paradox at the end of the breath it might go positive again. At the same time the abdominal flow initially might be positive, then continue positive and, with the onset of expiration, become negative. Thus, there would be three situations for rib cage and abdomen:

If we look at the flows continuously throughout the breath it is possible to compute how much time of the breath is spent in paradox, as compared to how much time of the breath is spent in phase. This can be expressed as a percentage.

In the fully in-phase situation, the value would be zero, and in the isovolume situation the value would be 100%.

DR. STOTT: It is slightly more complex than the approach that I was suggesting. I think that the sensible thing would be to do both - they are sufficiently technically simple, so that even the simplest microprocessor could handle them both at the same time.

They are not providing quite the same information; they are complementary and it would be nice to have both. Either approach seems to me to be workable, useful and simple enough to be easily comprehensible. One would very quickly learn about the kind of application for which one or the other could be used.

DR. PHILLIPSON: If, say, an individual were completely, or perhaps partially obstructed at the onset of a breath so that his rib cage was paradoxing, if his drive was very high there might be a lot of magnitude of paradox - but happening very quickly because often the rib cage can be seen springing out - Mr. Watson's methods would have a time base.

MR. WATSON: Which is the indicator of how much work is expended during breath?

DR. STOTT: Both are needed. Probably it clarifies it to think what happens when we cough. We have talked previously about cough analysis, and we have had quite simple analog methods of recognising coughing. With this kind of system, if both those coefficients are taken, I think a cough could be completely categorised with a unique pair of values.

DR. COHN: The other point to be brought up again is why do we want to measure this? It is not just the sleep analysis, which is very interesting, but also its potential importance in terms of patients with respiratory failure, those on respirators and those being weaned from respirators. There is a lot of good evidence to indicate that paradoxing is a good prognostic sign in terms of coming off a respirator. What we really do not know is how good an indicator are minor degrees of paradoxing, in terms of those who will and who will not succeed in coming off a respirator without any problems. Obviously, that is a research question, but without the aid of this particular kind of analysis, nobody will be able to answer it.

DR. PHILLIPSON: But, as has been said, it has potential clinical application in the same sense that analysing muscle fatigue - diaphragmatic fatigue - may be a useful prognosticator of who can and who cannot come off a respirator, and who will switch from diaphragmatic to intercostal breathing. Once this has been developed, its clinical application might be much simpler to use as a clinical indicator than trying to measure the EMG and the fatigue pattern.

DR. SACKNER: Perhaps the next problem of great ethical concern is coming up with definitions for breathing that falls between good breathing and no breathing - that means "under-breathing" and "hypopnoeas" which are used a great deal in the literature with varying definitions. Looking at breath after breath after breath of respitrace-type signals under extremes of hypopnoeas, "central" hypopnoeas or "obstructive" hypopnoeas, the differentiation of the respitrace signal does not provide a clue about whether we are dealing with an upper airway problem that is reducing tidal volume to an ineffective level or a reduction in the central neurogenic output to the respiratory system. This is a very important problem.

There is pattern recognition, which I think I can see in a patient who is under-breathing because of increase in respiratory resistance, versus someone who is under-breathing because of decreased respiratory output to the muscles of respirator without upper airway obstruction. This is a problem with looking at long-term signals, that we must produce better definitions.

DR. PHILLIPSON: I agree - I do not have the answer, but it seems to me that not only do we require better definitions based on the pattern but also a physiological definition about whether it is really impairing gas exchange.

If we are talking at the clinical level, the pattern and certainly the respitrace are extremely useful in distinguishing central and obstructive, and indeed desaturation due to other causes, but in all this we should not lose trace of the fact that some measure of gas exchange is still extremely important in a clinical assessment. In the final analysis, in someone who has a partial degree of paradox, whether it is due to weak intercostals or upper airway muscle obstruction, but who has no desaturation, it is possible that he is headed for something. That is why I showed the slide of the man who clearly has outright obstruction - the question is where is he headed for? At least at the moment there are no cardiographic changes and no desaturation. I agree that in order to communicate with one another the terms must be defined and made more precise. If nothing else, we should agree that the term "sleep disordered breathing" should be outlawed. At the moment, that term includes a mish-mash of everything: apnoeas without desaturation, desaturation without apnoeas, hypopnoeas - everything gets thrown into a term, some mean number is arrived at, and I do not think that that is a useful way to go clinically.

DR. COHN: We should not lose sight of the fact that the respitrace is a sole monitor, even with oxygen saturation in terms of the particular individual just discussed - the 35-year old man who snored. Perhaps we should be measuring his blood pressure continuously because at that particular loading on his respiratory system catecholamine release might perhaps be causing systemic hypertension. Dr. Phillipson really said this in his introduction on clinical polycinemography - that other things have to be investigated in addition to respiration when monitoring is carried out. Personal judgement has to be used about when those measurements are made. Oesophageal pH, as was mentioned also, may be very important in terms of what is really occurring during sleep in patients.

We must get to the point where lots of parameters are being investigated easily, simply and non-invasively - and accurately, if possible - processing the records, but pre-selecting the kinds of tests that we want, based upon the respiratory patterns that are found. Incidentally, was his daytime blood pressure elevated?

DR. PHILLIPSON: Not during the day time - it was checked. But he may well be repeatedly elevating it during the night. It is known that patients with obstructive apnoeas develop sustained systemic hypertension, so presumably there is some point between the transient increases in blood pressure and the sustained increases...perhaps at this point he should be treated, in the sense that hypertension is a treatable disease and carries certain risk factors - but we do not know.

In fact, I would be interested to know what should that patient be told? He is a 40-year old man and he asked me how was his sleep study. What should I tell him?

DR. COHN: My approach to the patient is to tell him what I know - that is, that I do not know, but that it is a potential risk factor and that other risk factors can worsen the condition, such as weight gain, certain ingestion of various chemicals including alcohol, and that heshould be aware of the disease so that in the future if symptomswere to develop he would know what was wrong with him. At least at that level of education, it is important.

DR. PHILLIPSON: I agree - in fact, that is exactly what was done with that man. We warned him about not putting on weight, about not drinking in the evening - which, if one thinks about it, is a fairly serious handicap to put on an individual - and not to use any sleeping pills. The slide I showed was a 40-year old man who was perfectly healthy and who volunteered for a sleep study and who was found to be having periods of 20 to 30 seconds of outright, clear-cut obstructive apnoeas, with no desaturation and no heart rate disturbance. As Dr Sackner said, he may have blood pressure increases during the episodes but we do not know. It is a laboratory finding at the moment. What do you tell such people, Dr. Miles?

DR. MILES: Very similar to what has just been said. It can probably be added that he should not become sleep-deprived too much if he can avoid it, and should perhaps not live at high altitude. Also, he should be re-evaluated. We should keep an eye on those people.

DR. PHILLIPSON: Are there other burning issues, either related to those topics or to some of the papers presented today?

DR. STOTT: I would certainly like to take the opportunity to bring up another related topic, and to seek the opinions of all those who have done any work on arterial oxygen tension measurement and also on transcutaneous oxygen partial pressure measurement, together with the

relative advantages and disadvantages, which is thought usually the
more useful - or likely to be the more useful - and finally comments
about the existing hardware that is available for the job.
DR. PHILLIPSON: Does anyone use the transcutaneous oxygen
electrodes?
MR. WATSON: We have tried such a system. We carried out breath-
holding studies looking at response times simultaneously with
oxymetry. For breath-holding in acute changes, I found them very
good, with what to me would be clinically sufficient respnse time to
apply, for example, in patients with sleep apnoeas.
DR. STOTT: It is not as fast as the oxymeter, but it is sufficiently
fast to follow - generally, I would think - changes that occur
naturally, as opposed to the changes that are induced by artificial
means.
    Problems of accuracy, stability, reliability and acceptability:
how does everybody find these?   Presumably, if people are not using
that, they must be using the oxymeter. Is anybody using anything
other than the Hewlett-Packard?
DR. MILES: The Hewlett-Packard is a great machine, but it just about
kills the patients. We are testing a device from the Minolta camera
company. It is an oxymeter which has a fibreoptic system in it. It
has been put on people's fingers, babies' toes and so on, and it has
a fast response and it seems to be really good. It is certainly much
more painless than the Hewlett-Packard machine to have on.
    I have heard from other bioengineers that the technology is
available greatly to improve those machines.
DR. STOTT: The Hewlett-Packard is an excellent scientific
instrument, but a rather impractical clinical instrument.
DR. PHILLIPSON: I am sure that it is impractical. Certainly, it is
impractical for ambulatory monitoring because of its size and bulk.
For short-term awake studies, exercise studies and others it is very
useful at the clinical level - and even for sleep studies. I agree
with what has been said, that if patients complain about anything in
the whole array of transducers, it will be about the oxymeter - in
fact, I have made that comment previously. Our experience is that
the majority of patients fall asleep without any difficulty with it
on, but when they wake up 3 or 4 hours later (and they do not
necessarily wake up because of the oxymeter but perhaps for other
reasons) they will very often complain that their ear is too warm,
and we have to transfer it to the other ear. In any case, they want
to change position. However, I would say that in the 200-odd
patients in whom we have used the Hewlett-Packard it has probably had
to be removed completely after a few hours in not more than 10%.
DR. MILES: It is really no problem in the majority of patients. An
apnoeic is always sleeping so poorly and yet will have his apnoea.
But there are some people who have great symptoms from the Hewlett-
Packard and it really does disturb their sleep. They will often be
the rather milder cases. There are others who seem to have small
ears or small ear lobes so that it is virtually impossible to put on
the Hewlett-Packard. When there is a serious problem of that sort
with a patient sometimes a technician has held it on his ear to get
a recording.
DR. PHILLIPSON: There is an important practical point about the
application - that is, it is often put on incorrectly. Some time

must be spent in applying it to make sure that the ear is not being twisted. If the subject says that it is uncomfortable when it is first put on, you might as well stop because you can be sure that it will get worse. I have made the same comment earlier about the respitrace; if it is just slapped on and not calibrated, we might as well use a couple of rubber bands. The secret with all these devices is to take the time. If a patient is going to spend 8 hours having the study, it is worth taking 8 minutes to apply the equipment properly.

DR. MILES: That is certainly an important point with clinical sleep recording laboratories, to have a stable technician working in the place who has been there for more than just a few weeks. It is not always easy.

DR. ROYSTON: We have a slightly different problem because our patients are post-operative and they are usually in a low-flow state anyway because they have been on the operating table for however long the surgeon decides to operate on them. Many of the people in whom we are interested are old patients who tend to have more respiratory problems in the post-operative period. They have thin ears. No matter how well it is originally put on the ear, on people with thin ears it will come off with a very small amount of movement. That is the big problem, and we also sit there and hold it in place.

DR. PHILLIPSON: Perhaps I am just showing my naivety about post-operative anaesthesiology, but in that situation do you not really want blood gases? You are as much interested in their pH and their metabolic status as in their saturation.

DR. ROYSTON: We are looking at sleep and sleep apnoeas, whether obstructive or central, in the post-operative period, so we monitor continuously.

DR. PHILLIPSON: I did not understand that this was being done as a study of sleep apnoeas in the post-operative period. I thought it was just for routine post-operative monitoring.

DR. ROYSTON: This is to study respiratory depression post-operatively on a continuous basis.

DR. STOTT: In that application would the transcutaneous PO_2 electrodes serve equally well. They do not give quite the same information. It is important, again, that the physicians and physiologists make quite clear to the engineers which information it is that they want.

DR. PHILLIPSON: It depends on their response.

DR. STOTT: Oxygen arterial saturation and tissue PO_2 are not the same thing, and they are not necssarily even closely related.

DR. PHILLIPSON: But again, for this sort of problem, where a patient is obstructing in the post-anaesthetic state, it would depend on the response time of the transcutaneous electrode. If the time constant is 2 or 3 mins, it will clearly miss the whole event.

DR. ROYSTON: We have tried using a mass spectrometer for the transcutaneous PO_2 and the main problem with that is that the mass spectrometer acts like a 2 kW heater and the room becomes unbearable after about 2 hours. You want to keep the patients quiet and let them sleep, but they wake up dehydrated. With a long sampling line, response time is the problem; we need a fast response. There is still a real need for a better way of measuring oxygenation.

THE USE OF MECHANICAL PEDOMETERS IN THE MEASUREMENT OF PHYSICAL ACTIVITY

J.M. IRVING AND J.M. PATRICK

Department of Physiology and Pharmacology,
University Medical School, Clifton Boulevard,
Nottingham, UK

Summary

We have re-examined the possibility of using mechanical pedometers to
categorize large numbers of subjects in terms of their daily physical
activity. Pedometers are stable and sensitive in their response to
regular movements on test-rigs covering most of the range of maximum
accelerations reported at the hip in normal walking. During purposeful walking over courses of 1.5 km, pedometers over-estimate the
number of steps taken as recorded by a foot-pressure sensor with an
Oxford tape-recorder. There was no apparent effect of walking speed,
but the two measures of steps were highly correlated. Pedometer
records of normal activity lasting several hours show a better agreement with actual steps taken. Records collected daily for a full
week in 250 subjects show that the activity scores of industrial
workers, laboratory personnel, retired men and students differ appropriately and that weekday and weekend scores can be distinguished.
Pedometers appear to be useful devices for the rate of activity in
epidemological studies.

Introduction

Measurement of physical activity is an important application for
ambulatory monitoring. Day-long recording of some variable changing
with activity provides an indication of an individual's current
habitual or customary activity. Heart rate is the variable most
widely used for this purpose, sometimes with foot-fall in addition
(1), but the technology required for collection and analysis of this
data is both complex and expensive, limiting the number of subjects
that can be studied. However, in many epidemiological studies, e.g.
recent studies of the incidence of coronary heart disease (2) and the
maintenance of muscle bulk in the elderly (3), only broad categorisation of individuals into a few groups of lower or higher customary
physical activity was required. For this a simpler method seemed
sufficient and we have re-examined the possibility of using mechanical pedometers.
    Pedometers are cheap, easily available and designed for use by
the general public. Several reports of their use as scientific
instruments in activity studies are available (4, 5, 6) but rather
little validation has been published. We have examined the
performance of one type with subjects in several different occupations on the assumption that in most ordinary occupations, walking
comprises the main form of activity.

Description of the Pedometer

The Yamasa Digital Pedometer is small (25 mm radius by 20 mm depth) and light (28 gm) and has a good watch mechanism. It costs around 10 pounds sterling and can be worn clipped to a waist-belt on the right side without inconvenience.

The pedometer contains a two-gram mass suspended by a spring against the force of gravity. Upward accelerations of the body cause the mass to move up. Subsequent downward accelerations in combination with gravity displace it downwards against the spring tension. The downard perturbations are transmitted by a ratchet-and- worm-gear system to a 3-digit display, which accumulates the total distance moved by the pendulum. It records up to 99.9 arbitrary units and can be read to the nearest 0.05 unit, which represents about 100 maximal pendulum displacements.

A stock of 58 pedometers has been in regular use in this laboratory for 20 months. 28 have suffered minor damage which has been repaired, 9 on more than one occasion. 12 have been lost and 4 irretrievably damaged. Recalibration of 18 pedometers, after one week's normal use, showed a small non-significant change in the calibration constant from 0.67 (SE 0.05) to 0.65 (SE 0.06) units per thousand movements.

Hip Accelerations in Walking

The pedometers needed to be tested formally over an appropriate range of accelerations. Cavagna et al (7) measured vertical acceleration during treadmill walking with an accelerometer mounted at waist level on the subject's back. The pattern is shown in the inset of Figure 1. The second integral of acceleration gives a measure of the vertical displacement, and this agrees (to within 8%) with estimates made from cine-photography. Calculations of the vertical acceleration of the body's centre of gravity during walking at different speeds have also been made (8) from force platform recordings and produced a similar pattern.

Two groups (4, 9) have mechanically measured the vertical displacement of the hip during walking on the treadmill. From their records, the maximum acceleration of a point on the hip has been calculated, using the simplifying assumption of simple harmonic motion and plotted against walking speed (Figure 1). The relation is continuous over a wide range of speeds. So a pedometer attached to the hip needs to be sensitive to movements having maximum accelerations from 0.5 to 8 m/sec/sec/

Bench Testing

The pattern of acceleration of the hip in walking has been simulated in the laboratory. Two test-rigs spin or shake the pedometers with approximately simple harmonic motion: between them, they cover the range of maximum accelerations encountered in walking. One device, the rotating disc, was a vertically-mounted record turn-table, whose angular velocity was controlled by altering the radius of the drive wheel. Three pedometers at a time were mounted on the turn-table: they were pivoted on low-friction bearings and remained vertical as

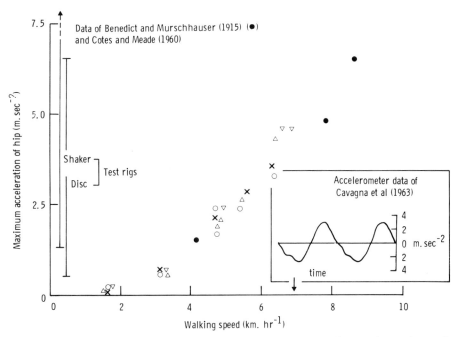

Fig. 1   Inset: Simplified trace showing vertical acceleration of
pelvis during two steps taken by a subject walking on treadmill (ref 7). Main figure: Maximum acceleration during
treadmill walking at various speeds, calculated from hip-
displacement data (refs 4 and 9).

the turntable rotated. The pedometer mechanism was activated once
per revolution. The amplitude of movement was controlled by altering
the position of the mount: i.e. the radius of revolution. A photo-
electric cell and shutter mechanism provided a count of the actual
number of movements, during a calibration procedure. The second
device was a standard laboratory flask-shaker, whose arms underwent a
displacement of 6mm   at a frequency between 200 and 600 movements
per minute.

For any given setting on either device, the pedometers responded
linearly to continued spinning or shaking (Figure 2(a)):   some of the
scatter about the line is reading error. The slope of the linear
regression, expressed as units per 1000 movements, is used to characterize the response.

The response depends on the size of the maximum acceleration
produced by the test-rig, but it is independent of the type of device
used. Figure 2(b) shows that, for maximum accelerations above 2.5
m/sec/sec/. the pedometer has a response that shows a small linear
increase with acceleration due to insufficient damping. Below that
value, the response quickly falls off towards zero because the pendulum is not being maximally displaced. Figure 3 shows that all the 9
pedometers, which were fully tested display a similar pattern with
flat linear portions above 3 m/sec/sec/ For routine testing, a
single maximum acceleration at about 4.5 m/sec/sec. has been used.

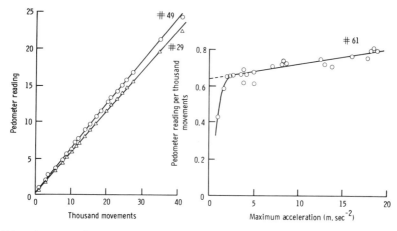

Fig. 2   a.   Response of 2 pedometers to simple harmonic motion on a
test-rig at same maximum acceleration.
b.   Relation between pedometer response to repeated movements and the maximum acceleration in simple harmonic
motion on test-rig. The inflexion occurs at the point where
the pendulum is just maximally displaced.

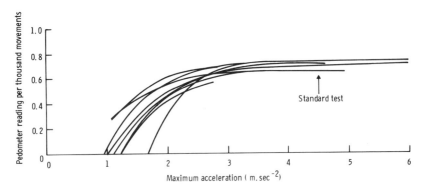

Fig. 3   As Fig. 2b, for 9 pedometers tested over a range of accelerations. In routine testing, calibration constants were
measured at 4.5 m/sec/sec.

The response at that value gives the calibration constant for the pedometer. In use, the pedometer reading divided by the calibration constant gives the number of movements registered, in thousands.

Formal Field Trials

On a laboratory test-rig, the pedometer registers regular movements, reasonably faithfully over the appropriate range of accelerations. On the treadmill, previous workers (6, 10) found that the pedometer count per step increased with walking speed, under-estimating at 2 and 4 km/hr respectively and over-estimating at speeds above 3 and 6 km/hr.

These findings were tested on 9 subjects during purposeful walking at three different speeds (about 4.5, 5.4 and 6.8 km/hr) around a measured level course of 1 to 1.5 km. The subjects also wore a foot-sensor (1), which enabled each right footfall to be recorded on an Oxford Medilog tape-recorder. On play-back, the steps were counted using an Advance digital counter, which accumulated the number of pulses generated by a Schmitt trigger. In the analysis, the step count has been doubled to represent the number of oscillations of the hip.

The results in Figure 4 show three interesting features. There is a high correlation (r=0.91, n-77) between the two measures of the number of steps taken. A little of the variation arises from the

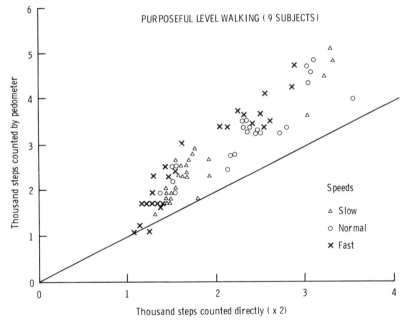

Fig. 4   Relation between pedometer reading (expressed as thousands of steps) and number of steps (one foot x 2) counted directly during purposeful walking at different speeds. The line of equality is shown.

imprecision involved in reading the pedometer, proportionally more important over short walks and some is probably from extra accelerations produced by insecure attachment to the pelvis. Seond, the relation is independent of walking speed: in a multiple regression analysis speed makes no significant contribution. This is a little surprising, in view of the direct relation between maximum acceleration of the hip and walking speed (Figure 2) and the positive relation between pedometer response and maximum acceleration (Figure 3(b). On the 'plateau' of the walking-speed curve, the effect of speed might be expected to be small, but below the shoulder it could be substantial. Third, the pedometer step count exceeds the direct step count by about 40%. This suggests that other trunk movements have made a material contribution, or that extra accelerations associated with heel-strike or insecure attachment have been registered.

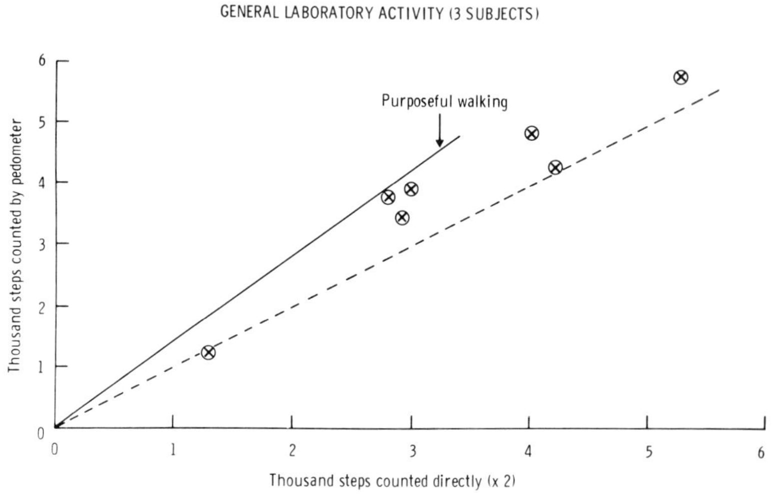

GENERAL LABORATORY ACTIVITY (3 SUBJECTS)

Fig. 5   Relation between pedometer reading and direct step-count during normal laboratory activities in 3 subjects. Axes as in Fig. 4, from which the regression line representing data obtained during purposeful walking is taken.

A few recordings have been made during several hours of general laboratory activity in 3 subjects, and pedometer step counts have again been compared with counts of directly-registered steps. Seven comparisons are shown in Figure 5 and the point again lie above the line of equality, but below the line (describing the data in Figure 4) for purposeful walking. This suggests that the slow 'pottering' movements that comprise a substantial part of walking during normal daily activity do not contribute many extra accelerations registered by the pedometer. If this is confirmed by further recordings, in a variety of occupations and environments, it will demonstrate that the pedometer gives a reasonably faithful estimate of the stepping movements of ambulant subjects, with a small over-estimate that might helpfully represent other trunk movements. No correction has been made to the pedometer readings obtained in ambulant subjects.

Application to Groups of Ambulant Subjects in Normal Life

A team in this laboratory has been investigating the contribution made by physical activity to the maintenance of body muscle in retired workers (3), and to the cardio-pulmonary fitness of middle-aged subjects (11). Large groups of subjects were needed and cheap, convenient and robust methods. It was sufficient to categorize subjects into broad activity bands, or to rank groups in order of activity.

250 subjects were given mechanical pedometers to wear for a week at a time, and asked to read and reset them each night on going to bed. Results from 5 different groups are shown in Figure 6, which gives the mean number of steps taken and the SE for each day of the week, in thousands. The larger groups, which have the smallest standard errors, show the greatest stability from weekday to weekday. The mean weekday activity is least for the retired men and almost twice as great for the students, who live on a large university campus. Laboratory workers are as active as those in light industry. and textile workers are the most active group.

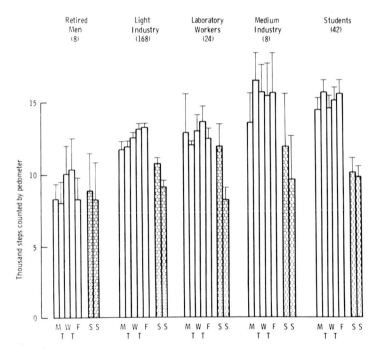

Fig. 6   Mean (± SEM) pedometer readings (thousands of steps) for weekdays and weekend days (shaded) in 5 occupational groups.

The non-retired subjects are less active on Saturdays than during the week, and on Sunday, they reduce their activity to the steady low level of the retired man.

These findings suggest that the pedometer can be used to obtain information about activity in sizeable groups of subjects; that students and workers are shown to be more active than retired men, and that the difference between weekday and weekend activity can be distinguished. However, we have by no means covered the whole range of activity expected in the population.

Acknowledgements

We are grateful for the financial support of the Medical Research Council and the Health and Safety Executive, and to many departmental colleagues, who contributed to the data-collection.

J.M. Patrick is grateful to the Wellcome Trust and the University of Nottingham for travel facilities.

References

1. Bassey E.J., Bryant J.C., Fentem P.H., Macdonald I.A. and Patrick J.M. (1980) ISAM 1979 Proc. of 3rd Int. Symp. on Amb. Mon. Eds: Stott F.D., Raftery E.B. & Goulding L. Academic Press, London, pp 425–4322.
2. Chave S.P.W., Morris J.N., Moss S. and Semmance A.M. (1978) J. of Epidemiology and Community Health 32, 239–243.
3. Patrick J.M., Bassey E.J., Jones P.R.M., Macdonald I.A. and Fentem P.H. (1981) Proceedings of the I.U.P.S. Satellite Symposium on 'Metabolic and functional changes during exercise'. Prague 1980 (in press).
4. Benedict F.G. and Murschhauser H. (1915) Carnegie Institute of Washington List Publications No. 231.
5. Stunkard A. (1960) Am. J. Clin. Nutr. 8, 595–601.
6. Saris W.H.M. and Binkhorst R.A. (1977) Europ. J. Appl. Physiol. 37, 219–235.
7. Cavagna G.A., Saibene F.G. and Margaria R. (1963) J. Appl. Physiol. 18, 1–9.
8. Cavagna G.A. and Margaria R. (1966) J. Appl. Physiol 21, 271–278
9. Cotes J.E. and Meade F. (1960) Ergonomics 3, 97–119.
10. Kemper H.C.G. and Verschur R. (1977) Europ. J. Appl. Physiol. 37, 72–82
11. Bassey E.J., Blecher A., Fentem P.H. and Patrick J.M. (1981) Walking Adults ISAM 1981 (in press).

METHODOLOGY OF HEART RATE AMBULATORY MONITORING RECORDINGS ANALYSIS, IN RELATION TO ACTIVITY: APPLICATIONS TO SPORTS' TRAINING AND WORKLOAD STUDIES

J.P. FOUILLOT*, T. DROZDOWSKI*, F. TEKAIA**, J. REGNARD*,
M-A. IZOU**, T. FOURNERON***, A. LEBLANC**** AND M. RIEU*

*Laboratoire de Physiologie, UER Cochin-Port-Royal,
St. Jacques, Paris, France
**INSEP Dept. Medical, Paris, France
***BEFIC, Silic, Rungis Cedex, France
**** Dept. d'Ingenierie, Universite du Quebec a Trois-
Rivieres, Quebec, Canada

Summary

Ambulatory monitoring ECG recordings in man at exercise are processed in synchronism with observed activity data. RR interval histograms are generated for each activity sequence.

Factorial analysis of correspondence between heart rate classes and activity sequences provides a macroscopic view of heart rate trends in relation to activities, for one subject or for a whole population. Heart rate variations of Airbus A300 crew members, during simulated flights are shown.

Introduction

The heart rate has been for a long time used for indirect measurement of energy for physical exercise, even though of oxygen consumption to heart rate raises doubt.

Nonetheless, heart rate provides good information on daily physical activity.

The complete autonomy provided by ambulatory monitoring systems allowed intensive applications in the cardiology field. It is now widely used in studies of man-at-work or during physical training.

In cardiology, ambulatory monitoring of the ECG is used mainly for the diagnosis of arrhythmias or ST segment depression. This does not require reference to an accurate chronology, but when one tries to study the relation between symptoms and ECG abnormalities. In ergonomy, the reference to physical activity events is compulsory and this is one of the reasons why our methodology had to differ slightly from the analysis of heart rate in cardiology.

Methods

1. ECG Recordings and Heart Rate Measurement

It is obviously essential to avoid EMG potentials from pectoral or deltoid muscles, which are often large in athletes and rowers. Heavy exercise is often associated with profuse sweating, sudden

acceleations and decelerations, and sometimes collisions, as when
playing football.

So perfection in ECG recordings is difficult to achieve.

We used the Medilog 4-24 miniature type recorder to register the
ECG at 2 mm/s, on standard C90 cassettes,(3) using one channel for
ECG and another for an event marker. A third channel is used for a
60 Hz timing pulse delivered by a crystal controlled oscillator with
its output directly recorded on the tape. This enables accurate real
time analysis independent of recording and play-back tape speeds.
The electrodes were applied to the manubrium sternum and the sixth
rib. The electrodes and wires we used were soldered together, completely waterproof and, after a good skin preparation, the adhesion
was good enough to allow the ECG recording of a swimming baby, a
swimmer training for two hours or an active windsurfer. In these
cases, the Medilog was waterproofed and we used special waterproof
bags. The latest model has been tested at 8 bars pressure.

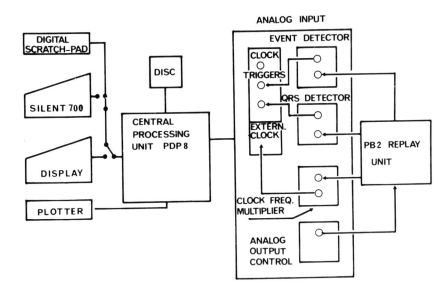

Fig. 1   General block-diagram of the system

The tapes were played back on a standard Medilog PB2 at sixty
times the recording speed (Fig.1) through an adjustable band pass
filter with a response equivalent to 18 Hz in real time. A triggered
puls originated from this filtered signal and was transmitted through
an interface to the central processing unit, a PDP8 computer[2]. The
60 Hz signal recorded simultaneously with the ECG was multiplied by
eight such as to obtain a 2 ms accuracy in real time, taking into
account RR intervals by time counting between two detection pulses of
complexes. The duration of these RR intervals was subject to different kinds of processing.

2. Synchronisation between the events and the recording

This was achieved with the event marker which simultaneously started the chronometer. Pitfalls occur with both the event marker and the 60 Hz time band, some of which can be avoided, but the observed duration of the activity has always to be compared with the recorded duration, and observations rejected when there is a difference.

If the physical activity sequence is heterogenous and associated with different types of exercise, the corresponding heart rate variation is of low significance. If the duration of activity is short, the heart rate variation will also be insignificant, so the observed sequences must be as homogenous and well detailed as possible.

In a study of wind surfers and yacht racers we have differentiated sequences according to the tack (against the wind, before the wind, tacking and veering...) according to the action of each crew member (sit down, trapeze, spinnaker handling...) to a total of 40 to 60 sequences per race and per crew member.

The observations were made by means of a grid to carry out a sequential study of heart rate. However, during training when sequences of physical activity were short and followed one another rapidly, it was tiresome to code observations and note the time of each sequence in this manner. Therefore, we not only tried to automatize the heart rate recording and ECG processing but also the collection of the coded observations. We used a digital autonomous, portable, scratch-pad Medicode Befic to measure the duration of each activity sequence and to characterise it by a 4-digit code. This unit is made up from a CMOS microprocessor system.

After starting up the program, the subject's identification number, time and date of recording was taped and the observer initiated the time counting and the event marking on the magnetic recorder.

While time was displayed on half the digital display, the observer displayed the four digit code of the activity on the other half. As soon as the sequential time counting stopped, the displayed data are stored and the chronometer moved to the start (zero) position ready to measure the time of the following sequence and so on. It is possible with this data storage to record about 300 observation code-time couples. Observations stored chronologically could be transferred by interface into the processor where they were transferred to disks.

3. Analysis of data

The heart rate was subjected to two kinds of processing per sequence of physical activity identified by the digital scratch-pad as well as for the whole recording.
i) Numeric or graphic printout of the mean heart rate calculated for periods of 5, 10, 15, 30 or 60 sec. in the course of all physical activity sequences.
ii) RR interval histogram which is an effective mean of condensing the heart rate data of a long recording into a simple diagram (i). An RR difference histogram was also generated and used as a quality test.

All these results for each activity sequence were stored on disk. The RR interval histogram provided us with a synthesis of the heart rate corresponding to an activity sequence, which is a microscopic view with regard to a training session or a day of work which contains hundreds of activity sequences.

Our aim was to evaluate the heart rate strain achieved by different types of exercise in a population, or the relationship between some characteristics of the population and the response to exercise. For that purpose we needed a macroscopic view of the relationship between exercise and heart rate. A simple way to do this was found by accumulating the RR interval histograms of the same exercise for one or several subjects. It is difficult to write more than 6 - 8 histograms on the same graph, so we used a mulitfactorial method, (the factorial analysis of correspondances) which is a good way to graphically represent the proximities between RR interval classes and the activity sequences (7).

Results

In this study, we report 8 mission simulations of a civil air transport scenario, and 2 real flights (Toulouse-Hamburg and return). The simulator and the aircraft used in this study were an Airbus A300B. The actions of the crews and the basic aircraft parameters were observed and heart rates were recorded. The participating aircrews were all volunteers from Airbus Industry. Each crew consisted of a captain, a first officer and a flight engineer. Each pilot was alternatiely captain or co-pilot.

When a pilot is taking off, landing, or going through a

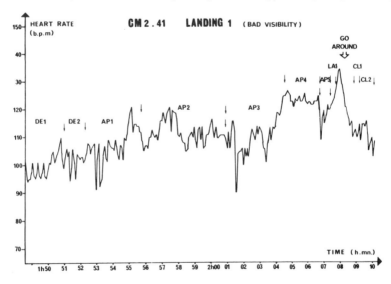

Fig. 2 Heart rate curve of an Airbus A300 second officer landing with bad visibility

difficult manoeuvre, his heart rate increases along with increased activity in other physiological systems.

This increased heart rate may be secondary to the increased physical workload during these tasks, but it could also be due to emotional states and increased vigilance concommitant to the danger involved in the manoeuvre (4,5,6). Fig. 2 shows the increasing heart rate curve of a second officer (CM2) acting as pilot during approach and landing with bad visibility.

Heart rate rises through the landing sequence, and reduces after the go round.

Fig. 3 shows RR interval histograms of these different flight sequences, approach (AP), landing (LA).

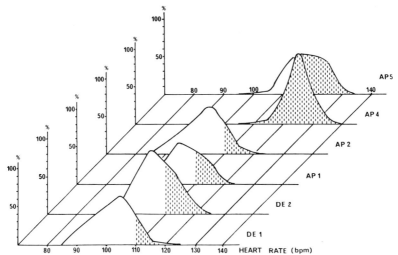

Fig. 3   RR interval histogram of the following flight sequences: descend (DE), approach (AP). The pilot recorded is an Airbus A300 second officer landing with bad visibility.

Fig. 4 shows a factorial analysis between heart rate and flight sequences which allows comparison of heart rate and 60 different flight sequences, only 9 being plotted on the graph. Heart rate studies can also be done on several subjects. Nineteen hundred and sixteen RR interval histograms have been generated from the ECG recordings of all crew members during 8 simulated flights. As we use a PDP 8 with a memory capacity of only 24 K, the data was reduced to 462 cumulated histograms corresponding to flight and incident sequences, and 20 cumulated histograms corresponding to the whole flight of each crew member.

Heart rate corresponding to the 462 sequences are plotted along a parabolic curve in Fig. 5. As it is impossible to plot 462 sequences on a graph, we have selected some flight and failure sequences.

Fig. 5 shows the correspondance between heart rate and the following sequences: take off (TO), climb (CL), air data computer failure (ADC fail), attitude and heading failure. The captain (CM1) is mainly concerned with these failures. During take off, CM1 heart

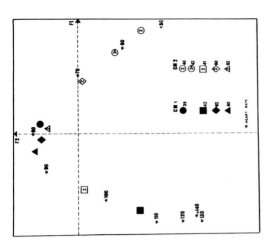

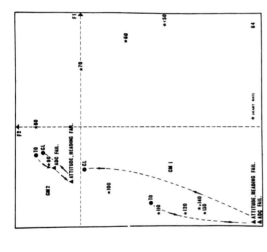

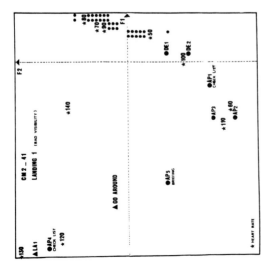

Fig. 4 (left)   Factorial analysis of correspondence between heart rate classes and flight sequences. The pilot recorded is an Airbus A300 second officer landing with bad visibility.

Fig. 5 (centre) Factorial analysis of correspondance between heart rate classes and flight, air data computer failure, attitude and heading failure sequences. Captain and second officer have been plotted on the graph.

Fig. 6 (right)   Factorial analysis of correspondence between heart rate classes and flight sequences. Heartrate classes and flight sequences barycentres are plotted. Each pilot is figured by a symbol and a flight number, dark symbol when he flies as a captain, light symbol when he flies as a second officer.

rate increased to 110 beats/min., and increased further when failure
occurred. During the following sequence (climb) failure was controlled, and heart rate decreased below 100 beats/min. This failure did
not affect the co-pilot (CM2) whose flight instruments were in working order. Take off and climb sequences showed the same heart rate,
and when failure occurred, it did not produce such a high heart rate
as for the captain.

Fig. 6 shows the relationship between heart rate and the whole
flight centre of gravity of each pilot, who were successively captain
(dark symbols), or second officer (light symbols). The barycentre
flight sequence produces a higher heart rate when the pilot is
captain (CM1) than when he is second officer (CM2).

In summary, this kind of heart rate processing provides a
macroscopic view of heart rate trends in relation to activities, for
one subject, or for a whole population, when there is a greater
number of data. This method will find application in a
multifactorial study of human work. The recording of heart rate and
other physiological parameters such as ventilation, temperature, rest
and activity indicators, should lead to a biological typology of
human activities. It should then be possible to present a
macroscopic view of the exercise strain in workers as well as in
athletes.

References

1.   Cashman, P.M. (1976) Postgrad Med. J. **52**, Suppl.7, 19-23.
2.   Drozdowski, T. Contribution a l'etude experimentale de
     phenomenes cardiaques chez le sportif, a l'aide de
     l'informatique. Memoire Universite Paris VIII.
3.   Fouillot, J-P., Rieu, M., Duvallet, A., Devars, J., Cocquerez,
     J.P., Klepping, J. (1978) 'Sports Cardiology' International
     Conference, Roma, Aulo Gaggi Ed., 231-240.
4.   Rubin, R.T., Miller, R.G., Clark, B.R., Poland, R.E., Arthur,
     R.J.(II (1970). Psychosom.Med. **32**: 589-597.
5.   Ruffel Smith, H.P. (1979) NASA Technical Memorandum, 78472.
6.   Schytte Blix, A., Stromme, S.B., Ursin, H. (1974), Aerospace
     Med. 1219-1222.
7.   Tekaia, F., Fouillot, J-P., Drozdowski, T., Rieu, M. (1981)
     (This vol. p.469)

AMBULANT MONITORING OF LIFTING AND CARRYING WORK

G.M. HAGG

Stockholm, Sweden

Summary

The physical strain caused by lifting and carrying heavy objects is
definitely related to low back pain and other physical disorders.
The "exposure" of workers to these strains has not been described in
quantitative terms. In order to measure the "exposure" of lifting
and carrying work on workers, in different situations, a measurement
system has been developed consisting of a pair of wooden shoes with
built in force transducers and a portable miniaturized tape recorder.
The recorded information is analysed by a computer to give the number
of liftings, amplitude of each lifting, balance between the legs,
lifting duration and number of steps during each lifting. In parallel physiological parameters, such as heart rate and respiration, are
recorded.

Introduction

In the field of occupational medicine, the concept "exposure" is
well-known when dealing with various chemical agents. However, when
it comes to physical stress in terms of forces and torques, little
has been done to measure them at different industrial work tasks and
relate this exposure to physiological responses and to various physical disorders.

One of the reasons for this is the complex biomechanical structure of the human body involved in a lifting task, which also implies
a difficult measurement problem.

The aim of this work has been to develop a measurement system,
which can collect and evaluate individual data from practical lifting
tasks in industry. The data collecting part of the system should be
worn by the worker and should not materially restrict freedom of
motion.

Data Collecting System

The fundamental variable of interest in this system is the load on
the floor caused by the worker and the object he is lifting. This
load is measured by four strain-gauge bridges built into a pair of
wooden shoes, two into each shoe (Figure 1). One gauge measures the
load on the toe and the other, the load on the heel.

Before recording the information on tape a signal processing is
done according to Figure 2. The four signals from the shoes (R=right,
L=left, t=toe, h=heel) are summed and converted into three signals Σ,
L/R and t/h. The Σ signal is the sum of our four signals, minus the
body weight B of the test subject. Hence Σ is at least static conditions the mass of the lifted object. Σ is fed through a low pass

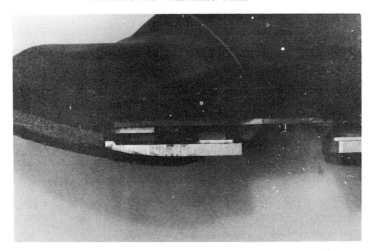

Fig. 1   Straingauge mounted into a wooden shoe.

filter with a time constant of 50 ms.

L/R gives the distribution of the total load between the left and right foot; t/h gives the distribution of the total load on toe and heel. These three signals are then fed to a Medilog recorder.

So far, only Σ and L/R are recorded in practice. The remaining two channels of the Medilog recorder are used for heart rate and pulmonary ventilation recordings.

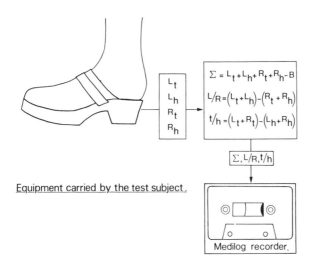

Equipment carried by the test subject.

$$\Sigma = L_t + L_h + R_t + R_h - B$$
$$L/R = (L_t + L_h) - (R_t + R_h)$$
$$t/h = (L_t + R_t) - (L_h + R_h)$$

$\Sigma, L/R, t/h$

Medilog recorder.

Fig. 2   Signal processing done before recording the information on tape.

Computer Evaluation

The computer used is a Swedish ABC-80, which is based on a Z-80
microprocessor. It has a total memory of 64 kbytes. 16 kbytes are
reserved for a BASIC-translater in ROM. Another 16 kbytes are reserved for various system tasks. Hence 32 kbytes are available for
programming and data.
    Most of the programming is done in BASIC, while the data sampl-
ing routine is written in assembler.
    The tapes are replayed on the RP-2 replay unit and the signals
e and L/R are sampled at a rate of 360 Hz each, corresponding to 6
samples/s in real time.
    The tape is replayed 15 s (15 min in real-time) at a time. This
is the maximum amount of raw data, which the computer can store at a
time. After the evaluation of these 15 s another 15 s are replayed
and evaluated.
    The setting of the identification criterion for a lifting was
quite delicate. Many different criteria were tested. The following
proved to be the best:
    A lifting starts when the $\geq$ signal exceeds a load corresponding
to 4 kg and is finished when the $\geq$ signal falls under 1/5 of the
maximum value. The signal is too noisy to detect lifts below 4 kg.
All durations less than 1 s are rejected. The maximum value is
stored as an amplitude measure.
    The L/R balance signal is measured at the start and at the end
of each identified lifting, and each value is put in one of three
classes, central, more than 80% of total load on left foot, more
than 80% on right foot. Hence the balance of the lifting has 9
possible combinations.
    The number of steps with the carried object is also evaluated
from the balance signal.
    All lifting data from each test-subject are stored on floppy
discs.
    The accuracy of the identified liftings was tested by letting
two test-subjects preform 16 lifts each of 4 boxes with a weight of
7, 12, 17 and 22 kg under different conditions. The outcome of the
test is shown in Figure 3. The mean values of the response at each
level falls very close to a linear regression line (R-0.999). It is
obvious the masses are over-estimated at higher levels and somewhat
under-estimated ar low levels. A linear correction is, therefore,
introduced in the evaluation programme.

Practical Experience and Results

So far, two studies of warehouse workers at two different plants have
been carried ouut.
    The large amount of gathered data is shown in one form in Figure
4. At the bottom, each lifting is plotted as a vertical line on a
time-scale. Above this, the corresponding heart rate and pulmonary
ventilation are plotted.
    The distribution of the masses of the lifted objects is shown in
Figure 5. It can be plotted for each individual or for a group of
individuals.

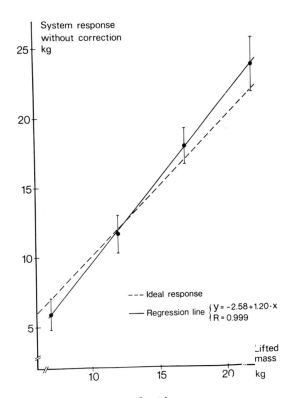

Fig. 3 Result of system evaluation.

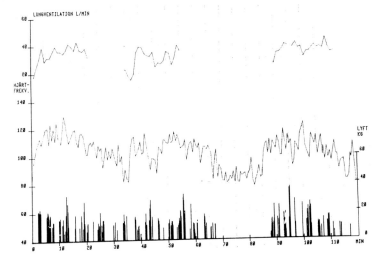

Fig. 4 Presentation of raw data.

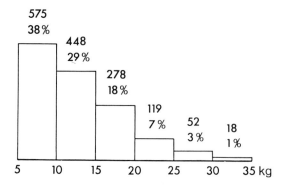

LIFTING PROFILE, PLANT 2.
TOTAL NUMBER OF LIFTINGS 1505.

Fig. 5   Lifting profile.

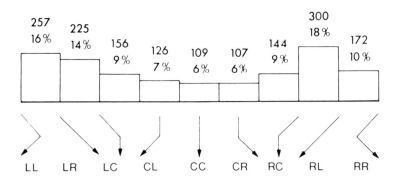

BALANCE PROFILE, PLANT 1.
TOTAL NUMBER OF LIFTINGS 1596.

Fig. 6   Balance profile.

The "balance profile" is shown in Figure 6. The percentages of each of the nine balance combinations are shown as vertical bars. C=central, R=right, L=left. Ideally, one should have a 100% bar in the middle CC position.

Conclusion

It is obvious that the accuracy of the data for each lifting is moderate. However, the aim of this system is not to study single liftings and when a large amount of data is put together, different kinds of statistical analysis give valuable information about the stress in manual material handling.
The statistical analysis of the data collected, so far, is not yet finished and the physiological conclusions will be presented later elsewhere.

Discussion

MR. EVANS: I cannot see how this particular method can assess back strain because there is no indication whether the lift is being performed with the knees bent or with a straight leg. Surely, something would also be needed to measure the angle of the back.
MR. SKOLDSTROM: That is correct. This is just the first step that has been taken in a large project determining lifting and carrying problems. We are just evaluating what the system could do. I fully agree that more information is required on that.

MEASUREMENT OF HEAT STRESS OF GLASSWORKERS USING PORTABLE MICROPROCESSOR-BASED DATA-COLLECTING EQUIPMENT

B. SKOLDSTROM AND I. HOLMER

Work Physiology Unit, National Board of Occupational
Safety and Health, S-171 84 Solna, Sweden

Summary

Heat stress has been measured on glassworkers, employing a new
portable data-collecting system based on a microprocessor. The
system can collect data from 16 different transducers, make a data-
reduction, and store the result in semiconductor memories containing
4000 data-words. In this study pulse rate, six skin temperatures and
one rectal temperature were measured and stored. The result was fed
into a minicomputer for evaluation and plotting.

Heat stress was measured on glass-workers at different working
sites and the obtained physiological result was compared with a
climate index; WBGT (Wet Bulb Gobe Temperature) was taken at the
same time and place.

The physiological strain and the climate index did not correlate
very well, but WBGT is difficult to measure correctly in a field
situation and more studies have to be done to verify this result.

Introduction

In many industrial sites, workers are periodically exposed to
extremes of heat: for instance, in steel plants and glass factories.
Hot weather conditions are often a problem in many industries, but
the problem is pronounced where there is already a hot environment.
The first thing usually done is to measure the heat exposure on the
worker, by either direct or indirect measurement.

In this study, at a glass factory, we have measured the heat
load both directly, with a man-carried equipment, and indirectly,
through a heat climate index and then compared the two methods.

Method and Material

Indirect Method

Equipment described by Kuehn and MacHattie (1) was used for
measurement of the climate index. Heat radiation was measured with
a 41 mm globe bulb, with a settling time of 5-minutes. Air temperature was measured with a heat radiation protected transducer. Globe
and air temperatures were measured simultaneously at four places
surrounding the working area. Wet temperature was measured at one
place only with a wetted temperature transducer.

The climate index WBGT (2) is calculated for each measured point
with the formula: WBGT = 0.7 WB + 0.3 gt ^{o}C , where WB is Wet

Bulb Temperature and gt is Globe Temperature for the small globe.

The signals from the nine temperature transducers were sampled by a microprocessor data logger and data were stored in semiconductor memories.

The results were plotted and the WBGT value calculated for the working period.

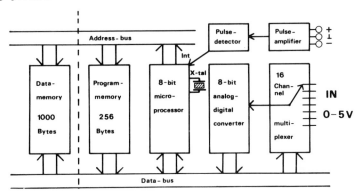

Fig. 1   Microprocessor based data collection system

Direct Method

For the measurements of the physiological variables a microprocessor based data collecting system was used (3). A system was put on each subject and the data collected was stored in semi-conductor memories for later evaluation. Heart beats were detected with a cardiometer (Exercentry) and each heart beat stored in the microprocessor. Each minute the accumulated heart beats were stored in the memory giving directly the heart rate . Deep body temperature was measured with a Yellow Spring rectal transducer (YSI 401). Skin temperature was measured with six temperature transducers (YSI 44004) taped to six different places on the subject with surgical tape (Blenderm 3M). The six values were weighted to give mean skin temperature. All temperatures were measured and stored each minute.

Results

Climate and physiological strain were measured at one working site where glass plates were made. The climate transducers were moved to follow the subject who worked at three different places in the work-ing area. After about 50 minutes, the subject took a break and rested for 25 minutes .

The climate measurement is showed in Figure 2. Calculated WBGT value weighted for 2 h was 28_oC, which is within recommended limits, with a peak value of almost 40_oC.

At the same time, the physiological variables were measured . As can be seen from (Figure 3), mean skin temperature is sometimes higher than the deep body temperature, which means that heat is transported into the body, heating the subject up. This can be verified as an increase in rectal temperature from 37.2_oC to 37.7_oC.

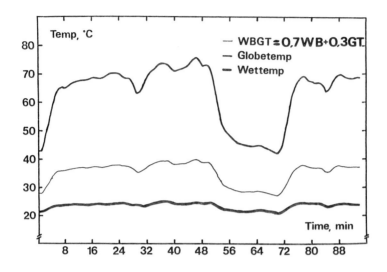

Fig. 2   Climate Measurements over 90 min period

Mean skin temperature was 37.3 with a peak temperature of $45^{\circ}C$ on the subject's chest as he worked in front of an oven. Mean heart rate was 86 beats/min. during the measured period with a peak value of 101.

Measurements taken in other work-stations showed, however, that deep body temperature sometimes exceeded $38^{\circ}C$ and the heart rate

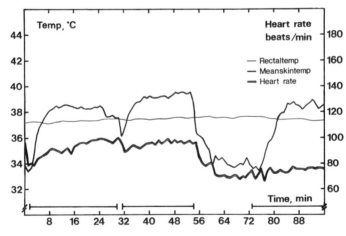

Fig. 3   Physiological measurements correspnding in time to climate measurements of Fig.2

exceeded 130 beats/min., both being recommended limits for hot work during one day. At the same time, the WBGT values were acceptable. Apparently under these conditions, the WBGT index is not a reliable predictor of the actual heat stress.

The climate index is difficult to measure, because the worker occupies the area where the WBGT-transducer should be located. One alternative is to place the transducers directly on the subject, but no such system has been constructed. The results in this study indicates that the direct measurement method gives the best correlation of the real heat exposure on the subject. This method should be used when an accurate measurement is required and especially when a climate index is difficult to obtain.

The microprocessor data collecting systems used worked well even under hard environmental and mechanical strain. The all-solid-state design makes it reliable and easy to use. The greatest advantage of such a system is the ease and speed of evaluation, since the data can be fed directly into a computer for listing, plotting, calculations and storing for later statistical analysis.

References

1.   Kuehn L.A., MacHattie L.E. (1975) Am. Ind. Hyg. Assoc. J.(May) 325-331.
2.   Occupational exposure to hot environments. U.S. Dept. of Health, Education and Welfare. Nat. Inst. for Occupational Safety and Health.
3.   Skoldstrom B., Holmer I.(1979) ISAM: Proceedings of the Inter-national Symposium on Ambulatory Monitoring.

Discussion

DR. MILES: May I congratulate Mr. Skoldstrom on a very nice system. Did I understand correctly that the memory is a separate small unit with its own battery in it, that it is plugged out and then put into a minicomputer?

MR. SKOLDSTROM: Yes, that is right. It was cheaper to build several RAM memories than severy whole systems, so I have built a lot of memories.

DR. MILES: In the EPROM programme is there any switch control of samples times or is the entire programme in the EPROM?

MR. SKOLDSTROM: I have the entire programme in EPROM - I just change the programme. That was the easiest way. By this means I can also change the battery of the system without losing the controlling programme.

MR. LOVELY: Mr. Skoldstrom showed a diagram of a multiplexer feeding into an A-to-D converter. Are there any filters on the front end of the multiplexer interfacing between the transducers and the multiplexer?

MR. SKOLDSTROM: No, I have not found it necessary to do that. I sample only very slow signals, and only once per minute - there is really no problem in doing that.

DAILY PHYSICAL ACTIVITY MONITORED BEFORE, DURING AND AFTER A WALKING-PROGRAMME IN MIDDLE-AGED SUBJECTS

E.J. BASSEY, A. BLECHER, P.H. FENTEM AND J.M. PATRICK

Department of Physiology & Pharmacology, University Medical School
Nottingham, UK

Summary

108 factory workers volunteered for an unsupervised 12-week walking-programme. After baseline measurements, the subjects were randomly divided into three groups, who entered the programme in series. This provided test and control subjects for a study of the effect of the programme on customary physical activity measured both immediately after the programme and 12 weeks later. Pedometers and body-borne tape-recorders provided complementary indices of activity.

One week after the walking-programme a consistent 15% increase in activity was found in participants. No decline in activity was seen in the 12 weeks after the programme. These findings suggest that a moderate exercise-programme can be of benefit in increasing customary activity levels in older people.

Introduction

Physical deterioration can be a serious problem for older people. The deliberate addition of 20 minutes' extra regular exercise on at least three days of the week is known to improve 'physical fitness' in middle-aged subjects (1). It is not known, however, whether an unsupervised walking-programme would be effective, nor to what extent such a programme changes the rest of the customary activity patterns. It is possible that participants may compensate for the extra exercise by doing less than they had done previously, or that they might feel more energetic as a result of the improved physical condition and do more. Customary activity is more difficult to measure than physical condition.

We have encouraged a group of middle-aged factory workers (half of them women) to participate in an unsupervised walking-programme, lasting 12 weeks. Customary physical activity was measured by two different methods, before and immediately after the programme, and again 12 weeks later in an attempt to answer these questions.

Methods

The subjects were 108 shift-workers from a light manufacturing industry in Nottingham. Measurements were made at the factory with the informed consent of the subjects and with the full co-operation of the management and the trades unions. The age range of the men and women subjects was 55 to 60 years and their mean weight and height were 72.5 and 63.8 kg, and 1.70 and 1.59 m. respectively.

The 12-week training programme consisted of five periods of

walking per week. The durations and speeds gradually increased over
the weeks until the subjects were walking for 40 minutes at 7 km/hr.
The programme was taken from Cooper (2) and subjects followed it in
their own time, keeping a log-card of what they achieved.

TABLE 1

Protocol for recruitment and testing of subjects and their
participation in the walking-programme. All subjects were
tested 4 times (T1 to T4): on each occasion a pedometer was
worn for a week, a day-long tape-recording of ECG and footfall was made, and a self-paced walking-test was performed.
In addition, a pedometer was worn for a week in the middle
of each subject's walking-programme.

PROTOCOL FOR WALK-PROGRAMME STUDY

(n = number of subjects at each test)

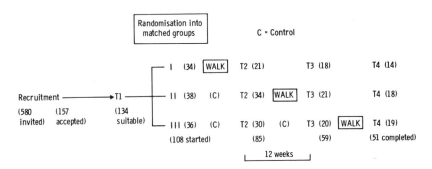

The protocol is outlined in Table 1. All subjects were tested
before entry into the programme, as shown in Table 2. They were then
randomly assigned to one of three groups and Group I started the
walking-programme immediately. After 12 weeks, all subjects were re-
tested and then Group II started the programme. After a further 12
weeks, all subjects were again re-tested and Group III started walking. All subjects were finally tested 12 weeks later. The numbers
of subjects remaining in the study at each stage are given in Table
1. This arrangement provided control subjects for those in Groups I
and II while they were on the walking-programme, and for subjects in
Group I in the 12 weeks after the programme.

Measurements of Customary Activity

We have used two different methods in the hope of detecting
changes in both intensity and duration of activity. We have relied
on repeated measurements with a simple instrument, and single measurements with a more sophisticated one.
1.   A mechanical pedometer which counts paces (Yamasa Digital Pedometer (3)) was worn at the hip for seven consecutive days, and the
subjects themselves recorded the day's accumulated reading when they
went to bed each night. The reading has been expressed as thousand
steps per day, using a calibration constant obtained for each instru-

ment (3), and the average over the whole week has been used as the
index of physical activity.
2.   An Oxford Instruments Medilog tape-recorder was used to record
the ECG and footfall signals during the whole of one waking day (the
first day on which the pedometer was worn). The subject's heart rate
while walking at 4.8 km/hr was measured using a self-paced walking-
test (4) on the same day. That heart rate (less 5 bt/min to allow
for variation in estimation) was used as the criterion of 'activity'.
The analysis was done in two ways: first, accumulating all periods
of heart-rate elevation above the walking heart-rate, no matter how
short: and second, accumulating only those periods of elevation
lasting at least two minutes, i.e. those likely to have some train-
ing-effect. The methods have been fully reported to ISAM previously
(5, 6). The self-paced walking test was also used to assess changes
in physical condition.

Results and Discussion

1.   Did the subjects actually carry out the walking-programme?
      Two sources of information are available to help answer this
question. First, the subjects were asked to complete a log-card of
the extra walking activity undertaken during each week of the programme. The log-cards were scored as shown in Table 2. It appears
as if the majority of the subjects achieved, or came near to achieving, the prescribed exercise.
      Second, pedometers were used to record a full week's activity in
the middle of each subject's walk-period. These results have been

Table 2

Subjects' compliance with walking programme

A.Evidence from subjects' own record cards

Score	Record	Criteria	No. of subjects
3	Complete	Achieved full programme	22
2]	Incomplete	[Failed to achieve required	
1]	"	[intensity	17
0	Not known	No log returned; or invalid	30

B.PedometerStep-Countinmid programme and before programme

Group	n	Steps in thousands Before (T1)	Mid Programme		Sig.
3	19	12.9	14.2	1.3	NS
1, 2	12	11.4	13.4	2.0	*
0	17	10.8	13.3	2.5	*
All	48	11.8	13.6	1.8	*

* = P < 0.05 in a paired t-test.

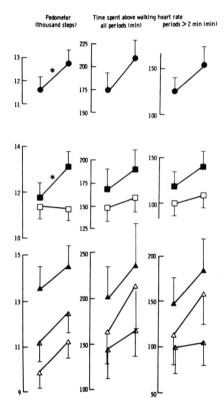

Fig. 1   Three indices (mean, SEM) of physical activity measured
          before and immediately after a 12-week walking-programme.
          Upper panels: all subjects.   Center panels: ■ subjects in
          Groups I and II, □   control subjects not yet started on the
          walking programme.   Lower panels : subjects scoring 3 (▲),
          1 or 2 (▲), and 0 (△) on their record cards of compliance.
          * indicates P < 0.05 in a paired t-test.

expressed in thousand steps per day, and in Table 2, the subjects are
grouped by the score given to their log cards.   The significant
increase of about 1800 steps roughly represents the equivalent of 20
minutes' walking on five days of the week, and again suggests that
the subjects, even those with unreliable log-cards, were indeed
participating in the walking-programme.

2.   Did the walking-programme alter activity?
      At the end of the walking-programme, the prescribed exercise
amounted to 22 km every week.   It was possible that they might have
compensated for this by reducing their other activities;   or they
might have maintained their other activities to give an increased
total, or they might even have increased their non-programme activities. The subjects were re-tested soon after completing the walking-

programme and their measured activity indices are, therefore, not
contaminated by the prescribed walking.

Values for the three indices are given in Figure 1. For the
group as a whole, the pedometer step-count increased significantly by
10%, while the time spent above walking heart-rates increased by 20%.
This latter finding might have been a chance one, but it parallels
rather closely the finding for the pedometer index. Some further
insight into these changes can be obtained from particular subgroups.

Comparison between walkers and controls indicates whether the
changes seen might have been due to factors (e.g. seasonal changes)
other than the walking-programme. The control subjects showed no
material or significant change in either direction for any of the
three variables, and the increase in the pedometer step-count for the
walking group was significantly greater than the change in the controls.

Comparison of changes among the groups classified by their log-
score might also have provided evidence about the effectiveness of
the walking-programme in changing total activity. It is noticeable
that the subjects who returned a complete log (score 3) started off
with higher values for all variables even before entering the programme. They went on to increase their activity on all counts, but
so did the other groups. It is possible that the first group might
have shown a greater increase if they had not already been more
active at the start of the programme.

The overall impression given by these findings is that participation in Cooper's 12-week walking-programme leads to a modest
increase in total spontaneous activity when measured soon afterwards.
There is no suggestion whatever of any reduction in other activity to
compensate for the time spent in the programme.

3. Did the activity fall off in the 12 weeks after the walking-
programme?

Thirty-six subjects (Groups I and II) returned for re-testing 12
weeks after completing the walking-programme. In these subjects,
there were no material or significant differences from the values
obtained immediately after the programme in any of the three activity
indices analysed (Figure 2). A control group of 20 subjects who had
not yet embarked on the programme is availale for comparison with the
18 subjects in Group I. In these smaller groups, the three variables
show a somewhat discrepant pattern, but in none do the changes differ
significantly between the test and control groups. The pedometer
data suggest that the walkers at least maintain their total activity
over the 12 weeks after the walking programme, but the other variables rather suggest a decline in the time spent at higher heart
rates. A possible explanation for this discrepancy is that by 12
weeks after the programme, any walking activity is of much shorter
duration with correspondingly lower average heart rates. However,
these groups are relatively small and the variation in the tape-
recorder indices is large, so no firm conclusions can be drawn.
Nevertheless, it is encouraging that there was no evidence of a large
fall in activity, which we would have expected to see if it had been
present.

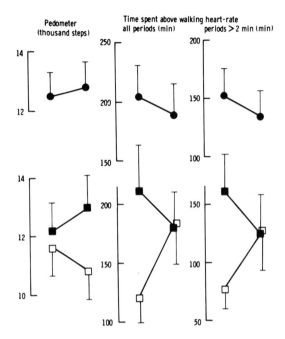

Fig. 2   Three indices (mean, SEM) of physical activity measured
immediately after, and 12 weeks after a 12 week walking-
programme. Symbols as in upper and centre panels of Fig.
1. No significant differences were found.

Conclusions

We were able to persuade one-third of the 55-60 year-olds in a
large local industry to volunteer for an unsupervised moderate exercise programme involving about 20 minutes' walking on five days per
week for 12 weeks. Questionnaire and pedometer records suggest that
the majority of the volunteers came close to completing the programme.
There was good evidence for a 15% increase in spontaneous customary
activity from pedometer and Oxford tape-recorder measurements one
week after the programme was finished. This change in activity is
roughly equivalent to half-an-hour's walking per day. The evidence
for the persistence of this increase over the subsequent 12 weeks is
less strong, but there is no suggestion of a significant decline in
activity. It is our hope that such an exercise-programme, introduced
in the years before retirement, might delay physical deterioration in
later years.

Acknowledgements

We are grateful for the financial support of the Medical Research
Council and the Health and Safety Executive. Christine Lewis, Julie
Beardsley, Martin Irving, Brenda Laurie and Janet Bryant gave
valuable assistance with the data collection and analysis.

References

1. Saltin B. and Rowell L.B. (1980). Federation Proceedings 39: 1506-1513.
2. Cooper K.H. (1970).New Aerobics. Bantam Books.
3. Irving J.M. and Patrick J.M. (1981) ISAM 1981 Gent.
4. Bassey E.J., Fentem P.H., MacDonald I.C. and Scriven P.M. (1976). Clin. Sci. and Mol. Med. **51**, 609-612.
5. Bassey E.J., Fentem P.H., Fitton D.L., MacDonald I.C., Patrick J.M.and Scriven P.M. In ISAM 1977. Proceedings of the Second International Symposium on Ambulatory Monitoring, Eds: F.D.Stott, B. Raftery, P. Sleight, L.Goulding, London Academic Press, 1978, 207-217.
6. Bassey E.J. Bryant J.C., Fentem P.H., Macdonald I.A. and Patrick J.M. In: ISAM 1979. Proceedings of the Third International Symposium on Ambulatory Monitoring, Eds: F.D. Stott, E.B. Raftery, and L. Goulding. London, Academic Press 1980, 425-432.

Discussion

DR. OJA: That was a very nicely executed programme, and I would like to congratulate Dr. Patrick on it. Were any differences observed in the work capacity and, if so, how large were they?

DR. PATRICK: I did not really want to report on that aspect of the study today, but the self-paced walk test was carried out as an index of physical condition, and overall a small, but significant improvement of the order of 5% was observed in physical condition in these subjects.

MR. S. DASHWOOD: Has this scheme been tried in other age groups, or is there an intention to do so?

DR. PATRICK: No, we do not intend to do that. The group with which I work is particularly interested in older people; 55-year-olds are the youngest we are prepared to study. We believe that there is plenty of work to do amongst older people.

PHYSIOLOGICAL STRAIN IN METAL MINE AND CONCENTRATION WORK AS DETERMINED BY 8-HOUR HEART RATE RECORDING

P.OJA*, T. SUURNAKKI* AND A.ZIEMBA**

*Institute of Occupational Health, Helsinki, Finland,
**Department of Aplied Physiology, Medical Research Centre,
Polish Academy of Sciences, Warsaw, Poland

Summary

Thirty jobs in a metal mine and concentration plant were subjected to
Ergonomic Job Description Questionaire analysis, 8-hour heart rate
measurement, and physical activity classification. According to the
heart rate data, physiological strain was apparent in only a few
cases. Underground work proved to be similar to other types of non-
office work, and maintenance work tended to be the most demanding
physiologically. With respect to the muscular work demands, work
heart rate response was logically dependent on the amount and intensity of both the dynamic and static effort required by the task. Work
heart rate correlated the best with the physical activity classification specific to the metabolic cost of work.

Introduction

New technology is making the ambulatory monitoring of physiological
response to work increasingly feasible. In order to understand
better the occupational significance of these data, it is important
to examine individual, environmental and job-related factors responsible for the obtained reactions. Of these, the job-related aspects
have thus far received relatively little attention. In this experiment, we have performed both heart rate and work study measurement in

TABLE 1

The Plant

Branches of Production	...	mining – iron ore
	...	concentration – iron pellets for further production
	...	end products – vanadium, ilmenite
Number of Employees	...	640 (565 men, 75 women)
Amount of Ore Produced per One Man Shift	...	50 tons
Depth of Mine	...	max 661 m
Work Shift	...	3-shift rotation.

a workplace comprised of a metal mine and concentration plant in an
attempt to gain experience in applying these methods, on one hand,
and in order to describe some task-specific determinants of the heart
rate response to work, on the other.

Material and Methods

Workplace and Subjects
     The mine and concentration plant are located in a rural area of
central Finland. They produce iron ore and iron pellets for further
concentration and vanadium and ilmenite are the end products (Table
1).
     Thirty men (Table 2) from four operational divisions of the
workplace comprised the subjects. They were selected to represent
typical jobs throughout the production line, including clerical work.
The selection resulted in two distinct age groups of 15 men each, one
between the ages of 20 and 33 years and the other between 38 and 54
years.

TABLE 2

Age of the Subjects and Two Weight Indices

| Subjects | Age (Years) | | | Body Weight | | | |
	Range	Mean	SD	Kilograms Mean	SD	Ponderal Index Mean	SD
Group 1 (15 men)	20-33	26.8	4.0				
Group 2 (15 men)	38-54	46.4	6.1				
All (30 men)	20-54	36.6	11.2	76.3	8.4	40.1	20.0

Work Studies
     The jobs were subjected to Ergonomic Job Description Question-
naire analysis, or AET, developed by Rohmert and Landau (1). The
standard AET cluster analysis resulted in the following three homogeneous groups of jobs: one with 19 jobs characterized by production and application of force, a second with 3 jobs characterized by
control and regulatory tasks, and a third with 6 jobs involving
clerical tasks. Underground and maintenance jobs typically fell into
the first group, machine- or process-tending jobs into the second and
office jobs and foremen into the third.
     The amount and type of muscular work was assessed from the
relevant AET items. Dynamic work was classified as "heavy" if more
than two-thirds of the work time involved dynamic muscle work of
either the upper or lower extremities or both. When dynamic work
appeared less than two-thirds of the work time, it was considered
"light". For static work, the classification was the same, i.e.,
"heavy" for more than two-thirds of the time and "light" for less,
when the effort was localized in any one of three anatomic areas,
finger-hand-forearm, upper arm-shoulder-back, leg-foot. For both
dynamic and static work, an additional classification was based on
the intensity of effort. It was classified as "high" if the applica-

tion of force was very high or high and as "low" if the force applied was average or small.

Energetic activity was assessed during work with the Edholm scale (2). The classification was performed on a minute-by-minute basis simultaneously with the heart rate recording.

Heart Rate

Each subject's heart rate was recorded continuously for one 8-hour day shift on a portable 2-channel Howel-Corder cassette recorder (3). After the read-out and editing of the raw heart rate data, the activity classification was synchronized with the heart rates. Computerized data processing provided descriptive statistics and graphic illustration on both individual and group bases.

Results

The mean heart rates across the shift were well under 100 beats/min for the workers from each division of the workplace (Table 3). The mean was the lowest for office work (72.7 beats/min). The difference between this value and those of the other divisions was statistically significant ($p < 0.05$). The concentration division included one man, the conveyor cleaner, whose mean heart rate for the 8-hour shift was 128 beats/min. With him excluded, the mean value for this division becomes 88.2 beats/min.

TABLE 3

Mean and Peak Heart Rates of the Subjects from Different Workplace Divisions

Division	n	Heart rate			
		Mean	SD	Peak (% of time)	
				>100 beats/min.	>120 beats/min.
Office	6	72.7	12.9	2.4	0.3
Mine	11	90.2	11.1	29.0	6.2
Maintenance	8	94.9	15.2	31.6	12.4
Concentration	5	94.3	17.7	29.8	10.6

In office work, heart rates of over 120 beats/min. were virtually non-existent, whereas peaks of this magnitude appeared, on average, 6% of the work time in the mine division and 11-12% in the maintenance and concentration divisions (Table 3). If the conveyor cleaner is again excluded, the corresponding value for the concentration division becomes 2.4%, and only the maintenance department is left wih a notable pecentage of peak heart rates.

The mean heart rates across the shift in the three AET groups, particularly for the clerical tasks, were also low and the standard deviation was large in all the groups (Figure 1). The highest mean heart rate was recorded for AET group 1, production and application of force. When the tasks were grouped according to those AET items specific to muscular work, the mean heart rates indicated a logical, but statistically non-significant pattern (Table 4). With respect to dynamic work, the mean heart rate was highest in the group in which dynamic work appeared often and the application of force was high. Conversely, the heart rate was lowest when there was little dynamic work and the application of force was low.

As for static work, the general impression was exactly the same, i.e., when both the amount and intensity of static effort were high, the heart rate was also high, and when both were low, the heart rate was low.

The Edholm scale classifies physical activity into seven classes based on the estimated metabolic cost of the activity. The first class equals 110% of the basal metabolic rate, and the seventh class 1000%. This material covered only classes 3 through 6. Heart rate systematically increased as the activity class increased (Figure 2). The large and statistically significant differences between the means and the relatively small standard deviations resulted in distinct activity classes with respect to heart rate.

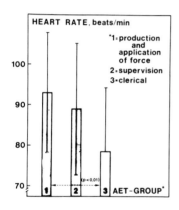

Fig. 1   Mean heart rates across
          the shift (with standard
          deviations) in the three
          AET groups determined by
          cluster analysis.

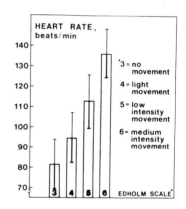

Fig. 2   Mean heart rates with
          standard deviations for
          minutes in different
          Edholm classes.

The mean heart rate across the shift in the older age group, i.e. those over 38 years of age, was 79.7 (±11.0) beats/min and that of the younger age group, 20 to 33 years of age, was 97.6 (±14.3) beats/min. This difference remained in the mean heart rates of the different Edholm classes.

TABLE 4

Mean Heart Rates across the Shift (with Standard Deviations)
for Eight Groups of Subjects According to the Dynamic and Static
Muscular Effort in the Work. The Criteria of Classificiation are
listed in the Text

Application	Dynamic Effort				Static Effort			
of force	Heavy		Light		Heavy		Light	
	Mean	SD	Mean	SD	Mean	SD	Mean	SD
High	92.0	14.9	90.5	6.7	93.9	14.4	85.7	19.5
	n=16		n=5		n=11		n=5	
Low	85.6	0.6	78.2	17.7	90.1	3.6	84.0	16.5
	n=2		n=6		n=2		n=11	

Conclusions

From the physiological point of view, the present results do not
reveal any particular overstrain in metal mine and concentration
work. In most jobs the mean heart rate across the shift was less
than 100 beats/min. In only five cases did the individual mean heart
rate exceed 100 beats/min, the highest individual mean heart rate
being 129. In comparison, Ilmarinen and Rutenfranz (4) reported mean
heart rates of 109 for building construction, 106 for iron and steel
work, 101 for the chemical industry, 86 for the retail trade, 88 for
civil service and 80 for sales work.
     The analysis based on workplace divisions indicated that the
underground work was not particularly straining, perhaps contrary to
common belief. This result must be, to a great extent, due to the
high level of mechanization in the mine. On the other hand, the fact
that maintenance work proved to be the most straining was apparently
due to the specific work demands in this particular workplace, i.e.,
the repair and maintenance of machinery and equipment on the spot, in
difficult locations and in unexpected circumstances.
     Combining the work study information with the physiological data
yielded meaningful results, which showed that the degree of physiological strain was logically dependent on the amount and intensity of
muscle work needed in the job. Yet the general work study technique
did not provide a sensitive indication of the physiological strain
involved in the jobs. Rather, the physiological observations served
as a rough validation of the work study data. A work study technique
specific to metabolic activity is required whenever possible physiological overstrain in work needs to be identified.

Acknowledgements

The AET analyses were kindly provided by Dr. Kurt Landau, REFA-
Institute, Darmstadt, Federal Republic of Germany.

References

1. Rohmert W. and Landau K. (1979) Das Arbeitswissenschaftliche
    Erhebungsverfahren zur Tätigkeitsanalyse (AET) Verlag Hans
    Huber, Bern.
2.   Edholm, O.G. (1966) In: Physical Activity in Health and
    Disease (Ed. K. Evang and K. Lange Andersen) pp 187-197,
    Universitets-forlaget, Oslo.
3. Rutenfranz J. et al (1977) Europ KJ. Appl. Physiol. **36**, 171-
    185.
4. Ilmarinen J. and Rutenfranz J. (1980) in: ISAM 1979, Proc.
    Third International Symposium on Ambulatory Monitoring (Ed.
    Stott F.D. et al) pp. 285-296, Academic Press, London.

Discussion

DR. MONSTER: Has Dr. Oja compared any of the groups in terms of the
overall physical conditions using a generally accepted test, for
example, a step test?

DR. OJA: No, not with this sample, but we are proceeding with another study on a rather larger number of subjects, during which the
work capacity will also be measured in addition to the physiological
response during work.

DR. MONSTER: What about the average age of the people in the different groups? Do people, who do relatively more heavy physical work,
live longer in the long run? There must be a fair amount of data
available from previous years.

DR. OJA: We do not have those data. It is hoped to get closer to
that kind of approach, but at the moment, we do not have such data.

DR. PATRICK: With regard to Dr. Monster's first point about physical
condition, it seems to me that the heart rate was being used as an
index of the strain on the subjects as part of the argument. But Dr.
Oja gave the example of a man, who played a lot of volleyball in the
evening. He would probably be what we would call "fitter", or he
would have a better physical condition, than his colleagues, who did
not have the activity. Therefore, his heart rate during exposure to
the same work will be less. Is it not possible to calibrate the
subjects in some way such as this in order to differentiate the high
heart rates due to the strain of the work from the high heart rates
due to the strain of lesser work in less fit subjects?

DR. OJA: That has not been done, partly because the heart rates in
general were rather low. Very few peaks were observed, so this group
was not particularly interesting in that regard. The effect of age
was analysed and I would suspect that there is a decrease in work
capacity with increasing age. For example, the heart rate response
to the Edholm classification showed a very clear difference between
the two age groups; in other words, the older age group was systematically lower than the younger age group and this difference persisted throughout the range of classification.

DR. PATRICK: We have done a similar sort of investigation and found
that for exactly the same work, older people have lower heart rates,
so it could be simply an ageing phenomenon, if you like, rather than
the fact that they do not participate so heartily in the harder
activities.

MONITORING GAIT OF PATIENTS WITH TOTAL KNEE PROSTHESIS BY VECTOR DIAGRAM TECHNIQUE

G. GUALTIERI, E. LUNA, G. NANNINI, A. PEDOTTI,*
R.RODANO.*

Istituto Ortopedico G. Pini, Centro di Chirurgia dell' Artrite
Reumatoide, P.za Cardinal Ferrari 1, 20100 Milano. * Centro di
Bioingegneria, Fondazione Don Gnocchi - Politecnico di Milano
20148 Milano, Italy

Summary

Usually, diagnosis of patients with different lower limb anomalies is
performed by the clinician through inspection of gait, x-ray records,
routine clinical examination and patient-response. However, a meaningful functional evaluation should also take into account the dynamic modifications introduced by the disorders. This evaluation involves a quite complicated procedure and is seldom performed in clinical
practice.

The common clinical procedure is to use a film or a TV recording
of gait; this, however, gives only a qualitative record of the
kinematics and does not provide any information on the load distribution characteristics. Moreover, the records obtained through this
procedure are difficult to store and to analyze in a normal clinical
environment.

The development of an efficient procedure to obtain quantitative
data on dynamic characteristics has attracted wide attention (1, 2,
3, 4). However, most of the procedures available so far are either
quite complicated to perform or require extensive data-processing to
obtain the requisite information.

In the present paper, we describe a vectogram technique which is
easy to perform and also provides immediate quantitative information
on the dynamic characteristics. This technique allows the clinician
to differentiate various lower limb anomalies, to assess the effect
of operative treatment and to evaluate the recovery process.

Method

During the stance phase of each step, the foot exerts a pressure on
the ground. The resultant force, termed 'ground reaction force', is
the resultant of all gravitional and inertial forces acting on the
various segments of the body and provides a synthesis of the whole
body dynamics (Figure 1a).

The vertical component of the ground reaction force has been
measured for normal and for some pathological gaits (5), but the
results obtained have not been conclusive.

When the subject goes through the stance phase on the

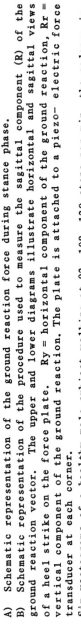

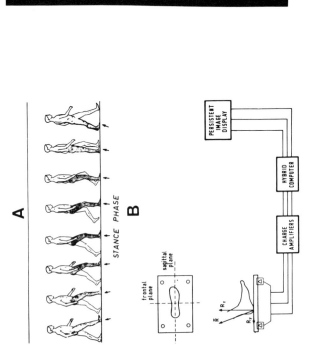

Fig. 1
(left)
A) Schematic representation of the ground reaction force during stance phase.
B) Schematic representation of the procedure used to measure the sagittal component (R) of the ground reaction vector. The upper and lower diagrams illustrate horizontal and sagittal views of a heel strike on the force plate.   Ry = horizontal component of the ground reaction, Rr = vertical component of the ground reaction. The plate is attached to a piezo- electric force transducer at each corner.

Fig. 2
(right))
Six vectograms of a healthy male subject walking at 92, 108, 120 steps per min, the cadence increasing from the top to the bottom. At left are the vectograms of the right foot. The direction of advance is from right (heel-strike) to left (toe-off).   Vectors are sampled at 20 msec intervals.

piezoelectric force plate, our instrumentation allows us to obtain
directly on-line, the spatial-temporal evolution of the ground reaction force projected on either the sagittal or the frontal plane.
The resultant diagram, named vectogram, is obtained through a special
purpose device that uses the electrical signals from the force plate
to compute the ground reaction force, and to display its amplitude,
inclination and point of application on a persistent-image display
(6).   In order to obtain the vectogram, the subject is required to
walk at a fixed cadence along a 15m. long pathway. The force plate
is placed at 2/3 of the pathway to ensure that the subject is in a
steady state condition.

    The advantages of this procedure with respect to clinical appli-
cations have been described in literature (7, 8). The main advantages
can be summarized as follows:

- The tests are easy to perform, even for subjects with severe
impairment of gait.
- It takes only a little time to perform these tests and
quantitative results are obtained immediately.
- The results are very reliable because of the high precision
devices available for measurement and also a large number of
vectograms can be easily generated.
- Clinical interpretation of the quantitative measurements
obtained is possible.

The typical pattern of vectograms for normal gait are well-known.
Figure 2 illustrates six vectograms obtained respectively from the
right and the left feet of a normal male subject walking at three
different speeds of 92, 108, 120 steps per minute. These typical
normal vectograms indicate that:

-    The force envelope has two maxima (at the impact and push-off
     phases) and a central minimum.
-    At each of the three speeds, the vectograms from the right
     and left are similar, indicating a symmetric gait.
-    The vectograms are modified by progressively increasing speed,
     with an increase of the maxima and a decrease of the minimum;
     moreover, at higher speed, the number of vectors decreases
     demonstrating the shorter time of the stance phase.

Results

The results reported here are based on a study of 15 patients with
problems induced by rheumatoid arthritis, localized in the knee
joint. In order to obtain information on the time of recovery, the
analysis has been carried out at the following times:

-    Immediately before the surgical treatment.
-    6-8 months after the treatment, when the subjects were able
     to walk without any external aid.
-    12-15 months after the treatment when a stabilized condition
     could be assumed.

Figure 3 shows the vectograms of six different subjects, walking at

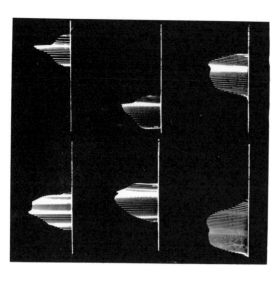

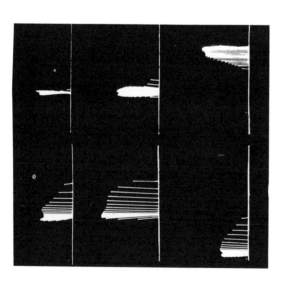

Fig. 3 (left)   Vectograms of six subjects affected by rheumatoid arthritis localised in the knee joint. On the right are the records of the subjects with bilateral diseases, the vectograms being obtained from the limb with the worse pathology. On the left are the records of three subjects with monolateral diseases, the vectograms being obtained from the pathological limb. The direction of advance is from right to left; the vectors are sampled at 34 msec intervals. The cadence of walk was free.

Fig. 4 (right)   Vectograms from a female subject with bilateral disease. The vectograms at the top were obtained immediately before surgery while the middle and bottom vectograms were obtained six and twelve months, respectively, after surgery. The vectograms on the right are from the limb with the worse pathology, which was under treatment. The direction of advance, sampling intervals and cadence are the same as in Fig. 3.

their typical cadence (the cadence imposed by the pain). The vectograms of the affected limb of each patient are shown here. It is
interesting to note from the vectograms that limitation in the knee
function gives rise to two different dynamical patterns.

All the vectograms on the left show a quick displacement of the
vectors from the heel to the toe, with a large concentration of
vectors in the toe region. These vectograms indicate a gait in which
the main loads are sustained by the anterior part of the feet. The
three subjects had monolateral diseases and they utilized compensatory mechanisms to permit a gait with the least pain in the suffering
leg. In fact, they overload the normal limb and give a remarkable
forward inclination to the trunk; in order to facilitate the forward
movement the support base is restricted, with all the significant
vectors being concentrated and quite vertical.

These patterns show a very slow gait with the foot utilized only
like a passive support. The subjects are not able to perform an
active push-off phase and all the loads are sustained by the central
part of the foot.

Since all the three patients have bilateral diseases, they cannot
use the other leg as a compensatory mechanism; therefore, these
patients have only a limited gait efficiency.

Figure 4 shows the vectograms of a subject with bilateral rheumatoid arthritis. The arthritic condition is more advanced in the left
limb (on the right side). The tests have been carried out before
surgery, and also six and twelve months after surgery. The subject
shows the typical initial patterns of patients with bilateral
diseases where the vectors assume low amplitudes and are concentrated in the centre of the support base. The second test shows a
modification in the treated limb, the modification being apparent in
the length of the support base and in the amplitude of forces, while
the shape remains practically the same. An improvement is evident in
the other limb as well. The situation after twelve months is largely
improved in both legs. All the parameters appear to be similar for
both legs. The central concentration of vectors on the right suggests the presence of some problems in the central support phase.
These are probably due to an incomplete adaptation of the subject to
the prosthesis.

Figure 5 shows the vectograms of a subject with monolateral
rheumatoid arthritis localized in the right limb. The tests have
been carried out before the treatment and at eighteen and twenty
seven months after it; unfortunately, a short-term evaluation is
missing. The initial vectogram of the painful leg shows the typical
monolateral pattern for the right limb (on the left) and this pattern
also influences the vectogram of the healthy limb. The first evaluation shows, possibly because of the period lapsed between analyses,
a situation that is almost stable. Both vectograms show improvement,
but the dynamic characteristics of the two legs are not similar. In
fact, for the right limb a quick passage of the load from the heel to
the toe is present and for the left, the concentration of vectors in
the impact phase has not disappeared. After twenty seven months a
very positive situation appears. The gait is similar for the two
legs, the vectogram patterns are practically normal except for some
minor differences present at the first impact. It is thus possible
to confirm the complete adaption of the subject to the prosthesis.

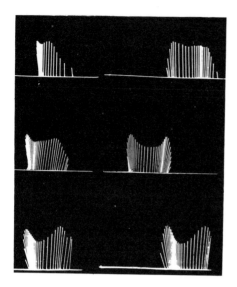 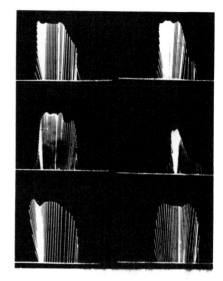

Fig. 5   Vectograms of a female subject with disease localised to the
(left)   right limb. The vectograms from this limb are shown on the
            left. The vectograms at the top were obtained before sur-
            gery while the middle and bottom vectograms were obtained
            six and twelve months, respectively, after surgery. The
            direction of advance, sampling interval and cadence are the
            same as in Fig. 3.

Fig. 6   Vectograms of a male subject with bilateral disease which is
(right)   more pronounced in the left limb. The vectograms from the
            left limb are shown on the right. The vectograms at the top
            were obtained before surgery while those in the middle were
            obtained six months later but immediately prior to the
            replacement of the knee prosthesis by a new one. The vecto-
            grams at the bottom were obtained six months after the
            second operation. The direction of advance, sampling inter-
            val and cadence are the same as in Fig. 3.

     The vectograms in Figure 6 refer to a subject with a bilateral
disease which is more pronounced in the left limb (on the right
side). The subject was tested before the treatment, six months later
when the prosthesis was replaced because of the yielding of the
tibial bone, and again six months after the second treatment.
     The evolution of the gait of this subject is very interesting.
At the beginning, there is the pattern which is typical of his class.
The func-tional loss is higher for the left limb, but the other
vectogram is pathological as well.
     The second test shows a deterioration of the situation. The
subject has a vectogram which has worsened by comparison with the
initial situation. The vectogram is still typical of patients with
bilateral diseases but it shows a large functional loss. The concentration of vectors has increasd while the maximal forces and the
stance phase duration have decreased. Also, the vectogram at right

is influenced by the increase in pain in the treated knee; the vectors have four maxima, probably due to the complex changes in the dynamic equilibrium of gait induced by the new and increased pain.

The last two diagrams suggest an interesting observation. It is possible to confirm that the replacement of the prosthesis has been carried out successfully by an inspection of the shape of the vectogram, on the right. The improved gait efficiency is underlined by the pattern of the non-treated limb; in fact, it shows the typical shape obtained from patients with monolateral diseases. Thus, it is reasonable to suppose that the prosthesis is able to furnish a dynamic support very similar to the natural joint.

Conclusions

The vectogram technique has been applied to fifteen subjects in order to analyze the efficiency of the replacement of the knee joint with the Lotus prosthesis.. Also the time-recovery of gait has been investigated from a dynamical point of view. On the basis of this research we can draw the following conclusions:

- A more rigorous analysis of clinical results is possible as compared with the inspective observation technique; moreover, the results are obtained under dynamic conditions so that they possess a high level of significance.

- A quantitative evaluation of the functional loss can be carried out before the treatment and the functional recovery can be verified carefully after the treatment, even if long periods of time are necessary to observe significant changes in the gait.

- The adaptation time to the prosthesis can be analyzed and, based on this, it is possible to set up optimal rehabilitative procedures.

Acknowledgement

This work has been partially supported by C.N.R. (National Research Council), Special Project on Biomedical Engineering, Contract No. 80.01186.86.

References

1. Stott J.R., Hutton W.C. and Stokes I.A.F. (1973) J. Bone & Joint Surg., 55B, 335-344.
2. Gyory A.N., Chao E.Y.S., & Stanfer R.N. (1976) Arch. Phys. Med. Rehab. 57, 571-577.
3. Sutherland D., Olsen R,, Cooper L. & Woo S.L.Y. (1980) J. Bone & Joint Surg. 62A, 336-353.
4. Jarret M.O., Moore P.R. & Swanson A.J.G. (1980) Med. & Biol. Engineering & Computing. 685-688.
5. Jacobs M.A., Storecky J. & Charnley J. (1972) J. Biomechanics. 5, 11-34.6. Boccardi S., Chiesa G. & Pedotti A. (1977) Am. J. of Phys. Med.56 No. 4. 163-182.
7. Pedotti A & Santambrogio G.C. (1979) VII Int. Congr. of Biomechanics. In Press.
8. Cova P., Pedotti A., Pozzolini M., Rodano R. & Santambrogio G.C. Acta Orthopaedica Belgica. In press.

A MEASUREMENT SYSTEM TO STUDY FREE RANGE LOWER LIMB PROSTHETIC LOADING

D.F. LOVELY, N. BERME, S.E. SOLOMONIDIS AND J.P. PAUL

Bioengineering Unit, University of Strathclyde, Glasgow
Scotland

Summary

An 8-channel cassette recorder suitable for ambulatory monitoring, of the loads developed in lower limb prostheses, has been developed at the Bioengineering Unit, University of Strathclyde, Scotland. By using C120 tapes, an uninterrupted recording time of one-hour is possible and this allows the acquisition of loading data from outside the artificial confines of the laboratory. The system has been used on subjects with both above and below knee amputations and the results obtained, so far, have shown some interesting effects.

Introduction

A prosthesis should have adequate strength to withstand the loads being applied to it by the patient during various activities, but it should be as light as possible to allow sufficient mobility and minimum physiological expenditure to the wearer. To obtain a compromise between these two conflicting factors of strength and weight, accurate loading information is required under all possible circumstances met in practice.

The strain gauged pylon transducer has been used, for many years, to obtain loading data from lower limb prostheses. (1, 2). However, in the past, several problems associated with the actual acquisition of the pylon data have been encountered, mainly related to the multicore cable, which was used to connect the transducer to the bridge amplifiers and the associated electronics. Overhead gantry systems, using sliding pulleys, were employed to keep the drag of this umbilical cable to a minimum (3). However, this has the disadvantage of restricting the subject to a defined area within the laboratory. At Strathclyde University, the cable was attached to the rear of the subject's belt and was held clear of locomotion by an assistant (4). This technique, while requiring an extra person to be present at a test, does allow locomotion anywhere within the restraints of the cable length. Even so, several meters of umbilical cable must have a detrimental effect on the S/N ratio of the signals appearing at the bridge amplifiers. Consequently, over the last three years, a recording system has been developed, at Strathclyde University, especially for use with the pylon transducer. The objectives of the system were to provide a small ambulatory recording system,, which would make the umbilical cable superfluous and free the amputee from the confines of the laboratory.

Methods

At present, there are three main methods available for recording
data. These are:
1. Telemetry
2. Magnetic tape
3. Solid state memories

As it was desirable to record timing information, as well as magnitude data, the solid state recorder becomes impractical. Consequently, the choice of recording system was limited to telemetry or
magnetic tape. Telemetry, in a noisy EM environment, such as in a
city-based university campus, can be troublesome, especially over
large distances. Therefore, it was decided to adapt an ambulatory
tape recording system to perform the required task.

A commercial 'dictaphone type' cassette recorder formed the
starting point of the overall design. The internal electronics of
the commercial machine were removed and replaced with custom-designed
circuits. The low quality single track recording head was replaced
by a high-quality four-track device, to enable the full width of the
tape to be used without needing to turn the cassette over.

Frequency modulation (FM) techniques were used to obtain a d.c.
to 40Hz bandwidth for each channel (-3dB). The eight data channels
were recorded onto two tracks of the tape by using a time dividion
multiplexing (TDM) scheme. The other two tracks were used for synchronisation of the data and to compensate for tape speed fluctuations on playback (flutter compensation). To accommodate the necessary electronics to perform the multiplexing, modulation and associated control functions, a package similar in size to the modified
commercial recorder was constructed. To complete the recording system, six bridge amplifiers are required to boost the signals from the
pylon transducer so that they are compatible with the FM electronics.
The signals from the transducer can be very small inded (30 uV typical); consequently, it was initially planned to mount the strain
gauge amplifiers on the pylon itself to keep any noise pick-up to a
minimum. However, due to the size of these amplifiers, only three
could be accommodated at the pylon level, while 3 had to be carried
with the electronics package and the tape unit.

The recording system, therefore, consists of the pylon transducer and three other packages; these being the tape unit, the
electronics package and the three strain gauge amplifiers, which
could not be mounted on the pylon. These three packages are carried
by the amputee on a belt and are connected together by a single
multicore cable. The connections to and from the pylon are made with
a similar cable to form a neat, compact system. The total weight of
the recording system is approximately 1 kg and imposes no restriction
on the gait of the amputee.

To complement this recording system, a playback unit was constructed to allow the data to be replayed in real-time. The reproduced data is in analogue form and can be recorded on UV sensitive
paper by means of an oscillograph recorder. The record is calibrated
by using a specially recorded calibration tape, which was produced by
recording the effect of loading all six channels of the pylon transducer in turn with known loads at specified bridge voltages. Consequently, if this tape is replayed immediately after replaying a test

tape, and the bridge voltages used during the test are taken into account, the sensitivities of all six channels and the associated cross-effects are known.

Clinical Trials

Now that a system had been developed to free the amputee from the artificial environment of the laboratory, it was decided to investigate the effects of terrain on the prosthesis loading patterns. A walking course around the university campus was chosen, which required the amputee to walk on several different gradients. These gradients were split up into five different categories:

1. Flat
2. Slight downhill
3. Steep downhill (1:9)
4. Slight uphill
5. Steep uphill (1:9)

It was felt that this route offered all the conditions that an active amputee would experience in everyday activities. The route was approximately 800m long and took on average 20 minutes to complete.

Typical waveforms, from three of the six recorded channels, are shown in Figure 1. The standard right-handed convention system has been adopted with the x-axis in the direction of locomotion and the y-axis vertical. Thus F_y represents the axial load while M_z is the plantarflexion/dorsiflexion moment. These waveforms are from an active BK amputee and are pylon level signals uncorrected for cross-effects. It is quite evident that the change of gradient has a dramatic effect on some of the loading profiles. In particular, the negative peak of M_z almost disappears on uphill locomotion, while the positive peak develops among a 'F_y' characteristic double peak. This effect could be the result of inertia as the load is present for a greater percentage of the walking cycle; it is also noticeable in the F_x channel together with a reduction of the positive peak.

To obtain some statistical representation of these results, blocks of 60 steps from each gradient category were considered. Measurements were performed on UV paper records and fed into a microcomputer so that cross-effect corrections could be made. Averages of the positive and negative peak loads developed in each category of terrain for $M_z F_x$ and F_y are shown in Figure 2. This diagram confirms the trend of decreasing dorsiflexion moment as gradient increases, as shown earlier in Figure 1. However the plantarflexion moment is about the same in going uphill and on the flat. Figure 2 also shows that there is a considerable decrease in the forward shear force, F_x, in going uphill, while the axial load remains relatively constant.

At present, only two subjects have been used so far for tests. It is not envisaged that many further tests will be conducted until a better scheme of analysis is adopted. The transcription of data from UV paper to the microcomputer is fraught with errors and is quite time-consuming. Therefore, direct playback to a PDP-11 computer is planned. This would enable more sophisticated analysis routines to be used on the data. Also, translations and rotations of the pylon reference system could be accomplished to produce loading information concerning the ankle, knee and hip joints.

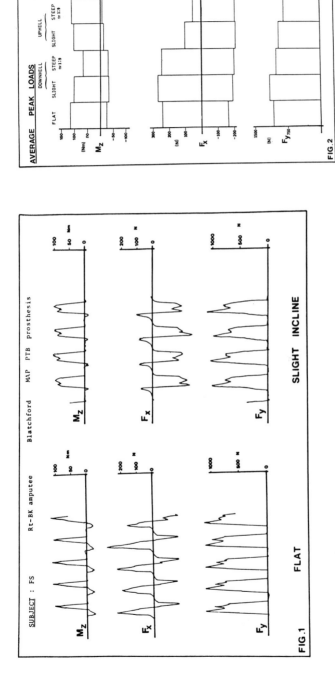

Fig. 1 (left)   Typical waveforms from three of the recorder channels
Fig. 2 (right) Average peak loads for each terrain category

Conclusions

An ambulatory system has been designed and built to record the loads
acting on lower limb prostheses.   Early clinical trials have shown
that the system operates as designed and loading data from various
terrains has been obtained.   Once the direct playback to the PDP-11
computer has been accomplished, the resultant system will be an
invaluable aid to the acquisition of loading data from outside the
confines of the laboratory.   Finally, a summary of the technical
features of the recording sytem are given in Table 1.

TABLE 1
Recording/Replay System Characteristics

No. of channels	8
Bandwidth (-3dB)	d.c. - 40Hz
S/N	> 40dB
Linearity	$\simeq 2\%$
FM deviation	30%
Carrier frequency	5k Hz
TDM sampling frequency	200 Hz / channel
Tape speed	4.76 cm/s
Weight of recording equipment	< 1 Kg.

References

1.   Cunningham D.M. and Brown G.W. (1952) Soc. Experimental Stress
     Analysis. Vol. IX No. 2.
2.   Berme N., Lawes P., Solomonidis S., Paul J.P. (1976) Engineering
     in Medicine Vol. 4 No. 4.
3.   Judge G.W., Murray D. (1973) Laboratory Studies of Amputee
     Loading Patterns. BRADU Report, Roehampton.
4.   Jones D. (1976) Data Handling in Amputee Data Analysis.
     University of Strathclyde Ph.D. Thesis.

Discussion

MR. OLDANO: Mr. Lovely will presumably know that in the use of a
prosthesis made up of modular parts, it is very important that the
technician is capable of adapting the prosthesis to the individual
patients. (Mr. Lovely agreed) Has any study been made of the analysis of these small variations?
MR. LOVELY: In our laboratory, there is a group working to carry out
an alignment study programme. At the moment, all their work is based
inside the laboratory using the old system. I feel, however, that
when this system is integrated into a computer, so that the analysis
becomes much easier, this would be an area to be investigated. The
patients tested so far are what we call "professional amputees", fit
people, who come into the laboratory, are at ease and know exactly
what is happening. When they get outside, though, they seem to

forget that they are on a test and their walking changes completely.
MR. OLDANO: Secondly, if I was not mistaken, the transducers are situated on the prosthesis near to the ankle joint? (Mr. Lovely agreed) Has the influence been evaluated of this weight placed in a position, where the velocity is very high in relation to the dynamics?
MR. LOVELY: The transducer is placed instead of the shin tube, which is removed, so that there is not very much difference in weight. The transducer that replaces the shin tube is only slightly heavier. I do not feel that it makes a great difference. The position of the pylon is measured so that the loads can be transferred from the pylon level up to joint levels, and the forces, for instance, on the hip can be measured. To get this going - returning in part to Mr. Oldano's first question - I expect that we may try to have this alignment to minimise the resultant joint forces. However, if a series of six prosthetists is asked to align a leg dynamically, each will align it differently - and yet, the patient will be quite happy with any of those alignments. Therefore, this is an area being investigated to see whether there is a quantitative method of alignment, rather than a method based purely on a prosthetist looking at a patient as he walks about.
MR. EVANS: Why did Mr. Lovely feel that he must completely re-design a system for his particular mode of measurement, when there are tape recorders on show at this meeting, which I feel would be perfectly adequate for these sort of measurements?
MR. LOVELY: I wanted an 8-channel device, and there is yet to appear on the market an 8-channel ambulatory tape recorder.
MR. EVANS: But I understand that you multiplex on to 4 channels anyway.
MR. LOVELY: There are two answers to the question. I started this work three years ago, at which time, there was nothing suitable available in the way of tape recorders. Secondly, even looking at the equipment available now, I still do not think that it is possible to multiplex on the available bandwidth that these recorders provide. Taking a single-channel recorder, the best figures that I have been given are 0.05 to 100 Hz. I think it would be impossible to attempt to cram all the multiplexing into that from eight data channels.
MR. EVANS: What is the bandwidth of your system?
MR. LOVELY: DC to 40 Hz on all 8 channels.

AMBULATORY MONITORING OF WALKING
USING A THIN CAPACITIVE FORCE TRANSDUCER

J.L.DION*, J.P. FOUILLOT** AND A. LEBLANC*

*Dept. d'Ingenierie,
Universite du Quebec a Trois-Rivieres, Quebec, Canada
**Laboratoire de Physiologie,
UER Cochin-Port Royal, Paris, France

Summary

A system has been designed and realized, which allows recording of
the vertical force component exerted by the foot heel during walking
over a 24-hour period. the ultra-thin capacitive force transducer is
inserted into an unobtrusive 2mm thick sole, which can be worn in any
type of shoe, with no effect at all on the gait. The FM signal is
transmitted by a mini-coax cable to the receiver and Medilog recorder
carried at the waist, for step counting and force measurement.

Introduction

The assessment and measurement of forces under the foot in static and
dynamic conditions has been a research subject of interest for several years, in relation with normal and pathological cases (1-6). The
various types of possible measurement may be of value in the areas of
work physiology, rehabilitation and physical training. However, it
seems that very few systems have been designed for recording forces
under the foot in normal work or play, or clinical situations for any
long period. The use of force plates or similar static devices (3,
4) considerably limits the possibilities of realistic evaluation of
forces. Various types of instrumented shoes have been developed for
dynamic measurements, but the problem with these is the bulkiness of
the attached transducers, which limit the number of applications and
modify the walking style of the subject (5, 7, 8).
     Our goal was to design and realise a force transducer system to
be carried by the subject, and record force signals over periods of
several hours. This system had to allow continuous measurements of
step frequencies, and furthermore, a qualitative study of human
locomotion by differentiating the various phases such as walking,
running and climbing. So the force signal was not required to be
linearly related to the force, but to be repeatable and give clear
indications of changes. The transducer had to be placed into any
type of shoe, be quite unobtrusive and have no effect at all on the
gait of the subject. We have built a suitable working system, based
on a thin capacitive force transducer placed into a foot sole. The
recording is presently done with a Medilog 4-24 cassette recorder;
however, any ordinary cassette recorder can be used.

Description of the System

The transducer outline is shown in Figure 1. The base electrode is made of sheet steel 20 x 15 x 0.62 mm. The second electrode, slightly recessed, is sheet steel 0.25mm thick. A 0.025mm thick brass screen is connected to the base electrode. Among all the dielectric materials tried so far, a better bonding to the electrodes was achieved by using 0.075mm cellulose acetate film with silicone cement. It is connected to the transmitter with a short length of mini-coax cable and the assembly has a capacity of about 100 pF. The transducer is mounted into a sole made with a few layers of soft materials glued together. The transducer is practically undetectable and weighs 26 grammes.

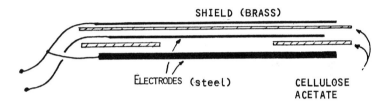

SHIELD (BRASS)

ELECTRODES (steel)   CELLULOSE ACETATE

Fig. 1   Outline of capacitive transducer

The transmitter is a simple multivibrator based on a RCA 4047 CMOS integrated circuit (Figure 2A). The transducer being placed in parallel with a 270 pF condenser gives a 55 kHz signal with no force applied. The frequency goes down to less than 50 kHz with a 100 kg-f load on the transducer. Power is supplied from the receiver, directly by the coaxial cable. It is moulded in epoxy and the weight is 28 grammes.

As a receiver, we use a phase-locked loop integrated circuit, the RCA 4046 CMOS (Figure 2B). A 5 kHz frequency deviation gives a signal variation of about 100 mV at pin 10, which is reduced to 3 mV for input to the medilog AD2 direct recording preamplifier.

The transmitter may be attached to the shoe or the ankle with a quickly attachable band ("Velcro" type). The receiver is carried at the belt, along with the recorder. A small 9 volts battery carried with the receiver powers both the transmitter and the receiver and delivers a current of about 4mA.

Experimental Results

The output of the receiver has a d.c. component, which is normally blocked with a condenser. We first measured the variable part V_s of the signal as a function of the weight in a static test by placing the transducer into a shoe, under the heel and stepping unto a scale. The graph is shown in Figure 3. Graph (a) shows the average values of 5 consecutive tests on the same subject in identical conditions.

Graph (b) shows the results obtained with the same subject after 135 hours of use. One can notice that V_s is not a linear function of the applied force; it is normal since the capacity variation is non-linear with force so as the frequency variation with capacity.However, it is felt that linearity has secondary importance as long as we are interested in the evaluation of pattern variations corresponding to changes in the way of walking and counting steps. The form of the signal given by a typical recording is shown in Figure 4, and can be easily processed by a computer system to give the step frequency and to identify the various sequencies of physical activity.

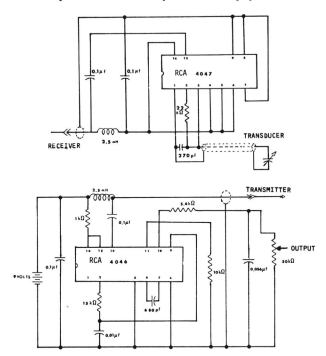

Fig. 2   A. Transmitter circuit
          B. Receiver circuit

Conclusion

The under-foot force measuring system we have built, gives good results as far as our needs are concerned. Consecutive test and re-test show good accuracy and reliability over long periods of use. It can be carried for many hours by any subject, without discomfort or changes in the normal gait.

At the present time, the system has been used for more than 60 hours, without significant changes in the results and any physical alteration of the transducer.

We are now evaluating the life-time of the transducer. These transducers are easily built at low cost and can be quickly inter-changed. This system provides valuable qualitative and quantitative information on the various phases of locomotion, without any discomfort for a variety of subjects, in almost any situation.

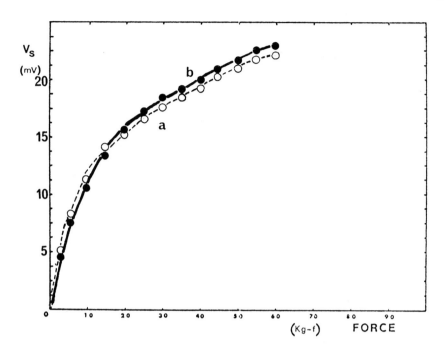

Fig. 3   Variable component of the receiver output as a function of
the applied force (a)   after 30 hours of use (O---O) (b)
after 135 hours of use (●——●).

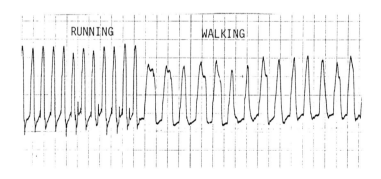

Fig. 4   Specimen of recorder signal corresponding to changing way
of walking or running

References

1.   Morton D.J. (1930) Amer. J. Surgery, 315-326.
2.   Elftman H. (1934) Anatomical Records **59**, 481-491
3   Ghosh A.K., Tibarewala D.N., Mukherjee P., Chakraborty S. and
      Ganguli S. (1979) Med. & Biol. Eng. & Comput. **17**, 737-741.
4.   Nicol K. and Henning, E.M. Johann Wolfgang Goethe-Universitat,
      Frankfurt/Main, 433-440.
5.   Miyazaki S. & Iwakura H. (1978) Med. & Biol. Eng. & Comput.**16**,
      429-436.
6.   Arvikar R. and Seireg A. (1980) MEP Ltd. Vol 9, No. 2, Mech. Eng.
      Dept. University of Wisconsin, U.S.A., 99-103.
7.   Spolek G.A., Day E.E., Lippert F.G. and Kerkpatrick G.S. (1975).
      Exp. Mech. **15**, 271-274.
8.   Lereim P. (1973) Bul. Prosth. Res., Fall.

Discussion

DR. MONSTER: I have considerable experience of this kind of
transducer and have found a closed-cell foam must be used; with any
sort of open-cell foam, its capacitance decreases very rapidly. This
kind of transducer goes bad very quickly if someone walks with it for
any distance.   Has Dr. Fouillot found this to be true?

DR. FOUILLOT: This transducer has been used for hours, without any
changes of capacitance. (Dr. Monster queried this) It has been used
by Dr. Dion for hours, and the signal is always there. The problem
that we find is not really in measuring the force, but mainly in
being able to differentiate between standing, walking and running and
to refer to other physiological parameters. With the pedometer that
I have described, such information can be obtained. With the sensor
in the foot, we expect to be able to obtain better informatin from
athletes and people at work.

DR. MONSTER: But that kind of question could be answered using he
kind of devices that Dr. Patrick has used in the past. I see an
application for this type of device if we are interested, for instance, in the distribution of load over the foot. Three or four of
these devices could be inserted into some type of insole in different
parts of the foot.   In fact, such devices are commercially available

DR. FOUILLOT: There are some very thin devices - but the problem is
that the energy consumption that they require is difficult to provide
in long-term ambulatory monitoring recordings.

DR. MONSTER: This device is available as an ambulatory recording
device. It is essentially similar to the device you have described.
The only difference that I can recall is that the commercially
available device contained some special precautions to eliminate
capacitance pick-up from the connecting cable - which is a big
problem in this kind of device.

BLOOD PRESSURE WORKSHOP

CHAIRMAN: M.W. MILLAR-CRAIG

A TEST TAPE FOR EVALUATION OF CONTINUOUS BLOOD PRESSURE ANALYSIS TECHNIQUES

P.A. CROSBY AND S.N. HUNYOR

Royal North Shore Hospital, St. Leonards, NSW 2065
Australia

Introduction

The Oxford Medilog equipment for recording continuous ambulatory blood pressure data over 24-hours has become the default standard. The recording apparatus has been the subject of technical evaluation from many aspects. Goldberg, Raftery and Green (1976) performed a careful evaluation of the original model with gas-powered infusion pump and found good agreement between recordings taken with the recorder and simultaneous recordings taken from a Millar catheter-tip pressure transducer in the same place. A similar study of the improved system with delta pump infusion unit was undertaken by Millar-Craig, Hawes and Whittington (1978), with comparable results. The long-term performance of the system in terms of drift, temperature stability and sensitivity to battery voltage have also been documented (4). Techniques for improving the accuracy and reliability of recordings have been suggested and methods for overcoming some of the limitations due to tape speed variations have been developed (7).

Analysis of long-term blood pressure records has been performed with a variety of methods. It is useful to consider a heirarchy of analysis methods, in order of decreasing complexity.
1. 'Brute force' computer data acquisition and analysis with digitization of the entire waveform (8, 9).
2. Beat-by-beat analogue pre-processing to extract systolic, diastolic and mean pressures, and perhaps rate, with subsequent computer analysis (1).
3. Longer term meaning pre-processors, which estimate mean pressures over some set time interval, such as 1 or 10 minutes, perhaps followed by subsequent computer analysis and generation of histograms.

Despite the attention focused on technical evaluation of the recording apparatus, evaluation of analysis methods has been relatively neglected. Analysis methods designed to estimate systolic, diastolic and mean pressures, and rate should be evaluated with attention to the following factors:

1.	Accuracy	of data values obtained compared to 'true values' (pressures and rate)
2.	Reliability	of estimating data values with different waveforms
3.	Specificity	at picking wanted details (e.g. coughs, ectopics and other artefacts)
4.	Resolution	of detail e.g. beat-to-beat variations
5.	Frequency response	to rapidly changing data (e.g. exercise valsalva)

6.   Repeatability   tape to tape: today and tomorrow
7.   Noise intolerance   ability to analyze data in the presence
                              of noise
8.   Noise generation   added noise due to analysis technique.

Methods and Techniques

The test tape contains real data taken from several different recordings. The generation of the test tapes is illustrated diagramatically in Figures 1 and 2.

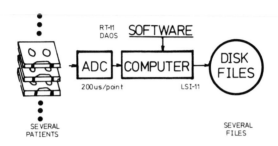

Fig. 1   Waveform Digitisation: Real data from several patients are
         digitised via a computer and stored as disk files.

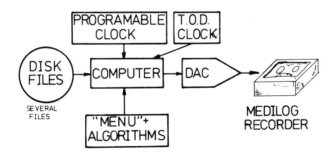

Fig. 2   Waveform synthesis: Data from several disk files are linked
         together in an order determined from a menu of possibili-
         ties. At predetermined times, different data may be output
         via a digital to analog convertor to a Medilog Recorder.
         The rate of waveform generation is controlled by a crystal
         locked programmable clock.

The computer system used is a LSI-11 computer with 32K words of
memory, KWV-11A programmable real-time clock, Datel Sine-Trac 12 bit
Analogue to Digital and Digital to Analogue convertors, and various
other peripherals.   The operating system is DEC standard RT-11 V3B,
and all the programmes were written in a programming language called

DAOS (Data Analysis Operating System, Laboratory Software Associates, Melbourne, Australia and Cambridge, U.K.), which is specifically designed for laboratory based real-time data management.

The first step in the process of tape generation is data acquisition. Recordings are replayed at 60 times real-time, and sampled at a rate of 5kHz, equivalent to about 83 Hz in real-time, and stored on disc files. These data files are then analyzed by the computer to estimate the systolic, diastolic and mean pressures and rate. The peak picking algorithm is similar to that described by Walsh and Goldberg (1979), but the faster sampling rate allows better accuracy. The amount of data recorded from each tape is generally only a few minutes, as the aim is not to get an entire 24-hour record, but extracts with particular characteristics and features.

The user is able to specify the sequence of events and types of data to be generated on the test tape in an interactive, menu driven dialogue with the computer programme. A large intermediate file is generated from this defined sequence and the previously recorded data. This file contains the data to be output to the test tape, along with other coded information such as time for events to occur, and data output clock rate.

Finally, the data is output to a Medilog recorder via a Digital to Analogue convertor, point by point, with the time between points controlled by the KWV-11 programmable clock. The electrical signal from the D to A convertor is first attentuated, and has added offset to match the input characteristics of the recorder. The rate at which data is output can be varied over a wide range with a temporal resolution of 1 micro-second per data point. A Time of Day clock allows scheduling of events.

The recorder is a standard Medilog recorder, with a modification to the power supply as previously reported (4). New Hitachi C120 cassettes are used and new batteries are used for generation of each tape. The whole apparatus is allowed to reach thermal stability for two hours before recording, and the recorder is run for 1 hour, without recording to allow the battery voltage to stabilize. It is possible to record simultaneously on several recorders. This allows a comparative check of recorder drift and facilitates the production of multiple copies of a tape.

Data Types

The data able to be recorded on the test tape are of five types at present. However, any data already recorded on a tape may be duplicated on a test tape, with manipulations as desired. The data types are:

Calibration Data
    The calibration is a staircase waveform from 0 to 300mmHg in 50mm steps, and about 2 minutes between steps. The calibration data may have different amounts of computer generated noise added, to evaluate the accuracy of the transfer of calibration to the analysis technique in the presence of noise. The calibration signal is repeated several times on the tape to allow an estimation of drift.

Normal Data

   Normal data is of 6 different types. The waveforms may be
scaled by multiplying and shifting to produce different systolic and
diastolic pressures. The mean pressure is obviously not independently variable. The rate can be altered at the time of tape generation, although at the moment, no attempt is made to change the dp/dt
with rate. The pressures may also be multiplied by a ramp, and
offset appropriately, to generate smooth transition regions between
data of different pressures. Various amounts of computer generated
noise can also be added as desired. These steps are summarized in
Figure 3.

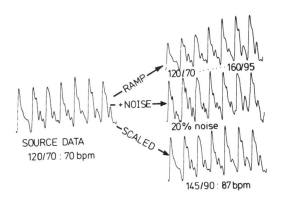

Fig. 3   Data Manipulation: Data from a variety of sources may be
          rescaled in both amplitude and frequency; may be turned into
          ascending or descending ramps of pressure; and may have
          various amounts of random noise added

Physiological Artefacts

   These include artefacts related to events such as fainting,
coughs, ectopic beats and exercise. These events may be peppered
through the tape as desired, and are useful in assessing the ability
of the analysis method to identify such artefacts.

External Artefacts

   These are true recordings of pressure from events, such as a
blocked infusion line, a tape recorder malfunction, or transducer
failure.

Added Variables

   To any of the data types (other than artefacts), computer generated noise may be added, and the rate may be changed at will.
   Care is taken to ensure that there are no discontinuities on the
tape when changing from one data type to another. One of the
problems encountered in developing the test tape generation process
was thermal drift. Although part of this is due to the recorder, the
main cause was found to be the attenuator between the D to A

convertor and the recorder, and this was redesigned more carefully to
eliminate drift and thermal instability.

Discussion

It may be said that the data on the test tapes do not look to be
'physiological'. Although true, the purpose of the test tape is not
to simulate a person, but to provide a selection of data types and
artefacts for evaluation of analysis techniques. All data recorded
on the tape is taken from previous recordings, so it is real in that
sense. The waveform of the blood pressure signal is not altered with
rate change, as is the case in real life, but this is not considered
a major drawback. In any case, the limited frequency response of the
recorder will tend to limit the rate of rise of pressure.

One of the most useful applications of the test tape is in the
assessment of sources of blood pressure variability. These are
summarized in Table 1. The basic problem is one of estimating the
primary noise source (i.e. the patient), from the data, which has
many other noise sources added to it.

Table 1: Variability (Noise) Sources: The physiological blood pressure variability in the patient is obscured by variability or noise
introduced at many other stages in the recording or playback process.

PATIENT	"True" blood pressure variability
HYDRAULICS	Waveform distortion
TRANSDUCER	Drift, Hysteresis, Non linearity
RECORDER	Tape speed, electronics
PLAYBACK	Tape speed, electronics
DATA ACQUISITION	Quantization noise
ANALYSIS	Computation noise

The test tape generation process by-passes the first three steps
in the chain, and allows estimates of other noise sources. A tape
was generated containing calibration sequence followed by a blood
pressure signal of 14 beats repeatedly endlessly. The data had an
average pressure of 120/70, and a periodic variation (i.e. repeated
every 14 beats) of about 10mmHg. It was clear that the noise added
by the recording and playback process is quite sinificant, and completely obscured the regular structure of the signal. Flutter compensation appeared to have no effect in reducing the noise. The
mplication of this observation is that low level long-term physio-

logical variability cannot be determined from taped data.

It might be suspected that the 'brute force' computer analysis technique would yield more accurate estimates of systolic and diastolic pressures than other methods. This is not necessarily so, as it has been shown (2) that there is a significant error in a unilateral direction in the estimation of peak values of a sampled data signal at low sampling rates. For example, with a pressure waveform at 100 beats per minute, a sampling rate of about 65 Hz is necessary to limit the maximum error in the estimation of the systolic pressure to 10%, if the waveform is assumed to have harmonics up to about 6 times the fundamental. The situation becomes progressively worse at high rates. It may be that a beat-by-beat analogue pre-processor will yield better results.

The test tape has been used in our laboratory to assess a brute force computer analysis method, and a meaning type pre-processor. Results of this assessment will be reported separately. An electronic beat-by-beat pre-processor is also under development and will be assessed.

The present system does not generate a pressure waveform directly, and thus it is not applicable for evaluation of the plumbing and transducer system. These aspects have been carefully studied in the past, and it is not necessary to duplicate this work. However, it should be possible to use this method to generate a pressure waveform directly for testing the entire Medilog recording and playback system, as well as analysis methods.

Conclusions

A system has been described for generating a test tape designed for evaluation of long-term blood pressure analysis techniques. The same technique may obviously be extended to other physiological signals (such as ECG, respiration, and EEG). As a by-product of this development, a technique has been found, whereby tapes, or portions of tapes may be duplicated.

Copies of the tape (or variations of it) may be made available to other workers for evaluation of their analysis techniques.

References

1. Cashmann P.M.M., Stott F.D. and Millar-Craig M.W. (1979) Med. & Biol. Eng. & Comput. 17, 629-635.
2. Crosby P.A. and Laird R.K.L. (1980) Australian J. Biomed. Eng. 1, 20-24.
3. Goldberg A.D., Raftery E.B. and Green H.L. (1976) Postgrad. Med J.52 (Suppl.) 104-109.
4. Kenny P. Hunyor S.N. and Renwick J.A. (1980) ISAM 1979 Proc. of 3rd Int. Symp. on Amb. Mon. Eds. Stott F.D., Raftery E.B. & Goulding L. Academic Press, London, 445-450.
5. Logan J.I. (1980) ISAM 1979 Proc. of 3rd Int. Symp. on Amb. Mon. Eds. Stott F.D., Raftery E.B. & Goulding L. Academic Press, London, 462-467.
6. Millar-Craig M.W., Hawes D. and Whittington J. (1978) Med. & Biol. Eng. & Comput. 16, 727-730.
7. Mitchell R.H., Ruff S. and Jenkins J.G. (1980) Med. & Biol. Eng.

& Comput. **18**, 353-357.
8.   Ruff S.C., Mitchell R.H. and Murnaghan G.A. (1980) ISAM 1979
      Proc. of 3rd Int. Symp. on Amb. Mon. Eds. Stott F.D., Raftery
      E.B. & Goulding L. Academic Press, London, 261-174.
9.   Walsh J.T. and Goldberg A.D. (1980) ISAM 1979 Procx. of 3rd Int.
      Symp. on Amb. Mon. Eds. Stott F.D., Raftery E.B. & Goulding L.
      Academic Press, London, 451-455.

Discussion

DR. GOLDBERG: Is Mr. Crosby taking an FM signal and turning it into
an analog signal on his computer, then putting it back to an FM, or
leaving it as AM?
MR. CROSBY: It is an analog signal taken from the playback unit of
the Oxford System...
DR. GOLDBERG: Much of the difference surely depends on the way that
the signal is detected at the computer head, what computer is used
and how the peak and trough are picked off, and how the signal is
picked off totally. Also, what is your frequency of detection?
MR. CROSBY: It is 200/usec per point (5 kHz), with a playback speed
of 60 times (about 83 Hz) sampling rate.
DR. MONSTER: Hs Mr.Crosby tried putting this same signal on a good
quality instrumentation tape recorder to see whether the same amount
of playback noise is obtained as was shown in his last slide?
MR. CROSBY: No, it has not been tried on an instrumentation tape
recorder, but the signal has been recorded as it goes on to the tape
recorder on a paper-chart recorder at the same time as recording.
The signal on the paper-chart recorder does not have as much noise
as the played back signal. We conclude from this that there is noise
added by the recording and replay process.
DR. MILLAR-CRAIG: The concept behind this important paper is certainly something about which I, and I am sure, others, have thought
about in the past. I think that the idea of producing a test tape,
copies of which could be available for analysis in different centres
worldwide, is excellent.
MR. CROSBY: We have a few copies here of the tape which we are
prepared to release under certain conditions if people are interested.

TEMPERATURE DEPENDENCE OF THE OXFORD-MEDILOG BLOOD PRESSURE MEASURING AMPLIFIER

C.A. GRIMBERGEN, G.A. VAN MONTFRANS, M. POS, C. BORST AND A.J. DUNNING

Medical Physics Laboratory and University Hospital, University of Amsterdam, Holland

Summary

The influence of the temperature of the blood pressure measuring electronics on the blood pressure recordings was studied. A method was developed to measure the contribution of parts of the measuring amplifier to the temperature dependence. The magnitude and the source of errors are presented and possible improvements are discussed. The need to keep the temperature of the recording amplifier as constant as possible is stressed, as errors in the order of 1mmHg/$^{\circ}$C seems to be inevitable with this system. Recommendations are given to obtain a blood pressure recording system with better performance in the future.

Introduction

The Oxford-Medilog blood pressure recording system has been used for ambulatory monitoring of the intra-arterial pressure since 1972. Inconsistent data on the temperature dependence of this system have been reported (1, 2, 3, 4, 5).

The pressure transducer bridge contained in the transducer perfusion unit is known to be temperature dependent and this should be checked for the individual pressure transducers (about 0.8mmHg$^{\circ}$C according to specifications of the Akers transducer).

The blood pressure measuring amplifier (AM-4) is contained in the Medilog recorder module and is also sensitive to temperature variation. This temperature sensitivity will be treated here.

System

The blood pressure measuring electronics consist of the pressure transducer bridge, a reference generator and a comparator (6). The output of the comparator is a pulse width modulated signal containing the blood pressure information and this signal is after differentiation led to the magnetic head of the recorder. This results in the following relation between the interval ratio (t_m/t_c) of the pulse width modulated signal and the pressure bridge voltage, reference voltage and comparator offset voltage (6).

$$\frac{t_m}{t_c} - \frac{1}{2} = \frac{V_B(T_1) + V_{co}(T_2)}{2V_{RM}(T_2)} \quad \text{--------------------(1)}$$

It should be remembered that the bridge voltage is dependent on the temperature T_1 of the transducer/perfusion unit and that the amplitude of the reference generator voltage and of the comparator offset voltage is dependent on the temperature T_2 of the AM-4 electronics board inside the recorder module.

The influence of T_2 on the blood pressure measurement is the subject of our investigation; in our first recordings the recorder module was worn on the waist in an unisolated bag, in contrast to the transducer perfusion unit worn on the breast.

Measurements and Results

For the measurement of the recorder module temperature dependence, the recorder module was placed in an open polystyrene box and heated to about $50^{\circ}C$ in a furnace. After half-an-hour, the box was closed and exposed to room temperature resulting in a slow cooling of the recorder module. Through the wall of the polystyrene box a constant voltage replacing the battery supply, an external input voltage replacing the pressure transducer bridge and an external reference voltage were connected. The internal reference voltage, the pulse width modulated signal and the thermistor signal were led to the outside of the box. In this way, the temperature dependence of the pressure transducer was excluded, as was the influence of the temperature dependence of the amplitude of the internal reference voltage. The interval ratio (t_m/t_c) of the pulse width modulated signal was measured using a timer/counter (HP 5300A) and the amplitude of the interval reference voltage was measured using a digital voltmeter. The temperature was measured using the resistance of a thermistor inside the recorder module near the AM-4 electronics board.

The results are shown in Figure 1 for two AM-4 amplifiers. The influence of the temperature on the ratio t_m/t_c is seen to be about constant and in the order of $1mmHg/^{\circ}C$ in the temperature region of interest for both systems. The sign of this dependence is opposite, however.

The temperature influence on the amplitude of the internal reference generator (Figure 2) is seen to be equal for both systems and in the order of $0.2\%/^{\circ}C$ at $30^{\circ}C$.

The temperature dependence on the resulting blood pressure, measured in the same way as described in Figure 1, is presented in Figure 3 for different values of te input voltage, corresponding to different pressure values at the pressure transducer bridge.

Discussion

The results of the temperature influence can be explained by considering the transfer function of the pulse width modulated signal (eq.1). Differentiation with respect to temperature leads to:

$$\frac{d(t_m/t_c)}{dT} = \frac{V_B + V_{co}}{2V_{RM}}\left[\frac{1}{V_B + V_{co}}\left(\frac{dV_B}{dT} + \frac{dV_{co}}{dT}\right) - \frac{1}{V_{RM}}\frac{dV_{RM}}{dT}\right]$$

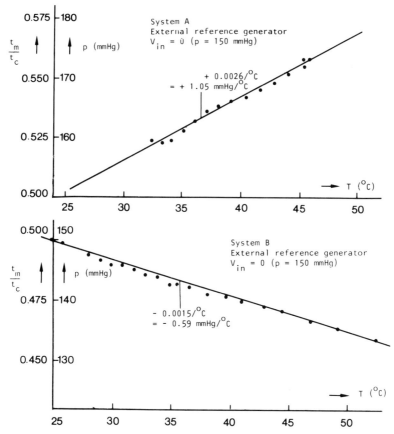

Fig. 1   The temperature dependence of the p.w.m. signal for two
AM-4 amplifiers. $p - p_0 = 150$ mmHg.

In this equation, the three terms playing a role in the temperature dependence can be recognized. The temperature on the bridge
voltage was excluded in this measurement. The influence on the
reference voltage amplitude was excluded too, but was seen (Figure 2)
to be small (0.2%/°C) leading to errors of 0.2mmHg/°C at the edges of
the blood pressure region of interest (50 and 250mmHg). The drift of
the comparator offset voltage appears to be the main cause of the
temperature dependence of the blood pressure measurement. The comparator offset voltage drift is a property of the comparator integrated circuit (offset voltage and offset current), which explains
the different sign and magnitude of the temperature dependence for
both systems.

The temperature influence was seen to be hardly dependent on
the input voltage in Figure 3, this in contrast to the results of
Logan (5), who used a shifted input voltage region to compensate the
pressure transducer temperature influence.

As an error in the blood pressure measurement of about 1mmHg/°C

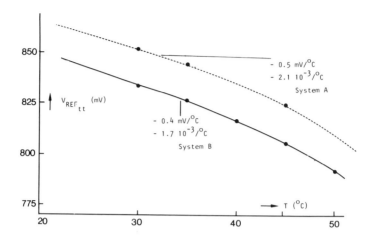

Fig. 2   The temperature dependence of the amplitude of the
           reference generator voltage.

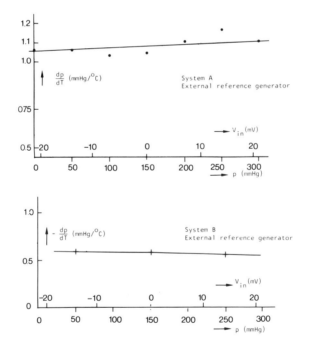

Fig. 3   The temperature dependence of the p.w.m. signal as a
           function of input voltage for two AM-4 amplifiers.

seems unavoidable, the strategy should be to keep the variations in the recorder module temperature to a minimum, just like the variations in the temperature of the transducer perfusion unit (the temperature dependence has the same order of magnitude). This can be done by wearing the recorder module on the body isolated from external environment just like the transducer perfusion unit (2, 4)) (a solution known as the 'Mae West System'). In this way, the temperature variations were measured to be smaller than 3ºC (29-31ºC) and the error in the blood pressure recording can be reduced to be less than 3mmHg.

Conclusion

It is shown that the Oxford-Medilog blood pressure system is sensitive to temperature variations of the recorder module, containing the measuring elecronics. A temperature influence in the order of 1mmHg/ºC, dependent on individual systems, seems inevitable. Therefore, attention must be paid to maintaining a constant temperature of the recorder module during calibration and the 24-hour recording. This can be obtained by wearing the recorder module on the body isolated from the outside environment.

Most ideally, the temperature influence should be excluded by an electronic temperature compensation of the pressure transducer bridge and by improving the measuring electronics. The demands on small dimensions of this portable system stand in the way of a simple solution; the development of a special purpose thick film circuit or even a special purpose integrated circuit seems indicated.

References

1. Millar-Craig M.W., Hawes P. & Whittington J. (1978) Med. & Eng. & Comput.16, 727-731.
2. Goldberg A.D., Green H.L. & Raftery E.B. (1976) Postgrad. Med. J. 52 (suppl. 7) 104-109.
3. Kenny P., Hunyor S.N. & Renwick J.A. in: ISAM 1979 Academic Press, London (1980) 445-450.
4. Murray A. and Sanders G.L. in: ISAM 1979 Academic Press, London (1980) 456-461.
5. Logan J.I. in: ISAM 1979 Academic Press, London (1980) 462-467.
6. Grimbergen C.A., van Montfrans G.A., Pos M., Borst C.& Dunning, A.J. Battery Voltage Dependence of the Oxford-Medilog Blood Pressure System. These Proceedings.

BATTERY VOLTAGE DEPENDENCE OF THE OXFORD-MEDILOG BLOOD PRESSURE SYSTEM

C.A. GRIMBERGEN, G.A. VAN MONTFRANS, M. POS, C. BORST AND
A.J. DUNNING

Medical Physics Laboratory and University Hospital, University of
Amsterdam, Holland

Summary

The influence of the varying supply voltage on the blood pressure
recordings was studied. A discrimination was made between errors
originating in the transducer bridge, reference oscillator and comparator of the measuring amplifier. The measured errors are presented
and the error sources are explained.

The main source of error is the unstabilized supply voltage of
the transducer bridge, which inevitably results in 5 to 10% errors
in pressure relative to 150mmHg.

A new solution is presented for supply voltage stabilization
built into the recorder module.

Introduction

Various sources of drift and linearity problems of the Oxford-Medilog
blood pressure recording system have been identified by other workers
(1, 2, 3, 4, 5). One of the major drift sources is recognized to be
the battery supply driving the recorder, the blood pressure measuring
amplifier and the transducer bridge.

The battery supply voltage (5.4 volts, 4 mercury cells)
typically decays 5 to 10% per 24-hour period, with the first three
hours a decay rate of about three times the average.

The consequences of this supply voltage decay for the blood
pressure recordings will be treated here.

System

The block diagram of the blood pressure measuring and recording
system is depicted in Figure 1. From the four mercury cells a mean
(zero) voltage is derived, leading to a plus and minus 2.7 Volts
supply. These voltages drive the recorder motor and the electronics.
The blood pressure measuring electronics consist of the pressure
transducer bridge in the pressure transducer module, and a reference
generator and comparator in the recorder module (AM-4). The output
of the comparator is a pulse width modulated signal containing the
blood pressure information, which is after differentiation led to the
magnetic head of the recorder.

In Figure 2, the various waveforms are presented. The bridge
Voltage VB linearly related to the blood pressure, is added to the

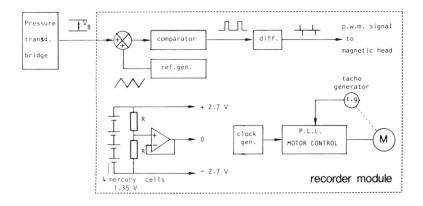

Fig. 1   Block diagram of the Oxford Medilog System.

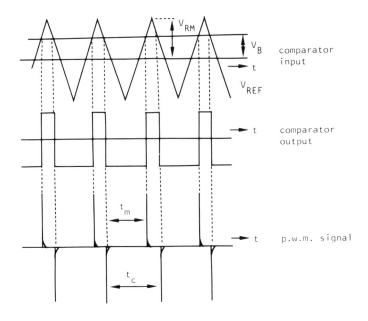

Fig. 2   The waveforms of the blood pressure measuring amplifier.

reference voltage at the comparator input. The amplitude of the
triangular reference voltage (frequency about 40Hz) determines the
blood pressure range and can be adjusted (V_{RM})The pulse width modulated signal at the comparator output is elated to the bridge voltage
and the amplitude of the reference generator:

$$\frac{t_m}{t_c} - \frac{1}{2} = \frac{V_B + V_{co}}{2V_{RM}} \quad \text{--} \quad \text{with } V_{co} \text{ the comparator offset voltage}$$

Pressure Transducer Bridge

The Oxford transducer bridge produces an output Voltage V_B which is
proportional to the excitation voltage of the bridge and the pressure
dependent resistance variation of the strain gauges (AE831B).

$$V_B = \frac{V_{BATT} \cdot \Delta R(p-p_o)}{R_{p_o}} \quad \text{--------------------------------------}$$

The excitation voltage of the Pressure transducer bridge is the
battery voltage V_{BATT}; p_o is the blood pressure at bridge balance,
which can be adjusted and is chosen in the middle of the blood
pressure region of interest (p_o= 150mmHg) because of the bipolar
character of the reference voltage (see Figure 2). R_{p_o} is the transducer resistance at bridge balance. For a 5.4 volt excitation voltage this leads to a 0.14 mV/mmHg sensitivity.*, dependent on variation
in the battery voltage.

* The system, as delivered, had an excitation voltage of half the
battery voltage leading to half the sensitivity of the bridge (70
/uV/mmHg). This has been modified with the help of Dr. Cashmann.

Reference Generator

Variations in the amplitude of the reference voltage lead to variations in the scale factor of the p.w.m. signal (see eq. 1) which can
partly compensate the variations in the bridge voltage caused by the
supply voltage decay (if these variations have an equal sign). In
the system, the variations are kept small by an amplitude stabilizing
circuit.

Comparator

At the comparator input there exists an offset voltage, caused by the
bias current and offset voltage of the comparator integrated circuit,
which is sensitive to supply voltage variations (indicated by the
power supply rejection ratio).

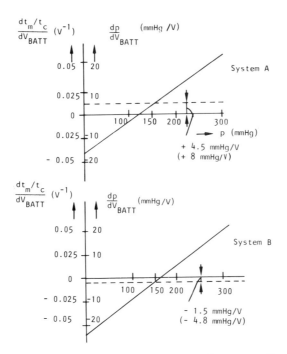

Fig. 3   The influence of the battery voltage on the blood pressure measurement as a function of blood pressure p_o = 150 mmhg $p - p_o = t_m t_c$.   400 mmHg.

Results

In Figure 3, the variation in t_m/t_c by the battery voltage variation is presented for two systems (AM-4). The pulse intervals t_m and t_c of the p.w.n. signal were measured using a timer/counter (HP 5300A) at the monitor output; the battery voltage was replaced by a variable voltage source. The error in the pressure measurement is linearly dependent on the blood pressure for both systems. At p_o (150mmHg) the influence of the battery voltage is non zero and of opposite sign for both systems (dotted line). (Between brackets the values are indicated for an excitation voltage of half the battery voltage).
   These results can be explained by considering the transfer function of the measuring amplifier (eq. 1). Differentiation to the battery voltage leads to:

$$\frac{dt_m/t_c}{dV_{BATT}} = \frac{V_B + V_{co}}{2V_{RM}} \left[\frac{1}{V_B + V_{co}} \left(\frac{dV_B}{dV_{BATT}} + \frac{dV_{co}}{dV_{BATT}} \right) - \frac{1}{V_{RM}} \frac{dV_{RM}}{dV_{BATT}} \right]$$

The three terms in this equation represent the influence of the battery voltage on the bridge voltage, on the comparator offset voltage and on the reference voltage amplitude. The first and last mentioned term cause the error to be linearly dependent on the blood pressure mainly determined by the bridge voltage, which is proportional to the battery excitation voltage. The second term causes the error to be non zero at p_0 and is dependent on the individual properties of the comparator integrated circuit, which explains the different sign and value of this term for both systems.

Stabilization

As can be seen from Figure 3, considerable errors in the blood pressure measurement are caused by the battery voltage decay. Per 24-hour period a 10% (0.5 V) decay is normal, causing errors of about 10mmHg at the edges of the blood pressure region of interest (50 and 250mmHg)

Stabilization was therefore thought to be essential, as reported by other workers (4, 5). A stabilizing circuit needs a considerable extra voltage and extra current and should have small dimensions to be built in. We have chosen a modern integrated circuit (LM10) as a stabilizing element, which has a current consumption of 0.27 mA (about 2% of the total current consumption) and needs an extra voltage of 0.3 Volt (about 6% of the battery voltage) avoiding the use of an external battery pack (see Figure 4).

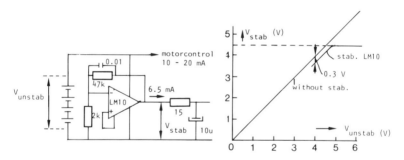

Fig. 4   The stabilisation circuit I_{so} = 0.27 mA, V_s = 0.3 V.

The integrated circuit is built into the recorder module itself together with 5 passive components. The maximum current from the stabilizing circuit is 15 mA, enough for the electronics (6.5 mA), but not enough for the total current (17 - 22 mA). Therefore, the motor control circuit was separated from the AM4 electronics with the advantage of less motor related noise on the supply voltage.

The stabilized voltage chosen was 4.5 Volts, which is maintained for battery voltages exceeding 4.8 Volts (See Figure 4), a voltage level normally reached after more than 36 hours battery life. In the blood pressure measuring procedure, battery voltage is measured after 24 hours to check this.

Conclusion

We have shown that the Oxford-Medilog blood pressure system is sensitive to the battery voltage decay during a 24-hour period. The main cause is the unstabilized excitation voltage of the transducer bridge. A stabilizing circuit has been built in in the recorder module using the LM10 integrated circuit. This stabilizing circuit delivers a stabilization without the need for an external battery pack, making the Oxford-Medilog system independent of the battery supply voltage.

References

1. Millar-Craig M.W., Hawes P. and Whittington J. (1978) Med. & Biol. Eng. &Comput. **16**, 727-31.
2. Goldberg A.D., Green H.L. and Raftery E.B. (1976) Postgrad. Med. J. **52**, (Suppl. 7) 104-9.
3. Millar-Craig M.W. In: ISAM 1977. Academic Press, London (1978) 305-10.
4. Kenny P. Hunyor W.N. and Renwick J.A. In: ISAM 1979. Academic Press, London (1980) 445-50.
5. Murray A. and Sanders G.L. in ISAM 1979, Academic Press, London (1980) 456-61.

Discussion

DR. MILLAR-CRAIG: The decay characteristics were very similar to findings made by us looking at drift of the total recording system. Does Dr. Grimbergen advocate turning on his equipment and running it on the bench for a couple of hours before use, or does he feel that it can be turned on and used immediately?

DR. GRIMBERGEN: We have tried this, but think that even then the error due to battery instability is relatively large compared to the noise in the system. The battery voltage is an unknown variable because we cannot be certain of the quality of the batteries and this gives a large possibility of error.

DR. MILLAR-CRAIG: It certainly was remarkable in our experience that at least 10% of the batteries provided were clearly substandard. This marked positive offset which Dr. Grimbergen showed so well, was very much a feature of nearly all the batteries we studied.

A SEMI-AUTOMATIC BLOOD PRESSURE MACHINE

D. JULIEN, P. ADAME, N. LAFFAY, J. LAFFAY*

*Dept. Internal Medicine, A. Mignot Hospital,
Le Chesnay, France

Introduction

Semi-automatic sphygmomanometers have the advantage of no observer error. We have studied such an instrument, which has the additional advantages of being non-invasive and utilising the Korotkoff sounds, so that it can be easily compared with standard techniques of blood pressure measurement. We have studied the techniques of calibration, blood pressure measurement in man at rest, and made comparisons with intra-arterial measurements.

Material and Methods

The Korotkoff sounds are detected by a microphone built into the cuff and are converted into electric signals, amplified, and displayed as visible signals on a fluorescent screen. However, there is no indication whether diastolic pressure is given by Korotkoff IV or V.
    The apparatus (OMRON, HEM 77)is Japanese and is commercially available. It can be operated by the mains' supply or batteries and consists of a box, which bears the on/off control, the battery check, the live control and a two-part screen, where numbers are shown, systolic on the upper part, diastolic below. Another control allows a display of heart rate.
    The cuff has a built-in microphone with many receivers, so that one is always in front of the brachial artery. The cuff is connected to a pump, which is controlled by an automatic deflating valve that deflates by 1 to 3mmHg, with each cardiac pulsation. The net weight is 1 kg and the scale ranges from 0 to 300mmHg, the smallest unit being 1mmHg.
    The equipment is easy to use: the cuff is wrapped around the upper arm as usual and the apparatus is inflated about 30mmHg over the systolic pressure. The screen then lights and shows the decreasing numbers, while the cuff is deflating automatically. Systolic pressure is recorded, when the signal becomes visible on the upper screen. The diastolic pressure is given on the lower screen later.

Results

Calibration
    The cuff was fastened around a stand and inflated to 300mmHg. The semi-automatic sphygmomanometer and in the pilot measurement were connected together by a Y tube. The pressure decreased from 300 to 0mmHg by 2mm steps. Each measurement was performed twice.
    The result was a perfect correlation between the two sets of measurement, with a correlation coefficient close to 1. However,

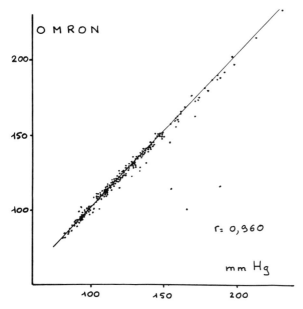

Fig. 1   Regression plot, Omron vs. sphygmomanometer, systolic
           pressures

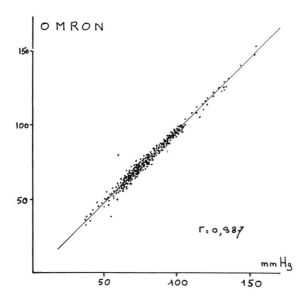

Fig. 2   Regression plot, Omron vs. sphygmomanometer, diastolic
           pressures

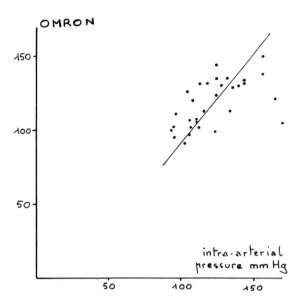

Fig. 3   Regression plot, Omron vs. intra-arterial, systolic pressures

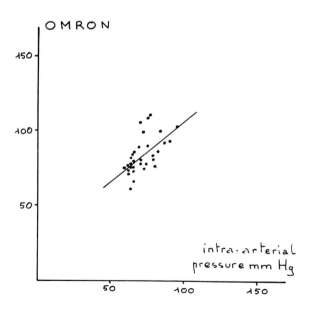

Fig. 4   Regression plot, Omron vs. intra-arterial, diastolic pressures

there was a systematic error of 2mmHg, the OMRON over-reading the mercury-in-glass pressure.

Blood Pressure Measurement in Man

   As previously, the semi-automatic sphygmomanometer was connected to a mercury manometer by a Y-tube. Systolic and diastolic values were recorded automatically, one observer taking down the corresponding values on the mercury manometer at the same time. 221 measurements were performed on both systolic and diastolic pressure in 69 patients.

   The mean systolic pressure (Figure 1) was observed to be 122.6mmHg by sphygmomanometer and 125.1mmHg by OMRON. There is no significant difference (F: 037, r = 0.96 and slope of linear regression is near 1.04).

   For diastolic pressure (Figure 2) the mean was found to be 79.1mmHg by sphygmomanometer and 82.2 by OMRON. Just as for systolic pressure, we found near-perfect correlation (r = 0.99 and slope near 1.05).

   Out of the 442 measurements, only 4 were in error, with systolic pressure by sphygmomanometer higher by 50mmHg and more. In other instances, the differences between the two types of measurement were less than 5mmHg.

   The role of the heart rate was examined, using a classification of systolic and diastolic pressure/differences and recorded heart rate. We observed that the lower the heart rate, the greater the differences betweeen techniques for diastolic pressure only. On these results, OMRON could be used instead of sphygmomanometer, using a correction (minus 33mHg).

Comparison with Intra-arterial Blood Pressure Measurement

   With the aid of the catheter laboratory, comparisons were performed during left heart catheterisation over as wide a range of values as possible. The catheter was passed into the axillary artery or just above the cuff of the OMRON equipment.

   The two measurements were performed at the same time by two observers, using a STATHAM pressure transducer and recorded on an Electronic for Medicine (VR 12).

   Thirty-two patients were studied. There was no significant difference in systolic pressure between OMRON (mean 122.4) and the intra-artrerial readings (mean 124.4) but correlation between measurements was poor (Spearman ρ = 68, r = 0.68). Differences ranged from -14 to +20 per cent (Figure 3). The mean diastolic pressure was 84.8 by OMRON, significantly higher than the intra-arterial mean (71.4). The difference was 13.4 mm (P < .001; ρ = 65 and r = 0.59) (Figure 4).

Conclusion

The OMRON semi-automatic sphygmomanometer cannot be considered as a scientific instrument for measuring blood pressure, because there are great discrepancies with simultaneous intra-arterial measurements. However, if it is required only to monitor changes in blood pressure following treatment, or to establish the normality of blood pressure, the OMRON manometer can be used safely.

Discussion

DR. G. SPERTI: During this study, how many patients were investigated and how many measurements were made comparing the Omeron indirect blood pressure system with intra-arterial blood pressure?

DR. LAFFAY: Sixty-nine patients were studied over six months. The number of measurements made in any individual patient varied; but usually, 3 or 4 measurements were made. These measurements were made during routine coronary arteriography and cardiac catheterisations.

DR. CASHMAN: Was there any indication from the Omeron at which particular cycle it was making its measurement to determine systolic pressure? If the intra-arterial pressure was varying rapidly between beats, the Omeron will require a significant time between measuring systolic and diastolic pressures.

DR. LAFFAY: During the procedure, the intra-arterial pressure measurement was made at the time the Omeron was recording systolic pressure.

DR. CASHMAN: I noticed, too, on the regression plot comparing the Omeron with the sphygmomanometer (by the human observer) that the systolic pressures were approximately 20mmHg higher, but there was still a correlation coefficient of 0.96, due partly to the substantial positive intercept.

DR. MILLAR-CRAIG: As Mr.Altman has pointed out, this shows some of the limitations of using correlation coefficients in the analysis of these data.

DR. MANN: We have already heard this morning about the differences between brachial artery and radial artery pressures. Dr. Laffay said that his intra-arterial pressures were measured during cardiac catheterisation. From where were these presures taken?

DR. LAFFAY: The catheter tip was usually positioned in the axillary artery. We were very careful to ensure that the catheter tip was not occluded by the blood pressure cuff.

DR. HUNYOR: I think that this is an important point. It seems strange, however, that the Omeron correlated with the standard sphygmomanometric blood pressure but not with the intra-arterial pressure, as intra-arterial and standard cuff blood pressures are known to correlate reasonably well. Is it possible that the presence of a catheter in the brachial artery might have created haemodynamic changes involving resistance, turbulent flow and other effects, which might have influenced the Omeron reading in that particular artery?

DR. LAFFAY: I think that question can be asked about all cuff methods of measuring blood pressure, not only about the Omeron. Surely, we are not measuring the same phenomena with an arm cuff as we are with an intra-lumenal catheter?

DR. STOTT: To some extent, I take issue here with Dr. Hunyor. Looking back over the literature, there have been many comparisons between cuff and intravascular measurements, from Steele (1942) onwards. I have been checking them out recently, and they all give about the same answer. The standard deviation of the difference between cuff and intra-arterial pressure is about 1 mm diastolic pressure and about 15 mm systolic. This means that there is a 5% chance of being about 30 mm out - that is about the same kind of scatter as shown here by Dr. Laffay.

Similar findings were presented at ISAM 1979 by Cowan, in which measurements made with the same cuff were compared by simultaneously reading them by two different methods. Not surprisingly, the measurements agreed very well. However, when the same instrument was compared with intravascular measurements, there was a big difference between the indirect and direct measurements, which was exactly what was demonstrated today by Dr. Laffay. Dr. Laffay's work confirms what has been done in the past, and is probably more reliable than what has been done previously because in some of the earlier work in this area, the intravascular transducers were not properly standardized. The sort of scatter that he has shown agrees very well with the scatter found by everybody else under similar conditions.

DR. GOULD: We have looked at indirect pressures, using an Aker's strain-gauge transducer linked directly to a chart write-out, in comparison with simultaneous intra-arterial pressure. While the mean of the discrepancy values for this comparison was quite good, in individual cases, the differences between indirect and intra-arterial blood pressures were up to 40mmHg. I would therefore support that it is certainly possible to get a good comparison between two different methods of indirect pressure measurement, but that there is a wide scatter if indirect pressures are compard with intra-arterial pressures.

DR. STOTT: It is very important that note is taken of this because another issue arises here. If we want to follow what is happening to the blood pressure in an individual patient, using indirect methods, in order to see whether therapy is doing any good, we need to know whether these observed discrepancies are systematic or random. I wish that somebody would take repeated measurements on the same patient at 10- or 15-minute intervals throughout the day and compare them with the intravascular measurements to see whether the scatter of the differences of the two readings is large and whether the indirect measurements track the direct measurements, which is what is important.

DR. GOLDBERG: When I worked with Dr. Stott, we reviewed the literature and found that there was a big discrepancy between intra-arterial and cuff measurement when these were compared. However, for the last five years, I have been using intra-arterial monitoring in cardiac and intensive care-units. In this situation, we have found that the cuff is a very good predictor of intra-arterial pressure. It is only at the very low pressures (below 60 or 70mmHg systolic) when it is almost impossible to hear the Karotkoff sounds, that there are problems. In most patients, the nurses do a very good job of predicting intra-arterial blood pressure.

DR. STOTT: The problem with saying that the cuff pressures agree with the intravascular ones, is that perhaps the clinican wants them to agree, so he notices when they do and rejects them when they do not. It is a random scatter, with quite a lot of points that lie more or less on the line of identity, but about 5% are wildly out. If the intention is to start treating patients by the million for half-a-lifetime with continuous drug therapy - 5% wrongly classified either way is just 4.999% to many.

DR. KANEKO: We have been measuring blood pressures in the same hypertensive patients using an indirect and a direct method. In our hands, there was a very high correlation with the values as determined by the indirect method being a very good indicator of the real intra-arterial blood pressure. We, therefore, think that measurement of blood pressure by the standard sphygmomanometer method is suitable for clinical use.

DR. O'BRIEN: While I agree with Dr. Stott, as a clinician, I would take grave exception to some of the strictures that he has passed on cuff measurement by the indirect technique. When looking back at various previous studies in which direct measurements have been compared against indirect measurements, it must be remembered that the finger might be pointed at some of the techniques for direct measurement just as much as it might be pointed at the indirect technique. Clinicians are becoming more aware in recent years that we have been, and still are, very careless in applying the indirect technique, however inaccurate it may be, and that it is certainly possible to perfect our methodology to a certain extent by taking care of certain empirical points. None the less, the Korotkoff technique remains probably the most valuable measurement tool in clinical medicine.

DR. HUNYOR: With all due respect to Dr. Stott, I am sorry but I have to take issue with most of what he said. It is surely all a question of range. I do not believe that in most of the comparisons of direct versus indirect measurement, the difference is as much as 15mmHg. If the difference was 3mmHg then the 5% who are more than 2 standard deviations from the mean, would not be regarded as "wildly" out.

Secondly, with regard to classiyfing the 5% wrongly, again it is all a question of magnitude. If they are classified wrongly by a level of 5mm or 3mmHg that is certainly less serious than classifying them wrongly by 30mmHg. The degree of reproducibility of indirect measurements has been discussed. There are parallels here in epidemiological data. It has been shown by Miall that if blood pressure is followed long-term in a population, individuals are found to track in blood pressure groups. If indirect blood pressure measurement was as poor as Dr. Stott said, it would not be found that the bottom decile stays in the bottom decile, year after year, and that the top decile stays in the top decile similarly.

Thirdly, with regard to the effects of drug treatment on blood pressure, if a group of patients are given a placebo tablet, their blood pressure decreases slightly and if they are given a known active anti-hypertensive agent, it decreases much more. We know that this is so, if the study is done in a randomised and blinded fashion. In this situation, the blood pressure change is not due to what the observer thinks or what he believes - but is shown subtly and accurately by the so-called indirect technique. If, as Dr. Stott said, the indirect technique is so unreliable, these differences would not be detected so clearly in study after study, involving groups of 10 or 12 patients.

Dr. O'Brien's point is also important. No doubt Dr. Stott has looked, much more critically than I, at all the past studies comparing indirect with direct readings. I am sure that with some of the earlier studies, as Dr. O'Brien pointed out, the direct techniques left much to be desired. O'Rourke and his colleagues in Sydney have shown, in an intensive care setting, that indirect and direct pressure measurements showed a surprisingly great degree of correspondence even down to pressures of 70mmHg systolic.

I say with all due respect and with a degree of humility that I also think that our study (Brit. Med. J., 1978 2, 159-162) was technically and measurement-wise quite a good one. I was advised by Dr. Stott's physicist colleagues about how to ensure that the measuring system was accurate. We used the regular mercury sphygmomanometer and the Hawkesley Random-Zero instrument, in a blinded, randomised fashion, in a small group of patients, who had widely differing blood pressures and showed that direct and indirect blood pressure measurements, carried out by trained observers, corresponded very closely.

DATA PROCESSING WORKSHOP

Chairman : D.G. Altman

THE EFFICIENT DIGITISATION OF 24-HOUR CONTINUOUSLY RECORDED BLOOD PRESSURE AND ELECTROCARDIOGRAM SIGNALS

R.H. MITCHELL*, S.C. RUFF* AND G.A. MURNAGHAN**

*School of Electrical and Electronic Engineering,
Ulster Polytechnic, N. Ireland
** Dept. Midwifery and Gynaecology, Queen's University,
N. Ireland

Summary

The computer analysis of 24-hour recordings of blood pressure and electrocardiograms requires, initially, a large storage capacity for the sampled data.

9-track magnetic tape is a reasonably cheap medium for storing data, and this has been used to store systolic and diastolic pressure values, R-R intervals and also complete blood pressure information.

In the interests of computing efficiency, systolic and diastolic pressure values and R-R intervals are obtained during the digitisation stage.

The software package also allows for editing and calibrating of the digitised data.

Introduction and Equipment

Digitisation is essential when it is required to insert the results of an experiment into a computer programme. This process might entail reading the values off a meter scale, or taking points of the tracing produced by a pen recorder. In many cases, the volume of data is too large to be dealt with by manual methods, because of the time involved and the possibility of errors arising.

In the application to be described here, blood pressure and electrocardiograms are continuously recorded over a 24-hour period and stored on cassette tape (1). The data stored on tape is analogue in nature and is converted to digital values by sampling the signals obtained from the playback system. The sampling is performed under programme control, using a PDP-11/34 minicomputer.

System Requirements

The first requirement for analysing ambulatory recordings is a programme, which will control the analogue-to-digital conversion procedure, so that it samples the incoming signals at a pre-determined rate and provides corresponding integer values. The sampling frequency will be governed by the expected spectral content of the signal (2).

The frequency spectrum of a section of blood pressure signal is shown in Figure 1. The frequency content is significant up to 15 Hz implying that a sampling frequency of at least 30 Hz is necessary in order to ensure accurate digitisation., Cost and efficiency of the system are important since sampling a 24-hour recording at 30 Hz would produce approximately 5×10^6 values. Floppy discs are imprac-

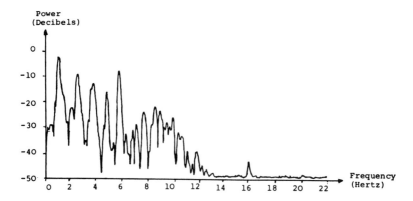

Fig. 1   Power Spectrum of a Blood Pressure Signal.

tical while hard discs are prohibitively expensive, especially for a
large population study. A reasonably cheap storage medium is 9-track
magnetic tape.

Since the three parameters, systolic and diastolic pressure and
R-R interval are of particular interest to the clinician, it could be
argued that it is unnecessary to store the entire sampled waveforms.
If all values are not stored, it will not be possible to determine
whether a certain value of (for example) systolic blood pressure is
outside the normal range due to artefact, or a genuine physiological
occurrence such as an ectopic beat. The possession of the raw,
digitised signals is also necessary for the calculation of other
parameters of interest such as maximum rate of rise of arterial
pressure, or the time between the systolic peak of pressure and the
dichrotic notch.

It is advantageous, in the interest of efficient use of computer
time, to be able to identify the systolic and diastolic values and to
measure the R-R intervals for each beat, during the digitisation
process. The R-R interval is measured by first feeding the ECG
signal into a peak detector circuit, which produces a TTL-compatible
signal, which can be directly interfaced with the computer (3, 4).
Software then times the interval between the peaks.

The PDP-11/34 computer used is equipped with an AR11 analogue
real-time sub-system (5), the essential features of which are the
following:

1. Programmable real-time clock (used to measure R-R intervals
or to initiate analogue-to-digital conversions).
2. A 16-channel, 10-bit analgoue-to-digital converter (used to
sample the blood pressure, ECG and marker channels).
3. An external interrupt line for causing processor interrupts.

Figure 2 shows how the hardware is arranged for the digitisation
process. Blood pressure and ECG signals from the Oxford Instruments
replay unit are sampled at 40 Hz real-time, which is 2.4 kHz at the

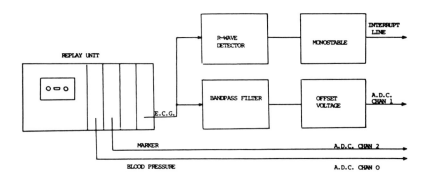

Fig. 2   Digitising Hardware Block Diagram.

60 replay speed.   This frequency was chosen to permit reasonable
resolution of the QRS complex of the ECG.

The 10-bit analogue-to-digital converter is used in a bipolar
mode with a range of - 2.5 to + 2.5 volts.   As only 8 bits are
required for a resolution of 1 part in 255, the gain and offset of
the blood pressure replay unit are adjusted, so that the normal range
of the signal is 0.0 to + 1.25 volts.

The ECG signal is first passed through a bandpass filter (30 to
700 Hz for x 60 replay) which removes the low frequency baseline
shifts and broadens the QRS complexes slightly.   The high frequency
cut-off is necessary because the 40 Hz sampling rate is a little low
for the ECG signal.   The removal of baseline shifts permits more gain
from the ECG replay amplifier and thus better analogue-to-digital
converter resolution can be obtained.   The signal is again kept in
the range 0.0 to + 1.25 volts by the adjustment of gain and offset
voltage.

Programme Description

Interrupts are used in the programme to allow a peripheral to be
serviced whenever it is ready, and irrespective of the stage that the
main segment has reached.   When a device causes an interrupt,   the
processor automatically jumps to a special sub-routine, called a
service routine, which executes the required operations before returning to the main programme.

In the sampling programme, three interrupts are used.   They are
as follows:
1.   Keyboard interrupts to allow the operator to start and stop
the sampling process by typing an appropriate letter on the
console keyboard.
2.   Clock interrupts, which initiate analogue-to-digital conversions at regular intervals, according to the sampling rate
required.
3.   External interrupts generated by R-waves of the ECG signal.

At the commencement of the programme, all the necessary locations are initialised. The processor then waits for a keyboard interrupt signifying that the operator has activated the replay unit and identified the start of the blood pressure and ECG signals. When this interrupt occurs, the AR11 clock is started and the clock overflow and external line (R-wave) interrupts are enabled. The programme then waits for an interrupt to occur, after which it tests to see if any data should be written to file. If this is the case, a request to write data is queued before the programme loops back to wait for the next interrupt. The programme is terminated via the keyboard interrupt routine, when the operator types the letter "S".

If an R-wave was responsible for the interrupt, the external interrupt flag is cleared, the R-wave software flag is set and the value of tthe R-R interval internal counter is stored before being cleared. A return from the service routine is then executed.

While this operation is proceeding, the last value from the blood pressure channel is compared with the current systolic and diastolic values. If the new value is greater than the systolic, or less than the diastolic, the appropriate updating action is taken. The value of the ECG channel is stored when the analogue-to-digital conversion is complete and, if the flag to sample the marker channel is not set, a return from the interrupt is made. The computer waveforms are shown in Figure 3.

Two 8192-byte sub-buffers are used to transfer the raw data to storage on 9-track magnetic tape. The derived data also uses two sub-buffers. These are of 1300 bytes permitting up to 325 systolic, diastolic, R-R interval and marker values to be accommodated. Each time an 8192 sub-buffer is stored, the corresponding derived information is also stored. Because it is unlikely that there will be 325 beats in the 102.4 seconds (4096 samples at 40 Hz), the first pair of unused values are zero-filled to facilitate their detection upon subsequent analysis. Figure 4 shows a flow chart of the main programme segment.

Editing the Data

After the ambulatory recording has been digitised and stored, it is necessary to provide some form of verification procedure to ensure that the data does not contain any gross artefacts. This is achieved by displaying the signals on a VDU and allowing the operator to accept or reject the data blocks. The unsuitable blocks are labelled in an array, where each element corresponds to one block. Subsequent programmes can interrogate this file to determine the location of bad data.

Calibration of Digitised Blood Pressure Values

After digitising an ambulatory recording and identifying the systolic, diastolic and pulse interval values, it is necessary to convert the pressures from integers produced by the conversion process into millimetres of mercury,

As seen in Figure 5, the characteristics of the pressure transducer and recording system are non-linear. The calibration programme digitises the calibration signals and fits a second-order polynomial

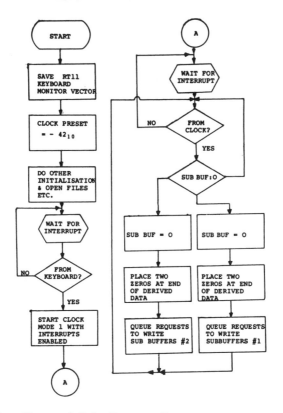

Fig. 4   Flow Chart of Main Program Segment.

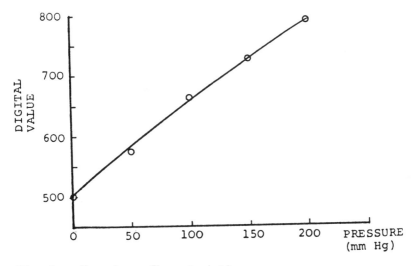

Fig. 5   Transducer Characteristics.

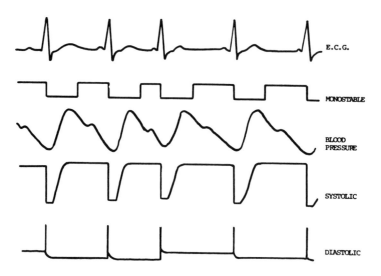

E.C.G.

MONOSTABLE

BLOOD
PRESSURE

SYSTOLIC

DIASTOLIC

Fig. 3   Computer Waveforms.

to the points by the method of Least Squares (5).
    Rather than take each value from the record of digitised samples
and compute the corresponding pressure by solving a quadratic equation, a look-up table is generated for all the numbers possible with
an 8-bit analogue-to-digital conversion. Each sample is then converted by address-ing the appropriate element of the table.

Conclusion

The digitisation and storage of ambulatory recordings is best carried
out by a method, which suits the available hardware. It is best to
perform a complete digitisation and storage of the data, as this
allows much greater flexibility in the methods of analysis, that may
be subsequently employed.
    The method described in this paper enables continuous sampling
and storage of data, with simultaneous on-line processing to quantify
certain derived variables.

References

1. Murnaghan G.A. (1976) Postgrad. Med. Journ. (Suppl.7) **52**, 123-
    127.
2. Schwartz M. and Shaw L. (1975) Signal Processing. McGraw-Hill,
    126-221.
3. Mitchell R.H., Ruff S.C. and Jenkins J.G. (1980) Med. and Biol.
    Eng. and Comput. **18**, 353-357.
4. Shimizu H. (1978) Psychophysiology **15**, 499-501.
5. Digital Equipment Corporation (1975) Processor Handbook 2.1-11
6. Schield F. (1968) Schaum Outline Series. McGraw-Hill. 235-236.

DISCUSSION

DR. GOLDBERG: I was very intrigued by the slide about the power spectrum because we found a very similar power spectrum when we looked at the output from the Oxford system. In comparison with the power spectrum that would be obtained from ordinary blood pressure wave form recorded on a scientific-type recorder it is found that there is a peak at 8 Hz. The gear box on the Oxford recorder produces an 8 Hz ripple which is very difficult to eliminate in all tapes. We have spent a lot of time trying to get rid of it, but unsuccessfully. I am currently looking at other tape recorders to see whether they are any better. If anyone has any information on this problem, I would like to hear it?

DR. MITCHELL: Other people have also reported that. Perhaps somebody here has some comments to make?

DR. CASHMAN: On Monday Dr. Davies presented some results which he obtained using the Medilog Mark II for recording blood pressure. At the moment, it is a dedicated recorder designed for 2 channels of ECG, but with a certain amount of modification it is possible to get blood pressure on to one channel. It uses a completely difference form of tape transport in which the gear-tooth frequencies have been moved way outside the carrier frequencies and this sort of artefact does not occur. There is artefact, but it is spikey and at a frequency, that is not in the blood pressure band.

MR. CROSBY: First, Dr. Mitchell uses a real-time clock in his computer for calculating the R-R interval. Does he use the crystal-locked clock on the tape or the one inside the computer and, if the latter, how does he compensate for variation in tape speed?

DR. MITCHELL: There is no compensation for tape speed variation. The clock in the AR-11 is used.

MR. CROSBY: Secondly, how well does the analog preprocessor that Dr. Mitchell described track rapid changes in pressure? Thirdly, he is recording data from the analog preprocessor as well as continuous digitised data. Has the correlation been looked at between the preprocessor systolic and diastolic values and the data actually recorded continuously in the computer?

DR. MITCHELL: The preprocessor does not track blood pressure - there is no preprocessor on the blood pressure channel. The blood pressure goes directly into the computer; it is digitised, and then software calculates the systolic and diastolic values. The circuit that I showed with the preprocessor is to detect R wave peaks, simply from the point of view that the output of that particular circuit goes directly on to the interrupter line with the PDP-11, and the sharp rising pulse and the sharp falling pulse allow the program to detect the interrupt and to start counting.

DR. MANN: Dr. Mitchell has defended his use of a rapid sampling technique of the whole signal by saying that if the lot is thrown out the baby gets thrown out with the bath water. As a humble clinician, I have two objections to that. First, we have already been presented with such a vast amount of systolic and diastolic pressures and heart rate data that interpreting it all is a fundamental feat even at the moment, and to look at any more would be extremely difficult.

Secondly, does the high-frequency artefact of the recording

system allow any meaningful interpretations to be made of this sort of data?

DR. MITCHELL: We have been looking at the information contained in the material that we are putting on to tape. It is felt that we may as well obtain it at the same time as we get systolic and diastolic pressures and heart rate. We will be presenting some data later in this meeting. At the moment, we are only looking at 24-hour systolic and diastolic values and the cyclical variations that take place within the 24 hours, and not at the significance or non-significance of the rates of rise of the blood pressure or the difference between the peak in blood pressure and the dicrotic notch, for example, which might be important. All we are doing is producing data which may eventually be important.

The frequency characteristics of the recording system are within the range of our sampling, so we think they should allow meaningful interpretations to be made.

DR. HUNYOR: Perhaps with our obsession with the blood pressure signal in Sydney we find that the blood pressure signal is much more robust than is the ECG signal. Perhaps much more attention should be devoted to good ECG recording, but even with considerable attention to detail we find that there are often poor quality ECGs, or the ECG decreases while there is a perfectly good blood pressure signal. It seems to me that if the blood pressure detection and analysis are linked to the ECG signal if, for any reason, 30 mins, 1 hour or 4 hours of ECG signal are lost, it would be impossible to assay perfectly good blood pressure data. Am I right about that?

DR. MITCHELL: No, that is not correct. Having obtained the blood pressure at the same time as the ECG, if ECG information is lost the blood pressure information is still there, the heart rate can still be extracted, and therefore heart rate variability too if that is what we are interested in having. In terms of detecting the peaks in blood pressure, some slides were shown earlier demonstrating the difficulty of detecting the right point at which to read the peak systolic value. By using the ECG as an interrupt, we have found this to be more efficient.

THE SKEWNESS OF THE R-R INTERVAL HISTOGRAM AS AN INDICATION OF ATRIAL FIBRILLATION

L. GOULDING

Department of Cardiovascular Medicine, John Radcliffe Hospital,
Oxford, UK

Introduction

Heart rate data have been displayed in the form of an R-R interval histogram for more than 50 years. Arnoldi used the method in 1927 for his study of the influence of digitalis on the heart rate. He and subsequent workers, until the early 1960's, measured the R-R interval by hand and manually plotted the histogram - an intimidating task! Since the mid-1960's, digital electronics has made it possible to use either a general purpose computer or a dedicated histogram generator to process the data in minutes rather than hours. As a result, the histogram and its extension, the difference histogram, have been much more commonly used in cardiac arrhythmia analysis.
It is customary to divide a horizontal axis of the histogram into units, or bins, each of some 10 to 30 mS wide and covering the range of 200 to 2000 mS. The vertical axis represents frequency and each bin has a capacity of 4K or more R-R intervals. Using this format, sinus rhythm produces a virtually normal distribution, whilst atrial fibrillation generates one, which is strongly positively skewed. Many investigators have described this phenomenon, but none apears to have quantified the degree of skewness.
Analysis of P-wave activity is difficult in ambulatory electrocardiography, unless one has recourse to the somewhat socially unacceptable oesophageal or intra-atrial electrode. It seemed possible, therefore, that the degree of skewness of the R-R interval histogram might prove to be a useful indication of the presence of atrial fibrillation.

Method

Medilog I recorders, manufactured by Oxford Medical Systems, were used to record 24-hour electrocardiograms from 50 patients in sinus rhythm and 50 patients with atrial fibrillation. The records were replayed x 25 on a type PB2 tape deck which incorporated the pulse interval timer and standard amplifiers. The values of the R-R interval were digitised and stored in a Data General S 200 Eclipse computer, which also generated histograms, difference histograms and heart-rate trends from one-hour, two-hour, four-hour, eight-hour and twelve-hour periods. Permanent records of these were produced by a Tektronix type 431 hard copier via a type 4006-1 computer display terminal.

Results

The 12-hour data were discarded because basic heart rate variation over such a long period tended to obscure the pattern due to atrial fibrillation. Also, processing times became protracted due to the volume of data. For patients in sinus rhythm, the mean values of histogram skewness were:

One-hour	-0.1995	S.D. 0.5874
Two-hour	-0.1228	S.D. 0.4771
Four-hour	-0.1352	S.D. 0.4156
Eight-hour	-0.0337	S.D. 0.4616

For patients with atrial fibrillation, the mean values were:

One-hour	1.1526	S.D. 0.4643
Two-hour	1.1185	S.D. 0.3615
Four-hour	1.0626	S.D. 0.3451
Eight-hour	1.0586	S.D. 0.3868

Conclusion

Comparison of the sinus rhythm and atrial fibrillation histograms collected over each period shows a statistically significant difference, but no advantage appears to be gained by the use of the longer duration results. Serial estimations of the skewness of the one-hour histogram might, therefore, be useful as a means of detecting atrial fibrillation in ambulant subjects, without the need for specialised and rather unpleasant electrodes.

DISCUSSION

DR. CASHMAN: I recognise the shape of some of those histograms from atrial fibrillation, but I think I should perhaps introduce a note of warning that it is possible to have highly skewed R-R interval histograms in sinus rhythm when the rate is changing according to some pattern. It is vital also to have an interval difference histogram to make quite sure that what is being seen is a disordered rhythm that jumps from beat to beat, not a smooth rhythm which changes. I think that a pair of histograms are needed to be absolutely sure.

DR. GOULDING: I have wondered about that. It is obvious that the R-R difference histogram in atrial fibrillation is wide compared with the normal. I wondered whether it would even be possible to concentrate on the difference histogram to the exclusion of the R-R interval histogram.

DR. CASHMAN: The difference histogram tends to be symmetric and triangular in a variety of conditions, so it does not help all that much on its own. But the pair together with skewness and possibly hgher moments, may give something quite useful.

PROF. FELDMAN: Has Dr. Goulding looked at the differencial diagnosis of this problem which is certainly important from our point of view?

With this kind of histogram plus the difference histogram it is possible to distinguish sinus rhythm from sinus arrhythmia from atrial fibrillation. The other things that come into that - the supraventricular arrhythmias that tend to confound the issue, the frequent SVP beats (which normally have no shape information) and also a second-degree block such as Wenckebach's syndrome; are they distinguishable with these techniques?

DR. GOULDING: In our limited numbers it was a problem to find a significant number of patients with one abnormal rhythm only over a long enough period to get enough information.

PROF. PINCIROLI: There are four points on which to focus with regard to the use of histograms for R-R intervals: first, what is the quantity to be used for the histograms? I feel that we can use R-R intervals and difference histograms, as used (and published) by Dr. Cashman. The use of ratio histograms may also be considered. For example, I had the same results working with ratios.

Secondly, how is it possible to save some dynamic information using histograms? I have tried to solve this problem by considering not only the R-R interval but also four ratios: the ratio between the value of the present R-R interval and the first, second, third and fourth previous R-R intervals.

Thirdly, how to use histograms in such a way that the events which occur only a few times are outlined and magnified in relation to the large number of normal events which occur. I tried to solve this problem by the use of logarithmic scales instead of linear scales.

Fourthly, how to save more dynamic information from histograms that necessarily eliminate all dynamic and time information. For this, I tried to use the area of logarithmic histograms plotted over time.

I suggest, therefore, that the use of histograms may maintain an important and interesting position for the investigations that we want to make with electrocardiograms only if used in a sophisticated way.

DR. MONSTER: I see no advantages in the use of these histograms as long as shortened patterns such as atrial fibrillation, bigeminy and trigeminy can readily be detected by simple means at high speed by looking at the prematurity or the lateness of successive beats.

DR. CASHMAN: One possible advantage is that it provides a very quick way of seeing what proportion of the time is spent in an abnormal rhythm if the histograms are divided up into, say, hourly or half-hourly sections.

DR. MONSTER: That can be done just as well by counting the number of bigeminy or trigeminy beats that there are, and saying how many in one hour and how many in another hour.

PROF. PINCIROLI: I had a positive result with regard to detecting bigeminy by plotting the area of the logarithmic histogram of the four ratios mentioned previously during time.

NEAR-SENSOR REDUCTION OF PHYSIOLOGICAL DATA BY USE OF A PORTABLE MICROPROCESSOR-SYSTEM

B. KUNZ, K. MERTENS, AND B. OESTE

DFVLR-Institut für Nachrichtentechnik
D-8031 Oberpfaffenhofen

Summary

A portable microprocessor-based data collection system for long-term registration of physiological data is presented. The problems arising while implementing near-sensor data reduction are discussed using this system as a reference.

Introduction

Analogue collection of physiological data over long periods of time presents considerable problems of data storage and retrieval. These can be overcome by using data-reduction at the point of acquisition, a technique which can only be used by accepting that only certain aspects of the data which are considered to be essential can be retained. As an example, take the electrocardiogram under different conditions:
1. Clinic: Analysis of Shape.   300 kbit.
2. Work Medicine: Heart rate.   Each R-R interval (8h) 400 kbit.
                                Mean Value per min (8h) 4 kbit.
3. Preventive Medicine: S-T change. One datum per QRS-complex : 400 kbit.

Problems of near-sensor data-reduction

We have designed and developed a portable data collection system for physiological signals and have already published the basic concepts (1, 2). The main features are:
1. Up to 10 channels available for data
2. Digital storage.
3. Microprocessor based data-processing.
4. Analogue pre-processing.
5. Modular construction of hard- and soft-ware.
6. Possibility of action - criteria based upon data.
These features allow long-term registration in the field on a number of patients without the disadvantage of creating an abundance of data, which cannot be processed later. Because of the modular construction different measurement profiles can be realized.
    When estimating the mathematical expense for performing such extraction of information out of the original signal, all deviations of the signal from the normal have to be considered whether of natural origin or externally induced and which are summed up under the term "artefact'. Taking the heart-rate measurement as an example, each QRS-complex within the ECG has to be recognized and its occur-

rence has to be correlated with time.

Expressed mathematically, the correlation $\int u(t-\tau)s(\tau)d\tau$ has to be executed when u(t) is the signal and $s(\tau)$ is the QRS-complex. The evaluation of the integral suffers from the fact that $s(\tau)$ cannot be expressed in close form because the QRS-complex varies individually and differs from person to person. When visually evaluating the ECG the experience of the physician takes this into account, but when using a computer, adaptive methods have to be used which sometimes incorporate repeating algorithms and are therefore not real-time. Another point to consider is the time consumption of software-controlled multiplication in a microprocessor-based computer system, which lies in the msec region.

It is obvious that a software-driven QRS-complex extraction will exhaust the capabilities of a microprocessor.

Similar estimations apply to the other physiological signals. It can, therefore, be stated that multi-channel data reduction by means of a conventional microcomputer is not possible.

Another point is the size of today's storage integrated circuits. Fast-Fourier and correlation-algorithms need a lot of storage room, which leads to a great number of integrated circuits and as a consequence of that, to larger size and weight of the overall system.

Hybrid data-processing

One way to solve the problem of limited computational power of the microcomputer is to process parts of the job in parallel branches, which are independent of each other. Furthermore, tasks which can better be done in an analog manner, such as filtering, should be carried out in this way. In our system, each physiological channel has its own analog pre-processing module, which transforms the signal tk one of the two inTerfaces of the microcomputer. In the example of the heart rate channel, the analog module performs the recognition of the QRS-complex of the ECG-signal. In the case of the EMG, bandwidth limitation and a first integration is carried out in the analog module.

The partitioning into analog and software-based processing is optimized regarding expense, weight and power consumption of the overall system. Obviously, it is heavily dependent on the progress in technology and will, therefore, move to more application of software with the development of more powerful microprocessors and related peripheral integrated circuits.

Validation of information

When data reduction is performed at the sensor, a valuable part of the information contained in the original signal is lost; that is the quality of the signal. From this value, the level of confidence of the measurement value can be derived. The traditional method used in stationary computer systems, to replay the recording and to apply a visual check when encountering a faulty processing, cannot be applied any longer. Other methods which have to be developed in order to make the information processing reliable, include:

1. Stable sensors/electrodes
2. Near-sensor preamplifiers (EMI)

3. Visualcontrol of the original signal ahead of the measurement.
4. Suppression of artefact (hard- and soft-ware) specifically
      tailored to the signal.
In addition, values indicating the quality of the signal have to be
derived, viz:
     1. By generating additional information: e.g., the number of
           RR-intervals used for calculating the mean heart-rate
     2. Recognition and counting of artefacts: e.g., during heart-
           rate measurements, 'triggers' declared faulty by the soft-
           ware, are counted and stored
     In the figures, part of the results of a first comparative study
are presented, which was carried out at the Forschungsgruppe Psycho-
physiologie in Freiburg (3). The investigation comprised analog tape
recordings of 14 patients with non-pathological ECG's, in 10 different situations of a psychophysiological study. The deviations of
the heart rate are less than 1 beat per minute, except for the last
but one situation. The differences in the values, especially in
sign, can be explained by the differences in the methods of evaluation (time resolution, trigger point, "noise handling") (4).
     Even with patients with a great number of triggering losses,
(Pat. 11, 12, 13), the values of the M2P-system and conventional
methods agree very well.

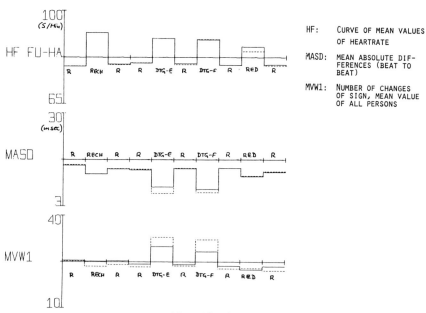

Fig. 1   Mean values over all patients :
          HF : Heartrate
          MASD : Absolute differences beat to beat
          MVW1 : Number of changes of sign

Conclusions

Unlike analog recording of the original signal, data reduction at the sensor requires thorough planning of the experiment with clear definition of the information wanted. Stable sensors or electrodes, with known accuracy and time-resolution, must be available. Artefacts and their influence should be estimated and criteria describing the quality of the signal have to be developed. With this in mind, one gains several advantages. The number of parallel channels is increased, the secondary data-processing becomes faster, with high accuracy and flexibility concerning type of signals, processing and storage. Going beyond data reduction, real data-processing is possible in the sense of recognition of hazardous situations for the patient, or remarkable events, which can be reported back to the patient. Another point of future investigation could be extensive artefact suppression by software and correlation of different physiological signals in order to make new physiological values accessible (e.g., pulse wave velocity).

TABLE 1

MEAN VALUES OVER ALL SITUATIONS FOR EACH PERSON

FU: M2P-SYSTEM
HA: EVALUATION BY HAND
LB: LABORATORY COMPUTER
ARR: PERCENTAGE OF NON-RECOGNIZED RR-INTERVALS

PROBAND (NR.)	HERZFREQUENZ			MASD		MVW1		MVW2		ARR=(0/0)	
	FU	HA	LB	FU	LB	FU	LB	FU	LB	FU	LB
1	89	89	89	9	9	23*	26	27	30	0	1
2	91	91	91	11	11	25	26	28	29	0	0
3	81	81	81	15	15	32	33	40	42	0	0
4	107	107	107	6	5	24	31	23	28	1	2
5	84	84	84	11	12	27	31	34	39	0	0
6	74	74	74	11	11	29	29	39	40	0	0
7	92	92	92	5	5	16	20	18	22	0	0
8	90	90	90	10	11	33	34	38	39	0	0
9	90	90	90	8	8	25	25	29	28	4	0
10	94	93	94	4	3	13*	23	14*	25	2	0
11	84	85	85	17	7	33	21	43	25	20	0
12	68	67	68	26	23	27	21	40	34	24	1
13	84	85	84	7	6	24	25	29	31	27	14
14	97	97	98	7	7	35	37	36	38	6	1

References

1. Kunz B., Mertens K., Oeste B. In: Proc. ISAM 1979, Ed: Stott F.D., Raftery E.B., Goulding L., Academic Press, London 1980, p.487,
2. Kunz B., Mertens K., Oeste B.(1979) Vortrag 13. Jarhestagung Dt. Gesellschaft für Biomedi. Technik, Kiel. Biomedizin. Technik, Bd. 24. Ergänzungsband 1979, 132-133.

3.   Foerster F., Müller W., Schneider H.J. Vergleich von EKG-Parame-
      tern des Funktionsmodells "M2P" der DFVLR mit Labor- und
      Handauswerteverfahren, Bericht der Forschungsgruppe Psychophys-
      iologie and die DFVLR-NE-NT.
4.   Oeste B., et al. (1980) Biomedizin. Technik, Bd. 25, Ergän-
      zungsband, 89-91.

METHODOLOGY OF HEART RATE HISTOGRAMS ANALYSIS BY MEAN OF FACTOR ANALYSIS OF CORRESPONDENCE

F. TEKAIA* AND M. RIEU**

*Laboratoire de Statistique, Universite P.& M. Curie, and
**Laboratoire de Physiologie CHU Cochin, Paris, France

Summary

The factor analysis of correspondence aims at synthesising the information contained in a data table and visualising the relations between the elements of two sets I and J. Its main characteristic properties are:
- The analysis of a table of profiles;
- The distance used between profiles in the distributional distance;
- The possibility of: representing the elements of two sets I and J simultaneously on the same factorial plane.
: adding individuals or variables as supplementary elements.

To apply this method to the study of Heart Rate (HR), we propose a methodology for processing HR histograms associated with activity sequences; it consists in constructing and analysing correspondence tables according to various criteria: chronology of sequences, accumulation of sequences, HR and modes of parameters characteristic of the subject's activity.

To realise this methodology, a chain of programmes has been written in FORTRAN IV language on a PDP8. Its different applications show the swiftness and flexibility of action it provides by giving the user an easy mean of establishing the relations between sequences and heart rate.

Principle of the Factor Analysis of Correspondence

The FAC method was developed by Professor Benzecri; here we shall merely present its general outlines. (For more details see 1, 2, 5).

The table to be processed by FAC must be homogeneous, i.e. the numbers represent enumerations of associations between the elements of two sets I and J. The method aims at obtaining a planar representation of each of these two sets I and J and, what is characteristic of FAC, of these two sets simultaneously.

Tables of Profiles

Let k_{IJ} be the correspondence table of positive numbers k (i, j), where I is the set of individuals (also referred to a rows or observations) and J the set of variables (or columns, or parameters).

Let k_i, k_j and k be respectively the sum of row iofI, of column j of J and the total sum of table k_{IJ}.

We have:

$$k_i = {\textstyle\sum_{j\epsilon J}} k(i,j), \quad k_j = {\textstyle\sum_{i\epsilon I}} k(i,j) \text{ and } k = {\textstyle\sum_{\substack{i\epsilon I\\j\epsilon J}}} k(i,j) = {\textstyle\sum_{i\epsilon I}} k_i = {\textstyle\sum_{j\epsilon J}} k_j$$

We obtain the profile of each row i of I according to set J by dividing every number of this row by the total of the same row:

$$\text{Profile of } i = \{k(i,1)/k_1 \dots \dots k(i,j)/k_i \dots \dots k(i,p)/k_i\}$$

The sum of the ratios defining this profile equals 1. The profile of i expresses, in terms of percentages, the distribution of i over the set J. Likewise, we obtain the profile of a column j of J on set I by dividing each number in this column by the total of the same column.

$$\text{Profile of } j = \{k(1,j)/k_j \dots \dots k(i,j)/k_j \dots \dots k(n,j)/k_j$$

Again, we note that the sum of the ratios of this profile equals 1. The profile of j expresses, in terms of percentages, the distribution of j over set I. The value $k(i,j)$, which is the number of associations of elements i and j, has value only in relation to the total of the associations of i with the elements of set J, and in relation to the total number of the associations of j with the elements of set I.

Masses

The notion of profile is interesting, as we have just seen, but we must not lose the size of the row or of the column; therefore, we associate it with every profile. Here also, the total of a row i or of a column j in the table k_{IJ}, has value only in relation to the total k of this table. The mass of the profile of i is the ratio of the sum of this row to the total of the table.

Mass of the profile $i = k_i/k$.

Likewise the mass of the profile $j = k_j/k$.

We note that the sum of the profile masses of the elements of I, as well as the sum of the profile masses of the elements of J, equals 1.

Notations

$f_{ij} = k(i,j)/k$ frequency associated with (i, j)

$f_i = k_i/k = {\textstyle\sum_{j\epsilon J}} k(i,j)/k = \{f_{ij}, j\epsilon J\}$ mass of the profile of i.

$f_j = k_j/k = {\textstyle\sum_{i\epsilon I}} k(i,j)/k = \{f_{ij}, i\epsilon I\}$ mass of the profile of j.

Whence we deduce: ${\textstyle\sum_{\substack{i\epsilon I\\j\epsilon J}}} f_{ij} = {\textstyle\sum_{i\epsilon I}} f_i = {\textstyle\sum_{j\epsilon J}} f_j = 1.$

$f^i_J = \{f^i_j = k(i,j)/k_i; j\epsilon J\}$ is the profile of i on J.

$f^j_I = \{f^j_i = k(i,j)/k_j; i\epsilon I\}$ is the profile of j on I.

Let us note that $f^i_j = j_{ij}/j_i$ and $f^j_i = f_{ij}/f_j$.

In particular, these formulae show the symmetry of the roles of individuals i and the columns j.

We denote $N_j(I) = \{(f_j^i, f_i), i \epsilon I\}$, the cloud of the profiles of the rows on J associated with their masses f_i. Likewise, we denote $N_I(J) = \{(f_I^j, f_j), j \epsilon J\}$, the cloud of the profiles of the columns on

I associated with their masses f_j.

How to Choose the Best Plane of Projection of a Cloud:

We determine the centre of gravity of the cloud, through which we draw the·line from which the cloud deviates the least and along which it is dispersed the most. The deviation and dispersion are measured in terms of inertia, which is a function of the mass and square of the distance. Line Δ_1 will be the 1st factorial axis or principal axis of expansion of the cloud, then we resolve the surrounding space into line Δ_1 and the supplementary sub-space orthogonal to Δ_1, passing through the centre; we project the cloud on to this sub-space and, for this projection, we once again try to find the principal axis of expansion, which will be the 2nd factorial axis of the cloud, and so on.

Centre of Gravity

The jth co-ordinate of the centre of gravity of the indivual's cloud is defined by $g_j = \underset{i \epsilon I}{\Sigma} f_j^i . f_i = \underset{i \epsilon I}{\Sigma} f_{ij} . f_i / f_i = \underset{i \epsilon I}{\Sigma} f_{ij} = f_j$.

Thus the centre of gravity of the cloud of individuals is the row of the profile masses of the elements in set J. Likewise, we demonstrate that the centre of gravity of the cloud of variables is the column of the masses of the profiles of the elements of I.

x^2 Distance or Distributional Distance

The distance between the profile of two rows is expressed as follows:
$$d^2(f_j^i, f_j^{i'}) = d^2(i, i') = \underset{j \epsilon J}{\Sigma} (f_j^i - f_j^{i'})^2 / f_j.$$

In the same way, the distance between the profile of two columns is:
$$d^2(f_I^j, f_I^{j'}) = d^2(j, j') = \underset{i \epsilon I}{\Sigma} (f_I^j - f_I^{j'})^2 / f_i.$$

The advantage of this distance, which is characteristic of FAC, lies in its obeying the principle of distributional equivalence, namely: several proportional rows (or columns), can be replaced by a single row (or column) whose profile is the common profile and whose mass is the sum of masses of rows (or columns), without modifying the distances between the columns of J (or rows of I).

Total Inertia of Cloud N(I) relative to its Centre of Gravity and Factorial Axes or Principal Axes of Inertia

The total inertia of the cloud relative to its centre of gravity G is: $I(N) = \underset{i \epsilon I}{\Sigma} f_i . d^2(i, G)$

Let Δ and $\Delta^{\perp}$ be two orthogonal axes passing through G.; according to Pythagoras' theorem, the total inertia of the cloud relative to G is resolved as follows: $I(N) = I (N)_{\Delta} + I_{\Delta^{\perp}}(N)$,   where $I_{\Delta}(N)$, $I(N)$ respectively denote the inertia of the cloud along axis Δ and axis $\Delta^{\perp}$.

Finding the 1st factorial axis is the same as determining axis Δ so that $I_{\Delta}(N)$ is maximum. (i.e. $I_{\Delta^{\perp}}(N)$ is minimum). To find the 2nd factorial axis, we consider a resolution of $I_{\Delta^{\perp}}(N) = I_{\Delta_2}(N) + I_{\Delta_2^{\perp}}(N)$ and we determine axis Δ_2 so that $I_{\Delta_2}(N)$ is maximum and so on.

In fact, the process is made easier by demonstrating that the principal axes of inertia of cloud $N_J(I)$ are the eigen vectors of Table YX obtained by multiplying the two matrices X and Y whose rows are the profiles on J (f_j^i) and the profiles on I (f_i^j).   In the same way, we define the principal factors of cloud $N_I(J)$ as eigen vectors of Table XY and we have:

$$XYu_{\alpha} = \lambda_{\alpha}u_{\alpha}$$
$$YXv_{\alpha} = \lambda_{\alpha}v_{\alpha}$$

The inertia of each cloud along the axis of order α (u_{α} or v_{α}) equals λ_{α} , which is the eigen value associated with u_{α} and v_{α} .

Basic Formulae

We denote $F_{\alpha}(i)$ the co-ordinate of the ith individual and $G_{\alpha}(j)$ the co-ordinate of the jth variable on the α factorial axis. These co-ordinattes verify he following properties:

$$\sum_{i \in I} f_i \cdot F_{\alpha}(i) = 0 \qquad \text{respectively} \quad \sum_{j \in J} f_j \cdot G_{\alpha}(j) = 0$$

$$\sum_{i \in I} f_i \cdot F_{\alpha}(i)^2 = \lambda_{\alpha} \quad \text{respectively} \quad \sum_{j \in J} f_j \cdot G_{\alpha}(j)^2 = \lambda_{\alpha}$$

These formulae indicate that the variance of $F_{\alpha}(i)$ respectively $G_{\alpha}(j)$ equals λ_{α} and finally $\sum_{i \in I} f_i \cdot F_{\alpha}(i) \cdot F_{\beta}(i) = 0$ $(\alpha \neq \beta)$

Transition formulae and barycentric principle

Given the symmetry of clouds, the transition formulae enable us to go from the factors of one to the factors of the other :

$$F_{\alpha}(i) = \frac{1}{\sqrt{\lambda_{\alpha}}} \cdot \sum_{j \in J} f_j^i \cdot G_{\alpha}(j)$$

$$G_{\alpha}(j) = \frac{1}{\sqrt{\lambda_{\alpha}}} \cdot \sum_{i \in I} f_i^j \cdot F_{\alpha}(i)$$

We note that, aside from coefficient $1/\sqrt{\lambda_{\alpha}}$, $F(i)$ appears as the barycentre of the $G_{\alpha}(j)$, weighted by the masses f_j^i since $\sum_{j \in J} f_j^i = 1$

In the same way, aside from coefficient $1/\sqrt{\lambda_{\alpha}}$, $G_{\alpha}(j)$ appears as the barycentre of the $F_{\alpha}(i)$ weighted by the masses f_i^j, since $\sum_{i \in I} f_i^j = 1$

With these formulae, we can harmonize the selection of the orientation of the axis and, above all, obtain a diagram, in which are superimposed the projection of the points of could $N_J(I)$ and the projection of the points of $N_I(J)$.

Formula of Data Reconstitution

Starting from the co-ordinates of points i and j on set A of factors, we can reconstitute the initial data using the following formula:

$$f_{ij} = f_i f_j (1 + \sum_{\alpha \in A} \frac{1}{\sqrt{\lambda_\alpha}} \cdot F_\alpha(i).G_\alpha(j)) \quad \text{Hence: } k_{ij} = k.f_{ij}.$$

Supplementary elements

These terms are used to denote an individual or a variable in the data table, which does not participate in the determination of axes. Let j_s be a supplementary column in a table of data; the profile of j_s on the set of individuals is:

$$f_I^{j_s} = \{f_i^{j_s}, i\epsilon I\} = \{f_{ijs}/f_{js}, i\epsilon I\} = \{k_{ijs}/k_j, i\epsilon I\}.$$

We compute its co-ordinates over the system of factorial axes

established by the principal elements : $G_\alpha(j_s) = 1 \quad \sum_{i\epsilon I}^{j_s} f^i.F_\alpha(i)$

In the same way if i_s denotes a supplementary row, we have

$$f_J^{i_s} = \{f_j^{i_s}, j\epsilon J\} = \{f_{isj}/f_{is}, j\epsilon J\} = \{k_{isJ}/k_{is}, j\epsilon J\},$$

and we have $F_{\alpha'}(i) = \frac{1}{\sqrt{\lambda_\alpha}} \quad \sum_{j\epsilon J}^{i_s} f_j.G_\alpha(j).$

In practice, adding individuals or variables as supplmentary elements has an explanatory value since the proximity or the distance, for instance, of a supplementary individual in relation to other principal individuals, illustrates the proximity or the divergence of their behaviours in relation to all variables.

Application of FAC to the Study of Heart Rate

With the development of miniaturized equipment, we can now record the electro-cardiogram (ECG) of a subject, while observing his activity simultaneously for long eriods and in situations he is used to (see 4). T. Drozdowski has written a programme, which allows the ECG signal to be processed according to the various activity sequences, which are observed, having in particular, constructed a histogram of heart rates for each of the sequences. This histogram is presented according to 24 classes of HR (from 10 to 240 beats/minute) and gives, for each class, the number of the detected QRS complexes. With this easily performed recording and processing of the ECG signal, we can obtain numerous histogrms of activity sequences. The resulting table of data, where I denotes the set of activity sequences and J the set of HR classes, is suited to FAC since this analysis allows the correspondence between te elements of te two sets I and J to be represented. The analysis of such a table, provided that we have a considerable number of sequences (card I>400) and we add the generally light extreme classes to the nearest heavy classes, allows set J of the HR classes to be arranged on a parabolic-like curve , on the factorial plane 1 x 2, which shows a considerable percentage of inertia. In relation to this curve, all points representing the activity sequences are placed according to the barycentric principle.

Thus on the plane 1 x 2 (Figure 1), if a seauence presents high values in the highest HR classes, it will be placed on the side of the highest classes; if, on the contrary, it presents high values for the lowest HR classes, it will be placed on the side of the low HR classes. On the plane 1 x 2, we obtain the representation of the set of activity sequences and HR classes:

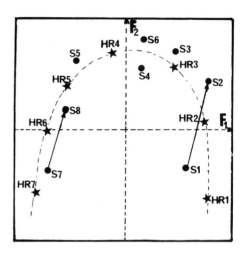

Fig. 1   Heart rate as related to activity plotted on the F1-F2 plane

there we are able to follow the HR variation according to the activity sequence, thus, as in this figure, the change from sequence s1 to sequence s2 brings about an increase in heart rates, whereas the change from sequence s7 to sequence s8 decreases the HR. The parabolic curve HR1 to HR7 reflects the deviation of the HR increase; a change in the activity sequences in the direction of the HR curve reflects a tendency towards an increase, while a change in the opposite directon reflects a tendency towards a decrease in HR.

Constructing Correspondence Tables

The barycentric representation allows the position of each sequence in relation to the HR classes to be determined. Each row of set I represents a histogram j, which may be either the associated with an activity sequence or rather the cumulative histograms associated with a class of sequences defined according to various criteria, for instance, according to the subject, the subject's role, the nature of the activity, etc.

The table may only include information about the activity of a single subject, or, on the contrary, brings together all the sequences relative to all subjects. It is possible, of course, to select the rows considered as principal elements differently, as well as those representing the supplementary elements. The analysis we may have to perform are of two types: analyses based on time, and analyses based on accumulation of activity sequences. Let us suppose set I is the set of HR histogram associated with activity sequences of several subjects (denoted by A, B, D, D, E and F).

Time-bases Analysis

This analysis lies in identifying the subject and the activity sequences by a sequential number corresponding to their order of occurrence. Therefore, this type of analysis allows HR variations to be followed according to time. It amounts to what is commonly done when the variation curves of mean HR are studied as a function of time.

Analysis based on Accumulation of Activity Sequences

A histogram accumulating other histograms of set I, added as a supplementary element is projected on to their centre of gravity; therefore, it can somehow be considered as representing them. Then, it is interesting, provided that the accumulation of sequences is meaningful in the study to be conducted to consider several types of accumulation.

Accumulation by Activiy

We construct a cumulative histogram of the histograms concerning a given activity for one or several subjects. Thus, for instance, if among the activity sequences of all subjects, there are sequences W (e.g. walking), it is possible to construct cumulative histograms of the whole of sequences W for each subject; then we will have cumulative histograms: AW (for subject A), BW (for subject B) and so on...and, for all subjects, the cumulative histogram W of all sequences W. Such an operation can be done for all of the various activities found in set I. It is naturally possible to suppose that the subjects belong to separate sub-groups; if, for instance, X denotes the sub-group of subjects A, B and C, while Y denotes the sub-group of subjects D, E and F, we calculate XW cumulative of AW, BW and CW and, in the same way, YW, cumulative of DW, EW and FW.

Accumulation by Activity Groups

As seen above, we can accumulate, by subject, group of subjects, or for all subjects, cumulative histograms of various activities, provided that the cumulative process is meaningful.

Accumulation by subject

It means constructing the histogram accumulating all the activity sequences of a subject: A (for subject A), B (for subject B) etc.

Which Table shall we Analyse?

It is preferable to take the histograms associated with initial sequences only as principal elements and to add, as supplementary elements, the cumulative histograms for the following reasons:
This procedure, on the one hand, gives us a means to check whether the cumulative histograms group homogenous sequence or, on the contrary, histograms differing from one another though associated

with the same type of activity;   on the other hand, to project the
cumulative histogram added as a supplementary element onto the centre
of gravity of the principal histograms it accumulates.   However, it
often happens that the number of simple histograms is too high;   in
this case, one can take the cumulative histograms as the set of the
principal elements.

In both cases, it is important only to have, as the principal
table, a set of histograms (card I>400) sufficient to obtain a
structure, shaped as a stable parabola, of set J of HR classes;   then
the principal or supplementary rows are placed satisfactorily.

Other Types of Analysis: HR and other Parameters

The processing of the ECG signal, according to the observed
activity, at the same time as it is recording, allows the HR to be
studied according to other parameters characteristic of the subject's
activity.   Thus, during a runner's training session, we can study his
heart rate as a function of the fractional distance, the rate at
which he covers it, the recovery time between exercises and the total
distance covered during the training session.

More generally, let us suppose that the activity sequence is
defined by the HR histogram, with which it is associated and by
parameters U, V... To homogenize these variables into a number of
modes, each delimited by boundary values and by assigning value 1 to
the sequence for the mode in which it is found and zero elsewhere.
Let JM be the set of modes corresponding to the variables U, V... In
this case, we propose to analyse the table crossing set JM of modes
with the set of HT classes by accumulating the histograms falling
into each variable mode.   Then we add, as supplementary elements to
this table, the table of sequences defined by the associated HR
histograms.   Such an analysis allows a typology of the modes of
variables to be obtained according to the HR classes.

Series of Analysis Programmes of Heart Rate Histograms

We have developed, on a PDP8, with 24 Kwords of 12 bits, a
series of programmes written in FORTRAN IV language, which performs
the various stages described above:
1.   A programme allowing the construction of the corresponding table
     according to the criterion or criteria above-mentioned;
2.   The programme (6) of factor analysis of correspondence allowing
     the cloud of sequences associated with the histograms and the
     cloud of HR classes to be constructed, as well as a guiding list
     for interpreting results;
3.   A programme (7) of graphical editing of clouds, of points on the
     factorial planes selected (1 x 2, 1 x 3, etc...).
With this programme, we can obtain:
     (a) A complete editing, that is to say, we can plot all the
          points, sequences and HR classes, or
     (b) A partial editing, i.d., we can include, on the selected
     factorial plane, the HR classes only and some points of the
     sequence cloud, which are of special interest.   In both cases,
     the graph is followed by the list of multiple points, which have
     not appeared as well as their locations.
In practice, we often have to use partial editing to show the HR
variations of a subject engaged in various activity situations, or of

several subjects engaged in the same activity, etc... Partial editing is especially helpful to the user since it gives him the possiblity of viewing only the points he wants to study.

This methodology has received application, with the analysis of heart rate histograms in relation with physical activity, during sport's training and workload studies (8).

Conclusion

The Advantage of FAC for the Study of Heart Rate

The factor analysis of correspondence provides a synthetic view of the activity sequences and HR classes by presenting planar images, which are easier to read than the mean HR variation curves used up to now. Moreover, this method prompts the construction of histograms associated with situations and activities of interest to the user, which was not usually feasible.

Finally, the FAC principal advantage lies in the swiftness and flexibility of action it provides by giving the user an easy mean of establishing the relation between activity sequences and heart rates, and, if need be, the modes of other parameters characteristic of the activity.

Partial graphical editing makes it easier for him to study HR variations according to a given sub-set of activity sequences.

References

1.   Benzecri F. (1980) Introduction a l'analyse des correspondances d'apres un exemple de donnees medicales. Les cahiers de l'analyse des connees: Vol v. No. 3. p. 283-310. Dunod Paris.
2.   Benzecri J.P. (1980) Pratique de l'analyse des donnees: Analyse des correspondances. Dunod 1980.
3.   Drozdowski T. (1979) (Mona. FC) Programme de traitement du monotorage ambulatoire de la frequence caediaque a partir de l'ECG Lab. Physiologie CHU Cohin Port Royal, Paris.
4.   Fouillot J.P. Rieu M., Duvallet A., Devars J., Coquerez J.P., Klepping J. (1978) Automatic analysis of electrocardiogram long-term recording during training and daily activity events. "Sports Cardiology" international conference Rom 1978. p.231.
5.   Lebart L., Morineau A., Tabard N. (1977) Techniques de la description statistique. DUNOD Paris.
6.   Tekaia F. (1977) Programme BENTAB d'analyse factorielle des correspondances Version PDP8.
7.   Tekaia F. (1980) (Sous-Graphe) Programme d'edition d'un graphe verifiant des contraintes a partir du'un graphe construit par l'AFC.
8.   Tekaia F., Fouillot J.P., Drozdowski T., Regnard J., Speyer J.J., Rieu M. (1980) (Freq. Card) Incidence des contraintes psychique et intellectuelle sur la frequence cardiaque. Les cahiers de l'analyse des donnes, Vol. VI No. 2. Dunod Paris.

STATISTICAL PITFALLS IN COMPARING TWO MEASUREMENT TECHNIQUES

D.G. ALTMAN

There is a frequent need to compare statistically alternative methods of measuring the same quantity. Most often data such as these are analysed by means of the correlation coefficient, but this approach is totally inappropriate. The correlation coefficient is just a measure of linear association, which is something that we expect with such data. It does not assess agreement, which is what is wanted.

Regression is also used quite often, but this method too has serious drawbacks. Notably the regression slope will be underestimated, and interpretation of the coefficients is difficult.

If it is reasonable to consider that the between-method differences are reasonably constant for all values of the variable being measured, the simplest way of looking at such data is to calculate the mean and standard deviation of the between-method differences (for each individual). The mean is called the relative bias, and the standard deviation measures the relative error. Both measures are needed to describe the comparison adequately.

In the context of ambulatory monitoring this approach would be used for example to compare two automatic blood pressure measuring machines.

These ideas are discussed at length in a recent paper[1].

References

1. Altman, D.G. and Bland, J.M. Measurement in medicine: the analysis of method comparison studies. Submitted for publication.

DISCUSSION

DR. CASHMAN: Let us suppose, then, that we have all been naively doing regression analysis and getting a correlation coefficient, we also have a slope and an intersept. Does not the slope of that line provide the same information as that obtained from the differences?

MR. ALTMAN: For regression it is assumed that the x variable is measured without error. That is a fundamental assumption of regression analysis. We clearly do not have it in this sort of case. If calibration analysis is being done in which there is one very accurate measurement and something which we want to test against it, regression is a good technique. But here where, for example, we want to compare two automatic blood pressure analysers, that does not happen. They are both equally unreliable, and therefore the usual assumptions of least-squares regression do not hold. In any case, I still think that the within-subject differences are much more informative.

PROF. PINCIROLI: When data are collected, for example, dealing with blood pressure, sometimes we analyse it with a fast Fourier transform. An example of this was shown this morning in one of the slides. What is the relationship between the errors that are present in the data that I collect and the maximum resolution of my frequency spectrum that I am able to provide and to demonstrate?

MR. CROSBY: There are several contributions to the noise which will be carried over into the frequency spectrum. First, if the noise is random - what is called Gaussian noise - effectively what happens is that Gaussian noise is added across the whole spectrum.

There is another source of error which is quantisation error due to the fact that a continuous signal is looked at in discrete levels. If sufficient bits are used, the quantisation error is quite significant compared to the other factors of noise.

Of the other types of error that are found one significant one is due to sampling not fast enough. In particular, if we are looking at peaks of pressure, systolic and diastolic pressure, although there may be enough sampling by Shannon's sampling theorem to get all the required frequencies, it is possible from the data points obtained to calculate the peak values of the pressure.

A NEW DEVICE FOR RECORDING BLOOD PRESSURE SEMI-CONTINUOUSLY: ADVANTAGES AND DRAWBACKS

B. DIEBOLD, J.B. VERCKEN, P. CORVOL

Hopital Broussais, 96 rue Didot 75014, Paris, France

Introduction

Although many systems have been designed for non-invasive ambulatory monitoring of blood pressure, none has yet shown a reasonable accuracy. The aim of this study was to test the performance of a simplified system developed for semi-continuous ambulatory assessment of blood pressure.

Materials and Methods

The method is based upon the occluding cuff technique and uses the Korotkoff sounds detected by means of a piezoelectric microphone. The system is composed of two parts: a recorder and an analyser. The recorder consists of a magnetic tape unit, an inflation and deflation mechanism connected to the cuff, a pressure transducer and electronic circuits allowing adjustment of the timing and the maximum pressure of inflation, to filter and to code the pressure signal and the Korotkoff sounds detected by the microphone. The latter is positioned in front of the brachial artery and fixed to the arm skin so that it is covered by the lower part of the cuff. As this positioning is critical, it has to be tested and adjusted using earphones.

The analyser consists of a magnetic tape recorder, electronic circuits and a strip chart recorder. When the tapes are played, the pressure and sound signals are detected, a switch allowing the use of different filters for the systolic and the diastolic sounds and the information is presented on paper as shown in Figure 1. Each cycle of measurement starts with a calibration, which is of 200 or 100mmHg depending whether the apparatus has been triggered internally by its timer or externally by the patient. Then the zero of pressure is displayed followed by inflation appearing as a rapid rise of the pressure curve. Deflation corresponds to the slow fall of the pressure curve. The sounds are superimposed on to the pressure curve and appear as transients whose amplitude varies with the intensity of sound.

The pressures are read directly from the pressure curve according to the sounds. It may be preceded by pre-systolic sounds of low amplitude. The diastolic is detected after switching in filter with a cut-off frequency of 35Hz. It corresponds to the rapid decrease in amplitude of the sounds. This type of presentation and analysis of the signal allows detection of artefacts related to external sounds or muscular contraction and the low amplitude sounds due to displace-

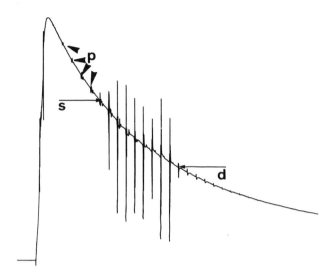

Fig. 1   Example of recording.

This study was performed to compare the values given by the apparatus to standard auscultatory measurements. For the diastolic pressure, we took the fifth phase of the Korotkoff sounds. For this purpose, the pressure circuit was connected to a mercury monometer by a T-connector so that the comparison was performed on the same arm at the same time. The evaluation was made using a series of four consecutive measurements.

Results

The results concerning the mean values of the series of four measurements are presented in Figures 2 and 3. They may be summarized as follows:

TABLE 1

		Systolic	Diastolic
Correlation coefficient	:	0.99	0.96
Slope	:	0.96	0.87
Ordinate at the origin (mmHg)	:	−0.01	6.27
Difference between the mean (mmHg)	:	6.76	6.75

These results emphasize the value of the technique as an accurate measurement of the mean pressure over a period of time. Nevertheless, if one considers separately all the measurements, the correlations are not so good as shown below and in Figures 4 and 5.

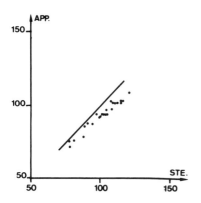

Fig. 2   Results for the
         diastolic pressures
         (mean values).

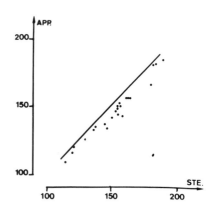

Fig. 3   Results for the
         systolic pressures
         (mean values).

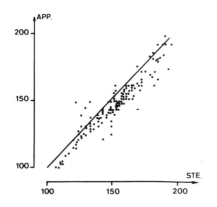

Fig. 4   Results for the
         diastolic pressures
         (all values)

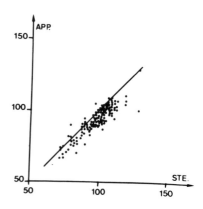

Fig. 5   Results for the
         systolic pressures
         (all values).

TABLE 2

	Systolic	Diastolic
Correlation coefficient :	0.93	0.86
Slope :	0.96	0.92
Ordinate at the origin (mmHg):	-0.92	20.24

Conclusions

The system evaluated in this study does not provide an accurate blood pressure profile with a high resolution. Nevertheless it allows a reasonable approach of the profile of mean values across the day provided the number of measurements is between three and five times the expected resolution.

REMLER M2000 SEMI-AUTOMATIC AMBULATORY BLOOD PRESSURE RECORDER

D.J. FITZGERALD, W.G. O'CALLAGHAN, K. O'MALLEY, E.O'BRIEN

The Hypertension Clinic, The Charitable Infirmary,
Jervis Street, Dublin 1
Department of Clinical Pharmacology, Royal of College Surgeons,
St. Stephen's Green, Dublin 2, Eire

Introduction

Blood pressure is highly variable and single clinic recordings may
not reflect the blood pressure status of many patients. Direct
invasive intra-arterial ambulatory monitoring has proved a useful
method of studying blood pressure behaviour, but it is not widely
applicable. Systems have been developed which record blood pressure
indirectly and which are small and light enough to be carried by the
patient. The Remler M2000 is a semi-automatic portable recorder
(Kain 1964) which consists of a cuff and microphone connected to a
pressure transducer and microcassette recorder worn on the patient's
waist. The cuff is inflated by the patient at prescribed intervals
and deflates automatically. During cuff deflation, the Korotkoff
sounds and cuff pressure are recorded on magnetic tape. A separate
decoder is used to analyse the tape and gives a strip-chart recording
of each blood pressure measurement in which the Korotkoff sounds,
superimposed on a tracing of cuff pressure, are displayed.
    In this paper, we discuss the accuracy and reliability of the
Remler M2000. Furthermore, we present our findings on the accuracy
of the London School of Hygiene Sphygmomanometer.

Accuracy of the Remler M2000

Previous studies on the accuracy of the Remler M2000 have given
conflicting results. Although accurate when compared with the standard mercury sphygmomanometer (Cowan 1980; Fong, 1979), the Remler
recordings were higher when compared with the London School of Hygiene Sphygmomanometer (LSHS) (Beevers, 1979; Fong 1979).
    We compared the Remler with the LSHS and Hawksley random zero
sphygmomanometer using simultaneous recordings in the same arm. The
Remler was first compared with the LSHS in twelve patients as part of
an inter-device variability study of three Remler recorders. Two
observers took part in the study. Paired LSHS-Remler recordings were
recorded in both arms, the two cuffs being connected to a common
inflation-deflation system. In this way, Remler recordings in opposite arms could be compared as could LSHS and Remler recordings in the
same arm. The order of machines and observers was randomised according to a Graeco-Latin square design. In the second part of the
study, the Remler was compared with the Hawksley in thirty-five

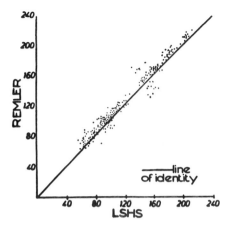

Fig. 1   Comparison of Remler
with the LSHS.

Table 1

Comparison of Remler, Hawksley and LSHS Blood Pressure Recordings

	SYSTOLIC		DIASTOLIC	
	Remler	LSHS	Remler	LSHS
N	153		153	
Mean	158.7	152.8	92.3	87.6
SD	32	30.6	13.1	12.9
Mean bias	+ 5.9		+ 4.7	
P	< 0.001		< 0.001	

	Remler	Hawksley	Remler	Hawksley
N	65		63	
Mean	159.3	159.8	99.8	99.5
SD	28.4	28	16.5	16.7
Mean bias	- 0.5		+ 0.3	
P	NS		NS	

	LSHS	Hawksley	LSHS	Hawksley
N	80		80	
Mean	133.3	140.4	82.4	86
SD	36.2	32.8	20.3	19.9
Mean bias	- 7.1		- 3.6	
P	< 0.001		< 0.001	

patients, two recordings being taken in each patient using one Remler device and one observer. All diastolic measurements were recorded at Phase V of the Korotkoff sounds.

There was no significant difference between observers or between Remler devices. The Remler recordings were higher than simultaneous LSHS recordings, (Figure 1; Table 1), the mean systolic differences being 5.9mmHg (P < 0.001) and mean diastolic difference 4.7 mmHg (P< 0001). Furthermore, the differences between the two devices were negatively correlated with heart rate both for systolic (r, - 0.24 P < 0.001) and diastolic (r, - 0.36 P < 0.001) blood pressures so that at higher heart rates the difference was less (Figure 2).

In contrast, there was no significant difference between paired Remler and Hawksley recordings which were highly correlated for systolic (r, 0.95) and diastolic (r, 0.92) blood pressures (Figure 3).

Accuracy of the LSHS

In view of these findings, we studied the accuracy of the LSHS. This is a mercury manometer incorporating special features to reduce observer bias and digit preference (Rose, 1964). When compared with a standard mercury manometer, the LSHS gave lower pressure recordings by an amount which increased with pressure so that at 200mmHg, the LSHS recorded 196mmHg. This error was found on repeated testing with two further standard mercury manometers and a second LSHS. By measuring the diameters of the reservoir and mercury column of the LSHS, this error was found to be consistent with a failure to calibrate the device for the fall of mercury in the reservoir when pressure is applied. However, the difference between the Remler and the LSHS is greater than can be explained by a calibration error alone. We therefore compared the LSHS with the Hawkesly random-zero sphygmomanometer in twenty patients with a wide range of blood pressures. The LSHS and the Hawksley random zero sphygmomanometer were connected to a single cuff through a Y-connector. Two observers recorded simultaneous recordings in the same arm using a two-channel stethescope, one recording with the LSHS and the other with the Hawksley. Four paired recordings were made in each patient and the order of observers was randomised between and within patients. Further, the observers were screened from each other to prevent manipulation of LSHS influencing the second observer. The LSHS recordings were lower than the Hawksley recordings (Table 1), the mean systolic difference being 7.1mmHg (P < 0.001) and the mean diastolic difference 3.6mmHg (P < 0.001) (Figure 4). These differences are greater than can be explained by the failure to calibrate the LSHS correctly. Furthermore, the difference between LSHS and Hawksley diastolic recordings were negatively correlated with heart rate (r, - 0.27 P < 0.02) after correction for the calibration error. This may reflect the different decision end points of the LSHS compared with the standard sphygmomanometer and the Remler M2000. As the measurement procedure with the LSHS is blind, the observer indicates systolic pressure after the first sound, often at the second sound as only at this point can the observer be certain that the systolic point has been recorded. Similarly, the diastolic end-point is indicated after the last sound, that point where a sound is expected but fails to occur. This is

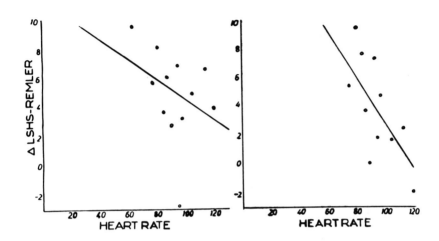

Fig. 2   Correlation between mean LSHS-Remler differences for each
          patient and heart rate for systolic (right) and diastolic
          (left) blood pressure.

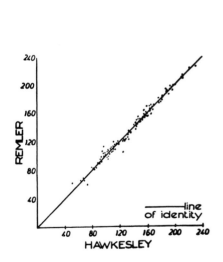

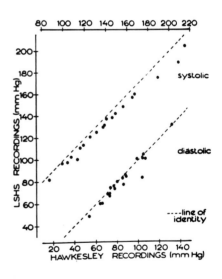

Fig. 3   Comparison of Remler
          with the Hawkesley
          random zero sphyg-
          momanometer.

Fig. 4   Comparison of mean
          LSHS and Hawkesley
          recordings in 20
          patients.

confirmed by the negative correlation between heart rate and the differences between the LSHS and the Remler recordings and between the LSHS and the Hawksley recordings.

Reliability of the Remler M2000

Reliability was tested by noting the number of undecodable recordings and their causes in all sixty-nine Remler day recordings from one of our studies. Of these, five failed totally, three because the microphone lead broke at its connection with the case and two because the machine failed to switch itself off despite normal deflation. Of the remaining 64 tapes, 1129 blood pressure recordings were attempted and 104 (9.2%) were uncodable. In thirty-five of these, no sounds were detected during recording. The remainder resulted from interference due to patient movement and incorrect settings of the inflation-deflation switches so that the machine began recording before the systolic point had been reached.

Conclusion

The Remler M2000 semi-automatic recorder was found to be accurate when compared with the Hawksley Random zero sphygmomanometer. As in previous studies (Beevers 1979; Fong 1979), the Remler gave higher recordings than the LSHS. However, the LSHS under-estimates blood pressure partly due to incorrect calibration, but also because of a difference in its decision end-points compared with other methods of blood pressure measurement. The conflicting results of previous accuracy studies reflects the different standards used for comparison and are not due to inaccuracy of the Remler M2000.

The reliability of the Remler is good but can be improved upon by improvements in the microphone-cassette connection. Frequent servicing will also prevent failure of the pressure switch.

In conclusion, the Remler M2000 is an accurate and reliable method of indirect ambulatory blood pressure recording. Furthermore, the London School of Hygiene sphygmomanometer should not be used as a reference standard in the assessment of new methods of recording blood pressure.

References

1. Kain H.K., Hinman A.T., Sokolow M. (1964) Circulation, 30, 882-892.
2. Beevers D.G., Bloxham C.A., Blackhorse C.I., Lim C.C., Watson R.D.S. (1979) Brit. Heart. J. 42, 366
3. Cowan R., Sokolow M., Perloff D. (1980) Brit. Heart J. 43, 715-6.
4. Fong P.L., Wilson L.C., Richardson E.J., O'Halloran M. (1979) Med. J. Aust. 3, 312.
5. Rose G.A., Holland W.W., Crowley B. (1964) Lancet 1, 296.
6. Malindzak G.S., Rapela C.E., Green H.D. (1968) Med. Res. Eng. 3, 39-42.

A VALIDATION OF HOME BLOOD PRESSURES, THE REMLER M2000 AND THE AVIONICS 1978 PRESSUROMETER WITH CLINIC AND INTRA-ARTERIAL AMBULATORY BLOOD PRESSURE MEASUREMENTS

B. GOULD, R. HORNUNG, H.A. KIESO, D.G. ALTMAN,
P.M.M. CASHMAN, E.B. RAFTERY

Department of Cardiology and
Divisions of Bioengineering, Clinical Chemistry,
Computing and Statistics,
Northwick Park Hospital and Clinical Research Centre,
Harrow, Middlesex, UK

Summary

Serial measurements of the blood pressure have been advised to improve precision in diagnosis of hypertension. These measurements
have been obtained either by patient recorded blood pressures or with
automated recorders such as the Remler M2000 and Avionics 1978 Pres-
sureometer. We have validated these techniques against indirect
pressures measured with the random zero sphygmomanometer and intra-
arterial blood pressures recorded with the 'Oxford System' for ambulatory monitoring. The mean discrepancy 'Home BP-Intra-arterial BP'
was 0/3 mmHg whilst for 'clinic BP-Intra-arterial BP' it was -13/1
mmHg. There was a mean error of 3/2 mmHg 'Remler-Intra-arterial
BP' and of -2/4 'Clinic BP-Remler'. There was a mean error of -2/11
mmHg 'Avionics-Intra-arterial BP' and of 3/8 mmHg 'Clinic BP-Avionics'. A wide scatter of data was found on comparing all non-invasive measurements against intra-arterial pressures. All indirect
methods over-estimated the diastolic blood pressure. Of the three
methods, patient recorded pressures showed closest agreement with
standard indirect measurements indicating that automated machines
have little advantage over self-recorded pressures.

Introduction

Numerous validations of the accuracy of indirect blood pressure
measurements compared to intra-arterial pressures(1-3) have shown a
wide range of pressure differences. The technique of serial blood
pressure measurement has been advised (4) to improve precision in
measuring blood pressure. One method of obtaining serial blood
pressure measurements is from patient-recorded pressures which may be
collected free of the anxiety associated with clinic visits. The
accuracy and reliability of patient-recorded blood pressures have
been tested by comparing these recordings with simultaneous measurements recorded by the observing physician(5,6). However, trained
observers may vary widely in their interpretations of the blood
pressure (7). To reduce observer variability, non-invasive automated
devices have been developed to measure the indirect blood pressure.
    We have evaluated patient recorded blood pressures, the Remler
M2000, and Avionics 1978 Pressurometer against clinic measurements
and against intra-arterial blood pressures.

Methods

Each method of non-invasive measurement was assessed separately.

Home Blood Pressures

Fifty-five patients with essential hypertension were recruited; 35 were on no medication. The group included 17 females, 38 males with a mean age of 51.8 years (range 23-70).

Patients attended a special session of the hypertension clinic where an indirect measurement was recorded using the Hawksley random zero spygmomanometer (Gelman Ltd). Patients were taught the technique of self-recording using a previously calibrated anaeroid gauge and standard techniques of measurement (8) but using phase V for diastolic pressure. Two other patients found difficulty in mastering the technique and did not enter the study. The patients' recordings were checked using a double-listening stethoscope but none were excluded from the study on the grounds of inaccurate recordings. Home blood pressures were recorded after five minutes' rest in the sitting position four times daily at 8-9 am, 1-2 pm, 5-7 pm, and at bedtime for ten days.

During this period intra-arterial ambulatory blood pressure monitoring was performed over two days (9) only, attending hospital at 12-hourly intervals for calibration and equipment checks. During these visits indirect recordings of the blood pressure were made by the physician using a random zero sphygmomanometer, followed by a check on the patient's technique using a double listening stethoscope.

The intra-arterial tape recording was marked with an event signal whenever an indirect reading was taken, both at home and in the hospital. Indirect measurements were made on the dominant arm and intra-arterial recordings on the contra-lateral arm. The pressure difference between the arms was assessed by two observers recording the pressure in each arm simultaneously. One random zero sphygmomanometer was connected to two blood pressure cuffs. A series of paired readings on each arm were recorded and repeated after switching the cuffs providing a total of eight paired readings.

Remler M2000

Twenty-eight patients volunteered to wear the Remler M2000 for one day in addition to the Oxford system for ambulatory intra-arterial recording. There were 7 females and 21 males with a mean age of 50 years (range 23-67). Ten patients were receiving anti-hypertensive therapy.

Simultaneous readings of intra-arterial, clinic and Remler M2000 pressures were recorded on three occasions in the hospital. The Remler M2000 was linked via a Y connector to a random zero sphygmomanometer and the clinic pressure ausculated using a standard stethoscope in the usual position. Thus simultaneous clinic and Remler pressures were recorded from the same arm whilst intra-arterial pressures were recorded on the contra-lateral arm.

Pressures were recorded hourly at home in the sitting position and the intra arterial tape was marked with an event signal.

Avionics 1978 Pressurometer

Twenty patients were recruited from those undergoing intra-arterial recording. The only difference in the protocol from that for the Remler was that a standard mercury sphygmomanometer was used in place of the random zero sphygmomanometer, which could not be used with the Avionics Pressurometer as this instrument 'searched for' the systolic pressure.

Data Analysis

A hybrid computer was used to compute hourly mean pressure values (10), and also a one minute average intra-arterial systolic diastolic pressure at each selected time marked by the event signal.

Analysis was divided into assessment of pressures recorded away from hospital and clinic pressures recorded whilst attending hospital. A system to mark events on the intra-arterial tape was added mid-way through the home blood pressure study, enabling 27 patients to have clearly identifiable event marks corresponding to the exact time they recorded their blood pressure at home. In the laboratory, event marks were initially produced by disconnecting the intra-arterial transducer from the tape-recorder for a short period immediately prior to the indirect measurement.

The analysis of the Remler and Avionics recorders followed similar lines. Three pressures were selected at random from the home recordings and the corresponding one minute mean intra-arterial pressure was found by the computer. The scope of this paper limits us to presenting data from the first of these three recordings. For each comparison the following information was calculated: mean and standard deviation of measurements by each method; mean, standard deviation and frequency distributions of between method differences. (The mean difference is referred to as the mean discrepancy). Only the lines of identity are shown on the scatter plots; regression lines and correlation coefficients are not presented. Correlation coefficients are not presented; these are a measure of association only, and by definition the different methods of recording the blood pressure must be associated. Correlation gives no measure of the agreement of the different methods of blood pressure measurement nor information on precision or accuracy, and if misused may give misleading results (11). Differences between two methods were also assessed by Student's paired (t) test.

Results

Analysis of the intra-arm difference showed that no patient had a mean difference greater than 10 mmHg and most had differences less than 5 mmHg.

In order to assess our technique of validation we took records from 28 patients and for each patient a single reading was randomly selected and compared with intra-arterial systolic peak and diastolic trough with the average intra-arterial pressure over one minute from which they were selected. The mean discrepancy was -2/2 mmHg (Table 1). The scatter plot (Fig.1) showed good agreement over a wide pressure range and the frequency distribution graph of differences

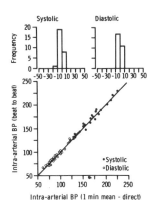

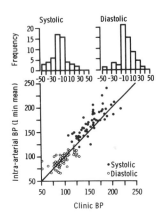

Fig. 1   Scatter plot, line of identity and frequency histogram of
(left)   intra-arterial BP (1 minute mean) – Intra-arterialBP (systo-
          lic peak and diastolic trough). Systolic – 64% within ± 4 mm
          Hg. Diastolic – 100% within ± 10 mm Hg.

Fig. 2   Scatter plot, line of identity and frequency histogram of
(right)   Clinic BP–Intra-arterial BP (1πmean).   Systolic – 36% within
          ± 10 mm Hg.   Diastolic – 65% within ± 10 mm Hg

between the methods showed that in only one of the 28 comparisons
there was a difference greater than 10 mmHg.

        Note that the frequency histogram of the between-method dif-
ferences (in this figure and all subsequent figures) has been constructed by substracting the value of the method shown on the
abscissa from the value of the method shown on the ordinate for each
patient.   In all cases the line shown on the scatter plot is the line
of identity.

Clinic Blood Pressure–Intra-arterial Blood Pressure

The mean discrepancy for this comparison was -13/1 mmHg (Table 1).
The scatter plot (Fig.2) showed that the majority of systolic points
is the above line of identity whilst the diastolic points were more
evenly distributed.

Home Blood Pressures

Blood pressures recorded by patients at home ('Home BP-Intra-arterial
BP') compared to simultaneous intra-arterial blood pressure gave a
mean discrepancy value of 0/3 mmHg (Table 1).   The plot of 'Home BP-
Intra-arterial' (Fig.3) showed a wide scatter of the points.   The
number of patients included in this analysis was limited to 27, due
to the late addition of the event marking systems.

        Comparison of the physician and patient recorded pressure (using
a double listening stethoscope and anaeroid gauge) showed generally
very good agreement with a mean discrepancy value 'Patient BP-Clinic
BP' of -2/2 mmHg (Table 1) with the scatter plot (Fig.4) showing good
agreement.

TABLE 1

Comparison of home, clinic and intra-arterial blood pressures (IABP)

	Mean	SD	Mean Diff. A-B	SD of Diff.	P	N	Fig No
SYSTOLIC							
A. IABP (1'mean)	162	28.7	-2	2.9	<0.001	28	1
B. IABP (Beat-to beat)	164	28.8					
A. Clinic BP	156	25.6	-13	16.2	<0.001	55	2
B. IABP	169	26.6					
A. Home BP	164	37.8	0	23.0	>0.9	27	3
B. IABP	164	32.6					
A. Patient BP	171	34.3	-2	5.9	>0.5	31	4
B. Clinic BP	173	35.2					
DIASTOLIC							
A. IABP (1'mean)	88	15.4	-2	2.1	<0.001	28	1
B. IABP (beat to beat)	90	15.2					
A. Clinic BP	95	17.7	1	13.0	>0.5	55	2
B. IABP	94						
A. Home BP	97	14.4	3	16.7	>0.2	27	3
B. IABP	94	16.5					
A. Patient BP	103	21.6	2	7.0	>0.1	31	4
B. Clinic BP	101	19.4					

NB. Mean values have been rounded to whole number thus difference between mean values in column one may not correspond exactly with mean difference in column 3.

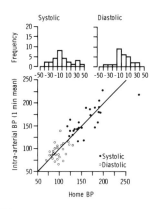 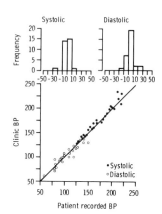

Fig. 3   Scatter plot, line of identity and frequency histogram of
(left)   Home BP–Intra-arterial BP (1πmean).   Systolic – 47% within ±
             10 mm Hg.   Diastolic – 55% within ± 10 mm Hg.
Fig. 4   Scatter plot, line of identity and frequency histogram of
(right) patient recorded BP–Clinic BP. Systolic – 93% within ± 10 mm
             Hg.   Diastolic – 83% within ± 10 mm Hg.

Remler M2000

Away from the hospital environment the mean discrepancy 'Intra-
arterial BP–Remler was 1/.2 mmHg (Table 2). The scatter plot (Fig.5)
showed wide deviation of the points from the line of identity but
diastolic points were distributed more evenly. The mean discrepancy
'Clinic BP–Remler' was -2/4 mmHg (Table 2). The plot (Fig.6) showed
modest scatter around the line of identity with the majority of
diastolic points lying below the line.

Avionics 1978 Pressurometer

The pressurometer over-estimated intra-arterial diastolic pressures
(at home) with mean discrepancy values of -2/-11 mmHg (Table 2). The
scatter plot (Fig.7) showed even distribution of the systolic points
around the line of identity but diastolic points lay above the line
of identity indicating higher Avionic diastolic pressures.
     The pressurometer over-estimated aortic pressures. Table 2
shows that the mean discrepancy of the 'Avionics presurometer BP-
Clinic BP' was 3/8 mmHg (Table 2). The scatter plot (Fig.8) showed
fairly close grouping but there were 2 systolic and 3 diastolic
points which deviated widely.

Discussion

The use of home blood pressure recording is increasingly being
advocated(5,6) but the accuracy of this method of recording has been
subjected to limited validation as have the Remler M2000 and Avionics
1978 Pressurometer. None of these methods has been assessed for

TABLE 2

Comparison of Remler M2000, Avionics 1978 Pressurometer and intra-arterial blood pressure

	Mean	SD	Mean Diff. A-B	SD of Diff.	P	N	Fig. No.
SYSTOLIC							
A. IABP	159	31.2	−1	15.5	>0.5	28	5
B. Remler	158	32.6					
A. Clinic BP	163	27.8	−2	9.9	>0.05	28	6
B. Remler	163	30.3					
A. IABP	148	25.7	−2	15.9	>0.05	18	7
B. Avionics	150	28.0					
A. Clinic BP	165	28.2	3	12.6	>0.1	18	8
B. Avionics	162	32.3					
DIASTOLIC							
A. IABP	93	22.4	2	11.6	>0.2	28	5
B. Remler	92	17.8					
A. Clinic BP	99	15.6	4	5.9	<0.001	28	6
B. Remler	95	14.1					
A. IABP	88	17.6	−11	12.3	<0.01	18	7
B. Avionics	99	18.1					
A. Clinic BP	102	13.2	8	18.3	>0.05	18	8
B. Avionics							
94	16.9						

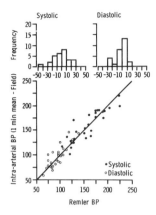
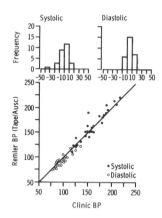

Fig. 5   Scatter plot, line of identity and frequency histogram of
(left)   Remler M2000-Intra-arterial BP.   Systolic – 54% within ± 10
          mm Hg.   Diastolic – 78% within ± 10 mm Hg

Fig. 6   Scatter plot, line of identity and frequency histogram Clinic
(right)   BP-Remler M2000.   Systolic – 75% within ± 10 mm Hg.   Dia-
          stolic – 75% within ± 10 mm Hg.

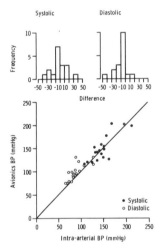
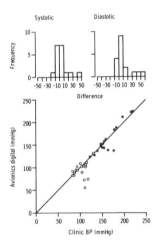

Fig. 7   Scatter plot, line of identity and frequency histogram of
(left)   Intra-arterial BP-Avionics BP.   Systolic – 56% within ± 10 mm
          Hg.   Diastolic – 61% within ± 10 mm Hg.

Fig. 8   Scatter plot, line of identity and frequency histogram of
(right)   Clinic BP-Avionics BP.   Systolic – 78% within ± 10 mm Hg.
          Diastolic – 72% within ± 10 mm Hg.

accuracy away from the hospital environment.

Because it would be difficult (if not impossible) to compare indirect with direct measurements away from hospital on a precise beat-by-beat basis we used one-minute averages of intra-arterial systolic and diastolic pressures for comparison with simultaneous indirect readings. Our results indicated that the one-minute average is a reliable estimate of intra-arterial blood pressure provided the patient is at rest preceding and during the measurement.

Home blood pressures have been assessed for accuracy in other studies only after excluding patients who were unable to read the blood pressures to within 5 mmHg of the observing physician during simultaneous auscultation. In our study no patients were excluded.

The most marked finding was the wide scatter of data on the scatter plots and frequency histograms when comparing indirect and intra-arterial blood pressures, with occasional individual differences up to 50 mmHg being recorded. The comparison of standard indirect clinic pressures and the other indirect methods showed fair agreement, the best being for the home recorded pressures. Similar close association ws reported by Joosens et al (12) who reported a mean discrepancy 'Physician-Home BP' of 0.19/-4 mmHg. Julius et al (5) reported a discrepancy of 3/-7 mmHg and Laughlin et al (13) reported a discrepancy of 11/5 mmHg.

Our data also showed close agreement between patient and clinic pressures with a mean difference of -2/2 mmHg and standard deviation about the mean discrepancy of 5.9/7.0 mmHg. Whilst there ws also good agreement for mean discrepancy 'Home-Intra-arterial BP' of 0/3 mmHg. This belies the wide individual mean differences which is better reflected by the standard deviation about the mean discrepancy of 23.0/16.7 mmHg.

The findings with the 'Remler-Clinic BP' comparison were closer than that reported by Beevers et al (14) but not nearly as good as that reported by Cowan et al (15). Discrepancy values in those studies were 8.3/8.1 mmHg and 0.06/0.24 mmHg respectively. In our study the mean difference of 'Clinic-Remler' was -2/4 mmHg with a standard deviation of 9.9/5.9 which compares favourably with the same comparison for home blood pressures. There was better agreement with intra-arterial blood pressures with less scatter as shown by the standard deviation about the mean discrepancy of 15.5/11.6 mmHg. The 'Avionics-Clinic BP' comparison as assessed by Harshfield et al (16) gave a discrepancy of 2/2 mmHg at rest whilst our study found a difference of 3/8 mmHg with a standard deviation about the mean discrepancy of 12.6/18.3 mmHg.

In conclusion, these data have demonstrated that indirect methods give estimates of intra-arterial pressure which may be inaccurate and that indirect diastolic pressures can seriously overestimate intra-arterial pressures. Of the three methods the home recorded pressures showed closest agreement with standard indirect pressures indicating that automated machines provide little advantage over home recorded blood pressures. However, comparison of indirect methods of monitoring and intra-arterial pressure showed wide individual mean differences for home blood presures with similar scatter for Remler and Avionics recorders. All indirect ambulatory methods are subject to the same constraints as clinic pressures. The variable nature of these pressures make indirect ambulatory methods an inappropriate method for assessing blood pressure variability. An accurate indirect method of ambulatory blood pressure recording remains to be described.

References

1. Regan C., Bordley J.(1941), Bull John Hopkins Hosp **69**: 504-528
2. Holland W.W., Humerfeld S. (1964), Brit.Med J.**2**, 1241-1243.
3. Raftery E.B., Ward A.P. (1968), Cardiovasc.Res.**2**, 210-218.
4. Dunne J.F. (1969), Lancet **1**, 391-392.
5. Julius S., Ellis C.N., Paseaul A.V., Matice M., Hansson L., Hunyor S.N., Sandler L.N. (1974), J.Am.Med.Assoc. **229**, 663-666.
6. Laughlin K.D., Fisher L., Sherrard D.J. (1979), Am. Heart J. **98**, 629-634.
7. Wilcox J. (1962), J.Am.Med.Assoc. **179**, 53.
8. Kirkendall W.M., Burton A.C., Epstein F.H., Freis, E.D. (1967), Circulation **36**, 980-988.
9. Millar-Craig M.W., Hawes D., Whittington J. (1978), Med.Biol.Eng & Comput. **16**, 727-731.
10. Cashman P.M.M., Stott F.D., Millar-Craig M.W. (1979), Med. & Biol.Eng. & Comput. **17**, 629-635.
11. Altman D.G. (1980), Brit.Med.J. **2**, 1473-1475.
12. Joossens J.V., Brems-Heyns E., Claessens J. (1974), In: Commission of the European Communities Biological Sciences - Medical Research. Methodology and standardisation of non-invasive blood pressure measurement in epidemiological studies. Proceeding of a workshop in Leuven (Belgium), Edited by Kesteloof W.
13. Laughlin K.D., Sherrard D.J., Fisher L. (1980), J. Chron.Dis. **33**, 197-206.
14. Beevers D.G., Lim C.C., Badhouse C.I., Watson R.D.S., Bloxham C.A. (1980), Proceedings of 3rd International Symposium on Ambulatory Monitoring. Ed. Stott F.D., Raftery E.B., Goulding, L. Academic Press, 223-233.
15. Cowan R.M., Sokalow M., Perloff D. (1980), Proceedings of 3rd International Symposium on Ambulatory Monitoring. Ed. Stott F.D., Raftery E.B., Goulding L., Academic Press, 241-247.
16. Harshfield G.A., Pickering T.G., Laugh J.H. (1979), Ambulatory Electro-Cardiology **1**, 7-12.

COMPARISON BETWEEN AN INDIRECT AND A DIRECT METHOD OF AMBULATORY BLOOD PRESSURE MONITORING

P. PALATINI, A.C. PESSINA, G. SPERTI, P. MORMINO,
V. AGNOLETTO, E. VENTURA, A. SEMPLICINI AND C. DAL PALÙ

Istituto di Medicina Clinica - Cattedra di Clinica Medica 2
University of Padua

Summary

To assess the validity of the Del Mar Avionics Pressurometer III ambulatory ECG and blood pressure recording system, eleven non-obese hypertensive patients were concomitantly studied with the Pressurometer and with the intra-arterial Oxford system.
    During the day, the correlations between the readings given by the two techniques were, in all but one patient, statistically significant for both systolic and diastolic blood pressure. During the night a poor correlation was found. Despite this limitation, the Del Mar Avionics system seems sufficiently reliable and therefore useful for clinical trials. Furthermore, because of its safety it can be widely and repeatedly applied.

Introduction

The validity of the Oxford system for continuous blood pressure monitoring is well established (1, 2, 3). During the last 5 years, we have been using this technique for studying spontaneous blood pressure variability and the response to various pressor tests in borderline and established hypertension (4, 5). It has, however, the limitation that it involves putting a catheter in the radial or brachial artery, and therefore, is not easily acceptable by the patient and requires specially trained personnel. For these reasons, a non-invasive method for monitoring blood pressure seems preferable.
    In this paper, we assess the validity of one of such methods, the Del Mar Avionics Pressurometer III Blood Pressure Recording System.

Materials and Methods

The study was conducted in 11 non-obese mild hypertensive in-patients. Before starting the continuous blood pressure monitoring with the invasive Oxford system on one arm and the Pressurometer III system on the other, blood pressure was measured on each arm with a Riva-Rocci sphygmomanometer.
    The Del Mar Avionics Pressurometer III ambulatory recorder operates at preset intervals by automatic inflations and deflations of a cuff (6). It is portable and consists of a Pressurometer with a solid state memory, an auscultatory cuff and microphone and a 3-lead electrode system for recording heart rate. Once the Pressurometer is in operation, it is possible to verify through a specially designed

valve whether the blood pressure readings through the microphone are the same as those through the stethoscope. In our study, blood pressure was measured at 7.5 minutes' intervals. On the opposite arm, blood pressure was continuously monitored by the Oxford method described in previous studies (4, 5). The blood pressure values obtained with the Pressurometer every 7.5 minutes were compared with those concomitantly recorded by the Oxford system. In order to do so, the patient was requested to keep the arm still and to press the Event Marker of the Oxford system when the cuff of the Pressurometer started to deflate. The Event Marker was obviously pressed only during the day, while during the night the detection of the 7.5 minutes interval on the Oxford tapes was obtained starting from the last marker pressed before sleep.

The minitapes recorded with the Oxford system were automatically analysed as previously described (5) and the means of the blood pressure values obtained during the 20 seconds following the signal of the Event Marker were compared wioth the single values given by the Pressurometer.

The Bravet Pearson r correlation coefficient wAs used. Only levels of 0.5 or less were considered as statistically significant.

Results

Table 1 summarises the average number of blood pressure readings recorded in our 11 patients by the Pressurometer III. 7% of these readings were eliminated by a microcomputer because they were grossly incorrect. Another 2.8% were considered unreliable because they were outside the individual's trend pattern and were not included in the final analysis. Two correlation matrixes for both day and night were automatically calculated for each patient: each one of ten variables was matched against all the others.

Table 1

Average Number of Readings given by the Pressurometer III[o]

Average No. Readings in 24 hr.	% Automatically Excluded Readings	% Readings Outside the Trend	Average Number Reliable Readings		
			Day	Night	24 hr
187	7.0	2.8	120	49.2	169.2

In the correlation matrix shown in Table 2, it can be seen that the blood pressure recorded by the Pressurometer III correlates almost equally with the mean of the systolic and diastolic blood pressures recorded over 20 seconds and with the Minimum and Maximum Systolic and diastolic blood pressures recorded during these same periods.

Table 3 shows the correlation coefficients between the blood pressures obtained with the Pressurometer III and those obtained with the Oxford system for each subject during the day. Systolic blood pressure correlates in all but one patient at the 0.001 probability level, while diastolic blood pressure correlates at a lower level,

TABLE 2

CORRELATION MATRIX

	1	2	3	4	5	6	7	8	9	10
1 SBP P3	1.00									
2 DBP P3	0.67	1.00								
3 HR P3	0.72	0.59	1.00							
4 SBP OX	→0.78	0.67	0.77	1.00						
5 DBP OX	0.71 →0.64		0.75	0.92	1.00					
6 HR OX	0.69	0.55	0.84	0.81	0.81	1.00				
7 MxSBP OX	→0.78	0.68	0.78	0.97	0.91	0.81	1.00			
8 MnSBP OX	→0.74	0.64	0.71	0.95	0.86	0.75	0.90	1.00		
9 MxDBP OX	0.71 →0.61		0.73	0.89	0.97	0.80	0.92	0.80	1.00	
10 MnDBP OX	0.65 →0.62		0.67	0.85	0.94	0.74	0.83	0.86	0.87	1.00

Table 3

Correlation coefficients between Pressurometer III° and Oxford System
Readings During the Day

PATIENT	READINGS	SPB	DBP	HR
1 M.Z.	96	0.78***	0.64***	0.84***
2 A.B.	121	0.18	0.54***	0.66***
3 F.S.	108	0.52***	0.37***	0.67***
4 M.L.	97	0.51***	0.52***	0.60***
5 C.F.	86	0.47***	0.24*	0.63***
6 M.D.	108	0.70***	0.63***	0.63***
7 L.B.	125	0.51***	0.40***	0.62***
8 G.C.	119	0.43***	0.25***	0.36***
9 A.C.	27	0.62***	0.32	0.54**
10 S.P.	128	0.37***	0.64***	0.74***
11 N.C.	115	0.52***	0.42***	0.42***

SBP = Systolic blood pressure   DBP = Diastolic blood pressure
HR = Heart rate   Readings = Total number of readings
  *p<0.05   ** p<0.01   *** p<0.001

level, while diastolic blood pressure correlates at a lower level,
which, however, is still significant in ten patients. Contrary to
the results obtained during the day, the correlations found during
the night are in most cases not significant, particularly for
diastolic blood pressure, where in one patient, there even is a
negative correlation (Table 4). During the night, heart rate also
shows poor correlation.

Table 4

Correlation coefficients between Pressurometer III° and Oxford
System Readings During the Night

PATIENT		READINGS	SBP	DPB	HR
1	M.Z	22	0.53**	0.24	0.39
2	A.B.	53	0.31*	0.15	-0.05
3	F.S.	39	0.08	0.13	0.22
4	M.L.	50	0.24	-0.31*	0.20
5	C.F.	41	0.18	0.08	0.36*
6	M.D.	65	0.41***	-0.02	0.26*
7	L.B.	51	0.27	0.47***	0.31*
8	G.C.	8	0.55	-0.08	0.55
9	A.C	48	0.75***	-0.02	0.59***
10	S.P.	54	0.47***	0.22	0.30*

Footnotes as in Table 3

Discussion

The Purpose of this study was to assess the validity of the Del Mar
Avionics Pressurometer III system against the intra-arterial Oxford
system. Only non-obese subjects were chosen because, in our experience, the Pressurometer III is not reliable in people with big
arms.
        The main object of our trial was to assess whether there was
agreement between blood pressure values given by the   Pressurometer
III and those given by the Oxford system. A significant correlation
was found during the day for both systolic and diastolic blood pressures although it is lower than that found by some other Authors, who
limited this comparison to a much shorter period of time (6, 7). On
the contrary, a low and even negative correlation was found during
the night, suggesting that the Pressurometer III does not operate
correctly during sleep, when the microphone can easily be displaced.
        As for the analysis of the data, the choice of the 20 seconds
periods in the intra-arterial tracings for the comparison with
indirect readings, is an arbitrary one. This choice, however, was
proved not to be incorrect by the results given by the correlation
matrixes, where it clearly appears that indirect blood pressure
correlates equally with the mean and with the Minimum and the Maximum
of the pressure values recorded during the 20 seconds periods.
        In agreement with other Authors (6, 8) we can conclude that the
Del Mar Avionics Pressurometer III provides reliable blood pressure
readings during the day, while during sleep it is not sufficiently
accurate. Despite these limitations, it appears of useful application, especially for monitoring hypotensive therapy since, contrary
to the direct method, it causes only minor discomfort to the patient
and therefore can be repeatedly applied.

References

1. Littler W.A., Honour A.J., Sleight P and Stott F.D. (1972). Br.Med. J. 3 76.
2. Goldberg A.D., Raftery E.B., Green H.L. (1976). Postgraduate Med. J. 52 Suppl. 7, 104.
3. Raftery E.B. (1978) Br. J. Clin. Pharm. 6, 193.
4. Palatini P., Pessina A.C., Ardigo'A., Veronese P. and Dal Paulu C. (1977). Boll. Soc. It. Cardiol. 22, 1477.
5. Pessina A.C., Palatini P., Semplicini A., Mormino P., Casiglia E., Hlede M. and Dal Palu' C. (1980) Biotelemetry Patient Monitg. 7, 96.
6. Harshfield G.A., Pickering T.G. and Laragh J.H. (1979). Ambulatory Electrocardiology 1, 4, 7.
7. Hunyor S.N., Flynn J.M. and Cochineas C. (1978). Br. Med. J. 2,15.
8. Kennedy H.L., Padgett N.E. and Horan M.J. (1979). Ambulatory Electrocardiology 1, 4, 13.

HOW TO IDENTIFY CUFF-RESPONDERS;
CONTRIBUTION OF ARTERIOSONDE, CASUAL AND HOME BLOOD PRESSURE WITH CONTINUOUS INTRA-ARTERIAL REGISTRATION AT HOME AS REFERENCE

G.A. VAN MONTFRANS, C.A. GRIMBERGEN, M. POS, C. BORST AND
A.J. DUNNING

University Hospital of Amsterdam and Medical Physics
Laboratory, University of Amsterdam

Summary

We investigated the contribution of Arteriosonde, casual and home
blood pressure measurements to the identification of "cuff
responders" - subjects showing a pressor reaction evoked by the
measurement itself - in 14 patients with mild hypertension without
signs of organ damage or non-compliance. On clinical grounds, patients were classified as "cuff-responders" (8) and hypertensives (6).
Mean age was 40 years. Twelve patients were on treatment for about
five years. Investigations were done 5 weeks after having stopped
the treatment.
    Intra-arterial pressure recorded with the Oxford-Medilog system
at home while the patients were watching television or reading,
served as reference. Patients with a normal intra-arterial pressure
were subsequently classified as true "cuff-responders" (7); those
with high intra-arterial pressures as true hypertensives (6).
    From the 8 predicted "cuff-responders", 4 were true "cuff-
responders" and 4 had under-treated hypertension. From the 6
predicted hypertensives, 3 were true "cuff-responders", 2 true hypertensives and 1 patient was neither "cuff-responder" nor hypertensive,
as he had a markedly higher indirect pressure as compared to direct
measurement.
    Stopping treatment, Arteriosonde and home measurements all con-
tributed in part to the correct diagnosis. Stopping treatment alone
was diagnostic in the true hypertensives; the three methods together
were necessary to identify the true "cuff-responders".
    In 4 patients, home readings proved to evoke even more stress
than casual measurements.
    As a result, in 9 of the 14 patients, management was drastically
changed.

Introduction

As long as blood pressure is measured, we know that certain people
find this procedure very stressful. Pickering (1) pointed out how
well the concept of the curiosity reflex, or its exaggeration the
defence reflex, known from animal physiology, explains this universal
human behaviour. Most doctors are familiar with the patient whose
initial high blood pressure becomes normal on subsequent measurements. In the Charlottesville blood pressure survey (2) of 12,371
adults screened for hypertension, 20% had a high blood pressure on

first screening;   after repeated measurements only 9% was still hypertensive, while in 11%, blood pressure fell to normal. These people were called "labile hypertensives". Most certainly, defence reactions were to a great extent responsible for this observation. Perhaps it is more appropriate to call them "cuff-responders", as this term better describes the underlying mechanisms.

While many people need more than two visits to have these reflexes extinguished, others never become habituated to clinic sur-roundings and the doctor's dilemma whether to stop or increase medi-cation is clear. Various approaches have been suggested to eliminate the doctor as principal stimulus to the defence reaction. Home blood pressure readings have proved their value in a number of studies (3) - (6).

However, patients may be biased just as doctors and a high pressure at home does not discriminate between true hypertension or persisting defence reactions.

The Arteriosonde is an example of a reliable automatic cuff method (7) (8). However, this type of registration has serious disadvantages.   Subjects are completely restricted in their activity and they are still within the hospital environment. The level of physical activity greatly influences arterial pressure and variabili-ty (9) and, therefore, the question remains whether Arteriosonde readings are truly representative.

Continuous intra-arterial ambulatory registration with the Oxford-Medilog system clearly is the most reliable method to identify cuff-responders, but its invasive character and complicated technology restricts its use to a few centres.

In this study, we investigated how cuff-responders could be identified best with various non-invasive measurement methods. We co}pared the contribution of home blood pressure readings, Arteriosonde and clinic pressure taken by nurses in a group of presumed cuff-responders and hypertensives to the eventual diagnosis, which was based on continuous intra-arterial registration at home.

Patients and Methods

Fourteen patients with mild hypertension were selected from the general out-patient department, 12 male, 2 female, with an average age of 40 years (28-57 years). Twelve patients were on treatment for about 5 years. Two were known with repeated elevated pressures for more than 9 months and had been referred to the hospital recently.

Hypertension was defined as a blood pressure higher than 160/100mmHg on three separate occasions. Causes for secondary hyper-tension were ruled out by clinical examination, measurement of creat-inine, electrolytes and excretion urography or renography.

Patients with evidence of target organ involvement were ex-cluded, defined as history or signs of ischemic heart disease or peripheral vascular disease; left ventricular hypertrophy on the ECG or a cor/thorax ratio larger than 50%; impaired renal function and/or proteinuria; retinal changes greater than grade 2 Keith-Wagener classification.

All patients were tested for absence of Hb_{sAg}.

On clinical criteria, patients were divided by the referring

physician in cuff-responders and hypertensives. Selection criteria suggesting the former were one or more of the following:
1.   When being treated for more than 1 year, persistently elevated blood pressure without signs of non-compliance, as judged by the referring physician.
2.   Inconsistent Arteriosonde readings, sometimes low, or discrepancy with clinic pressure.
3.   Striking nervous disposition or stressful social conditions, as judged by the referring physician.

According to these criteria, 8 patients were classified as cuff-responders, most with more than one criterion; their blood pressure was 131/101mmHg. The other 6 patients were considered as having mild hypertension; their blood pressure was 137/93mmHg. No patients had marked left/right arm blood pressure differences.

The nature and purpose of the study were explained and consent obtained. The investigations were approved by the hospital ethics committee.

Continuous ambulatory intra-arterial pressure

Five weeks after having stopped treatment, continuous ambulatory intra-arterial blood pressure was recorded with the Oxford-Medilog system, which does not need to be described here. Arterial cannulation was performed in the left brachial artery. Nine patients left the hospital to do their normal jobs, 5 patients had taken the day off. All slept at home. Activities were noted in a diary and marked with an event-marker on the tape, with special attention to periods spent "sitting at home".

Calibrations were applied in the afternoon and the following morning. The temperature of the measuring amplifier in the recorder was measured with a built-in thermistor. When calibration prior to the cannulation was done at 30° recorder temperature, changes on subsequent calibrations did not exceed 3°. In our systems, a temperature change of 1° caused 1mmHg zero drift.

Tapes were replayed at 25 times recording speed and written out on an Elema paper recorder.

Five- minute blood pressure samples of the whole registration were analysed manually, with adjustments for zero drift.

As clinic pressure is taken under more or less standardized conditions - patients awake and sitting - we took as the "reference" intra-arterial pressure at home periods when patients were watching television or reading, as indicated by their notes and marks on the tape. Duration of these periods varied; most patients did not remain seated for more than 45 minutes. We therefore selected, if possible, 45 minutes of leisure in the afternoon and in the evening. These 90 minutes were averaged to give the :"intra-arterial pressure at home".

Because of damping, 2 patients had recorded only 10 and 15 minutes of quiet sitting; however, it was evident how variability decreased within minutes once subjects stopped moving around.

Patients were then divided into two groups; those with a reference intra-arterial pressure lower thanb 140/90mmHg were called true cuff-responders. The others were diagnosed as true hypertensives.

Home Blood Pressure Measurements

Detailed instruction was given on the use of the Speidel-Keller aneroid manometer. This instrument has a conventional stethoscope diaphragm built in the cuff. After 2 hours' training, patients did not differ more than 4mmHg with the investigator. Diastolic pressure was determined on phase 5. Technique was checked on repeat visits. Patients took their pressure twice a day during $\pm$ 6 weeks. Readings of the last 2 weeks - 5 weeks after having stopped treatment - were averaged and presented as "home blood pressure".

Arteriosonde

The Arteriosonde 1216 was used. Before removal of the arterial cannula, a 1-hour registration was done with 5-minute measurement intervals, which were averaged.

Clinic Pressure

All clinic pressures were taken with the Random-Zero sphygmomanometer. Two treated anf three untreated measurements were taken by the same nurse and invgstigator in a random order.

Statistics

Significance between different measurement methods were tested for true cuff-responders and true hypertensives with the paired Student's t-test. P-values > 0.05 were considered insignificant.

Results

Table 1 shows prediction on clinical grounds and outcome, based on continuous intra-arterial pressure when quietly sitting at home in 14 patients.

Table 1

Prediction		Outcome		
		Cuff Responder	Hypertension	Cuff Hypertension
Cuff Responder	8	4	4	-
Hypertensionn	6	3	2	Arm 29 cm.
Total	14	7	6	1

Table 2 shows results of the various measurement methods of the true cuff-responders.
Table 3 gives the findings in the true hypertensives.

TABLE 2

TRUE CUFF-RESPONDERS, Home, Arteriosonde, casual and continuous bloodpressure untreated

patients no	age	sex	prediction	treatment in years	Oxford seated at home S	D	Home BP S	D	Arteriosonde 1217 S	D	HT-clinic BP S	D	difference untreated-treated HT-clinic S	D
1	42	M	CR	3	129.5	84	142	92	157	116	171	97	+10	-3
2	47	M	HT	7	121	78	137	95	137	81	138	87	+11	+1
3	57	M	CR	1	131	78	141	95	136	90	125	92	+15	+20
4	46	M	CR	1	145	86	132	92	112.5	87	140	89	-10	-13
5	28	F	HT	10	129	75	119	78.5	118	74	129	92	-4	-1
6	38	M	HT	-	137	80	144	90.5	133	87	136	82		
7	33	M	CR	-	125.5	76.5	141	90	136	82	144	88		
MEAN	41.5 (28-57)			3.8 (3/4-10)	131	80	137	90.5	131	88	140	89.5	+4.4	+0.8
SEM					±2.9	1.5	3.2	2.1	5.4	5.0	5.6	1.7	5.3	6.0

Of the 8 predicted cuff-responders, 4 patients were diagnosed as true cuff-responders (patients no. 1, 3, 4 and 7). Predicted cuff-responders no. 8, 9, 10 and 11, turned out to be true hypertensives. Of the 6 predicted hypertensives, 3 patients were to mutual surprise true cuff-responders (nos. 2, 5 and 6; Table 2). Two patients had a correctly predicted true hypertension (no. 12 and 13).

One patient with an arm circumference of 29 cm had a marked difference between simultaneous direct and indirect blood pressure measurements. Therefore, he simply had "cuff-hypertension"/ He had been on treatment for six years. Consequently, he was excluded from further analysis.

Figure 1 shows means ± SEM of the 7 true cuff-responders and 6 true hypertensives for treated and untreated clinic pressure, home readings, Arteriosonde and intra-arterial pressure at home.

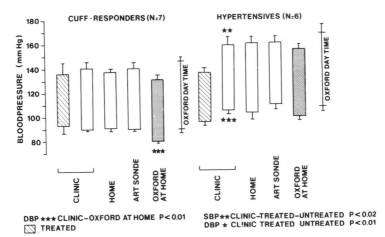

DBP ★★★ CLINIC-OXFORD AT HOME P<0.01   SBP★★CLINIC-TREATED-UNTREATED P<0.02
▨ TREATED   DBP ★ CLINIC TREATED UNTREATED P<0.01

Fig. 1   Means ± SEM of clinic, home, Arteriosonde and intra-arterial continuous pressure at home in 7 true cuff – responders and 6 true hypertensive patients.

When comparisons were made between the various methods without treatment, for the true cuffresponders only clinic diastolic pressure differed significantly from intraarterial pressure at home: 89.5 ± 1.7 and 80 ± 1.5mmHg respectiely, p < 0.001.

After stopping treatment in the 5 treated true cuffresponders, blood pressure did not change significantly: from 136/93 ± 8.9/6.5 to 140/91 ± 8.0/1.6mmHg.   Mean daytime pressure, averaged for all waking hours, was 146/90 ± 3.3/2.9mmHg.

Differences between untreated clinic, home, Arteriosonde and intraarterial pressures at home in the 6 true hypertensive patients were all insigificant.   However, 5 weeks after having stopped treatment, blood pressure rose in 5 patients from 136.5/95 ± 3.6/3.7mmHg to 161/108 ± 8.0/2.9mmHg.   Their mean daytime average was 169/108 ± 1.03/3.6mmHg.

Comparison of these various group measurements clearly

TABLE 3.

TRUE HYPERTENSIVES - Home, Arteriosonde, casual and continuous blood pressure untreated

patients no	age	sex	pre-diction	treatment years	Oxford cont-inous seated at home		Home BP		Arterio-sonde 1217		HT-clinic BP		Difference untreated-treated HT-clinic	
					S	D	S	D	S	D	S	D	S	D
8	34	M	CR	3	141	104	154	115.5	159	114	152	109	+13.5	+11
9	45	F	CR	12	171	94	181	116	185	117	188.5	117	+47.5	+20
10	44	M	CR	2	164	110	165	101	187	111	169	108	+25	+3
11	28	M	CR	4	145	87	142	80.5	152	91	149	95	–	–
12	33	F	HT	12	156	105.5	149	106	143	107	143	99	+20	+17
13	50	M	HT	1/3	160	100	169	87	164	117	153	105	+17	+11
MEAN: 39 (28-50)				5.5 (1/3-12)	156	100	160.5	103	160.5	109.5	159	105.5	+24.6	+12.4
SEM				±	4.7	3.3	5.9	5.3	5.7	4.0	6.8	3.1	6.7	3.2

demonstrated certain trends, but the small sample size and the wide ranges did not allow definition of useful probability limits.

Therefore to evaluate the contribution of the various non-invasive measurement methods to the eventual diagnosis in individual patients, data were analysed per patient (Tables 2 and 3).   The value of each measurement method was scrutinized and called either "misleading" or "diagnostic".   Results of this exercise are given in Table 4.

Stopping Treatment

In 2 treated true cuffresponders, pressure remained at the same hypertensive level after stopping treatment.   Hence, discrimination from true noncompliant hypertensive patients remained impossible. Therefore, in these 2 cases stopping treatment was called misleading. Other possibilities followed similar considerations.   In all true hypertensives pressure rose markedly after stopping treatment, as could be expected.   This was obviously diagnostic.

In some true cuffresponders presure decreased after stopping treatment; in patient no. 4 this finding was called diagnostic; in patient no. 5, misleading, as her pressure was still in the borderline range and previous noncompliance could not be ruled out.

Results in Table 4 refer to the 10 analysed patients who were being treated before the study started.

Home Blood Pressure

When home readings were substantially higher than intraarterial pressures, systolic blood pressure and/or diastolic blood pressure > 20/10mmHg, especially when clinic pressures were lower, home readings were not considered to have diagnostic value and were thus called misleading.   This was the case in patients no. 2, 3, 6 and 7, all true cuffresponders.   In all other patients, this method yielded useful information.

Arteriosonde

In 2 true cuffresponders, these registrations gave conflicting results; 1 patient fell asleep and produced a very low, clearly unrepresentative result (patient no. 4).   Patient no. 1 showed a marked reaction while connected to the machine.   In all other patients, results were in line with intraarterial pressures at home.

Patient no. 6 had normal clinic and Arteriosonde pressures; he was a predicted hypertensive, with a blood pressure of 147/98mmHg averaged for 3 visits before he was included in the study.   His results demonstrate the value of repeated measurements, although here pressure fell only after 6 months.   It was of interest that pressure dropped markedly in V5-10 minutes after connectin to the machine in true cuffresponders no. 2, 3, 6 and 7, the same patients who had elevated home pressures.   In all other patients, pressure decreased more gradually or not at all.

Comparison of clinical pressures between nurse and investigator did not add any information; averages for all patients, treated or untreated or according to groups, were correlating very well.

All patients: 144/95 ± 3.6/2.1mmHg investigator's readings;
144/98 ± 3.5/2.1mmHg measured by the nurse.   Systolic blood pressure
r = 0.95, p < 0.001; diastolic blood pressure r = 0.88, p < 0.001.
The clinical relevance of these results is also shown in Table
4.   Obviously, consequences for further management were in line with
the findings.   The patient with the cuff-hypertension was left out,
but of course his treatment was stopped.

Table 4

Contribution of non-invasive measurements to eventual outcome and
clinical relevance, in 13 patients

	Misleading	Diagnostic	Relevance	to treatment	
				Stop	Increase	No Change
Stop treatment	2	8	Stop CR(8) 3	3	2
Home BP	4	9	HT(5) 2	0	3
Arteriosonde	2	11	total(13) 5	3	5

Reliability of home blood pressure determination

Eight patients managed to record simultaneously their blood pressure
at home with the Speidel-Keller on the right arm while having the
arterial cannula in the left arm.
Figure 2 shows results for systolic pressures with the line of
identity.

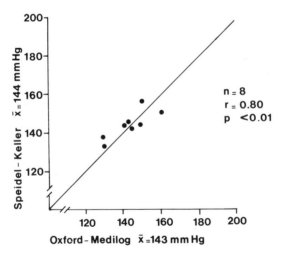

Fig. 2   Simultaneous measurements of indirect and direct systolic
blood pressure with the Speidel-Keller aneroid manometer
and the Oxford Medilog system.

For systolic pressures a very significant correlation was found: r = 80, p < 0.001.   Correlation for diastolic pressures was not so good: r = 0.65, 0.05 < p < 01.   In 3 patients who had 10mmHg or more higher diastolic pressures with the home readings compared to the intra-arterial "reference" pressure, simultaneous measurements with these two methods showed only a 2.1mmHg higher diastolic pressure of the Speidel-Keller compared to the Oxford-Medilog system.   Because of the scatter, we found no constant measuring error between the Speidel-Keller method and intra-arterial pressure.

With the Random-Zero meter consistently lower systolic pressures were measured compared to intra-arterial pressure with the Oxford-Medilog system on simultaneous measurements.   Random-Zero systolic pressure in 9 patients: 143 ± 6.9 versus 156 ± 6.8mmHg with the Oxford-Medilog system.   There was a highly significant correlation: r = 0.97, p< 0.001.

Discussion

The quantitative relationship between arterial pressure amd morbidity is appreciated, but, as is commonly agreed, management of the individual hypertensive patient needs an arbitrarily chosen dividing line.   Controversy stems from this wish to classify patients, for example, the matter of "labile" hypertension.   According to the WHO classification (10), labile hypertensives are subjects in whom arterial pressure oscillates around 140/90mmHg.   The term "labile" implies that these people have a greater blood pressure variability than normotensives.   In fact, great variability probably hs nothing to do with this condition; variability increases with height of arterial pressure and physical activity.   Systolic variability increases with progressive impairment of sino-aortic baroreflexes, diastolic variability with plasma-norepinephrine levels (9).   The WHO definition of "labile" hypertension is often used to indicate people who have a high initial pressure and lower readings on subsequent measurements, which is a common finding in population screening studies (11).   We feel that the majority of these labile hypertensives are more appropriately called "cuff responders", a term that exactly describes the responsible physiological mechanisms.

Arterial pressure varies widely with the circumstances of measurement; the common curiosity or defence reflex tends to diminish by repeated measurements. (12).

According to the 1980 recommendatins of the Joint National Committee (13), two diastolic readings of 90mmHg or more on successive examinations confirm the diagnosis of hypertension.   The Charlottesville survey results imply, in our opinion, that more than two readings are better practice; there is no justification to rush to a diagnosis of mild hypertension based on only two elevated clinic pressures with all practical consequences.

As shown by our small study, stopping treatment, Arteriosonde an home readings all contributed in part to a correct diagnosis of "cuff responder" or true hypertension in a group of subjects who either were difficult to control or were for other reasons suspected to react on blood pressure measurement.   Patients took this home reading very seriously and it was of interest to find a substantial number getting markedly stressed during this daily exercise, even after more than a month's practice.

On the other hand, there were cases where the physician ws misled by the patient's behaviour, resulting in clear under-treatment. Finally, when a patient with mild hypertension is a suspected "cuff responder", the first step to take is to withdraw all medication. When doubt remains, home readings together with an automatic cuff method, should give the correct diagnosis. Continuous intra-arterial ambulatory registration may still have a place when all non-invasive methods fail to discriminate, but it is felt that this will be a rare finding.

References

1   Pickering G: High Blood Pressure (1968); 2nd ed. New York, Grune and Stratton.

2.   Carey R.M., Reid R.A., Ayers C.R., Lynch S.S., McLain III W.L., (1976) JAMA **236**, 847.

3.   Freis E.D. The discrepancy between home and office recordings of pressure in patients under treatment with pentapoyrroidinium; importance of home recordings in adjusting dosages. (1954), Med. Ann. District of Columbia **XXIII**, 363.

4.   Ayman D., Goldshine A.D. (1940) Am. J. Med. Sci. **200**, 465.

5.   Laughlin D.K., Fisher L., Sherrard D.J. (1979) Am. Heart J., **98**, 629.

6.   Julius S., Ellis C.N., Pascual A.V., Matice M., Hansson L., Hunyor S.N., Sandler L.N. (1974) JAMA., **229**, 663.

7.   George C.F., Lewis P.J., Petrie A. (1975) Br. Heart J., **37**, 804.

8.   Hochberg H.M., Salomon H. (1971) Curr. Ther. Res. **13**, 129.

9.   Watson R.D.S., Stallard T.J., Flinn R.M., Littler W.A. (1980) Hypertension, **2**, 333.

10. Brod J., Hilleboc H.E., Kimura N. et al. Arterial hypertension ischemic heart disease: preventative aspects; report of an ex-pert committee. (1961) WHO Techn. Rep. Service, **3**.

11. Carey R.M., Ayers C.R. (1976) Am. J. Med., **61**, 811.

12. Pickering G. (1978) Am. J. Med. **65**, 561.

13. Report on the Joint National Committee on the Detection, Evaluation and Treatment of High Blood Pressure; a co-operative study, (19/7) **237**, 255.

DIFFERENCES BETWEEN CUFF AND DIRECT AMBULATORY BLOOD PRESSURES IN PATIENTS WITH ESSENTIAL HYPERTENSION

J.S. FLORAS, J.V. JONES, M.O. HASSAN, B.A. OSIKOWSKA,
P.S. SEVER, P. SLEIGHT

Department of Cardiovascular Medicine,
John Radcliffe Hospital, Oxford, and
Department of Clinical Pharmacology, St.Mary's Hospital, London, UK

Summary

Clinic cuff blood pressures, obtained on at least three occasions, were compared with mean arterial pressures in 59 patients with essential hypertension who underwent direct ambulatory monitoring of blood pressure. Cuff pressures were, on the whole, significantly higher and by more than 10mmHg mean arterial pressure in more than half of the patients. This latter group could not be otherwise identified by clinical examination, indices of sympathetic nerve activity, blood pressure variability or by recorded pressure rises during physical and mental exercise. They had less evidence of cardiovascular complications from hypertension and had better baroreflex sensitivity. The integrated blood pressure load, measured by ambulatory monitoring, bears greater relationship to the cardiovascular complications of hypertension than do cuff readings, which may be falsely high.

Introduction

The risks of developing cardiovascular complications of hypertension should be highest amongst those patients whose blood pressures are consistently elevated throughout the day and night (1). It is difficult to assess the pressure load on the circulation, integrated over time, from the limited number of measurements from a series of clinic visits, especially as these cuff measurements may be erroneous. To this end, some patients and their families have been instructed in home blood pressure recording (2) , (5); others have undergone continuous direct ambulatory monitoring of blood pressure (6), (7). Home blood pressures have been consistently lower than clinic pressures in some hypertensive patients, but there seems to be no way of distinguishing this subgroup from the others on clinical (3) or psychological criteria (5). Sokolow and his co-workers (8) noted that the ambulatory blood pressure, obtained with a semiautomatic recording device, was more consistently related to the presence and extent of target organ damage than were clinic cuff blood pressures, particularly in borderline hypertension. With this apparatus, movement is limited and only a minute portion of the day's blood pressure can be recorded. A marked discrepancy between clinic and direct ambulatory monitored blood pressure has been noted in some patients during 24-hour monitoring of blood pressure (7), (9). We propose to investigate this difference further.

Methods : Patient Selection

General practitioners referred patients to our clinic for the investigation of hypertension. Cuff blood pressures of 140/90mmHg or
greater were obtained on at least three occasions in all patients;
in a few cases, blood pressure readings below 140/90 were also noted.
The patients were examined clinically by two of us (JVJ, PS) for
retinal changes (10), and left ventricular hypertrophy, either by
standard voltage criteria on the electrocardiogram (11), or by an
increased cardiothoracic ratio on the chest radiograph (12).
Secondary hypertension was excluded by the appropriate investigations. The nature of the proposed study was explained to all patients and informed consent was obtained. The protocol was approved
by the Ethics Committee of the Hospital.

Fifty-nine patients (43 men and 16 women) agreed to participate.
Their mean age was 45.6 years (S.D. 11.3, range 16-69). All patients
had essential hypertension.

Protocol

A teflon cannula 11 cm long (Seldicath) was inserted percutaneously
into the left brachial artery under local anaesthesia. The arterial
catheter was connected to a strain gauge transducer (Statham P23 Gb)
and blood pressure was recorded from this simultaneously on to magnetic tape and directly into a minicomputer (Data General Eclipse S-
200). A second cannula (Medicut) was inserted into an adjacent
antecubital vein.

Blood pressure and heart rate were recorded before, during and
after mental arithmetic (subtraction of serial 7's from 300) and a
submaximal bicycle exercise (5 minutes at 50 watts, 5 minutes at 75
watts). Beat-to-beat blood pressure and pulse interval during these
procedures were calculated by the computer. In 44 of these 59 patients, 10 ml of venous blood was obtained before (after 15 minutes of
quiet rest) and in the last minute of bicycle exercise. After 10
minutes of centrifugation, the plasma was drawn off and frozen in
liquid nitrogen at approximately- 40°C. Plasma noradrenaline concentrations were determined from these samples by a modification of the
radioenzymatic method of Henry et al (13).

Baroreflex sensitivity was assessed in each of these patients
according to the method of Gribbin et al (14). A small amount of
phenylephrine (40 ug to 100 ug), an alpha-adrenergic agonist with no
direct cardiac effects, was injected intravenously and the slope of
the line relating the pulse interval to the systolic blood pressure
during the rise (ms/mmHg) was used as an index of baroreflex sensitivity.

Between 4 to 6 injections were given to each individual and a
weighted mean slope calculated for each patient (15).

The patients then underwent direct arterial recording of blood
pressure with the Oxford Medilog System (6,16). A digital watch and
a voice recorder were supplied and patients were asked to keep an
accurate log of their activities. A 24-hour period was spent away
from hospital, except for a brief visit in the evening for recalibration of the pressure transducer, refilling of the perfusion reservoir and flushing of the arterial line.

   The 24-hour record was replayed into the mini-computer from the
cassette (Oxford Instruments Replay Unit) at 25 times real time. The
60 Hz crystal time marker on one channel of the Medilog unit was
monitored at replay to ensure tape speed accuracy. The blood pressure signal was sampled by an analogue-to-digital converter and
dumped on to disc buffers in 8-hour samples. The input was displayed
on an oscilloscope and validated by a trained operator, who was able
to interrogate the disc buffer at variable speeds. This allowed for
editing of any damped pulses or pulse wave artefact from the record.
Edited data and analyzed data were stored separately on a secondary
disc (17). A frequency histogram, describing the mean and standard
deviation of all mean arterial pressure measurements during the
waking period, was obtained for each patient with an indication of
the percentage of edited beats eliminated (Figure 1).

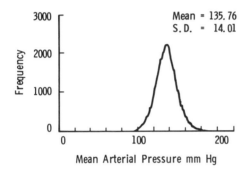

Fig. 1   Frequency histogram of all waking pressures, showing mean
          of mean arterial blood pressure, and its standard deviation
          in one patient.

Results

Cuff Pressures

The arithmetic means of systolic and diastolic cuff blood pressures
obtained on the clinic visits were calculated for each patient.
From these values an average mean arterial pressure (mean diastolic
plus 1/3 (mean systolic - mean diastolic) was derived. These mean
cuff blood pressures ranged from 99.7 to 162.3mmHg (Mean 129.1, S.D.
11.5).

Ambulatory Pressures

The average ambulatory mean arterial pressure for each patient was
derived from the frequency histogram for his waking period only.
These values ranged from 89.5 to 159.5mmHg (mean 119.1, S.D.
17.8mmHg). Mean ambulatory blood pressures ranged from 14.3mmHg mean
arterial pressure higher than the cuff readings to 41.7mmHg mean
arterial pressure lower. The overall difference between cuff and
ambulatory mean blood pressure{ 10mmHg, was significant (P<0.001)
(Figure 2).

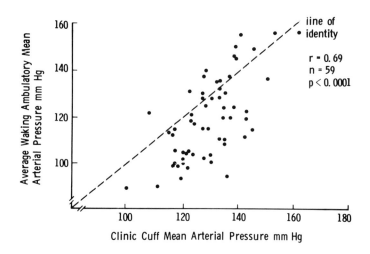

Fig. 2   Comparison of intra-arterial v. cuff mean arterial pressures.

In 22 patients (37%) ambulatory mean arterial pressure accurately reflected cuff mean arterial pressure to within ±10mmHg (Group 1). In 32 patients (54%) cuff mean pressures exceeded mean ambulatory blood pressures by more than 10mmHg (Group II). Twenty of these 32 patients in fact had ambulatory mean blood pressures of less than 108mmHg (i.e., equivalent to less than 140/90mmHg) despite elevated cuff readings. In the remaining 5 patients (9%) the mean ambulatory blood pressure was in fact greater than the clinic cuff pressures by 10mmHg or more (Group III).

Comparison of Sub-groups

Groups I and II were compared (Table 1).Although clinic cuff mean arterial pressures were identical in the two groups (131.9 ± 11.7mmHg v. 127.1 ± 11.1mmHg), the mean waking intra-arterial blood pressure was significantly higher in Group I (131.7 ± 13.2mmHG v. 107.0 ± 10.9mmHg, p<0.0001). The groups were otherwise similar in age and resting heart rate.
Bicycle exercise increased mean arterial pressure more than mental arithmetic in both subgroups. This difference was not as

Table 1

n	Group I 22	Group II 32	p
Cuff mean arterial pressure (mmHg)	131.9 ± 11.7	127.1 ± 11.1	n.s.
Ambulatory mean arterial pressure (mm Hg)	131.7 ± 13.21	107.0 ± 10.9	0.001
Age (years)	47.1 ± 11.7	75.0 ± 11.3	n.s.
Resting heart rate (bpm)	73.4 ± 11.2	75.0 ± 12.4	n.s.
Variability (S.D.) of mean arterial pressure (mm Hg)	14.8 ± 2.7	13.5 ± 2.6	n.s.
Baroreflex sensitivity (ms/mm Hg)	5.64 ± 3.08	10.06 ± 9.59	0.02
Evidence of end-organ damage	15 (64%)	6 (19%)	0.001

pronounced in the discordant group (II) but was nonetheless significant (29.8 ± 12mmHg v. 24.0 ± 10.5mmHg, p<0.05). Mental arithmetic
provoked a similar rise in each group (26.5 ± 10.4mmHg v. 24. ±
10.5mmHg, n.s.), but bicycle exercise evoked a greater increase in
mean arterial pressure in those patients who showed a good correlation between cuff and ambulatory blood pressures (36.1 ± 12.4mmHg v.
29.8 ± 12.3mmHg, p<0.001).

Plasma noradrenaline concentrations in Group I and II were
similar at rest (685 ± 282 pg/ml v. 623 ± 192 pg/ml) in the sitting
position and during bicycling (1143 ± 400 pg/ml v.1146 ± 521 pg/ml).

The standard deviation around the mean of the frequency histogram for waking mean arterial pressure was used as an index of blood
pressure variability (18). This was similar in both groups of subjects (14.8 ± 2.7mmHg v. 13.5 ± 2.6 mmHg.)(Table 1).

Baroreflex sensitivity was lower in those patients who had
good correspondence between cuff and ambulatory blood pressures
(5.636 ± 3.084 ms/mmHg v. 10.057 ± 9.587 ms/mmHg, p<0.02).

In Group I, in whom the high clinic pressures persisted during
the waking portion of the 24 hour record, 15 patients (64%) exhibited
one or more of Grade II fundal changes, or left ventricular hypertrophy by voltage on the electrocardiogram or chest radiograph. In
contrast, only 6 (19%) of the patients in Group II showed these
changes (p<0.001 x^2) (Table 1). Four out of the five patients in
Group III showed such changes.

Discussion

The distinction between patients whose cuff pressures accurately reflected their ambulatory records (Group I) and those in whom a significant discrepancy exists (Group II) could not be made on clinical criteria. They were of similar age and clinic cuff blood pressures, but the ambulatory mean arterial pressure was 25mmHg lower in Group II. The patients in Group II had no evidence of greater sympathetic activity as their resting heart rates and plasma noradrenaline concentrations were identical; nor could they be called more "reactive" to stimuli. The increase in mean arterial pressure during mental arithmetic and bicycle exercise was in fact lower in Group II and plasma noradrenaline concentration was identical in the two groups during bicycling. Evidence for increased 'lability' of blood pressure was also absent; the beat-to-beat variability (or standard deviation) was slightly lower in these subjects. The patients with good correlation between their cuff and ambulatory mean pressures showed more retinal and cardiac changes. The lower baroreflex sensitivity seen in the patients in Group I is consistent with their high ambulatory mean arterial pressures (14). The integrated blood pressure load, as measured by ambulatory monitoring, bore a greater relationship to the cardiovascular complications of hypertension than did the clinic cuff readings.

Differences between clinic and home blood pressure records have been noted previously (2) (5). In one study, this applied only to patients with borderline hypertension, and not to normal subjects (3). Lower pressures obtained from a semiautomatic portable indirect recorder appear to be related to a smaller risk of cardiovascular disease (8), but with this device measurements were taken at half-hourly intervals under essentially resting conditions and might not reflect the full range of beat-to-beat variation of blood pressure during physical activity and exercise in these subjects. Littler et al (9) noted a discrepancy between indirect clinic pressures and ambulatory records in eight treated patients with hypertension, but the individuals were selected for study because their indirect pressure readings seemed inappropriately high when considered against a general absence of target organ damage; in the same study, a good correlation was observed between intra-arterial blood pressures and cuff pressures as obtained by the general practitioner or in the hospital setting in unselected, untreated subjects with hypertension. Thus, the reason for the discrepancy between cuff and ambulatory readings is not clear from these data. Although the hypothesis of an 'alerting response' or 'defence reaction' towards the clinic setting in some of these patients is attractive, there appeared to be no evidence of increased reactivity in these patients in the laboratory. Perhaps their psychological reaction to the stress of day-to-day events is somehow different, but this cannot be ascertained from these data.

Some of these subjects may have exhibited a difference between simultaneous cuff and intra-arterial blood pressure measurements, although this was not formally studied. Raftery and Ward (19) found good agreement between direct and indirect measurement taken simultaneously from the same limb, but noted that a single indirect reading might be as much as 18mmHg higher, or 30mmHg lower than the direct one. This difference seems unrelated to arm circumference (20).

The ambulatory record thus provides additional information, but in turn poses a clinical dilemma: in 20 out of the 59 patients, all of whom fulfilled the conventional definition of hypertension, the average mean arterial pressure through the waking day was less than 108mmHg (i.e. equivalent to 140/90mmHg) and even lower during sleep, when the average mean arterial pressure fell approximately 25% from waking levels. Should these patients be classified as borderline hypertensives and treated, or as 'pre-hypertensive', or as normal, to be followed closely? This information cannot be related to epidemiological studies which have used either basal or casual cuff blood pressures to estimate the risk of developing the complications of hypertension (21), (22).

References

1. Folkow B., (1978) Clin. Sci. Mol. Med. **55**, 3s–22s.
2. Ayman D., Goldshine A.D., (1940) Am.J. Med. Sci. **200**, 465–474.
3. Julius S., Ellis E.N., Pascual A.V. et al (1974) JAMA **229**, 663–666.
4. Editorial. (1975) Lancet **1**, 259–260.
5. Laughlin K.D., Sherrard D.J., Fisher L. (1980) J.Chron. Dis. **33**, 197–206.
6. Littler W.A., Honour A.J., Sleight P., Stott F.D. (1972) Br. Med.J **3**, 76–78.
7. Millar-Craig M.W., Bishop C.N., Raftery E.B. (1978) Lancet **1**, 795–797.
8. Sokolow M., Werdegar D., Kain H.K., Hinman A.T. (1966) Circulation **34**, 279–289.
9. Littler W.A., Honour A.J., Pugsley D.J., Sleight P. (1975) Circulation **34** 1101–1106.
10. Keith N.H., Wagener H.P., Barker N.W. (1939) Am. J. Med. Sci.**197**, 332–343.
11. McPhie J. (1958) Aust. Ann. Med. **7**, 317–27..
12. Ungerleider H.E., Gubner R. (1942) Amer. Heart J. **24**, 494–510..
13. Henry D.P., Starman B.J., Johnston D.G., Williams R.H. (1975) Life Sci. **16**, 375–384.
14. Gribbin B., Pickering T.G., Sleight P. (1971) Circulation Research **29**, 424–431.
15. Floras J.S., Hassan M.O., Jones J.V. et al. In: Arterial baroreceptors and hypertension, ed. by Sleight P. Oxford University Press, 1980, 470–475.
16. Stott F.D. In: Blood Pressure Variability, ed. by Clement D.L., Lancaster, MTP Press, 1979, 55–60.
17. Sleight P., Floras J.S., Jones J.V. Automatic analysis of continuous intra-arterial blood pressure recordings. Ibid.61–66.
18. Watson R.D., Stallard T.J., Flinn R.M., Littler W.A. (1980) Hypertension **2**, 333–341.
19. Raftery E.G., Ward A.P. (1968) Cardiovasc. Research, **2**, 210–218.
20. Nielsen P.E., Janniche H., (1974) Acta. Med. Scand. **195** 403–409.
21. Kannel W.B. (1974) Progress Cardiovasc. Dis. **17**, 5–24.
22. Smirk F.H., Veale A.M.O., Alstead R.K. (1959) New Zealand Med.J. **58**, 711–755.

AUTOMATIC AMBULATORY NON-INVASIVE BLOOD PRESURE RECORDING METHOD, METHODOLOGY, CLINICAL APPLICATIONS

J.M. MALLION, R. DE GAUDEMARIS, P. VILLEMAIN *,
H. DAVER*, J.L. DEBRU*, G. CAU

*Laboratoire d'Application de la Micro-informatique
(L.A.M.I.) de l'Universite Scientifique et Medicale
de Grenoble, France

Summary

The authors report the consistency and reliability of BP values as measured by an instrument, which performs automatic ambulatory BP measurements. The clinical applications of the instrument are described, and the practical applications of the method to diagnosis, therapy and prognosis are studied.

They conclude that this method of ambulatory BP measurements should lead to a re-thinking of our definition of hypertension, which has been based on resting measurements until now. They also point out the possiblity of studying what can be referred to as blood pressure load.

Introduction

The study of ambulatory blood pressure (BP) has already proven itself both for the determination of physiological circadian BP variations in normotensive subjects, and for the differentiation of different population types of hypertensive subjects.

Until now, these measures could only be performed by invasive methods, so that their use was limited by the constraints and risks to the patients.

The possibility of an ambulatory non-invasive BP recording method should increase investigative possibilities, provided the method used gives reliable and reproducible results.

We present a method of ambulatory BP recordings measured with a new automatic device (Del Mar Avionics Ambulatory Pressurometer II System).

Apparatus

(1) Avionics apparatus consisting of:

 - A standard sphygmomanometric cuff coupled with a flexible microphonic sensor applied over the humeral artery.

 - An arterial manometer, 1977 model, weighing 1.5 Kg, worn over the shoulder, with:

        A electro-pneumatic pump for cuff inflation, which can be activated at pre-selected time-intervals, or by manual switching.

        An electronic unit.

        A liquid crystal digital display for systolic blood

pressure (SBP) and diastolic blood pressure (DBP) values in mmHg.

A re-chargeable nickel cadmium battery pack.

- A two-channel band electro-cardio recorder, model 446A, weighing 750 g and fastened to the patient's belt, hooked up to the sphygmomanometer as well as to 3 or 5 electrodes placed on the patient's chest. The instrument records SBP values, DBP values as well as ECG leads.

- A dynamic electro-cardiographic scanner, model 640 A comprising:

An oscilloscope, which displays the ECG leads (by a Holter system) as well as the heart rate (HR) variations

A digital display for: * time clock
                       * arrhythmias
                       * heart rate (QRS/mn)
                       * SBP and DBP valuers

A printer, which not only registers the preceding data on graph paper (1 mm = 1 min), but also automatically plots 2 separate curves: HR vs time curve and an ST depression vs time curve.

2. A Computerized Readout Data Processing System Consisting of:

- A micro-computer Apple II Plus, with two disc memory units, one print out and one video.

- An interface chart: composed of electronic components permitting the connection between the Avionics unit and the microprocessor.

- An assembly of floppy discs for storage of individual BP and HR values for further comparative statistical studies.

Consistency and Reliability of the Measurements

This study was carried out on 28 normotensive subjects, 13 during physical activity and 15 during normal activity (ambulatory).

There is no significant difference between values recorded man-

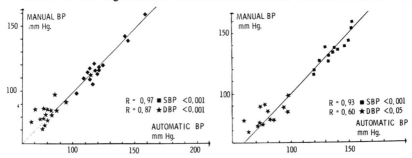

Fig. 1   Correlation between averages of 12 ambulatory measurements
(left)   on 15 subjects by manual and automatic methods.

Fig. 2   Correlation between average BP values for 13 subjects, at
(right) rest and under physical stress, using manual and automatic
         methods.

ually and those recorded by the automatic procedure (Figures 1 and 2)There is statistically significant correlation between the manual and the automatic values for all measurements.

For each subject considered separately, the correlation coefficients are not all of the same order of magnitude, and do not all have the same significance. However, overall, the values obtained by the two methods correlate well.

Reliability studies show that only 3.4% of the 672 ambulatory measures are aberrant. The values, during stress testing, particularly the DBP values, become aberrant for HR greater than 150.

Functioning of the System and Expression of the Results

1. BP Measurement

SBP and DBP values are analysed by the microphonic sensor to the nearest mm of Hg. The captor detects Korotkow sounds during a preset time period and will only register those sounds synchronized with the "R" wave on the ECG.

This method has its limitations. The subject must cease all activity and let his arm hang loosely by his side during the BP measurements. The subject's co-operation and the necessity for perfect positioning of the microphonic captor are the two imperative conditions for meaningful recordings.

2. Display of the Results

The computer printout records:
(a) All the SBP and DBP values as well as the time and HR corresponding to each value.
(b) A BP vs time profile, where time is plotted on the abcissa (hours) and BP on the ordinate (mmHG). Each BP value is drawn as a vertical line whose length is proportional to the differential BP (Figure 3).
(c) A histogram expressing those BP measurements within a pre-

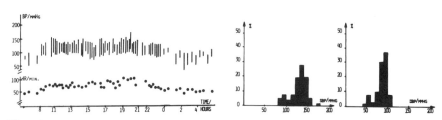

Fig. 3   Variation in blood pressure and heart rate throughout
(left)   24-hour period in normotensive subject in activity.

Fig. 4   Same subject : SBP and DBP expressed as % histograms.
(right)

determined range. These are plotted as a percentage of the total
number of measurement. Two separate graphs are drawn, one for the DBP
and one for the SBP. The abcissa represents the BP, the ordinate represents the percentage. Columns representing the calculated percentage are drawn for every 10 mmHg (Figure 4).
(d) A histogram expressing work-load vs time: during the first
step, the mean resting SBP is established over the first 15 minutes
with the subject in a sitting position away from any physical or
psychological stress. The computer then calculates the difference
between the resting SBP and the mean SBP during successive predetermined time intervals (Figure 5). The results are displayed on a
histogram: calculated difference vs time.

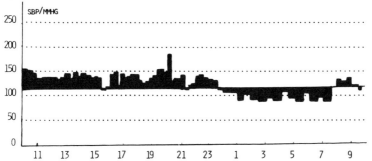

Fig. 5   Variations in SBP throughout 24 hours, relative to resting
value (120 mmHg), in normotensive subject.

Practical Applications

This method of automatic ambulatory BP measurement has diagnostic,
prognostic and therapeutic implications.

A. Diagnostic Implications

Ambulatory BP study allows a better diagnostic approach by
recognizing those subjects, who are not necessarily hypertensive, and
differentiating them from the others.
(a) Hyperemotive Subjects: Sometimes, certain emotive subjects
even after an extended period of time in the supine position are not
in a state of true relaxation. The ambulatory BP recording away from
the stressful atmosphere of the physician's office, allows a more
accurate evaluation of the BP and HR values. Figure 6 illustrates
the case of a subject, whose BP and HR values are abnormally high,
only during physical examination.
(b) Hyperkinetic Subjects: Measurement of the ambulatory HR of
these subjects throughout the day, demonstrates the constantly
elevated HR, even outside of any stressful situation. In this case,
elevated BP values are not necessarily abnormal considering the
increase HR values (Figure 7).
(c) True Hypertensive Subjects: The recorded ambulatory values
show that at whatever time of the day the measurements are made and
no matter what the stress situation is, the BP values are constantly
higher than the norm, whereas the HR is variable (Figure 8).

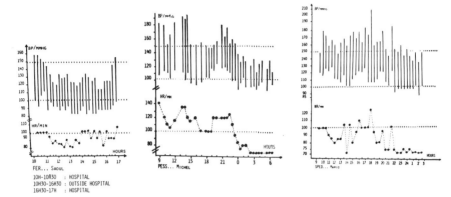

Fig. 6 (left)   Blood pressure profile in hyperemotive subject.
Fig. 7 (centre) Blood pressure profile in hyperkinetic subject.
Fig. 8 (right) Blood pressure profile in true hypertensive.

B.   Prognostic Implications

Ambulatory BP measurements allow the study of an activity pressure profile as well as blood pressure load versus time.

It can be considered that a subject has a high BP load, if his BP values are elevated over a prolonged period during the day. It is clear that those subjects, who have an elevated BP at rest, generally have the largest BP loads. But similar loads can be seen in normotensive subjects at rest, who repeatedly are under stress. In the long run, we consider that such a BP load is not without cardiovascular effects.

Figure 9 shows the magnitude of the BP load of a switchboard operator while at work. The recording performed at rest enables us to determine that this subject is not hypertensive.

C.   Therapeutic Implications

The effectiveness of any hypotensive treatment is generally evaluated during successive measurements of resting BP (measured while the patient is either supine or standing). Sometimes occasional measurements are taken by the physician or the subject himself. Standardized stress-testing enables us to measure the BP variations and the cardiovascular adaptation to a work load.

However, none of these techniques allows us to determine whether or not the treatment is effective throughout the day, what variations occur when the subject is under stress, or what is the most appropriate medication schedule, e.g. the effectiveness of once a day medication as compared to a multi-dose schedule.

For example, it would be interesting to study the therapeutic implications of the ambulatory treatment method on a series of hypertensive subjects recorded over 24 hours, before treatment and after treatment with Metoprolol (SELOKEN, Servier Lab., 1 tablet=100mg) prescribed either twice a day (100mg at 7 and 19H) or once a day

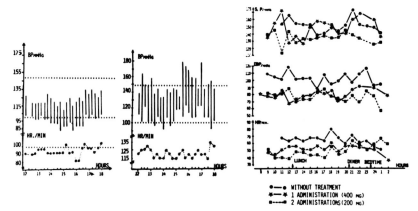

Fig.9 (left and centre) Blood pressure load in a switchboard operator, in hospital and at work.

Fig.10 (right)   Variation of DBP with time in predominantly
diastolic hypertension: effect of treatment.

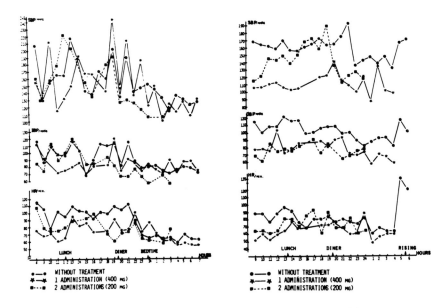

Fig. 11 (left)   Effect of treatment on hyperkinetic subject.
Fig. 12 (right) Effect of treatment on predominantly systolic hypertension.

(a) Therapeutic Effectiveness Throughout the Day:
Figure 10 shows the variation of the DBP with time in a 51-year cleaning lady presenting a predominantly diastolic hypertension.The values after treatment are always lower than the values before treatment. This is the case, whatever the treatment protocol, and over long periods of standardized time intervals. This could be predicted by the resting values.

Figure 11 concerns a 18-year old hyperkinetic hypertensive physiotherapist. The effectiveness of treament is beyond doubt, beneficial to the resting SBP. However, under stress, the BP values vary greatly and the pressure load is not modified by treatment. Resting BP alone would not reveal this information. Indeed, it seems that this subject is truly at rest only at night; true HR and BP values do not differ whether or not the subject is under treatment.

B. The Possibility of Real Chronotherapy:
Epidemiological studies point out that patient compliance varies inversely with the number of times the medication must be taken during the day. Ideally, a-once-a-day medication would be desirable, provided this decreased dosage schedule does not produce a decrease in the effectiveness of the medication.

Figure 12 shows that the hypotensive effect seems to be identical whatever the dosage schedule. However, slightly higher BP values are observed from 21.00 hours, on with a single dose schedule. This observation is, however, not noted in all subjects (Figure 10).

Figure 12 shows the BP values of 27-year old nurse presenting a predominantly systolic hypertension. The decrease in BP values is smaller when the dosage schedule is twice a day; we note an "escape phenomenon" beginning at the 8th-9th hour, precisely when this woman has important house-work to do.

The results given by these examples show the arbitrary character of the BP measurements, which are taken most often in a totally random fashion, at different moments of the day, from one consultation to the other and of course at rest.

A prescription must take into account at what time meals are eaten. It should also take into account the type of stress that the subject undergoes and at what time of the day it occurs.

Finally, in order to judge the hypotensive effect of a medication, it would be important to check BP values only at those times of the day determined to be important with respect to the time of ingestion of the medication and the daily activity of the patient.

PANEL DISCUSSION

DR. S. MANN: One of the first things we should do is to grasp this nettle of the correlation coefficient and any other mathematical indices that we might want to use for comparing two methods of measuring blood pressure. We heard the objections from Mr. Altman this morning.

The problem is, that if we do not accept it what easily understood method is left to decide whether two methods agree or not? There must be some method whereby the accuracy of different machines can be compared.

MR. ALTMAN: Because a method is simple and gives a nice answer it does not mean that it should be used. Dr. Gould's paper was rather complicated because it is not easy to reduce the answers to a single number. But if I had to choose a single quantity, I would choose the standard deviation of the differences within subjects between the methods being compared.

A further point which I did not make this morning is that when two methods are being compared with a correlation coefficient, this is very largely influenced by the variability of the measurement between subjects. The importance of this is that because systolic pressures vary more between subjects than do the diastolic pressures, there are always higher correlations between systolic pressures than between diastolic pressures. This has been demonstrated in about four papers presented this afternoon. I suspect that the low correlations in heart rate could be due just to a small amount of variability in heart rate between subjects, or within subjects in the Italan paper.

With regard to Dr. Sperti's paper, it seems to me that the lack of correlation at night-time within one subject is a pure statistical artefact, because the blood pressure would scarcely be changing, and therefore, there will be a whole lot of pairs of values where both methods may, or may not, be agreeing. Because the blood pressure is not changing no correlation will be observed.

DR. BALASUBRAMANIAN: We are measuring intra-arterial blood pressure by the Oxford Medilog system. Is there anything better with which to compare this? It was clear from Dr. Gould's paper that most of the lack of correlation occurred at the higher end of the curve where the blood pressure was above about 200mmHg.

DR. GOULD: In fact, if our data are studied carefully, while I accept that at the top end of the scale, there was quite a wide scatter of the data, in fact that also happened all the way through.

DR. HUNYOR: Several groups have presented calibration data, and the earlier feared lack of linearity of the system does not appear to be present in practice. Certainly, all our calibration curves are highly linear and reproducible. Having standardized or allowed for voltage fluctuation, and having corrected for it, we do not find the sigmoid sort of calibration curve that should be described according to the original characteristics of the system.

DR. van MONTFRANS: ...as long as we remain between 50 and 250mmHg - that is the range.

DR. GOULD: Once we start to get much over 250mm, that is getting beyond the region of accuracy.

DR. HUNYOR: A number of papers compared resting readings with resting readings under ideal circumstances, comparing indirect methods in which the cuff and the pick-up are known to be subject to movement with exercise. The Northwick Park group was one of the few groups seriously to address itself to trying to grapple with the situation during activity and during movement. We are comparing various groups of patients.

No one has mentioned the possibility of auscultatory gaps. Where the indirect methods are looking for the appearance of sounds and the disappearance of sounds, how do these methods handle the question of the silent gap (or auscultatory gap)?

I was very surprised at the total lack of heart rate correlation between two methods. I would return to something mentioned at the beginning of the day, something about which I am slightly chauvinistic. Those of us who are using continuous direct intra-arterial monitoring (I have identified at least 8 groups here today) need to find out whether our method is as good as we think it is. The front end of the system, the hydraulics, the frequency response characteristics and similar things have been well-documented. We know their limitations and their degree of accuracy. Our analysis techniques, however, is a different matter. None of us knows the accuracy of our analysis techniques. It has been looked at visevis these other standards, mainly at rest, but there is no real basis of comparison. I would like us to be able to analyse and assess blood pressure from the direct system to a degree of accuracy, which would allow us to come back in ISAM 83 and say that the method is accurate.

THE DISSOCIATION BETWEEN BLOOD PRESSURE AND HEART RATE CHANGES PRIOR TO WAKING

M.W. MILLAR-CRAIG, S. MANN, D.G. ALTMAN, AND E.B. RAFTERY

Department of Cardiology and
Divisions of Clinical Science and Computing and Statistics,
Northwick Park Hospital and Clinical Research Centre,
Harrow, Middlesex, UK

Summary

Ambulatory 24-hour intra-arterial blood pressure recordings were
obtained from 97 untreated hypertensive and 20 normotensive subjects,
using the "Oxford" recording technique. Analysis of hourly data in
relation to the time of waking showed that in both groups, blood
pressure was lowest four hours prior to waking, whereas heart rate
continued to fall until the hour before waking. During the 3-hour
period prior to waking, there was a statistically (but small) increase in blood pressure in both groups, but in the hypertensive
group, there was a fall in heart rate. Analysis of the times of
minimum heart rate and blood pressure in the hypertensive subjects
confirmed that the time of minimum heart rate was significantly later
than the minimum blood pressure.

Introduction

Physiological changes occurring during sleep have been studied both
in the sleep laboratory and the home using ambulatory monitoring. In
a previous study (1) on a small number of subjects, we found that
blood pressure was lowest at about 3.0 a.m. and gradually increased
until the time of awakening. However, heart rate in the same subjects did not increase until shortly before the time of awakening
(about 6.0 a.m.) This apparent dissociation between changes in blood
pressure and heart rate was in keeping with the findings of Snyder et
al (2), who used non-invasive blood pressure measurement in a sleep
laboratory. Because of the undoubted effects of awakening on both
blood pressure and heart rate, it is important that analyses of sleep
data are performed with reference to the time of awakening. Subsequent studies by Flores et al (3) and Littler (4) using ambulatory
intra-arterial monitoring showed little change in blood pressure,
prior to awakening. However, both of these studies involved even
small numbers of patients.
   We have, therefore, investigated the changes in blood pressure
and heart rate in a large group of hypertensive subjects to examine
in detail the changes in blood pressure and heart rate occurring
prior to awakening and to determine the times at which blood pressure
and heart rate are lowest during the period of sleep.

Patients and Methods

Ninety-seven patients with untreated hypertension, who had been referred to the Harrow Hypertension Clinic, were studied.   In each
case, secondary hypertension and evidence of target organ damage were
excluded by routine screening investigations. Data were also obtained from a second group of twenty subjects referred for ambulatory
monitoring because of possible mild hypertension. These patients had
a mean day-time intra-arterial ambulatory diastolic blood pressure of
less than 90mmHg; they were regarded as normotensive and have not
been treated.   The use of invasive intra-arterial recording has not
been possible on a truly 'normal' population, so those subjects who
were considered to be normotensive at the time of study have been
regarded as a control group.   None of the subjects in either group
was on treatment at the time of the study. Details of the subjects'
age, sex and clinic sphygmomanometric blood pressures are given in
Table 1.

TABLE 1

Patient Data

	Sex	Age	Clinic BP	Day-time Ambulatory BP
Hypertensives	78M, 19F	49 (12)	172 (21) 107 (13)	>95mmHg mean diastolic
Normotensives	18M, 2F	40 (14)	156 (19) 98 (13)	<90mmHG mean diastolic
mean (SD)				

     For each subject, fully ambulatory intra-arterial blood pressure
and ECG recordings were performed on an out-patient basis, using the
'Oxford' recording technique (5).   We used a modified transducer
perfusion unit (6) and the data were recorded on magnetic tape using
the 'Medilog' miniature cassette recorder (Oxford Medical Systems
Ltd.) The recordings were continued for 24-48 hours (32 hours in the
majority of cases). Informed consent was obtained from each patient
and approval for the project, as a whole, was obtained from the
Hospital Ethical Committee. During the study, the patients kept
diary cards and noted the timing of their activities during the
recording, including the times of waking and rising. In the latter
part of the project, the diary cards were replaced by miniature
cassette dictating recorders.
     Initial analysis of the twenty-four hour tapes was carried out
using a specially developed hybrid computer system (7) for each hour
of the twenty-four hours, using clock time. Hourly mean systolic
pressure, mean diastolic pressure and mean heart rate data were
subsequently stored on punched cards and further analysis was performed, using an ICL 1903A computer.

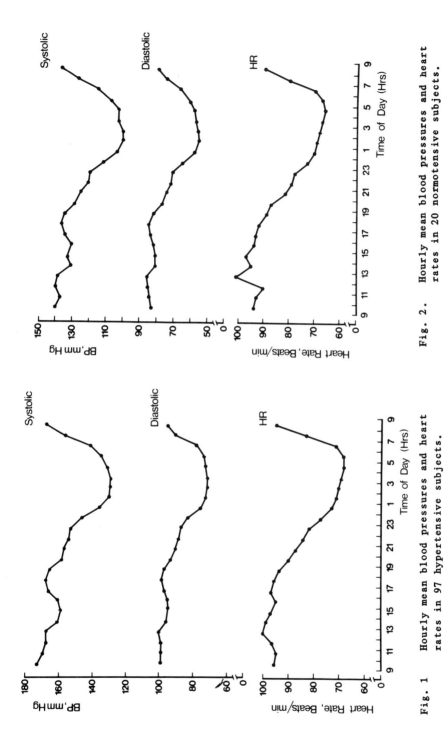

Fig. 1   Hourly mean blood pressures and heart rates in 97 hypertensive subjects.

Fig. 2.   Hourly mean blood pressures and heart rates in 20 normotensive subjects.

Results

The hourly blood pressure and heart rate data for the two groups were first analysed with reference to clock time. In the hypertensive group (Figure 1) systolic and diastolic pressure were highest during the morning, with the suggestion of a second peak at 17.00 hours. Blood pressure then progressively fell during the evening to reach a nadir during sleep at about 03.00 hours. There was then a gradual increase in pressure, which became more rapid at about 07.00 hours, which corresponded to the time of waking and dressing. The changes in heart rate were similar, the main difference being a progressive fall during sleep to a nadir at approximately 05.00 hours.

The changes in blood pressure and heart rate in the normotensive group (Figure 2) were very similar to those observed in the hypertensive subjects,. the main difference being that the pressures were lower. Again blood pressure fell in the late afternoon and evening to reach a nadir at about 02.00 hours, whereas heart rate for the group continued to fall until 05.00 hours. The mean blood pressure for the group at the nadir was 101/56.

The blood pressure and heart rate data were re-examined in each subject in relation to the hour of waking recorded in the diary. In the hypertensive group (Figure 3) there was evidence of a progressive increase in blood pressure during he four hours prior to waking but a fall in the heart rate. Both increased rapidly from the hour of waking. In the normotensive group (Figure 4) there was again evidence of a pre-waking increase in pressure, but no change in heart rate.

All of the preceding comments refer to the mean blood pressure and heart rate within each group. It is important to examine more closely the data for individuals. Each patient's blood pressure and heart rate one hour and four hours prior to waking were compared, using Student's paired t test (Table 2).

This confirmed a small but significant increase in blood pressure (3.0/1.8mmHg) but a fall in heart rate (-1.8 beats/min) in the hypertensive patients. In the 'normotensive' group, there was a significant pre-waking increase in blood pressure (5.9/3.8mmHg) but

TABLE 2

Changes in Blood Presure and Heart Rate Prior To Waking

		Mean	SD	P
Hypertensives	BP Syst	3.04	10.68	<0.01
(97)	Diast	1.81	7.82	<0.05
	HR	-1.78	4.19	<0.001
'Normotensives'	BP Syst	5.85	7.72	<0.005
(20)		3.80	6.01	<0.02
	HR	0.90	4.56	>0.25

P values refer to a paired t test comparing pressure and heart rate one hour and four hours prior to waking.

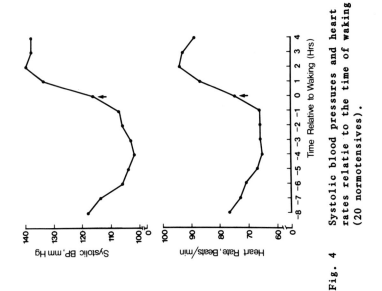

Fig. 3 Systolic blood pressures and heart rates relative to the time of waking (97 hypertensives). The hour within which the subject awoke was taken as 0.

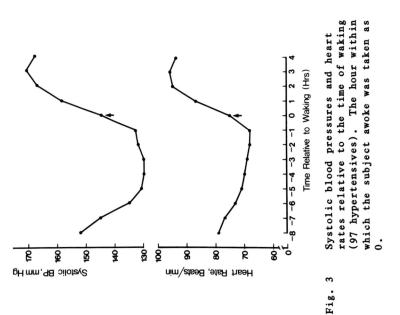

Fig. 4 Systolic blood pressures and heart rates relatie to the time of waking (20 normotensives).

no significant change in heart rate.

The hours of the systolic, diastolic and heart rate nadirs (taking only the hourly data between 22.00 and 08.00 hours) were obtained for each subject. A frequency distribution by clock time for the 97 hypertensives (Figure 5) shows that in this large patient group, there was considerable variation. However, for the group as a whole, the blood pressure nadirs occurred before the heart rate nadir (mean times of nadirs, systolic BP 2:50 hours; diastolic BP 2:55 hours; heart rate 4:10 hours). The timing of systolic and heart rate nadirs in each of the 97 hypertensive subjects were compared by a paired t test; the mean difference was 1.31 hours (S.E. 0.26) which was highly significant (P <0.0001). The between-patient variability is best appreciated by examining this data as a frequency distribution (Figure 6). A similar comparison of diastolic and heart rate nadirs was also performed and confirmed a difference of 1.21 hours (S.E. 0.25) which was also highly significant (P <0.0001).

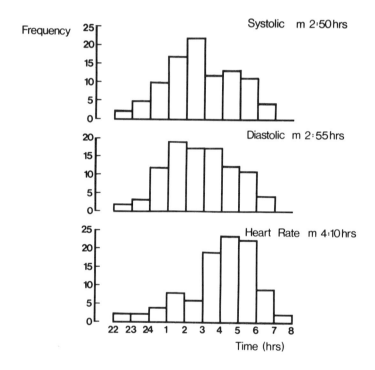

Fig. 5   Times of blood pressure and heart rate nadirs (97 hypertensives).

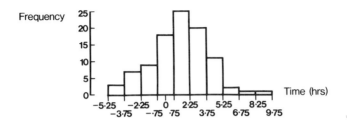

Fig. 6   Time between systolic and heart rate nadirs in 97 hypertensives (hours). The mean difference was + 1.31 hours
(s.e. 0.26) P<0.0001.

Discussion

The blood pressure and heart rate changes that we have observed in
this study are in keeping with our previous findings (1).   Snyder (8)
has suggested that there are two main rhythms occurring during sleep,
a "metabolic curve" involving heart rate, temperature, O_2 consumption
and respiratory rate and a "sleep curve" involving blood pressure,
body movement, EEG depth, arousal threshold, skin temperature and CO_2
tension.   The "metabolic curve" shows a progressive fall throughout
the sleep period with a nadir and rise just prior to waking, whereas
the "sleep curve" exhibits a relatively rapid fall shortly after the
onset of sleep with the nadir occurring after about 3 hours and then
a gradual and progressive rise.

It has been suggested that blood pressure changes during sleep
are dependent on physical activity (9), but this would appear to be
an over-simplification.   Detailed studies in our laboratory have
shown that circadian blood pressure changes in small groups of patients are repeatable from one day to the next (10) and that similar
changes occur in subjects confined to bed (11). Although the con-
troling mechanisms of circadian blood pressure changes remain uncertain, it would seem likely that two major factors are, firstly
neuro-hormonal changes acting through the sympathetic nervous system,
the ACTH-cortisol system and the renin-angiotensin system, and sec-
condly, the additive effects of physical activity and emotional and
environmental stress.   It has been shown that blood corticosteroid
levels are maximal at 06.00 hours, falling progressively throughout
the day to reach a nadir at 24.00 hours and increasing rapidly between 02.00 and 06.00 hours (12).   Ketosteroids differ in that the
nadir is at 02.00 hours, followed by a rise with the maximum at 08.00
hours (13).   Plasma renin and aldosterone production is also increased at night and detailed studies by Stumpe et al (14) have shown
a progressive increase in plasma renin from 24.00 hours to a maxiumum
at 03.00 hours.   However, catecholamines in the blood and CSF are
reduced during sleep until the time of waking (15, 16), and there is
also a decline in the adrenergic vascular response with a nadir
occurring at 03.00 hours (17).

The pre-waking rise in blood pressure that we have observed
occurring at a time when heart rate is continuing to fall could be

explained by changes in renin and angiotensin levels occurring at that time. An alternative explanation would be a pre-waking increase in adrenergical vascular response to noradrenaline occurring at a time when circulating catecholamine activity is unchanged.

References

1. Millar-Craig M.W., Bishop C.N., Raftery E.B. (1978) Lancet 1, 795-797.
2. Snyder F., Hobson KJ.A. Morrison D.F., Goldfrank F. (1964) J. Appl. Physiol., 19, 417-422.
3. Floras J.S., Jones J.V., Johnston J.A., Brooks D.E., Hassan M.O. and Sleight P. (1978) Clin. Sci and Mol. Med., 55, 395s-397s.
4. Littler W.A. (1979) Am. Heart J., 97, 35-37.
5. Bevan A. Honour A.J., Stott F.H. (1969) Clin. Sci., 36, 329-344.
6. Millar-Craig M.W., Hawes D., Whittington J. (1978) Med. & Biol.Eng. & Comput., 17, 629-635.
7. Cashman P.M.M., Millar-Craig M.W., Stott F.D. (1979) Med. & Biol. Eng. & Comput., 17, 629-635.
8. Snyder F. (1969) Biol. Psych., 1, 271-281
9. Rowlands D.B., Stallard T.J., Watson R.D.S., Littler W.A. (1980) Clin. Sci., 58, 115-117.
10. Mann S., Millar-Craig M.W., Melville D.I., Balasubramanian V., Raftery E.B. (1979) Clin. Sci., 57, 291s-294s.
11. Mann S., Millar-Craig M.W., Balasubramanian V. Cashman P.M.M., Raftery E.B. (1980) Clin. Sci., 59, 497-500.
12. Migeon C.J., Tyler F.H., Mahoney J.P., Florentin A.A., Castle H., Bliss E.L., Samuels L.T. (1956). J. Clin. Endocrinol and Metab., 16, 622-633.
13. Migeon C.J., Keller A.R., Lawrence B., Sheppard T.H. (1957) J. Clin. Endocrinol. and Metab., 17, 1051-1062.
14. Stumpe K.O., Kolloch R., Vetter H., Gramann W., Kruch F., Ressel C., Higuchi M. (1976) Am. J. Med., 60, 853-865.
15. Turton M.B., Deegan T. (1974) Clinica Chimica Acta, 55, 389-397.
16. Perlow M., Ebert M.H., Gordon E.K., Ziegler M.G., Lake C.R., Chase T.N. (1978) Brain Res., 139, 101-113.
17. Hossmann V., Fitzgerald G.A., Dollery C. (1980) Cardiovasc. Res., 14, 125-129.

CIRCADIAN VARIABILITY OF HEART RATE AND BLOOD PRESSURE IN AUTONOMIC FAILURE

S. MANN, M.W. MILLAR-CRAIG, E.B. RAFTERY AND R. BANNISTER

Department of Cardiology & Division of Clinical Sciences,
Northwick Park Hospital & Clinical Research Centre, Harrow, Middlesex
and Department of Neurology, St. Mary's Hospital, London, UK

Summary

The circadian variability of blood pressure and heart rate was studied in six subjects with autonomic failure and symptomatic postural
hypotension. The 'Oxford' system of ambulatory monitoring of intra-
arterial pressure was used and circadian curves plotted from computed hourly mean values of heart rate, systolic and diastolic
pressure. Heart rate variation was found to be normal in pattern,
but reduced in amplitude. Blood pressure followed a consistent
circadian trend inverted from the normal pattern with lowest pressures in the morning rising to peak levels shortly after retiring to
bed at night. The pattern was largely unaltered during 24 hours of
bed-rest or by the effects of waking and rising in the morning. The
nadir of pressure corresponded with the peak circadian incidence of
symptoms in this condition.

Introduction

Primary control of changes in heart rate and blood pressure is exerted by the autonomic nervous system. Study of these changes, where
this system is impaired, leads, therefore, to an appreciation of its
contribution and also to speculation about the role of other controlling mechanisms. Examples of this disorder are rare; they are known
to exhibit a fixed heart rate, but widely fluctuating blood pressure,
the latter largely due to rapid falls in pressure on standing (1, 2).
There is, however, evidence that some blood pressure changes are not
directly related to posture and that there is a circadian periodicity
in the symptoms of orthostatic hypotension. The earliest (3) and
subsequent case reports (4, 5), have referred to a peak incidence of
symptoms in the morning.
    Previous work from this department has demonstrated the presence
of a circadian cycle of blood pressure, with the highest values
occurring in the morning (6, 7, 8). The contribution of the autonomic nervous system to the physiological mechanisms controlling this
cycle is unknown and the incidence of symptoms in patients, where it
is diseased, suggests an abnormal cycle. We have, therefore, studied
a group of such patients, using established techniques.

Patients and Methods

Six subjects were studied, all of whom suffered from symptoms of
chronic postural hypotension, proven during at least one previous

intra-arterial study. In three, the autonomic failure was an isolated condition and the others had evidence of accompanying central
nervous system disease, either Parkinsonism or 'Multiple System
Atrophy' (Shy-Drager syndrome (9)). Details are given in Table 1.
Current medication was continued throughout the study, but nocturnal
head-up tilt was discontinued 48 hours previously.

     Intra-arterial pressure and electrocardiogram were monitored,
using the 'Oxford' system (10). All patients kept a written or
recorded diary of their activities, synchronised digital watches
being used to ensure precise timing of important events such as
awakening and rising. All six subjects were studied during 24 hours
of free ambulation, for geographical reasons only one was able to
leave the hospital to pursue her normal job. Four of the six (numbers 3-6) continued the recording for a further 24 hours, during
which they were confined to bed.

     The recordings were analysed by a hybrid computer system (11)
to yield hourly mean values of heart rate, systolic and diastolic
pressures, and circadian curves constructed from these values.

Results

Heart Rate
     Inspection of individual circadian curves revealed that two
subjects (numbers 4 and 6) exhibited a normal pattern and amplitude
of circadian variability. The other four showed little variation
during the whole period and in one patient, (number 5), heart rate
actually rose at night. The combined curve (upper part of Figure 1),
therefore, showed an essentially normal pattern with high day-time
pulse rate falling during the night, but a low overall amplitude of
change.

Blood Pressure
     Individual circadian curves showed great variability in hour-to-
hour pressures, but all showed a consistent trend with lowest pressures occurring in the morning, rising gradually during the day to
reach a peak shortly after the subjects retired to bed. Thereafter,
pressures fell steadily throughout the night to reach the nadir again
about 2 to 4 hours after the time cf awakening and rising. The
combined curve for systolic and diastolic pressures (lower part of
Figure 1) illustrates these features clearly.

Bed-rest and the Time of Awakening
     The combined circadian curves for heart rate, systolic and
diastolic pressures for the 4 patients, who completed both ambulant
and bed-rest phases, are shown (contrasting these periods) in Figure
2. Heart rate was similar at night on both occasions, but was lower
during the day of bed-rest. By contrast, day-time blood pressure
curves were remarkably similar on each day, although pressure was
higher during the night following the day of bed-rest.

     Re-aligning the curves for each patient around the time of
awakening as indicated in their diaries, revealed that, whereas heart
rate rose briskly from its lowest level at this point, the steady
fall in blood pressure was undisturbed, continuing for a further 2 to
4 hours with no alteration in rate of fall.

TABLE 1

Patient No.	Sex	Age (y)	Duration of Orthostatic Symptoms (y)	Other Conditions	Therapy	Orthostatic Hypotension			
						Supine		60° Tilt	
						HR	BP	HR	BP
1.	F	74	2	-	-	67	203/86	71	88/44
2.	M	57	5	Parkinsonism M.S.A.	9aF 0.1 mg/day	63	166/84	81	70/41
3.	M	61	8	Parkinsonism Severe MSA	Artane 2 mg/ t.d.s.	77	144/76	88	40/15
4.	F	54	2	-	-	71	141/78	91	90/56
5.	F	65	4	-	9aF 0.2 mg/day	76	198/86	80	88/44
6.	M	40	1	Severe Parkinsonism	Sinemet 110, 7 tabs daily	88	96/51	103	56/32

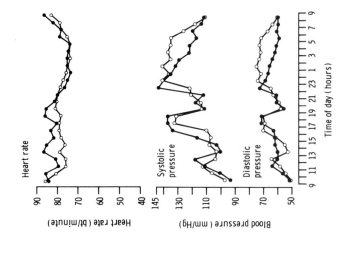

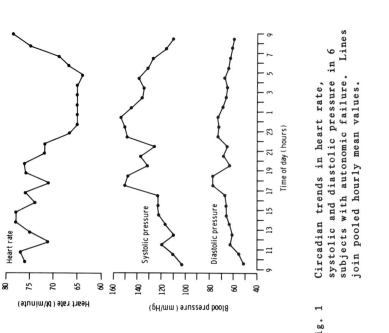

Fig. 1   Circadian trends in heart rate, systolic and diastolic pressure in 6 subjects with autonomic failure. Lines join pooled hourly mean values.

Fig. 2   Circadian trends in heart rate, systolic and diastolic pressure in 4 subjects with autonomic failure during a normally ambulant day (●——●) and a day of bed rest (0——0).

Conclusion

As early as 1941, Stead and Ebert (4) drew attention to the possibility of a consistent circadian cycle of blood pressure in subjects with autonomic failure. However, little subsequent work has taken this into account. Those, who have tried to examine the problem (5, 12, 13), have generally had inconsistent results probably due to the errors of non-invasive measurement and inadequate frequency of sampling of a highly variable signal. The pattern shown in the present study does, however, reflect those found by observations on individual cases by Browne and Horton (5) and Bannister, Ardill and Fentem (13).

By analysing continuous recordings on freely ambulant patients, we have demonstrated a consistent circadian pattern, which is an almost complete inversion of the normal cycle. It is, therefore, clear that the normal pattern is dependent on an intact autonomic nervous system, and in the absence of this, other factors come into play. Subjects with orthostatic hypotension show an inverted circadian pattern of urine output with oliguria during the day and a diuresis at night (1, 15). Changes in plasma volume may well follow this cycle and, in the absence of autonomic control, may play a more fundamental role in determining arterial pressure levels.

Somewhat paradoxically, those hypertensives treated with adrenergic neurone blocking agents (which produce a short-term blood pressure response closely resembling that in autonomic failure (16) show an expansion of plasma volume (17). The circadian blood pressure pattern has not been reported in these subjects.

The remarkable similarity of day-time blood pressure, during the phase of bed-rest, is difficult to explain. Certainly, one of the four subjects was limited by his symptoms during his 'ambulant' phase to sitting in a chair (but two others were active round the hospital and one went to work) and none were restricted to the supine position during bed-rest. Unfortunately, the cycle of urine output was not studied. The higher night-time pressures, after the day of bed-rest, reflected an exactly similar finding in normal and hypertensive subjects (8) but the mechanisms are again obscure. The lack of effect of awakening and rising on the blood pressure curve again suggests that physical activity is not of fundamental importance in determining the circadian blood pressure cycle derived by these methods.

The findings of this study are also of practical importance. The correlation in circadian pattern of peak incidence of symptoms with trough of blood pressure suggests that therapeutic endeavours should be directed specifically here. Nocturnal head-up tilt is one of the most effective measures (13, 18) and may help particularly at this time; therapy with pressor agents and plasma-expanding methods could be directed here too. Delaying mobilisation until later in the day may help in resistant cases. Supine hypertension is often a feature of this condition, especially after pressor therapy (19). Efforts to detect and ameliorate the problem should be directed towards the early part of the night.

One conclusion of importance, for those who study subjects with autonomic failure, is that physiological measurements should be made at standard times of day, preferably including both peak and trough periods. Perhaps the confusion over the possible benefits of various therapies for orthostatic hypotension results from a lack of attention to this phenomenon.

Acknowledgements

We should like to thank Mrs. Tarlika Vadgama and Mr. Stuart Dashwood for skilled technical assistance and Mrs. Paula Lacey for secretarial help.

References

1. Wagner H.N. Jr. (1959) Bull Johns Hopk Hosp. **105**, 322-359.
2. Bannister R. (1979) Lancet 2 404-406.
3. Bradbury S., Eggleston C. (1925) Am. Heart J. **1**, 73-86.
4. Stead E.A. Jr., Ebert R.V. (1941) Arch. Intern, Med. **67** 546-562.
5. Drenick E.H. (1957) Ann. Intern. Med. **47**, 124-131.
6. Millar-Craig M.W., Bishop C.N., Raftery E.G. (1978) Lancet **1**, 795-797.
7. Millar-Craig M.W., Mann S., Balasubramanian V., Raftery E.B. (1978) Clin. Sci. Mol. Med. **55**, (Suppl 4) 391s-393s.
8. Mann S., Millar-Craig M.W., Melville D.I., Altman D.G., Cashman P.M.M., Raftery E.B. (1980) ISAM 1979 : Proceedings of 3rd Inter   national Symposium on Ambulatory Monitoring, Academic Press, London. 167-176
9. Shy G.M., Drager G.A. (1960) Arch. Neurol. **2**, 511-527.
10. Millar-Craig M.W., Hawes D.W.C., Whittington J.R. (1978) Med. Biol. Eng. Comput. **16**, 727-731.
11. Cashman P.M.M., Millar Craig M.W., Stott F.D. (1979) Med. Biol. Eng. Comput. **17**, 629-635.
12. Browne H.C., Horton B.T. (1939) Minnesota Med. **22**, 302-305.
13. Bannister R., Ardill L., Fentem P. (1969) Quart. J. Med. (NS) **38**, 377-395.
14. Niarchos A.F., Magrini F., Tarazi R.C., Bravo E.L. (1978) Am. J. Med. **65**, 547-552.
15. Bachman D.M. Youmans W.B. (1953) Circulation **7**, 413-421.
16. Goldberg A.D., Raftery E.B. (1976) Lancet **2**, 1052-1054.
17. Weil J.V., Chidsey C.A. (1968) Circulation **37**, 54-61.
18. Maclean A.R., Allen E.V. (1940) JAMA **45**, 2162-2167.
19. Chobanian A.V., Volicer L., Tift C.P., Gavras M., Liang C.S. Faxon D.(1979) N. Eng. J. Med. **201**, 68-73.

Discussion

DR. ROWLANDS: Has Dr. Mann any further data on the baroreflexes or other cardiovascular reflexes in these patients?
DR. MANN: The patients' short-term physiological changes had all been studied previously. We also carried out a number of experiments as part of the study. All 6 patients had profoundly abnormal Valsalva responses and also definite and profound orthostatic hypotension. They had different degrees of their autnnomic lesions obviously, and also different distributions - 2 of them showing the preserved heart rate variability - but certainly they were all markedly abnormal. I have no data on baroreflex sensitivity.

CONTINUOUS AMBULATORY OFFICE AND HOME
BLOOD PRESSURE LEVELS IN NORMOTENSIVES AND MATCHED
BORDERLINE HYPERTENSIVES

S.N.HUNYOR, H. LARKIN, D. ROFFE, J. MASSANG & P. KENNY *

Cardiovascular Research Unit, Department of Cardiology,
Royal North Shore Hospital, St. Leonards, NSW 2065,
*NSW Institute of Technology, Grove Hill, NSW, Australia

Summary

The levels and variation of blood pressure (BP) in normotensive (NT) individuals during the course of a day have not been previously defined. While borderline hypertensives (BHT) have been shown to maintain significantly higher BP home measurement than their NT counterparts, the possible effect of non-invasive measurement has not been taken into account.

We have measured continuous ambulatory 24-hour BP as well as office and home BP in 11 young normotensive males and in 16 age-matched BHT (122/70mmHg) p < 0.01, but the latter was still clearly in the commonly accepted "normal" range. The difference between the two groups was greater for night time (6/4mmHg) than daytime values (3/2mmHg).

Nearly all NT and BHT exceeded 160mm systolic (SP) during the day, the former for approximately half an hour and the latter for more than two hours. Diastolic pressure (DP) of 100mm was exceeded ony in 4 NT and in 8 of the BHT for 19 and 75 minutes respectively. The 24-hour BP pattern was very similar in the two groups with a clear nocturnal decline to about 80% of daytime values.

It is concluded that NT maintain a lower BP than BHT during a continuous 24-hour ambulatory out-patient period and that the difference is more marked during the night time when activity patterns can be assumed to be similar. The difference between the two groups is far greater on office and home BP readings.

Introduction

It has been shown that normotensives as a group maintain a lower BP at home than borderline hypertensives, even though the decline in SP from office to home was much greater in BHT. At home, approximately one third of BHT were found to have abnormally high BP, being greater than 2 SD outside the NT mean, while only one third were clearly NT (less than 1 SD from the NT mean). The home BP technique excluded the influence of office visits and medical personnnel, but it did not examine the effect of the physical and mental effort involved in BP measurement. Home BP measurements only provided 14 readings in the resting state and night time values remained unassessed.

Early publications dealing with continuous direct ambulatory BP monitoring (2) had included individual normotensive patient data, but there had been no concerted attempt until the work of Millar-Craig and colleagues (3) to define the overall range and variability of

normotensive BP during a 24-hour cycle. The latter group studied 5
young "normotensive" males who had initially been referred for a
suspected hypertension and the criteria for categorisation included a
mean clinic diastolic pressure (DP) of < 100mmHG. The authors themselves expressed reservations about their "normotensive" population
and while they graphically displayed mean hourly values throughout a
24-hour period, little quantitative information was provided.

In this study, we have obtained continuous 24-hour BP data in 11
young normotensive and 16 age-matched BHT males after categorisation
on the basis of strict BP criteria (4). We have examined the waking
versus the sleeping periods of the day and we have compared office
and home BP measurements with the continuous data.

Patients and Methods

The 11 NT and 16 BHT were well matched for age and height but BHT
were significantly heavier (Table 1), although skinfolds (mean of

Table 1

Characteristics of Study Population

	Normotensive (n = 11)	Borderline Hypertensive (n = 16)	
Age (years)	24.1+-4.25	25.4+-4.38	ns
Height (cm)	182 +-5.5	180 +-5.6	ns
Weight (Kg)	74.8+-4.12	78.9+-9.24	p < 0.01
Skinfolds (mm)	29	32	
Heart Rate (b.p.m)	65	66	

triceps, subscapular and mid thigh) were only marginally greater in
BHT. The sitting heart rate was similar for the two groups.

Office blood pressure measurement was performed according to the
protocol of the Australian National Blood Pressure (Study (5) and
involved duplicate readings after five minutes rest in the sitting
position using korotkov V as the diastolic end-point. All measurements were obtained with the Hawksley random zero sphygmomanometer
(6).

Subjects were taken to be normotensive if of three readings over
three months none exceeded 140mm systolic or 90mm diastolic. They
were categorised as BHT if of three such readings at least one exceeded these limits while one fell below them.

BHT were recruited predominantly among clerical workers where BP
screening was conducted during the course of the Australian National
Blood Pressure Study (7). Normotensives were obtained from the same
source as well as from a tertiary education institute. The level of
activity and fitness was generally high in both groups and they did
not differ in this regard nor according to alcohol or salt intake or
environmental stress exposure.

Home BP was measured twice daily for a week using a sphygmomanometer with an inbuilt stethoscope head and with straps allowing easy
and snug cuff application. The aneroid instruments were regularly

calibrated against a mercury standard.

Accuracy of measurement was assured by an initial period of instruction with a trained observer using an interconnected stethoscope and by a further check when the home record was returned. The subject's readings in each case corresponded to within 2mmHg of that obtained by the instructor.

Ambulatory 24-hour BP was recorded in all subjects with an Oxford-Medilog instrument (8, 9) modified to stabilise recorder voltage (10), using the perfusion/transducer system developed at Northwick Park (11). Brachial artery cannulation was performed in the non-dominant arm, well up from the cubital fossa, under local anaesthesia, with insertion of a 3F Grandjean teflon cannula by the Seldinger technique. All patients were out-patients and engaged in routine activities at work and at home.

A least squares regression line was computer-fitted to the three calibration sets and from this the overall calibration factor was derived. The replayed BP signal was fed to a pre-processor (12) whose accuracy was checked with a series of known simulated pressure signals. The average BP (systolic, diastolic, mean) over one minute was taken as the unit of measurement and from this 10 minute and 60 minute averages were derived. Beat to beat analysis was only performed on regions of specific interest.

The digitized values for SP,DP and mean pressure were stored on computer (PDP - 11/103) and the time course of BP levels as well as BP incidence histograms (1mmHg class intervals) were plotted by a Hewlett-Packard HP7221S graphics plotter.

The study was approved by our Institutional Ethics Review Committee, patients gave their informed consent and no complications arose.

Results

Normotensives had a 24-hour global BP of 117/6 ±3/3 SEM mmHg with the night time level (0100-0400 hours) being 81% of the corresponding day time value. Peak readings of 162/96 ±12/13 SD occurred between 10.00 and 11.00 hours whereas troughs of 88/43 ±9/8mmHg occurred at 01.00/5.00 hours. The major qualitative changes in 24 hour BP pattern occurred at 22.00 and 07.00 hours.

In BHT 24hour BP was only slightly but significantly higher, 122/7 ±2/2 p < 0.01, with a night time level at 85% of the daytime value. The times of BP peaks, troughs and qualitative changes were identical to those in normotensives.

The comparative BP's of the normotensives and BHT's on 24-hour ambulatory monitoring, office and home readings are shown on Table 2. No difference is seen between office and home values in either group. The daytime component of the 24-hour value is comparable to that obtained by the other measurement techniques, except for lower DP's which may be partly a measurement problem with the indirect techniques. The similarity of our home and office BP results with those obtained on a larger group of normotensives and borderline hypertensives by Julius et al (1) is striking. The only significant difference is in the office and home readings found in BHT by Julius and colleagues.

Table 2

Blood Ppressure Levels in Normotensives (NT) & Borderline
Hypertensives (BHT) on 24hour Monitoring in the Office and at home –
Comparison with Julius et al (1)

	Hunyor et al 1981		Julius et al 1974	
	NT(n=11)	BHT(n=16)	NT(n=49)	BHT(n=112)
Office	121/70	134/84	122/73	146/88
Home	122/77	132/83	121/76	131/84
24–hour BP	117/67	122/70		
Daytime				
(13.00–16.00 hrs)	125/71	128/73		
Night time				
(01.00–04.00 hrs)	100/58	106/62		

The overall difference of 5/3mmHg betweeen the 24 hour BP of BHT
and NT was small but significant (p < 0.01) and BHT exceeded NT
levels for 17 of the 24 one hour periods. The most marked cluster of
differences was from 07.00 to 12.00 hours and from 02.00 to 04.00
hours. The main period of similarity was between 13.00 and 17.00
hours.

BP frequency histograms in BHT compared to NT showed a
small shift to the right with a noticeable rightsided skew. Table 3
shows the number and % of subjects in each group who exceeded certain
pressure limits throughout the 24hour period and it also gives the
time spent at these levels.

Table 3

Proportion of Normotensive and Borderline Hypertensive Subjects Who
exceeded "Normal" Pressure Limits, and Time Spent at "High" BP
Levels, during 24hours Ambulant Recording

	Normotensive (N=11)			Borderline Hypertensive (N=16)		
	Number subjects	Time %	(min)	Number subjects	Time %	(min)
SP > 160mmHg	9	82	29	14	88	134
> 150	10	91	81	14	88	201
> 140	10	91	219	16	100	314
DP > 110	2	18	6	2	13	7
> 100	4	36	19	8	50	75
> 90	7	64	97	14	88	161

The same proportion of each group reaches the higher systolic levels
but the time spent at these levels is far greater in BHT. There is a
greater proportion of BHT who achieve high diastolic pressures and
they spend significantly more time at these levels. Among the NT,

eight had clearly bimodal 24-hour BP distribution on frequency histogram. Of the three without such a pattern, two were found to have the lowest of the 24hr NT blood pressures and the other the fourth lowest (the latter would have been far lower without the contribution of two one- hour periods of table tennis). The average 24hr BP of the three without bimodal BP was 105/55mmHg, whereas the other eight normotensives had a BP of 122/72mmHg.

Discussion

The paucity of continuous 24-hour ambulatory blood pressure information in normotensives has deprived discussion dealing with absolute BP levels or variability/lability patterns of a comparative baseline. Thus it has been concludedd that BHT do not show BP "lability" when compared to essential hypertensives (13) despite earlier comparisons with normotensives (using only home and office cuff readings) which had revealed excessive systolic pressure lability (1). It could be expected that BP lability in BHT would be enhanced during ambulation due to the control system abnormalities already evident in this group (14).

Millar-Craig and colleagues (3) had made the only previous attempt at examining continuous ambulatory BP in normotensives, but their patient population consisted of 5 subjects whose categorisation could be criticised on at least three grounds: initial referral as hypertensives, mean clinic diastolic pressure of up to 100mmHg ,and average 24-hour BP of less than 140/95mmHg. The latter criterion seems liberal considering the effect of sleeping readings on the overall value, while the clinic limits are out of step with the World Health Organisation diastolic pressure limit of 90mmHg. The group of BHT studied by Pessina et al does not lend itself readily to comparative analysis as office BP levels are not given and the ambulatory BP recording was performed on hospital in-patients.

The distribution of BP levels over a 24-hour period is held to be bimodal unless distorted by changes in the "quality of sleep". We have found all our 16 BHT to show the bimodal pattern, but in three of the 11 normotensives it was absent. Anaysis of these three subjects leads us to the conclusion that their night time decline in blood pressure was not as marked because of the overall low daytime levels.

Thus bimodality of a given day's blood pressure readings is a function of daytime BP levels as well as "quality of sleep". This pattern is discernible also in pregnancy hypertension (15) where it is due to quite a different mechanism.

We have found that overall, 24-hour continuous ambulatory daytime BP, home BP and office BP levels correspond (allowing for probable cuff over-estimation of diastolic pressure), but that there is no significant correlation between them.

Nearly all the normotensive and borderline hypertensive subjects we studied exceeded systolic pressures of 160mm during the course of a typically active out-of-hospital day. However the time spent at these levels was far greater for BHT. Normotensives differed more from BHT during the night-time hours, which makes it unlikely that the 24-hour differences are related to differences in physical activity in the two groups. This conclusion is further strengthened by

the DP levels which should alter little during exercise.   BHT's
proportionately exceeded normal DP levels more often than NT and
stayed at these high levels far longer.

References

1.   Julius S., Ellis C.N. Pascual A.V., Matrice M., Hansson L.,
     Hunyor S.N. and Sandler L.N. (1974) JAMA, **229** 663-666.
2.   Littler W.A., West M.J., Honour A.J. and Sleight P. (1978)
     Am. Heart J. **98** 180-186.
3.   Millar-Craig M.W., Bishop C.N. and Raftery E.G. (1978) Lan
     cet 795-797.
4.   Julius S. (1977) Hypertension, Eds. Genest J., Koiw E. &
     Kuhel, O. McGraw-Hill, New York, 10.
5   Abernethy J.D. (1974) Med. J. Aust. **1**, 821-824.
6   Garrow J.S. (1963) Lancet, 1205.
7.   The Management Committee (1980) Lancet **1**, 1261-1267.
8.   Bevan A.T., Honour A.J. and Stott F.H. (1969) Cli. Sci. **36**,
     329-344.
9.   Goldberg A.D., Raftery E.B and Green H.L. (1976) Postgr.
     Med. J. **52**, (Suppl. 7): 104-109.
10, Kenny P., Hunyor S.N. and Renwick J.A. (1980) ISAM 1979.
     Proceedings of the third international symposium on ambu-
     latory monitoring. Eds. Stott, F.D., Raftery E.B. & Gould-
     ing L., Academic Press, London. 445-448.
11. Millar-Craig M.W., Hawes D. and Whittington J. (1978) Med. &
     Biol. Eng. and Comp. **16** 727-731.
12. Hunyor S.N., Larkin H. and Kenny P. (1980) ISAM 1979. (As
     above). pp. 189-196.
13. Pessina A.C., Mormino P., Semplicini A., Palatini E.,   Casi-
     glia E., Hlede M. and Dal Padu, C. ISAM 1979 Proceedings (As
     above), 253-259.
14. Julius S., Randall O.S., Ester M.D., Kashima T., Ellis C.
     and Bennet J. (1975) Circ. Research (Suppl. I) 36 and 37:
     1-199, 1-207.
15. Murnaghan G.A., Mitchell R.H. and Ruff S.C. (1980) ISAM 1979
     : Proceedings (As above) pp. 157-166.

CONTROL OF BLOOD PRESSURE WITH ONCE-DAILY TIMOLOL, ITS EFFECTS ON CARDIOVASCULAR REFLEXES AND ECHOCARDIOGRAPHICALLY ASSESSED LEFT VENTRICULAR MASS

D.B. ROWLANDS, D.R. GLOVER, M.A. IRELAND, T.J. STALLARD
AND W.A. LITTLER

Department of Cardiovascular Medicine, East Birmingham Hospital,
and University of Birmingham

Summary

Ten patients with mild-to-moderate essential hypertension underwent continuous intra-arterial monitoring of blood pressure (BP) and echocardiographic assessment of left ventricular (LV) mass. They were treated with once-daily Timolol and followed up at 2, 4, 8 and 12 weeks when dosage was titrated against BP control (indirect measurements) and degree of b-adrenoreceptor antagonism. At 16 weeks, 9 patients underwent repeat continuous monitoring together with echocardiography.

Blood pressure was well-controlled during the follow-up period, with once daily treatment. Continuous intra-arterial monitoring of BP at 16 weeks showed a reduction of BP throughout the 24 hours, although the reduction did not achieve statistical significance when sympathetic activity was low. Echocardiographic measurement of LV mass in 7 patients was significantly reduced after 16 weeks' treatment.

Timolol once daily reduces BP for at least 24 hours following its administration and after 16 weeks' treatment, is associated with a reduction in echocardiographically assessed LV mass.

Introduction

Timolol, the L-isomer of timolol maleate, is a non-selective beta-adrenoreceptor blocking agent, that does not have local anaesthetic, membrance-stabilising or sympathomimetic activity (1). Previous work has shown the value of this drug in the treatment of hypertension when given once daily with a diuretic (2) and when given twice daily without other anti-hypertensive agents (3). This study was carried out to assess the control of blood pressure (BP), and changes in echocardiographically determined left ventricular mass (LVM), in a group of patients with mild to moderate hypertension using Timolol once daily.

Patients and Methods

Ten patients (age range 29-58 years) with mild to moderate essential hypertension entered the study. Patients with evidence of target organ damage, diabetes mellitus, obstructive airways disease or females within the child-bearing years, were excluded. No patient had clinical, radiological or electrocardiographic evidence of left ventricular hypertrrophy (LHV). All patients gave informed consent and the study was approved by the Hospital Ethics Committee.

Patients underwent a 24-hour period of continuous intra-arterial ambulatory monitoring of BP (4) as hospital in-patients under standardised conditions (5). During this period, assessment was made of baroreflex sensitivity (6) and BP and heart rate (HR) response to sub-maximal bicycle ergometry (7) and sub-lingual glyceryl trinitrate (GTN) (8).

Immediately following the study, all patients underwent M-mode echocardiography and the LVM calculated as (total LV volume - LV cavity volume) x 1.05, where 1.05 is the specific gravity of cardiac muscle (9). Left ventricular cavity volume was calculated using the Teicholz formula, (10) the same formula being used for total LV volume, but here (D + 2 x left ventricular posterior wall thickness) was substituted for D. LVM was related to the build of individual patients by dividing by the body surface area to give the LV mass index (LVMI).

The patients were each initially started on a dose of 20 mg Timolol once daily and were followed up after 2, 4, 8 and 12 weeks during which time, the dose was titrated for each patient. The visits were at the same time of day, on each occasion, 24 hours following the previous dose of Timolol. Following 15 minutes' rest in a quiet room, the BP was measured by the same observer using a Hawksley random zero sphygmomanometer. Assessment of B-adrenoreceptor antagonism was made following BP recording by measuring HR response to sub-maximal bicycle exercise and to sublingual GTN, the latter being performed after a period of rest sufficient to allow the heart rate to return to control levels. After 16 weeks' treatment, 9 patients were re-admitted to hospital and 24-hour continuous ambulatory monitoring of BP repeated using the same protocol. In addition, assessment of b-adrenoreceptor antagonism was repeated a full 24 hours after the last dose of Timolol to correspond with assessment made during the titration and follow-up phase. M-mode echocardiography was again carried out immediately following the period of BP recording.

All results are expressed as mean ± standard deviation. The significance of differences between means was tested by Student's t-test. Where parametric statistics were not appropriate, the Mann-Whitney U test and the Wilcoxon matched-pairs signed-ranks test were used.

Results

Nine of the 10 patients completed all parts of the study, 1 patient refusing the second period of continuous ambulatory monitoring. All patients were free from serious side-effects due to Timolol although several complained of lethargy in the evenings especially shortly after starting treatment.

Blood Pressure and Heart Rate
Indirect measurement of both systolic BP (SBP) and diastolic BP (DBP) showed a significant reduction after 2 weeks' treatment, each patient taking 20 mg Timolol daily (Figure 1).

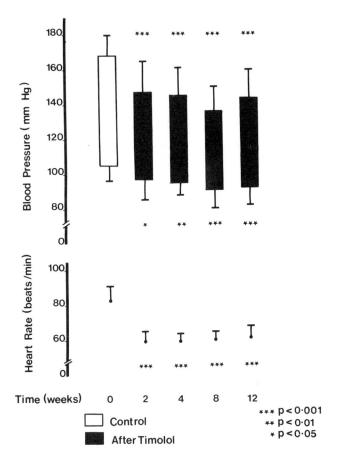

Fig. 1   Blood pressure (indirect measurement) and heart rate   during
         12 week titration and follow-up period.

The heart rate was significantly reduced over the same period. Titration of Timolol dosage (mean dose at 12 weeks = 29 ± 4.6 mg) based on
BP control and degree of B-adrenoreceptor antagonism resulted in a
significant lowering of BP and HR during the remainder of the follow-
up period.
     The results for the 9 patients who underwent a second period of
continuous ambulatory monitoring plotted on an hourly basis are
shown in Figure 2. This recording, at 16 weeks after starting treatment, shows a significant fall in SBP, DBP and HR throughout the day-
time period following administration of Timolol and extends well into
the early hours of the following morning. Between the hours of 04.00
and 09.00, the BP and HR was not always significantly lower, but
as soon as the patients became active SBP, DBP and HR were again
significantly lower than control values.

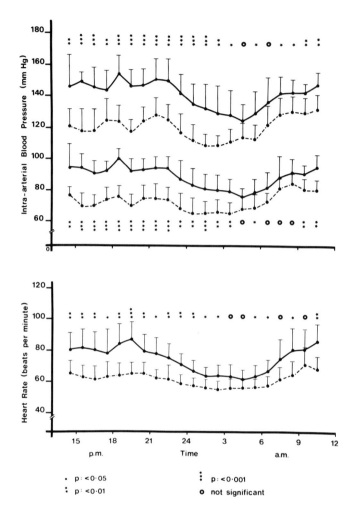

Fig. 2   **Hourly averages of BP and HR during 24 hour continuous
ambulatory monitoring before (solid line) and after (broken
line) treatment with Timolol.**

When data were averaged for timed periods (Figure 3) both BP and
HR were significantly lower for the whole 24-hour period, during Day
1, sleep and during Day 2.

Variability of BP during the total awake and sleep periods was
not significantly different before and after treatment. However,
variability of both SBP and DBP during activity was reduced after
treatment from a mean value of 17 ± 3 to 12 ± 2 mmHg in the case of
SBP ($p < 0.001$) and for DBP from 10 ± 1 to 8 ± 3 mmHg ($p < 0.01$).

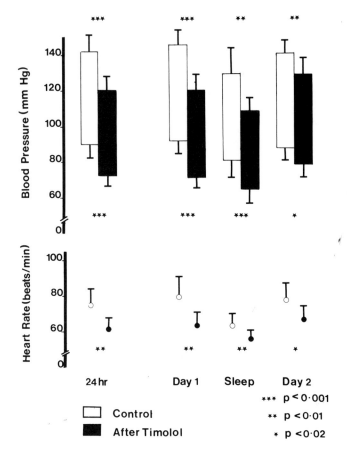

Fig. 3   Intra-arterial BP and HR averaged for timed periods before
and after 16 weeks treatment with Timolol.

Degree of b-adrenoreceptor antagonism
    Assessment of b-adrenoreceptor antagonism during the 12-week
follow-up period is shown in Figure 4.   The HR response to both sub-
maximal exercise and sub-lingual GTN was significantly reduced at 2
weeks and during the subsequent follow-up visits, all at least 24
hours following Timolol administration.
    Blood pressure and HR response to exercise, during the repeat
intra-arterial study, is shown in Figure 5. This shows that BP and
HR in response to the exercise were highly significantly reduced at 4
hours after Timolol administration and remained significantly reduced
at least 24 hours after the last dose of Timolol.
    The HR response to GTN was also significantly reduced from 109±
9 bpm to 74 ± 9 bpm (p < 0.001) at 4 hours and to 90 ± 11 bpm (p <
0.01) at 24 hours following Timolol.

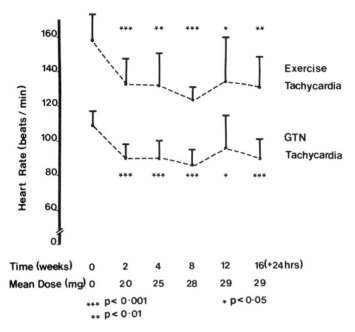

Fig. 4   HR response to exercise and sub-lingual GTN before and
during 16 weeks treatment with Timolol.   All measurements
were made at least 24 hours after drug administration.

Baroreflex Sensitivity
    Baroreflex sensitivity was measured on all patients before and
after treatment and although this rose from a median value of 6.8
msec/mmHg (range 2.5 to 13.5 msec/mmHg) to a value of 8.0 msec/mmHg
(range 1.2 to 21.5 msec/mmHg) this was not significant, $p = 0.1$
(mann-Whitney U test).
Echocardiographic LV mass
    Satisfactory echocardiograms showing continuous endocardial
echoes of the interventricular septum and LV posterior wall were seen
in 7 patients.   The LV mass was reduced in 6 of the 7 patients, in
the last patient, no change was seen.   Pre-treatment, the mean LVMI
was 73 ± 10 g/m^2 and after the treatment period of 16 weeks, this was
significantly reduced to 66 ± 9.5 g/m^2 ($p < 0.05$).

Discussion

Work using continuous ambulatory monitoring of BP has previously been
shown to be valuable in assessing control of hypertension over 24
hours, using once-daily drug dosage. (11, 12, 13).   This study shows
that Timolol once daily conmpares favourably with previous once daily
b-blocker studies, with respect to BP control (12, 13) and in
addition, exerts a significant b-blocking effect 24 hours after
treatment as shown by a reduction of heart rate response to sub-

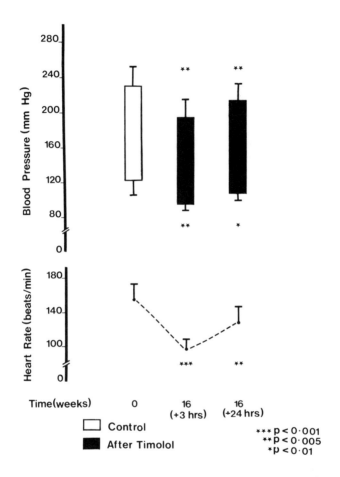

Fig. 5   BP and HR response to sub-maximal exercise before and after
          16 weeks after treatment with Timolol.

tion of activity, the reduction in BP again achieves statistical
significance.
     Reduction in variability of BP was seen following treatment, but
as previously reported (5) this was only during periods of activity
and not during rest or sleep.
     The mechanism of BP reduction by b-blockers is not well-defined.
Work has previously shown an increase in baroreflex sensitivity
following administration of b-blockers in patients under the age of
40 years, (14), but in this study, with a smaller number of patients,
we were unable to show a significant increase in baroreflex sensitivity.

Left ventricular hypertrophy has long been recognised as a complication of hypertension, although the genesis of the hypertrophy is uncertain and thought to be of multifactorial aetiology (15). The advent of echocardiography has provided a non-invasive means of assessing LV mass in hypertensive patients and a relationship has been shown between BP recorded during continuous intra-arterial ambulatory monitoring and echocardiographically assessed LV mass index (16). We have shown that good control of BP over a 24-hour period with Timolol results in a significant fall in LV mass index. In conclusion, once-daily Timolol lowered BP over the 24 hours following administration, although in this series of patients, the reduction is not always statistically significant during the hours when sympathetic activity is at its lowest. In addition, BP and heart rate response to exercise are significantly reduced by a fall 24 hours after treatment. Importantly, we have also shown a significant reduction in echocardiographically assessed LV mass in this group of hypertensive patients treated with Timolol.

Acknowledgements

We thank Miss A.M. Strong for secretarial asistance and Dr. A. Ferraro for technical assistance. Merck Sharp & Dohme (UK) kindly provided financial assistance and supplies of Blocardren.

References

1. Scribiane A., Torchiana M.L.,Stavorski J.M., Ludden C.T., Minsker D.H., Stone C.A. (1973) Arch. Int. Pharmaco Ther. **205**, 76.
2. Jennings G., Bobik A., Korner P. (1970) Med. J.Aust. 2, 263-265.
3. Rofman B.A., Kilaga S.F., Gabriel M.A., Thiyagarajan B., Nancarrow J.F., Abrams W.B. (1980) Hypertension, 2, 643-648.
4. Littler W.A., Honour A.J., Sleight P., Stott F.D., (1972) Brit. Med. J. 3, 76-78.
5. Watson R.D.S., Stallard T.J., Littler W.A. (1979) Lancet, **1**, 1210-1213.
6. Smyth H.S., Sleight P., Pickering T.G. (1969) Circ. Res. 24, 109-121.
7. Watson R.D.S., Stallard T.J., Flinn R.M., Littler W.A. (1980) Hypertension 2, 333-341.
8. Fitzgerald J.D. (1970) Int. J. Clin. Pharm. **4**, 125-130.
9. Devereux R.B., Reicheck N. (1977) Circulation, **55**, 613-618.
10. Techolz L.E., Kreulen T., Herman, M.V., Gorlin R. (1976), Am. J. Cardiol. **37**, 7-11.
11. Watson R.D.S., Stallard T.J., Littler W.A. (1980) Br. J. Clin. Pharmac. **9**, 209-212.
12. Mann S., Millar-Craig M.W., Balasubramanian V., Raftery E.B. (1980) Brit. J. Clin. Pharmac. **10**, 443-447.
13. Millar-Craig M.W., Mann S., Kenny D., Raftery E.B. (1979) Br. Med. J. **1**, 237-238.
14. Watson R.D.S., Stallard T.J., Littler W.A. (1979) Clin. Sci. **57**, 241-247.
15. Frohlich E.D., Tarazi R.C. (1979) Am. J. Cardiol. **44** 959-963.
16. Rowlands D.B., Ireland M.A., Littler W.A., Shiu M.F., Stallard T.J., Watson R.D.S. (1980) Clin. Sci. **59**, 17p.

TREATMENT OF ESSENTIAL HYPERTENSION WITH SINGLE DOSE OF BETA-BLOCKERS
ANALYSIS BY AMBULATORY MONITORING OF ARTERIAL PRESSURE

M. CARRAGETA, R. SOARES, A. MARTINS

Department of Cardiology, Clinical Medical Centre, Almada, Portugal

Summary

The hypotensive activity of Atenolol and Mepindolol was compared in a randomised cross-over trial of once-daily treatment of essential hypertension.

Clinical blood pressure measurements and ambulatory monitoring of arterial pressure was recorded over 24 hours in ten patients performing their normal activities, during placebo period and after four weeks' treatment with Atenolol or Mepindolol.

No difference was observed in the clinical standard measurements between the effects of both beta-blockers. However the 24 hours profile of blood pressure appears favourable to Mepindolol.

The ambulatory monitoring technique provides more meaningful and detailed quantification of blood pressure than that provided by casual readings.

Introduction

Clinical acceptance of beta-blockers in hypertension has led to the development of a larger number of these compounds for which various theoretical advantages have been claimed.

At the community level, low compliance has been the central issue in the management of hypertension (1). Ensuring that patients comply with their therapeutic regimen is a very difficult task. The simpler the regimen, the easier it should be for patients to comply.

Therefore, we decided to assess the anti-hypertensive effect of once-daily beta-blockers, comparing the results of casual measurements in an out-patient clinic study, with the 24 hour blood pressure ambulatory measurements in subjects exposed to their normal environment and activities (2-5).

This study was designed to investigate whether the same degree of blood pressure control could be obtained throughout the day with a once-daily dose of Atenolol and of Mepindolol.

Patients and Methods

We studied 10 patients (4 men, 6 women) with essential hypertension, aged 32 to 54 years (mean 44.5). Four other patients withdrew; two because they were not beta-blocker responders.

At the first visit, any antihypertensive therapy was stopped and then the patients were seen again after two weeks. If the standing blood pressure exceeded 150/95mmHg at the end of this period, the patients entered the study. For the next two weeks, they took placebo tablets one daily and thereafter, the patients were allocated by the random order method to Atenolol (100 mg once daily) or Mepindolol (10 mg once daily) for the next four weeks.

Blood pressure and heart rate were measured after lying supine for 5 minutes and after standing for 2 minutes. The mean of two readings in each position was recorded. All blood pressures were measured by the same observer with a Hawksley random zero sphygmomanometer taking phase V (disappearance) as the diastolic value. Patients were seen every two weeks. At the end of each treatment period, patients received the second beta-blocker for the next four weeks. The trial was single-blind, the observer being unaware of which drug the patient was taking.

We performed 24-hour blood pressure recording during the placebo period and during the last week of each treatment period, using the fully automatic portable and non-invasive Del Mar Avionics Pressurometer II equipment. (The instrument was set to take readings at 30-min. intervals) Tape records were analysed by a blood pressure and heart rate trend computer.

Statistical evaluation for significant difference of results was carried out by using Student's paired t-test.

Results

The relevant results are given in Table 1. Both Atenolol and Mepindolol produced similar reduction in systolic and diastolic blood pressures and heart rate; compared with values on placebo all differences were statistically significant. Differences between Atenolol and Mepindolol were not significant.

Ambulatory blood pressures monitoring during the placebo period (Figure 1), showed that peak pressures occurred around 1620 h. and 0811 h. There was a fall during the night, which increases after the patient retired to bed and the curves reached their nadir at about 0204 h. There was a rapid early morning rise which reached the highest levels at 0810 h.

With Atenolol, we see an effective reduction of blood pressure during the daytime, but not during the night or early morning period (Figure 1). Mepindolol produced an effective reduction of blood pressure, throughout both day and night, with an attenuation of the nocturnal fall (Figure 2).

Comment

No essential difference was observed in the clinical standard measurements between the effects of Atenolol and Mepindolol. However, noninvasive ambulatory monitoring showed that Atenolol taken once daily resulted in a reduction of the blood pressure throughout the day, with preservation of the overall shape of the basal curves.

This study illustrates the value of the ambulatory monitoring technique for examining the 24 hour profile of blood pressure reduction in hypertensive patients after chronic drug therapy (5, 6).

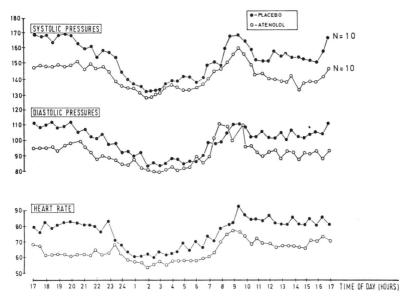

Fig. 1   Mean ambulatory blood pressure (mm Hg) and heart rate in 10
         hypertensive patients during placebo period (●--●), and
         after 4 weeks treatment with Atenolol 100 mg once daily at 8
         a.m. (0--0).

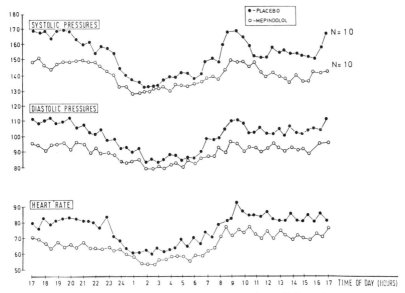

Fig. 2   Mean ambulatory blood pressure (mm Hg) and heart rate in
         ten hypertensive patients during placebo period (●--●), and
         after 4 weeks treatment with Mepindolol 10 mg once daily at
         8 a.m. (0--0).

Table 1

Comparison of the Effects of Atenolol and Mepindolol in Ten
Hypertensive Patients

Variable	Placebo 2 weeks	Atenolol 100 mg 4 weeks	Mepindolol 10 mg 4 weeks
L Y I N G			
Systolic BP	169 ± 6	147 ± 4*	148 ± 5*
Dyastolic BP	107 ± 3	94 ± 2+	94 ± 3+
Heart Rate	78 ± 6	63 ± 3*	62 ± 3*
S T A N D I N G			
Systolic BP	167 ± 5	145 ± 4*	146 ± 4*
Diastolic BP	109 ± 2	97 ± 3+	96 ± 4+
Heart Rate	83 ± 7	68 ± 4*	66 ± 5*

Mean (± SE of mean) blood pressure (BP; mmHg) and heart rate
(beats/min.)

+$P < 0.01$ as compared to placebo
*$P < 0.001$) as compared to placebo.

The technique appears to provide more meaningful and detailed
quantification, than that provided by casual readings. Differing
duration and amplitude of the effect of medication can be much better
assessed, looking at the 24 hours' blood pressure data in detail.

References

1. Report of the Joint National Committee (1978) Detection,
   evaluation and treatment of high blood pressure. U.S. Dept. of
   Health, Education and Welfare, Bethesda.
2. Sokolow M. (1979) In: Clement D.L., ed. Blood pressure
   variability, MTP Press, Lancaster, England. 25- 29.
3. Hashfield G.A., Pickering T.G., Laragh J.H. (1979) Ambulatory
   Electrocardiology 1, 7-12.
4. Kennedy H.L., Padgett N.E., Horan M.J. (1979) Ambulatory
   Electrocardiology 1, 13-18.
5. Priert R.T., Weber M.A., Brewer D.D., Winer E.I. (1979) Ambulatory Electrocardiology 1, 1-6.
6. MillarCraig M.W., Bishop C.N., Raftery E.B. (1978) Lancet 1,
   795-97.

PANEL DISCUSSION

DR. BALASUBRAMANIAN: We all know that for the past four years, there has been a controversy about whether or not there is a circadian rhythm to blood pressure. Recently, Prof. Littler's group has mentioned in their monograph on blood pressure measurement and ambulatory monitoring, that they do not agree with the Northwick Park group in this regard. Would Dr. Watson open the discussion?

DR. WATSON: The studies in Birmingham and in Oxford have failed to confirm that there is any increase in blood pressure prior to waking. We believe that the changes that occur early in the morning are related to changes in physical activity and the act of waking. Dr. Millar-Craig's presentation this afternoon has made quite clear the reasons for this disagreement. First, the changes that they observed are a rather inconsistent phenomenon. Secondly, the changes are very small in magnitude: 4mm for systolic blood pressure and 2mm for diastolic blood pressure.

How does Dr. Millar-Craig interpret the biological significance of these small pre-waking changes that he has observed?

DR. MILLAR-CRAIG: Having now analyzed a larger group of patients, I believe that the observed changes are real.

The analysis, that we have presented today, has not been done previously - when the data were shown four years ago, it had not been done. The idea of looking at data with reference to the time of waking is a very valid one. I believe that in the majority of people, there is a change in blood pressure prior to waking, although it is relatively small.

The curious thing, which has been alluded to previously in the literature, but as far as I know, on which there is no hard data, is why blood pressure should go up whereas heart rate goes down during this period. I suggest that it may be due to a change in renin secretion.

DR. MANN: Perhaps I may make a moderating comment. Certainly, it can be seen that the blood pressure rise in the morning is divided into two phases: first, one that is pre-waking. I believe, having been sceptical initially, that it is there, it is small, its clinical significance is possible dubious, but its physiological significance is interesting. If we are still arguing about whether or not this is present, perhaps a look at the cover of Sir George Pickering's textbook on hypertension, which was produced long before Northwick Park was thought of, would be interesting - showing that 24-hour curve and the changes in blood pressure during sleep that occurred.

DR. GOLDBERG: In support of Dr. Millar-Craig, we have also found in Detroit that the blood pressure dips around 3.0 a.m. and the heart rate keeps decreasing until the patient wakes up. I cannot reconcile that with the Oxford group's findings unless there is a difference in the analysis. I was interested to note that the placebo group presented from Birmingham also showed a dip in BP around 3.0 a.m.,

followed by the blood pressure starting to go up although the heart rate continued to decrease...
DR. ROWLANDS: (interrupting)... As I understand it, I think that Dr. Goldberg and Dr. Millar-Craig are perhaps describing different things. We do not disagree with the fact that blood pressure and heart rate decrease until waking...
DR. GOLDBERG: Yes, we do disagree, because we have observed that blood pressure plateaus and starts to increae again about 3.0 a.m. or 4.0 a.m., whereas the heart rate continues to drift downwards until there is a very sudden increase on awakening. This has been studied with 2-min. averaging, which gets away from the problem of 1-hour averaging. Our 2-min. and 5-min. averaging show exactly the same result, that the blood pressure appears to dip about 3 o'clock in the morning. At first, I thought it was due to temperature drift, but I know now that our system is stable.
DR. GOULD: In the past, Dr. Millar-Craig with Atenolol and Dr. Mann with other beta-blockers have shown that there is a lack of effect during the morning period before and after awakening. I think that Dr. Rowlands and Dr. Carruthers have also shown this same effect with Atenolol. When alpha-blockade alone is added, there is separation of the curves at those times. Would they like to speculate whether this rise - certainly after waking - might be due to alpha-mediated response?
DR. ROWLANDS: Certainly, some of the data published from Northwick Park in the British Medical Journal on Atenolol, and more recently, in the British Journal of Clinical Pharmacology on Propranolol LA, show a reduction in blood pressure. However, it is open to debate whether it is statistically significant for such long periods as has been shown with Timolol. That is my interpretation of the figures that are given.
    I agree that when the sympathetic activity is low, it has now been shown that there are significant levels of reduction. I do not know whether there is an alpha-mediated response involved.
DR. MANN: I think it would be accepted gnerally that of studies that have been presented both here and elsewhere, using data collected over the whole 24 hours, before and after beta-blockade, the reduction in the later part of the night and the early part of the morning, by the beta-blocker, has been less consistent than during the rest of the 24 hours. In some cases, there seems to be very little effect at all; in others, the effect is rather more profound. At the moment, it seems that the studies that have been done, using these techniques, on non-beta-blockers, alpha-blockers and diuretics, seem to show rather more effect at that time of the day.
DR. MILES: There has been a lot of interest in evaluating the significance of the changes in temperatue, and comparing the fall in the evening with other circadian variables. The first insight that has emerged from that has come from looking at the results in a time-isolation facility, which were published recently in 'Science'. It seems to me that many of these questions may well be answered by looking at some of the data from time-isolation facilities.

CYCLICAL VARIATIONS OF BLOOD PRESSURE
IN NORMOTENSIVE PREGNANCY AND PRE-ECLAMPSIA

R.H. MITCHELL*, G.A. MURNAGHAN**, AND S.C. RUFF**

*School of Electrical and Electronic Engineering,
Ulster Polytechnic, ** Dept. Midwifery and Gynaecology
Queen's University, Belfast, N. Ireland

Summary

Ambulatory blood pressure recordings have been made on normotensive pregnant women and on those suffering from pregnancy-induced hypertension (pre-eclampsia).

The circadian rhythm patterns have been analysed by fitting cosine wave to the 24-hour pattern.

The results show that, up to 30 weeks gestation, normotensive blood pressure has a period of 24 hours, is highest at about 1600 hours and is lowest during sleep. After 30 weeks, the period shortens, but the pattern remains "locked" to the 24-hour cycle.

In pre-eclampsia, the blood pressure pattern does not appear to synchronise with the 24-hour cycle, but tends to "free-run" at about 20 hours. This gives rise to maxiumum pressure values, which can occur at random times of night and day.

Introduction

It has been shown that blood pressure falls during sleep in both normotensive and hypertensive subjects (1, 2, 3). During pregnancy, similar patterns have been observed (4, 5).

Pre-eclampsia has been variously described as being associated with a reduction in the degree of fall in blood pressure during sleep (4), or to have a reversed circadian pattern when nocturnal hypertension becomes the predominant feature (5).

We have continuously recorded intra-arterial blood pressure in ambulant normotensive subjects and in subjects with severe pregnancy-induced hypertension (pre-eclampsia) (6). Fourier analysis was performed on 24-hour systolic and diastolic pressures, and the mean values and magnitude and phase of the first harmonic computed. (7). From these harmonic values, the acrophase and phase angle were obtained (8). For reference the results are reproduced in Tables 1 and 2. The results in these tables can be summarised as follows:

(A) Amplitude Spectra

(i) The mean values of the pre-eclampsia cases are higher than the normals.

(ii) In the normotensives, the amplitude of the first harmonic of diastolic pressure was typically 20% lower than the systolic

TABLE I : Chronobiological Analysis of Blood Pressure Variation in Normotensive Pregnancy
(by Fourier Analysis)

GESTATION WEEKS	PHASE ANGLE				D C		1st HARMONIC	
	SYSTOLIC ± SD		DIASTOLIC ± SD		SYS ± SD	DIAS ± SD	SYS ± SD	SD
	DEGREES	TIME	DEGREES	TIME				
8 – 20 n = 8	235.1 ± 17.5	15.40 ± 1.10	235.8 ± 17.6	15.43 ± 1.10	92.9 ± 8.9	61.8 ± 10.2	10.41 ± 2.65	7.4 ±
20 – 30 n = 6	240.3 ± 18.6	16.01 ± 1.14	241.9 ± 27.9	16.07 ± 1.04	91.9 ± 6.3	63.2 ± 9.2	13.37 ± 5.35	11.4 ± 6.86
30 – 38 n = 8	244.3 ± 13.1	16.17 ± .52	244.1 ± 15.3	16.16 ± 1.01	88.7 ± 12.3	58.4 ± 12.1	9.39 ± 1.69	7.0 ± 4.4

DIAS± 2.20

value. The relationship between the fundamental amplitudes of systolic and diastolic pressures in pre-eclampsia showed more variance with, in some cases, the diastolic amplitude being larger than the systolic one.

(B) Phase Spectra

(i) The phase spectra of the normotensive patients showed a large degree of similarity.
(ii) The phase spectra of the pre-eclampsia recordings showed a large degree of dispersion. The fundamental phase angles varied widely with some having values similar to normotensives and others having completely different patterns. Also, the phase information of systolic and diastolic pressures can show widely different values.
The results summarised above have been obtained by performing a Fourier analysis on 24-hour data. This method of analysis assumed a fundamental frequency of one cycle every 24 hours. Before concluding that the change in the fundamental component of blood pressure in pre-eclampsia is due to an alteration of phase angle alone, the 24-hour fundamental component was investigated by the Method of Least Squares

Chronobiological Analysis by Least Squares Method

It is first assumed that the data values of blood pressure are given by Y_i, i = 1 ....N, and the curve to be fitted is
$$y_i = a + b \sin (\omega i + \phi)$$
where
$$\begin{aligned} a &= \text{mean value} \\ b &= \text{amplitude} \\ \omega &= \text{frequency} \\ \phi &= \text{phase angle} \end{aligned}$$

The square of the sum of the errors is given by

$$E = \sum_{i=1}^{N} (Y_i - y_i)^2 = \sum_{i=1}^{N} (Y_i - (a + b \sin (\omega i + \phi))^2$$

The method requires the computing of a, b, ω and ϕ such that E is a minimum. These are obtained by differentiating E with respect to each of the four variables in turn, and then setting the derivataives equal to zero.

Results

The results obtained from the above method of analysis are presented in Tables 3 and 4.
     In normotensive pregnancy up to 30 weeks gestation, a good fit between the blood pressure data and a sinusoid having a period of approximately 24 hours, has been obtained. There is considerable variation about the 24-hour value, but as the phase information obtained by the Fourier method shows consistent values, it would suggest that the average period is 24 hours, although there may be

TABLE II : Chronobiological Analysis of Blood Pressure Variation in Pre-Eclampsia
(by Fourier Analysis)

PATIENT NO	AGE	PARA	H.T.	AT TIME OF STUDY GEST	Rx	PHASE ANGLE SYSTOLIC DEGREES	TIME	PHASE ANGLE DIASTOLIC DEGREES	TIME	BLOOD PRESSURE D.C. SYS	DIAS	1st HARMONIC SYS	DIAS
1	22	0	–	36	METHYL-DOPA	266.4	17:46	268.0	17:52	134	86	16.5	9.9
2	34	1	+	35	–	204.7	13:39	194.2	12:50	132	69	14.1	9.1
3	38	3	–	38	–	191.5	12:46	213.3	14:13	134	64	10.9	5.5
4	38	1	–	33	PROPRAN-OLOL	227.0	15:08	226.5	15:06	127	89	13.3	8.1
5	21	0	–	31	–	234.5	15:36	221.3	14:45	120	77	13.6	8.8
6	25	0+2	+	33	–	306.4	20:25	303:6	20.14	109	73	1.1	7.6
7	29	0	+	34	HYDRALL-AZINE	298.1	19:52	301.2	20:05	125	81	4.0	5.4
8	29	0	–	30	–	307.8	20.31	309.1	20:36	125	65	8.5	3.3
9	28	0	–	36	–	90.3	6:01	94.6	6:18	107	69	1.9	7.6
10	29	2	–	24	METHYL-DOPA	100.4	6:42	144.2	9:37	133	80	7.2	2.1
11	31	1	–	31	–	22.0	1:28	36.9	2:27	139	88	10.9	3.5

TABLE 3
Chronobiological Analysis of Systolic Blood Pressure in Pre-Eclampsia
(By Fourier Analysis)

Gestation (weeks)	DC (mm Hg)	1st Harmonic (mm Hg)	Period Hours
8 - 20 n = 8	92.61 ± 8.67	10.73 ± 2.35	23.22 ± 3.18
20 - 30 n = 6	93.13 ± 6.31	13.87 ± 4.99	23.69 ± 3.65.
30 - 38 n = 8	94.51± 7.4	10.38 ± 2.05	20.87±2.01

variations from day-to-day.   The average period for the pre-
eclampsia patients was found to be under 21 hours with a standard
deviation of nearly four and three quarter hours.   The behaviour of
blood pressure in normotensive pregnancy beyond 30 weeks gestation is
not so straight forward.   The phase information obtained by the
Fourier method is consistent, yet, by Least Squares the fundamental
period is less than 24 hours in all of the cases studied.
All the cases of pre-eclampsia, except one, were studied at more than
30 weeks' gestation.   The average period of these was similar to the
normotensive cases at 30+ weeks.

TABLE 4
Chronobiological Analysis of Systolic Blood Pressure in Pre-Eclampsia
(by Least Squares)

Patient No	D.C. (mmHg)	1st Harmonic (mmHG)	Period (Hours)
1	113.9	16.21	25.00
2	130.6	14.30	20.94
3	134.1	12.33	20.94
4	128.3	14.02	26.64
5	117.9	15.84	17.75
6	108.7	1.62	27.50
7	124.9	6.62	15.84
8	125.9	13.03	15.84
9	107.6	10.63	13.34
10	133.5	6.91	24.00
11	134.0	12.20	21.68
Mean ± S.D.	123.6 ± 10.0	11.25 ± 4.49	20.86 ± 4.71

Conclusions

The chronobiological analysis of 24-hour pressure recordings reveal
  hat, in normotensive pregnancies, up to approximately 30 weeks
gestation, blood pressure shows a strong periodicity of 24 hours.
After 30 weeks, this period is found to shorten to about 20 hours,
yet it still remains "locked" to the 24-hour cycle, because the time
of the occurrence of the maximum pressure values remains constant.

In pre-eclampsia (which generally arises after 30 weeks) the
blood pressure cycle does not appear to synchronise with the 24-hour
rhythm, but tends to "free-run" at about 20 hours. This gives rise
to maximum pressure values, which can occur at random times of the
day or night.

With confirmation of a change in circadian pressure rhythms,
avenues of investigation of the disordered patho-physiology are
opened up. Correlation between a disordered rhythm and blood
pressure-related steroid hormone outputs are being investigated.

References

1.   Bevan A.T., Honour A.J. and Stott F.D. (1969) Clin. Sci.36, 329.
2.   Millar-Craig M.W., Bishop C.N. and Raftery E.B. (1978) Lancet 1,
      795.
3.   Muller S.C. and Brown F. (1930) Ann. Intern. Med. 3, 1190.
4.   Seligman S.A. (1971) J. Obstet. Gynaecol. Br. Cwlth. 78, 417.
5.   Redman C.W.G., Beilin L.J. and Bonnar J. (1976) Hypertension in
      Pregnancy, ed: Lindheimer M.D., Katz A.I. and Zuspan F.L., Wiley
      Medical, New York, 53-59.
6.   Murnaghan G.A. (1976) Postgrad. Med. Journ. (Suppl. 7) 52, 123.
7.   Murnaghan G.A., Mitchell R.H. and Ruff S.C. (1979) ISAM 1979,
      157-166.
8.   Halberg F. et al., eds (1977) Glossary of Chronobiology, I 1
      Ponte, Milan.

Discussion

DR. MANN: Was there any difference with regard to the activity of
those patients as compared with the others?
DR. MURNAGHAN: Both the normotensive and the pre-eclamptic patients
are managed in hospital under the same conditions; they were allowed
up, ambulant, within the ward, but not allowed free-range within the
hospital.
DR. HUNYOR: In one of the cases, the nice sort of normal pattern
seemed to change at the onset of toxaemia to a suddenly disturbed or
flat cosine pattern. How do you define that condition?
DR. MURNAGHAN: I find it difficult to characterise this girl. I saw
her early in pregnancy. At that stage, she was characterised as
having borderline hypertension. She behaved unusually, in that she
had a notional indirect mid-trimester drop of her blood pressure,
which was followed by the development of well-established toxaemia.
This was the first lady we had seen, who apparently changed her
rhythm. After pregnancy, her pressure came down to borderline levels,
and was sometimes normotensive and sometimes hypertensive. She is

now normotensive again.

MR. CROSBY: It is not suprising that only frequencies of less than 24 hour are shown because there are no data of other frequencies.

DR. MITCHELL: No, that has not been done. I should say, first, that the 24-hour record and pattern are there until 30 weeks. We have only now started to look at 48-hour records, which we have not had previously.

THE ASSESSMENT OF BLOOD PRESSURE VARIABILITIY FROM HOURLY MEAN VALUES

S. MANN, M.W. MILLAR-CRAIG, B.A. GOULD, D.G. ALTMAN
AND E.B. RAFTERY

Department of Cardiology, Divisions of Clinical Science and
Computing and Statistics, Northwick Park Hospital and
Clinical Research Centre, Harrow, Middlesex, UK

Summary

A method is described of expressing aspects of circadian blood pressure variability using hourly mean values derived from continuous
intra-arterial recordings. It was applied to records from 142 normotensive or hypertensive subjects and six patients with autonomic
failure, all of whom were normally ambulant when studied. Hourly
variability was only weakly positively correlated with mean pressure
and borderline hypertensives did not show excessive variability.
There was a significant inverse correlation of nocturanal fall in
pressure and overall mean, but those with left ventricular hypertrophy did not form a distinct group. Subjects with autonomic failure showed low values for all indices of heart rate variability, an
inverted circadian trend of blood pressure and high hour-to-hour
blood pressure variability. No index of variability discriminated
groups stratified by sex or race but age and hourly variability were
positively correlated. The ability of the method to discriminate a
known abnormal group suggests its usefulness in the further study of
the importance of blood pressure variability.

Introduction

Intra-individual variability of blood pressure is of importance in
several respects: firstly, it may be used to qualify impressions
gained from single recordings in the office or clinic; secondly, it
may be related to disorders of blood pressure control including those
involved in the production of hypertension; and thirdly, it may play
a direct role in producing pathological cardiovascular events. The
search for valid indices of blood pressure variability is, therefore,
of importance, but many current methods are subject to overwhelming
measurement artefact, or are statistically unsound.
     Of those centres sustaining programmes of ambulatory intra-
arterial pressure monitoring, several, especially our own, have
chosen to describe each day in hourly segments from which are derived
mean values of heart rate and blood pressure, as a convenient means
of data reduction. This is a compromise between maximal use of data
and practicality, enabling comprehensible display and meaningful
statistical comparisons between different recordings. It has revealed underlying circadian trends, probably largely independent of
changes in physical activity (which produces short-term variation
about the hourly means). While it has been possible to compare

individual or pooled curves from the point of view of general shape or on an hour-to-hour basis, no general method for expression of the overall circadian trend or variability of the derived curve has been put forward.

In this paper, we describe such a method, which allows simple mathematical expression of some of these features, and have applied it to examine constitutional factors in a large group of unselected subjects. We have also contrasted the findings with those from a small group with a known severe disorder of circulatory control, reported elsewhere in this volume (1).

Methods

Patients

A consecutive series of 145 subjects was utilised for this ana- lysis, comprising five true normal subjects and 140, who had been referred to the hypertension clinic with suspected or established hypertension (all studied in the untreated state). Twenty subjects satisfied the criteria of Romhilt and Estes (2) for electrocardio- graphic left ventricular hypertrophy. Three hypertensives were later excluded: in two cases, data from the recordings were insufficient to derive the desired indices and in the other, night work had dis- turbed the usual circadian activity pattern. The remaining 137 hypertensives included 11 of Asian extraction (all male), 12 black subjects (2 female) and 114 caucasians (20 female) The mean age of the hypertensives was 48 years (range 19-72 years), the normals being slightly younger with a mean age of 34 years (range 29-44 years). The six subjects with autonomic failure have been described elsewhere (1).

Mode of Study

All subjects were studied for at least 24 hours using the 'Ox- ford' system of ambulatory recording (3, 4). Activity was not stand- ardised, subjects being asked to follow their normal daily routine as far as possible. Most went to work and all slept at home (except for five of the group with autonomic failure).

Data Analysis

Tapes were replayed and analysed (after excluding artefact) by a hybrid computer system (5) which derived hourly mean values of heart rate, systolic and diastolic pressure. These values were later transferred to a data file on the central Clinical Research Centre ICL computer. Three indices of circadian variability were then derived for each 24-hour recording for heart rate, systolic and diastolic pressure. These were as follows:

1. Day-Night Difference (DN Diff)

The mean value of each variable from midnight to 06.00 hours (a time when nearly all subjects were in bed and asleep) was subtracted from the corresponding mean taken from midday to 18.00 hours (when all were active outside the hospital). This gave a reflection of overall circadian change.

2. Standard Deviation (24 SD)

The standard deviation of the distribution of the 24-hourly

mean values about their overall mean was derived by conventional
statistical analysis. This provided a measure of the general
variability of the data.
3. Average Hourly Change (AHC)
     The rectified absolute differences between each hourly value
and the subsequent one were totalled and divided by the number
of observations (24 in each case). This gave a value reflecting
shorter-term variability.

     Where groups of subjects were compared (for example, stratified
by sex or race) the mean and standard deviation of each index was
calculated and results compared using parametric statistics (unpaired Student's 't' test). Where a relationship with a continuous
variable (e.g. age, mean pressure) was under study, correlation
analysis was performed.
     We felt justified in using parametric statistics in view of the
reasonably Gaussian distribution of the indices of variability although in some instances, there was a small positive skew (vide
infra).

Results

Mean Pressure, Borderline Hypertension and Left Ventricular Hypertrophy:
     The application of the derived variables in the mathematical
description of a circadian curve has been demonstrated using the data
in Figure 1.

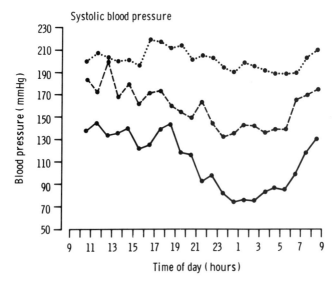

Fig. 1   **Circadian trends in systolic pressure in 3 individuals:**
upper trace – a subject with left ventricular hypertrophy
(LVH): middle trace – subject with essential hypertension
(HT): lower trace – a normotensive subject (NT).

These three curves of systolic pressure appeared to demonstrate a tendency for the nocturnal fall in pressure to be less with higher mean pressure, especially in those with left ventricular hypertrophy. The derived indices of variability were as follows:

	DN Diff	24SD	AHC
LVH	12.8	8.6	5.8
HT	36.0	17.8	10.7
NT	52.0	24.0	10.4

DN Diff and 24SD showed a progressive decrease with increase of mean pressure. Average hourly change, reflecting other aspects of variability, did not quite follow this pattern.

To explore this relationship in the larger groups DN Diff was plotted against 24 hour mean for systolic pressure in all 142 subjects (Figure 2). An inverse relationship was confirmed with a correlation coefficient of r = -0.28 (p < 0.001). The group with left ventricular hypertrophy, although tending to have the highest mean pressures (and the lowest values of DN Diff) were not distinctly separated from the others.

The full results of the correlation of means and variability indices are shown in Table 1. For blood pressure, while DN Diff had

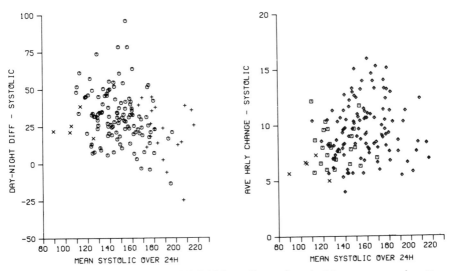

Fig. 2 (left)   Relationship of DN Diff v. Mean (systolic pressure). X = normal subject: (1) hypertensive: + = hypertensive with left ventricular hypertrophy (r = -0.28, p < 0.001).

Fig. 3 (right)   Relationship of AHC v. Mean (systolic pressure). X = normal subject: (1)= 'borderline' hypertensive: [1] = 'fixed' hypertensive (r = 0.21, p < 0.01).

TABLE I

Correlation coefficients relating variability indices to mean values and other indices (key in text)

	DN Diff	Systolic Pressure			Diastolic Pressure			Heart Rate	
		24SD	AHC	DN Diff	24SD	AHC	DN Diff	24SD	AHC
24h Mean	-0.28**	-0.10	0.23*	-0.16	-0.04	0.21	0.24*	0.27**	0.13
DN Diff		0.85**	0.34**		0.84**	0.33**		0.91**	0.60**
24SD			0.63**			0.61**			0.74**

* p = < 0.01m   ** p = < 0.001

an inverse relationship with mean, AHC correlated positively (although none of the correlations were particularly large). The negligible correlation with 24SD may reflect the opposing trends of the other two indices. Also shown in Table 1 is the generally good correlation of DN Diff and AHC with 24SD, whereas DN Diff and AHC correlated less well. For heart rate, all indices of variability correlated positively with the mean (although again, none of the correlations were particularly large).

The possibility of 'borderline' hypertension showing excessive 'lability' (6) was explored in Figure 3, where for systolic pressure, AHC has been plotted against the mean. Borderline hypertensives (those who had clinic readings sometimes above and sometimes below 140/90mmHg) were distinguished, but did not show generally high values.

Autonomic Failure

The indices of variability derived from these subjects' recordings were superimposed on the frequency histograms of the indices of the other (larger) group (Figure 4). Values are also given in Table II. All indices of heart rate variability in four of the subjects were very low, although the other two had values in the middle of the normal' range. As blood pressure followed a generally inverted circadian trend, DN Diff in systolic and diastolic pressure was low or negative. However, AHC in systolic pressure especially was very high, three subjects sharing values well outside the range of normal or hypertensive subjects. 24SD for blood pressure indices in autonomic failure seemed to show less deviation from normal, again possibly compromising between two opposing features demonstrated by the other indices.

Age, Sex and Race

Average hourly change in both systolic and diastolic pressure increased significantly with age (r = 0.43 and 0.31 respectivelyu). There was no significant correlation between age and other indices of blood pressure variability or any index of heart rate variability. The minority sex and racial groups were compared both with all others from the majority groups and with matched individuals. Results in both cases were similar in that no significant differences for any index of blood pressure variability were apparent. Day-time heart rate in black subjects appeared to be low giving values for all indices of heart rate variability significantly lower than those of either of the other racial categories. Results are given in Table II.

Discussion

Most previous work estimating blood pressure variability from intra-arterial recordings has been based on the variance of data points derived from individual beats (7-9). Two statistical problems apply to this form of analysis (10): first, these data points are not independent of previous values in the same recording and the number of degrees of freedom is much lower than the number of points; and second, continuous physiological variables do not necessarily constitute stationary data even when physical activity is controlled.

TABLE II

Sex, race and autonomic failure : values (mean and standard variation) of indices of variability in each group

	Caucasian (n=119)	Black (n=12)	Asian (n=11)	Male (n=120)	Female (n=22)	All NT/HT (n=142)	Autonomic Failure (n=6)
SYSTOLIC							
DN Diff	30.5 (18.3)	28.5 (15.1)	31.2 (15.6)	30.8 (17.8)	28.3 (18.3)	30.4 (17.8)	-15.7 (19.4)**
24SD	18.0 (5.9)	18.3 (4.1)	18.0 (5.5)	18.4 (5.8)	16.4 (4.9)	18.1 (5.7)	23.9 (8.7)*
AHC	9.2 (2.5)	10.8 (3.1)	8.4 (1.7)	9.3 (2.5)	9.0 (2.9)	9.2 (2.5)	18.7 (7.5)*
DIASTOLIC							
DN Diff	24.1 (12.2)	22.2 (10.6)	24.9 (10.6)	24.3 (11.9)	22.5 (12.1)	24.0 (11.9)	- 0.9 (13.6)**
24SD	31.2 (4.0)	13.2 (2.7)	13.5 (3.9)	13.4 (4.0)	12.6 (3.1)	13.3 (3.9)	11.5 (3.6)*
AHC	6.2 (1.7)	7.1 (1.5)	5.9 (1.6)	6.3 (1.6)	6.1 (2.0)	6.3 (1.7)	7.8 (2.5)
HEART RATE							
DN Diff	26.9 (11.1)	17.0 (8.2)++	28.3 (8.8)	26.5 (11.2)	24.1 (10.1)	26.2 (11.0)	11.1 (11.8)*
24SD	14.0 (4.0)	10.3 (3.1)**	13.7 (3.5)	13.8 (4.0)i	13.7 (4.0)	13.7 (4.0)	8.0 (4.1)**
AHC	6.7 (1.8)	5.6 (0.8)**	6.3 (1.6)	6.6 (1.8)	6.6 (1.7)	6.6 (1.7)	4.9 (1.8)

** p<0.001 wrt Caucasians
++ p<0.001 wrt Asians

Sex differences all p>0.05

* p<0.01 wrt all NT/HT
** p<0.001 wrt all NT/HT

Taking hourly means as the units of data overcomes the problem of temporal dependence; in all recordings so far analysed, statistical independence has been reached long before one hour from the previous point has elapsed. We have shown that grouped hourly mean values of heart rate and blood pressure in freely ambulant subjects are reasonably reproducible in both short-term (11) and long-term (12) studies, so that one may construct valid circadian curves from hourly mean values and derive from them indices of variability.

Some workers have assumed that there is a linear positive relationship between variability and mean pressure and feel that the former should be expressed only as a normalised 'coefficient of variation' (13). This method has also been applied to the examination of responses to standard stimuli, the responses being often expressed as percentage changes from 'baseline' level. Whereas measurement errors may well increase in direct proportion to the mean, little has been reported of the relationship of true variance and mean. Some indices (such as AHC) showed a direct relationship with mean blood pressure, but other aspects, such as nocturnal pressure fall (Figure 2) showed an inverse relationship. Hence night-time blood pressure may discriminate better between individuals than daytime values - a possible factor behind Smirk's finding (14) of improved correlation of 'basal' blood pressure with prognostic features of hypertension.

In the examination of borderline hypertension (Figure 3), we have confirmed other work using non-invasive measurement (15) and short-term intra-arterial variability (8), refuting the suggestion of greater blood pressure variabiltiy (6). Highest short-term variability (AHC) was seen in those with higher (though not the highest) pressures.

Subjects with autonomic failure have known major disorders of circulatory control (16) including low variability of heart rate, as observed here. Abnormally high short-term blood pressure variability may be due in part to profound changes occurring with alteration in posture, but his has also been observed in dogs, following baroreceptor denervation (17) and in supine measurements of subjects with autonomic impairment (18). The inverted circadian trend in these subjects (1) was accurately reflected in the abnormalities of DN Diff. The apparently normal values for 24SD here and the correlation results given in Table 1, suggest the importance of using the other two indices of variability and not merely the most statistically obvious one (24SD).

The increase of hourly variability with age may reflect an alteration in blood pressure control, as it may also in the subjects with autonomic failure. This is in keeping with previous findings that short-term variability correlated inversely with baroreflex sensitivity (7). Increasing age may, therefore, be the common factor behind these trends.

We feel we have developed useful indices with which to examine further the variability of blood pressure (and heart rate). Abnormalities have been clear in those with a known substantial defect in circulatory control mechanisms, and emphasise the validity of the technique. Further work, especially prognostic studies, is needed to establish the true clinical importance of blood presswre variability.

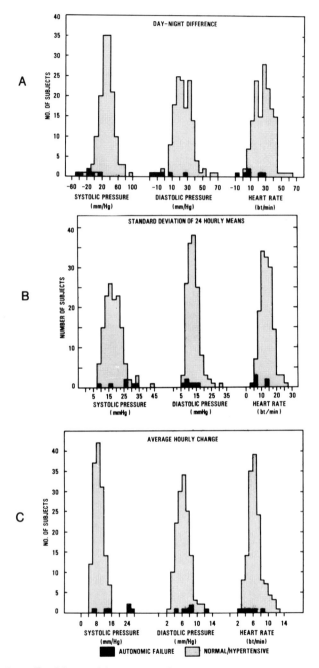

Fig. 4   Incidence histogram of variability indices – a) **DN Diff**, b) **24SD**, c) **AHC**.

We feel we have developed useful indices with which to examine further the variability of blood pressure (and heart rate). Abnormalities have been clear in those with a known substantial defect in circulatory control mechanisms, and emphasise the validity of the technique. Further work, especially prognostic studies, is needed to establish the true clinical importance of blood pressure variability.

Acknowledgements

We should like to thanks Mrs. Tarlika Vadgama and Mr. S.Dashwood for skilled technical assistance and Mrs. P. Lacey for secretarial help.

References

1. Mann S., Millar-Craig M.W., Raftery E.B., Bannister R. (This volume, 539-544).
2. Romhilt D.W., Estes E.M. (1968) Am. Heart J. **75**, 752-758.
3. Bevan A., Honour A.M. Stott F.D. (1966) J. Physiol. (Lond) **186**,3p.
4. Millar-Craig M.W., Hawes D.W.C., Whittington J.R. (1978) Med & Biol. Eng. & Comput. **16**, 727-731.
5. Cashman P.M.M., Millar-Craig M.W., Stott F.D., (1979) Med. & Biol. Eng. & Comput. **17**, 629-635.
6. Frohlich E., Kozul V.J., Tarazi R.C. Dustan H.P. (1970) Circ.Res. **27**, (Suppl. 1) 55-63.
7. Millar-Craig M.W., Mann S., Balasubramanian V., Raftery E.B. (1980) In: ISAM 1979, Proc. of the 3rd Int. Symp. on Amb. Mon. Eds: Stott F.D., Raftery E.B. Goulding L. Academic Press, London 147-155.
8. Pessina A.C. Mormino P., Demplicin A. Palatini P., Casiglia E., Hlede M., Dal Palu C. (1980) Ibid pp. 253-260.
9. Rowlands D.B., Watson R.D.S., Stallard T.J., Littler W.A. (1981). Clin. Sci. **60**, 24p.
10. Sayers B. McA., Ellis N.W., Green H.L. (1978) Pilot Study Report. Engineering in Medicine Laboratory. Imperial College, London.
11. Mann S., Millar Craig M.W., Balaslubramanian V., Cashman P.M.M., Raftery E.B. (1980) Clin. Sci. **59**, 497-500
12. Gould B.A., Mann S., Davies A.B., Altman D.G., Raftery E.B. Clin. Sci. (In press).
13. Goldberg A.D. (1980) (In discussion) ISAM 1979 Proc. of 3rd Int. Symp. on Amb. Mon. Eds: Stott F.D., Raftery E.B. and Goulding L., Academic Press, London, 445-448.
14. Smirk F.H., Veale A.M.D., Alstad K.S. (1959) N.Z. Med J. **53**, 711-735.
15. Kannel W.B., Dawber T.R.,Sorlie P., Wolf P.A. (1976) Stroke **7**, 327-331.
16. Ewing D.J. (1978) Clin. Sci. Mol. Med **55**, 321-327.
17. Cowley A.W., Liard J.F., Guyton A.C. (1973) Circ. Res. **32**, 564-576.
18. Niarchos A.F., Magrini F., Tarazi R.C. Bravo E.L. (1978) Am. J. Med. **65**, 547-552.

THE EFFECT OF A VENTRICULAR DEMAND PACEMAKER ON BLOOD PRESSURE

A.B. DAVIES, P.M.M. CASHMAN, V. BALASUBRAMANIAN, B. GOULD
D. ALTMAN, E.B. RAFTERY

Department of Cardiology and
Divisions of Bioengineering and Computing and Statistics,
Northwick Park Hospital and Clinical Research Centre,
Harrow, Middlesex, UK

Summary

We have investigated the variability of the intra-arterial blood pressure in a group of patients known to be dependent on their ventricular demand pacemaker, thus having lost the ability to alter their heart rate significantly. They have been shown to preserve the normal circadian blood pressure curve, although it is attenuated. This attenuation was not caused by any reduction in hour-to-hour variability.

The most significant finding was a marked beat-to-beat fluctuation in systolic pressures, which was due to atrio-ventricular asynchrony and ectopic beats. No patient was symptomatic during the study, but it is postulated that symptoms of lightheadedness or frank syncope may be related to more profound beat-to-beat changes of systolic blood pressure.

Introduction

Since the introduction of implantable cardiac pacemakers (1, 2), the treatment of intracardiac conduction defects and arrhythmias has been revolutionised. The life expectancy of patients presenting with complete heart block has been dramatically improved, and troublesome or dangerous cerebral disturbances due to cardiac arrhythmias can now be effectively controlled (3). Nonetheless, pacemaker clinics frequently deal with the difficult problem of patients who continue to suffer from cerebral disturbances; in the vast majority of cases, these are found to be related to pacing failure in some form. There remains a small group of patients who, as far as can be determined, have perfectly adequate pacemaker function, but who continue to have symptoms.

Little is known about blood pressure behaviour in patients who have lost the ability to alter their heart rate significantly. In particular, cerebral disturbances in the absence of pacemaker failure might be associated with rapid fluctuations of blood pressure.

Patients and Methods

We have investigated eleven patients (ages 52-83 years) who had been treated for symptomatic 'idiopathic' complete heart block with ventricular demand pacemakers, but who continued to suffer from symptoms of syncope, near-syncope or dizziness. Pacemaker failure could not be demonstrated in any of these patients and none was receiving any form of medication at the time of study.

All patients underwent brachial artery cannulation; using an Akers transducer the blood pressure signal was recorded together with one ECG lead on an Oxford Medilog Mark 1 recorder (4). Patients underwent a programme of cycle ergometry (3 min. stages of 200, 400, 700 watts), carotid sinus massage, 60° head-up tilt for 5 minutes after a period of supine rest, andfinally a formalised Valsalva manoeuvre. They were then allowed home for a full 24 hours of unrestricted activity. The data was analysed by computer enabling beat-by-beat extraction of systolic, diastolic blood pressures and heart rate (5). The results were then subjected to statistical analysis to assess short and long-term variability. Wherever possible, results were compared with age and sex matched controls, these being hypertensive subjects, whose mean clinic pressures were 186 ± 7 (S.E.) mmHg systolic and 109 ± 2mmHg diastolic.

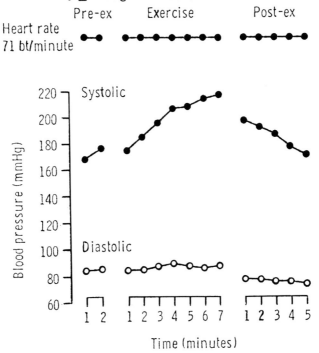

Fig. 1   The response of blood pressure to cycle ergometry in 6 patients with effectively a fixed heart rate.

Results

Cycle Ergometry
Figure 1 confirms that the paced patients were unable to change their heart rate in response to exercise, nor did they demonstrate the expected elevation of diastolic pressure; however all patients elevated their systolic pressures.

Carotid Sinus Massage

No patient exhibited a vasodepressor response (6) to vagal stimulation. As they were all dependent upon their pacemakers, no effect was seen on heart rate.

Head up Tilt

There was a small but definite postural fall in systolic and diastolic pressures; one patient became symptomatic as her pressures fell to 93/49mmHg.

Valsalva

A normal response to Valsalva manoeuvre for a period of 10 seconds was seen in the control group, in that there was an initial increase in arterial pressure followed by a fall associated with a reflex tachycardia. At the end of the manoeuvre, there was a marked overshoot of systolic pressure, which was absent in the paced group possibly explained by the inability to produce a reflex tachycardia.

Ambulant Period

Despite the apparently satisfactory paced rhythm, there was a marked beat to beat instability of blood pressure (Figure 2) mainly as a result of atrio-ventricular asynchrony, but also because of ectopic beats.

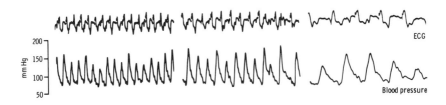

Fig. 2   Examples of blood pressure and ECG recording from the ambu-
          lant period demonstrating the beat to beat fluctuations
          caused by atrio-ventricular asynchrony and occasionally
          ectopic beats.

This is reflected in the circadian analysis of beat-to-beat variability (Figure 3), which clearly shows that the systolic pressures were significantly more unstable than in the control group. Beat-to-beat pulse interval was irregular in both groups because of ectopic activity. These effects were sustained over 24 hours.

Interestingly, the broad circadian pattern obtained from the hourly mean values (Figure 4) gives the opposite impression; systolic and diastolic values were less variable than in the controls as is shown more explicitly in Table 1, which lists the standard deviation of the hourly means.

In order to determine how much of this variation arises from hour-to-hour changes, these have been summed independent of direction and the results given in Table 2. They indicate that hour-to- hour changes do not contribute to the differences between the two groups and thus the overall flattening of the curve (Fig.4) predominates.

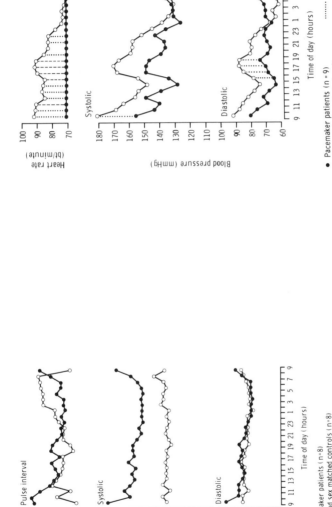

Fig. 3   Beat to beat changes plotted as their
standard deviations. The difference in
variability of systolic pressures is
marked and present throughout the 24
hours.

Fig. 4   Circadian representation of blood
pressure and heart rate is paced and
matched control patients.

TABLE 1

Standard Deviation of Hourly Mean Values of Blood Pressure

	Systolic			Diastolic	
Paced		Controls	Paced		Controls
7.7		24.4	7.7		13.6
21.6		13.4	10.6		6.9
13.3		13.7	4.9		11.6
19.4		21.4	9.4		11.4
17.0		17.8	15.7		12.2
16.0		23.5	11.0		15.7
9.3		23.9	6.2		15.4
19.0		21.9	7.6		17.0
10.7		23.3	8.3		15.4
Mean 14.9		20.3	9.0		13.2
Range 7.7		17.8	6.2		11.6
	– 21.6	– 24.4		– 15.7	–17.0
n 9		9	9		9
	p < 0.02			p < 0.02 (Mann-Whitney U test)	

TABLE 2

Mean Hour to Hour Change in Blood Pressure (Magnitude Only)

	Systolic			Diastolic	
Paced		Controls	Paced		Controls
7.2		12.7	3.7		7.1
12.5		6.6	7.3		4.9
12.6		11.2	5.0		8.0
11.3		9.0	5.1		4.2
8.1		9.8	5.2		6.0
13.4		12.6	6.2		8.2
8.3		10.6	4.3		7.5
13.1		14.2	6.1		12.5
6.4		16.4	3.1		10.2
Mean 10.3		11.4	5.1		7.6
Range 6.4		6.6	3.1		4.2
	–13.4	–16.4	–7.3		–10.2
n 9		9	9		9
	NS			p = 0.05 (Mann-Whitney U test)	

Conclusions

The circadian pattern of blood pressure has been the subject of much disagreement. Some workers have argued (7) that there may be an intrinsic regulatory mechanism causing this pattern whilst others (8) suggest that it merely reflects activity or heart rate changes.

By studying this particular group of patients, we have been able to eliminate the effect of heart rate changes. Activity levels, on the other hand, were not standardised in this study and objective measurements would have been difficult to obtain.

We have demonstrated that in these paced patients, the circadian pattern of blood pressure is present although 'flattened'. This could have been caused by either a suppression of normal heart rate response (also evidenced during Valsalva manoeuvres) or else possibly by a reduced level of activity in the paced patients. A criticism could be raised in that the control group were not in fact true normals, but hypertensive patients. Data on true normals was not available because of the advanced age of the paced group; however, it has been demonstrated that hypertensive patients have a reduction in day-night differences of blood pressure (9) and so the attenuation of the circadian blood pressure curve in the paced patients is even more significant.

We have also demonstrated that this attenuation is not substantially due to any change in hour-to-hour variability.

Ventricular pacing is recognised to be unphysiological and haemodynamically inefficient (10), and ideally the study should have been performed on patients with synchronous atrio-ventricular pacing. However, in our group of patients, this loss of synchrony was constant throughout the time of study and it is difficult to envisage any effect on long term variability.

On the other hand, when short-term or beat to beat fluctuations were scrutinised, it was clear that this atrio-ventricular asynchrony was extremely important and was responsible for as much as 50-60mmHg beat-to-beat differences of systolic pressure. This effect was also produced by ventricular ectopic beats and it was obviously important to differentiate and quantify the two; therefore, the recordings were further analysed with respect to the ECG signal by playback on u.v. paper and hand counting of ectopics. Only one patient from each group showed significant ectopic activity; these two were excluded from a repeated statistical analysis, with the result that pulse interval variability was reduced in each group, whilst the marked difference in variability of systolic pressures was maintained.

Physiological pacing has been fraught with practical difficulties, but recent advances in electrode technology have now made it a viable proposition (11). This form of therapy would probably remove the beat-to-beat instability and has been demonstrated to improve cardiac function and exercise tolerance in both long and short term.

The question of the aetiology of the persistent cerebral symptoms has not been fully answered. It is known that there is an autoregulatory mechanism which ensures preferential blood flow to the cerebrum and that the effectiveness of this control may be impaired in various pathological states (12). However, it is in any case unlikely that such a mechanism could respond fast enough to compensate for beat-to-beat fluctuations of much greater magnitude than we have encountered in these patients. Unfortunately, no patient exhibited symptoms during our study and it can, therefore, only be postulated that the symptoms may be related to an excessive beat to beat fluctuation of blood pressure and cerebral perfusion.

Acknowledgement

We would like to thank Reynolds Medical Equipment Ltd for their assistance with the ECG analysis in this study.

References

1.   Furman S., Robinson F. (1958) Surg.Forum, **9**, 245-248.
2.   Elmqvist R., Senning A. (1959) Proc. 2nd Int. Conference on Med. Electronics, 253-254.
3.   Parsonnet V. (1977) Am. J. Cardiol. **39**, 250-256.
4.   Millar-Craig M.W., Hawes D., Whittington J. (1978) Med. & Biol. Eng. & Comput., **16**, 727-731.
5.   Cashman P.M.M., Stott F.D. Millar-Craig M. W. (1979) Med. & Biol. Eng. & Comput. 629-635.
6.   Weiss S., Baker J.P. (1933) **12**, 297-354.
7.   Millar-Craig M.W., Bishop C.N., Raftery E.B. (1973) Lancet 795-797.
8.   Rowlands D.B., Stallard T.J., Watson R.D.S., Littler W.A. (1980) Clinical Science **58**, 115-117.
9.   Millar-Craig M.W., (1979) M.D. Thesis 173-254.
10. Joseph S.P., Taggart P., Pace (1979) **2**, A.40.
11. Sutton R., Citron P., (1979) Br. Heart J. **41**, 600-612.
12. Lassen N.A. (1959) Physiol. Rev. **2**, 183-238.

Discussion

DR. WATSON: How many 24-hour ECG tapes were done on these patients? In our experience, elderly patients who have recurrent symptoms not infrequently have tachyarrhythmias as a cause.

DR. DAVIES: This was a specially selected group of patients, who had been taken out of the pacemaker clinic and who were not prone to these tachyarrhythmias as far as we could tell.

DR. WATSON: It might be of interest to repeat some further ECG's on these patients because that would increase the chances of picking up possible tachyarrhythmias.

DR. DAVIES: I agree - as I said, it is a very attractive proposition to say that the beat-to-beat fluctuation might be responsible if it was more marked.   The problem with arrhythmias, though is that the arrhythmia cannot always be related to the cerebral disturbance.

DR. GOLDBERG: What was the cause of the bradycardia in these patients, who required pacemakers?

DR. DAVIES: They were all complete heart block due to degeneration of the conduction system.

DR. GOLDBERG: Was there any postural hypotension in these patients observed on the 24-hour recording?

DR. DAVIES: No, we did look closely for postural hypotension, but there were no profound drops.

REPRODUCIBILITY OF BLOOD PRESSURE MEASUREMENTS OBTAINED WITH SEMI-CONTINUOUS RECORDING DEVICES

G.O. VAN MAELE*, D.L. CLEMENT**

*Dept. Medical Informatics, ** Dept. Cardiovascular Diseases
University Hospital, Ghent-Belgium

Summary

The reproducibility of blood pressure measurements obtained with semi-continuous recording devices is studied as well for recordings made with ulrasonic method arteriosonde type 1217 as for the ambulatory recording device called portometer ("Remler M2000").

Introduction

The assumption that blood pressure measurements are normally distributed is questionable (1). Arguments against normality are that there are marked differences in the dispersion of individual distributions; moreover, many of the frequency distributions of systolic and diastolic blood presure values are bimodal or multimodal and many of the distributions are skewed towards higher values.

In the same study (1), it has been demonstrated that for blood pressure measurements, the value of a particular interval scale unit is not uniform throughout the measurement range; this means that the distance of a certain difference in blood pressure in the low area of the measurement scale is not comparable with the distance of the same difference in the highest area. Otherwise stated, one cannot presuppose that the difference between 190 and 170 mmHg is the same as the difference between 140 and 120 mmHg (systolic pressures). It is therefore recommended that non-parametric statistical methods should be used.

Reproducibility of Blood Pressure Measurements

Reproducibility of blood pressure measurements is expressed as the number of times significant differences are not observed between the frequency distribution of the blood pressure recordings obtained at two or more occasions in the same patient, expressed as a percentage.

Non-parametric statistical methods were used to test the hypothesis that the blood pressure does not differ from one occasion to another. The reproducibility is studied for recordings made with the Arteriosonde type 1217 in two patient groups and for recordings made with the ambulatory recording device (portometer) in one patient group.

Reproducibility of Blood Pressure Measurement with the Ultrasonic Method

In a group of 12 out-patients with moderate hypertension supine systolic and diastolic blood pressures were measured every five minutes during six hours' sessions, using arteriosonde. All patients have been examined at 4 or 5 occasions during a placebo treatment. For all patients, the systolic and diastolic blood pressure of each recording are compared by the Kruskal-Wallis one-way analysis of variance method. A highly significant difference ($p < 0.01$ or even lower) was found between successive recordings both for systolic and diastolic pressures. The difference in median systolic pressures varied between 8 and 32 mmHg and for diastolic pressures between 5 and 25 mmHg.

This rather discouraging result is also found in a second group of arteriosonde recordings obtained in a study (2) where the effect of β-Adrenergic blockade on blood pressure variation in patients with moderate hypertension has been investigated. This group consists of 10 out-patients with blood pressure measurements obtained with the same method of recording as in the previous study group.

Using this data material, the two placebo recordings, which were planned in a 12-week double-blind randomized cross-over study, have been compared.

Again the reproducibility of the Arteriosonde recordings appears to be very weak. Applying the Mann-Whitney U test for each patient, one obtains a reproducibility index of 30% for systolic and 20% for diastolic pressures. The differences between the median systolic pressures varies from 3 to 22 mmHg, and for diastolic pressures from 2 to 11 mmHg. This result is somewhat better than for the group of 12 patients with 4 or 5 recordings. However, even with these low reproducibility percentages, nevertheless, one is able to demonstrate in that study, a significant decrease of the arterial systolic and diastolic blood pressure after the administration of β-blockade (2).

Reproducibility of Blood Pressure Measurements obtained with the Portomer (Remler M 2000)

Another part of the study refers to the reproducibility of ambulatory recordings obtained with the portometer device, during an investigation of the effect of a daily dose of metroprolol on the continuously recorded blood pressure and heart rate.

The double blind randomized design of this study is organized in such a way that each patient had two placebo recordings and two recordings after administration of metoprolol.

The study group contains 18 patients with moderate essential hypertension, but one is excluded because of a recording failure.

Again the Mann-Whitney U test is used for the comparison of the two placebo recordings.

Although the differences between the two recordings are a little less pronounced than in the arteriosonde recordings, the number of times the patient has two different pressures is still large for the systolic pressure; for diastolic pressure, however, many more patients show reproducible recordings.

For systolic pressures, the reproducibility is 38% but for

diastolic pressures 62% while the differences of the median systolic pressures varies from 0 to 27 mmHg and for the diastolic pressures between 1 and 14 mmHg. As for the β-blockade study with arteriosonde recordings, in the metoprolol study, it is also possible to demonstrate an overall decrease of the blood pressure after the administration of a daily dose of metoprolol. Figure 1 shows clearly a shift to the left of the histogram after metoprolol. This is also represented in Figure 2, where blood pressure values are plotted as a function of time, and also shows a significant decrease of blood pressure for both systolic and diastolic pressures, throughout the period of observation.

Therefore, it should be stressed that even in situations where two placebo recordings produce data that are not reproducible, drug treatment can over-ride this effect and demonstrate a clear and significant change in blood pressure.

Reproducibility of Blood Pressure Variability

Reproducibility testing with regard to blood pressure variability expressed as the standard deviation of the measurements is difficult to perform because of the lack of an appropriate non-parametric statistical method. We have compared the variances of the two placebo recordings for arteriosonde and for portometer recordings, applying the variance ratio test, but the results of this test are given with reservations because this method is very sensitive to the requirement of normality, a requirement, which has already been questioned. Subject to these restrictions, one finds a significant change in variability for the gorup of 10 patients with arteriosonde in one case only for systolic and 2 for diastolic pressures (Table 1)

TABLE 1

Reproducibility with regard to Variability
Arteriosonde
F - Test or Variance Ratio Test

	Systolic Variance			Diastolic Variance		
1	87.4	85.8	NS	53.2	74.9	NS
2.	46.3	115.7	p<0.01	72.1	46.8	NS
3.	364.4	246.0	NS	124.2	88.6	NS
4.	109.5	109.3	NS	42.8	82.4	NS
5.	207.8	176.3	NS	111.9	47.9	p<0.001
6.	409.1	445.0	NS	343.3	106.6	p<0.001
7.	107.6	76.8	NS	60.0	64.2	NS
8.	229.0	313.3	NS	143.2	113.6	NS
9.	167.4	110.8	NS	67.5	73.6	NS
10.	45.9	24.6	NS	25.1	20.6	NS

The group of 17 patients, with portometer recordings, shows a significant difference in variability in five cases for systolic and in only one, for diastolic pressure in a total of 16 patients. So,

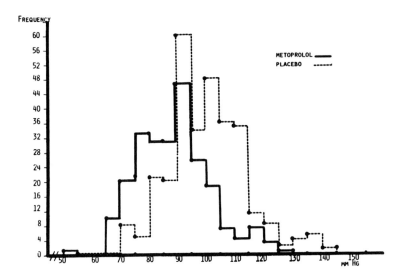

Fig. 1   The decrease of the systolic blood pressure after the
          administration of metoprolol.

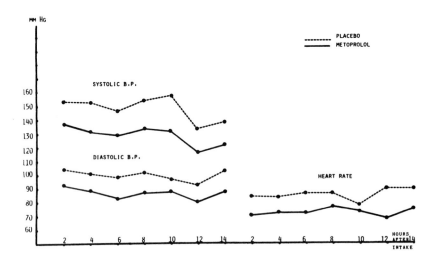

Fig. 2   Effect of metoprolol registrated with the   REMLER M 2000
          portometer.

this means that as far as variability is concerned reproducibility is
very satisfactory (Table 2).

TABLE 2

Reproducibility with Regard to Variability
Portometer
F - Test or Variance Ratio Test

	Systolic Variance			Diastolic Variance		
1.	33.7	93.4	p<0.05	86.8	62.4	NS
2.	148.5	91.4	NS	193.8	50.5	NS
3.	287.6	94.9	p<0.05	28.1	19.6	NS
4.	65.9	87.2	NS	36.5	88.9	NS
5.	101.7	161.9	NS	108.0	50.4	NS
6.	100.4	59.7	NS	37.4	39.3	NS
7.	197.8	118.9	NS	42.7	57.0	NS
8.	133.1	67.8	NS	71.5	98.5	NS
9.	849.4	552.6	NS	87.3	59.1	NS
10.	447.0	560.2	NS	120.1	89.8	NS
11.	507.1	249.8	NS	132.8	260.6	NS
12.	54.5	69.0	NS	42.4	35.7	NS
13	440.1	115.4	p<0.01	315.5	80.9	p<0.01
14	349.4	-	-	68.7	-	-
15.	135.2	57.9	NS	47.7	48.4	NS
16.	660.1	123.5	p<0.01	153.8	210.9	NS
17.	54.8	233.8	p<0.05	25.4	86.7	NS

Conclusion

We have found a rather poor reproducibility for arteriosonde; it was
better for portometer recordings, mainly as far as the diastolic
pressure is concerned; by contrast, variability appeared to be quite
reproducible.

In spite of the peculiar behaviour of blood pressure measurements, it still remains possible to demonstrate the effect of an
active drug in decreasing the blood pressure.

The small degree of reproducibility and the inherent variation
of blood pressure measurements once again affirms that the blood
pressure of a patient cannot be represented by one of his casual
readings, or even by a single point estimate such as the mean or the
median.

References

1.   Kantor S., Winkelstein W. (1969) Amer. J. Epid. **90**, 201-213.
2.   Clement D.L. Bogaert M.G., Pannier R. (1977) Europ. J. Clin.
     Pharmacol. **11**, 325-327.

Discussion

MR. COWAN: Would Dr.van Maele please briefly review the evidence of non-normality in these distributions?

DR. van MAELE: It is mainly because there is an important skew for systolic pressure towards the higher values. In addition, most of the histograms obtained have been bimodal, or even multimodal - which is another argument against normality.

MR. COWAN: We have examined individual patient distributions and have found that in perhaps 80 or 90% of them the distribution satisfied the test for normality.

DR. van MAELE: In individual distributions, we have also applied the Kolmogoroff test, which was unable to demonstrate significant differences. This means that it is not possible to demonstrate a significant difference between the distribution function of the individual patients and the normal distribution. It is rather difficult with this statistical test, which can show that there is no difference - but that does not prove that the frequency distribution is the same as the normal distribution.

PROF. MALLION: Does Dr. van Maele think that the arteriosonde should still be used clinically? It is important because if we want to use that apparatus, the subject has to be asked not to move his arm and to be very quiet. It is difficult to use it therefore.

DR. CLEMENT: It is no longer used a great deal - but we had the data so we thought that it could form part of the discussion. We do not use it as much as previously for various reasons, one of which is the one mentioned by Prof. Mallion, that the subject has to stay extremely quiet at the time of the recording. The method is useful if we want to compare the blood pressure level on two different days and it is not possible to standardise what that person does on the two days.

THE RELATIVE EFFECT OF MENTAL AND PHYSICAL ACTIVITY ON BLOOD PRESSURE AND HEART RATE DURING THE WAKING-UP PROCESS

A. CATTAERT, J. CONWAY*, A. AMERY, R. FAGARD

Department of Pathophysiology, University of Leuven, Belgium
*Cardiac Department, John Radcliffe Hospital, Oxford, UK

Summary

1. The morning rise in blood pressure and heart rate was studied in 18 patients with mild blood pressure elevation. Passing from sleep to the drowsy state raised blood pressure and heart rate very little, while the awake state (reading a newspaper sitting in bed) increased the mean blood pressure by 13.2mmHg and the heart rate by 5.7 beats per minute.
2. Subsequent application of mental stress (arithmetic) in one third of the patients or physical activity in the upright position in another third showed a different pattern of response. Mental stress mainly raised the blood pressure while physical activity in the upright position mainly raised the heart rate.
   KEY WORDS: Blood pressure, drowsy state, heart rate, mental stress, physical activity, sleep, waking-up.

Introduction

During sleep, blood pressure and heart rate fall and increase again in the morning (1, 3, 4, 6, 7, 11, 12). Also emotional stress (2, 8) and posture (9, 10) produced well-determined haemodynamic effects.

We have studied blood pressure and heart rate as the subject woke up and compared the responses to mental stress or physical activity with those of a control group.

Methods

Eighteen patients (9 males and 9 females) with slight blood pressure elevation but without cardiovascular complications were studied after interruption of all treatment for at least three weeks. Their age averaged 34.2 ± 2.6 years. The mean blood pressure recorded during sleep averaged $96.1 \pm .1$ mmHg and the heart rate was 67.9 ± 2.1 beats per minute.

Studies were conducted in hospitalized subjects after 2-3 nights in which they became accustomed to the apparatus and procedures. Indirect measurement of mean blood pressure and heart rate was made at 12 minute intervals with an oscillometric apparatus (Dinamap) from 10.0 p.m. when the patient retired until s(he) awoke

spontaneously. These recordings were continued for a   further
period of at least 30 minutes while the subject remained with the
eyes closed and without turning on room lights (drowsy period).
Thereafter, the frequency of blood pressure recordings was increased
to 2-minute intervals and the subject was allowed to read for 30
minutes with the head raised and the lights on. The subjects were
then divided at random into three groups:

    The 6 patients of Group 1 (Control Group) continued reading in
bed,   Group 2 (n=6) were asked to walk around the bed (physical
activity), and Group 3 (n=6) were given a test of mental arithmetic
while remaining in bed (mental stress).   After this 15-minute
intervention period, all 18 patients returned to reading for 30
minutes.   The entire sequence of blood pressure and heart rate
recordings is given in Figure 1.

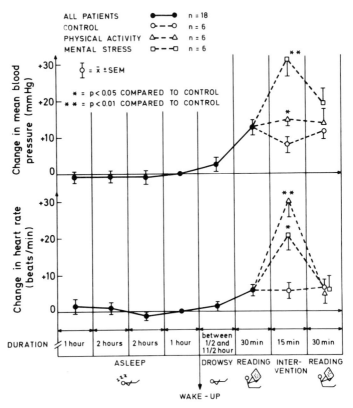

Fig. 1   Change in mean blood pressure (in mm Hg) and heart rate (in
        beats/min) compared to base line (average value during the
        hour before wake-up). Average values and   standard errors
        are given at night and during early morning in the total
        population (n = 18) and during the intervention period in
        the control, physical activity and mental stress group,
        each subgroup comprises 6 patients.

The results are expressed as changes in comparison to the readings obtained one hour before waking-up (base-line). During the intervention period, the results are compared to the values obtained in the control group, using an unpaired Student's t-test. The dispersion of data is given by the standard error of the mean.

Results

1. Observations at night and during early morning in the total population

During the 6 hours of the night the average blood pressure was stable. (Figure 1). It increased slowly ($p < 0.01$) by 2.9mmHg during the drowsy period and increased further ($p < 0.001$) by 13.2mmHg during relaxed reading.

During the hour before waking up (base line) the heart rate averaged 67.9 ± 2.1 for the 18 patients. During the drowsy period, the heart rate tended to rise ($p > 0.1$) but clearly increased ($p < 0.001$) by 5.7 beats per minute during relaxed reading.

2. Observations during the intervention period.

The patients in Group 1 (Control Group) continued their relaxed reading throughout the intervention period; the average mean blood pressure and heart rate did not change significantly (Figure 1).

Compared to Group 1, physical activity (Group 2) provoked a blood pressure increase ($p < 0.05$) of 7.3mmHg. This physical activity induced also a significant ($p < 0.01$) increase in heart rate of 25.0 beats per minute.

On the contrary, mental stress (Group 3), produced less tachycardia (15.1 beats per minute) but induced a more pronounced blood pressure increase ($p < 0.01$) of 23.4mmHg.

During the subsequent relaxed reading no significant differences in heart rate or blood pressure ($p > 0.1$) were observed between the three groups.

Discussion

Our results are in general accord with many others who have shown a rise in blood pressure and heart rate as the subject wakes up (1, 3, 4, 6, 7, 11, 12)

To study this in more detail, we standardized the waking-up procedure and separated the mental from the physical activity, which normally accompanies the "getting-up" sequence.

Thus, we were able to observe that passing from sleep to the drowsy state raised blood pressure and heart rate very little, while the awake state (reading a newspaper increased blood pressure by 13.2mmHg and heart rate by 5.7 beats per minute. These values are similar to those reported by others using intra-arterial blood pressure recordings (5, 9, 10).

The subjects who continued to read showed little progressive change in blood pressure and heart rate as the test proceeded. The two stress procedures produced differing responses. The mental arithmetic increased blood pressure by 23.4mmHg and heart rate by

15.1 beats per minute. On the other hand, physical activity in the upright posture increased heart rate by 25.0 beats per minute while blood pressure increased by only 7.3mmHg.

Thus it has been possible to show that activation of homeostatic reflexes by differing means produces a different pattern of response. However, the change in blood pressure on waking up appears to result mainly from mental activity, less from physical activity in upright position.

Acknowledgements

Work of this laboratory is supported by the Belgian Research Institute I.W.O.N.L. The secretarial help of Miss R. Nuyts is greatly appreciated.

References

1.   Birkenhager W.H., Van Es. L.A.,Houwing A. et al (1968) Clin.Sci. **35**, 445-456.
2.   Brod J., Fencl V., Hejl A. and Jirka J. (1959) Clin. Sci. **18**, 269-279.
3.   Coccagna G., Mantovani M., Brignoni et al (1971) Electroenceph. and Clin.Neur. **31**, 227-281.
4.   De Leeuw P.W., Wester A., Stienstra R and Birkenhager W.H.(1978) In: Blood pressure variability, pp. 37-41. Ed. Clement D.L., MTP Press Ltd.
5.   Floras J.S., Jones J.V. Johnston J.A. et al (1978) Clin. Sci.and Mol. Med. **55**, 395s-397s.
6.   Jouvet M. (1967) Phys.Reviews, **47**, 117-177.
7.   Khatri I.M., Freis E.D. (1967) J. Appl.Physiol. **22**, 867-873.
8.   Le Blanc J., Cote J., Jobin M. and Labrie A. (1979) J.Appl. Phys. **47**, 1207-1211.
9.   Littler W.A. (1979) Am. Heart J. **97**, 35-37.
10. Littler W.A. and Watson R.D.S. (1978) Lancet, **i**, 995-996.
11. Littler W.A., Honour A.J., Carter R.D. and Sleight P. (1975) Brit. Med. J., **ii**, 346-348.
12. Millar-Craig M.W., Bishop C.N. and Raftery E.B. (1978) Lancet, **i**, 795-797.

EFFECT OF HOSPITALIZATION ON SOME ASPECTS OF BLOOD PRESSURE VARIABILITY

P.W. de LEEUW, P.J. WILLEMSE AND W.H. BIRKENHÄGER

Dept. Internal Medicine, Zuiderziekenhuis, Rotterdam,
The Netherlands

Summary

To investigate whether hospitalization has any influence on daily variations in blood pressure, thirty patients with uncomplicated essential hypertension were admitted to a metabolic ward. Blood pressure was taken at frequent intervals over a period of five days. Average daily pressure, basal pressure (taken immediately after waking) and the highest pressure of each day, fell during the first three days of hospitalization and remained nearly constant thereafter. The coefficient of variation for the daily averages of blood pressure was unaffected throughout the whole period. Pressor range, defined as the difference between highest and basal pressure was also unaffected when expressed in mmHg. As a percentage of basal pressure, the pressor range increased with time; however, this increase was not statistically significant.

Introduction

The recent development of devices, which can monitor intra-arterial pressure over prolonged periods of time, has contributed greatly to the study of 24-hour blood pressure variations. Recordings have been made during day-time and during the night, during rest and during physical exercise, at home and in hospital. There is relatively little information, however, on the reproducibility of the results. Also, it is largely unknown to what extent hospitalization may affect the pattern of blood pressure variations. In a recent study, we found that the average daily blood pressure markedly fell during the first three days of hospitalization, concomitant with a reduction in adrenergic activity (1). In the present study, we investigated whether these changes would have any effect on pressor responses during ordinary day-time activities.

Patients and Methods

Thirty patients, with uncomplicated essential hypertension and aged 21 to 66 years, were admitted to hospital. Blood pressure taken at the out-patient department had ranged from 150 to 230mmHg systolic and from 92 to 140mmHg diastolic. At the time of admission, no patient had taken any medication for at least three weeks.

All studies were carried out in a metabolic ward, where sodium intake was restricted at 55 mmoles per day and checked by 24-hour urine collections. Blood pressure was measured upon admission and further at frequent intervals with an automatic device and, intermittently, also by sphygmomanometry. During day-time, patients were allowed to move freely.

Variations of blood pressure were analysed in several ways. First, we calculated the average and standard deviation of all blood pressure readings obtained during day-time for each day. From these data, the coefficient of variation could be calculated for each day. In addition, we noted on each morning, the so-called basal blood pressure, defined as the pressure taken immediately after waking. In accordance with the proposal of Birkenhäger and Schalekamp (2), we also spotted the highest blood pressure on each day and calculated a pressor range from the difference between this highest pressure and the basal blood pressure. For statistical analysis Student's t-test was applied; results are expressed as means ± S.E.M.

Results

Average daily blood pressure fell by 13 ± 3mmHg over the first 3 days of hospitalization to remain relatively stable over the next 2 days (Figure 1).

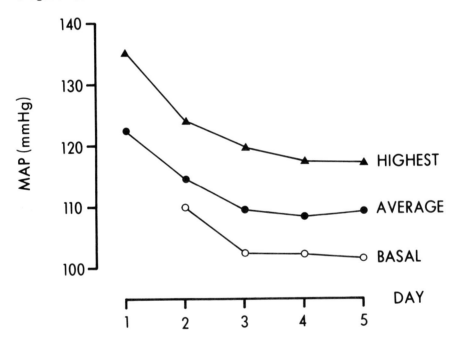

Fig. 1   Changes in basal, highest and average daily blood pressure during the first five days of hospitalisation.

The standard deviation of all blood pressure readings changed in concert with the average and as a result the coefficient of variation was nearly constant throughout the whole period. Basal blood pressure ran a parallel course to the daily average, albeit at a lower

level (obviously no basal blood pressure is available for the first
day of admission). The highest pressure of each day also fell with
the duration of hospitalization. Since blood pressure on admission
in many cases, was the highest pressure ever recorded, the decrement
in maximum daily blood pressures was most pronounced at the second
hospital day. When expressed as an absolute value, the pressor range
did not change with time. However, when the pressor range is taken
as a percentage of basal blood pressure, a slight increase is noted.
This increase did not reach statistical significance.

Discussion

The present study confirms once again that blood pressure falls
during hospitalization. It is rather difficult, however, to define
changes in blood pressure variability in such circumstances. The
conclusions reached depend heavily on the way that blood pressure
variations are analysed. We will not discuss here the merits of the
various methods to characterize the lability of blood pressure since
this will be dealt with elsewhere in this book.
     When we analysed our data in terms of averages and standard
deviations, there was a fall of both parameters during hospitalization, but the coefficient of variation remained constant. This
implies that only the distribution of blood pressure data shifted,
whereas variability in relation to the prevailing average level of
pressure was unaltered. Admittedly, our study was not designed to
record minute-to-minute variations of pressure and therefore, some
uncertainty still exists about the true distribution of pressure
levels. However, continuous recording of intra-arterial pressure has
shown a high degree of reproducibility when two consecutive days are
concerned (3, 4). Also Athanassiadis, using a semi-automatic cuff
machine in 10 hospitalized patients found a remarkable similarity in
blood pressure from day to day, not only in mean pressures, but also
in the range of pressures (5). Therefore, we feel more confident in
our conclusion that hospitalization only lowers the average level of
blood pressure without affecting its relative variations. We have
also analysed our data in another way, by plotting the upward excursions of blood pressure in relation to the basal pressure. Quite
interestingly, the latter parameter also fell during the first days
of hospitalization, indicating that one cannot determine reliably the
basal pressure of a patient from single 24- or even 48-hour recordings. Due to the change in basal blood pressure, one would expect
the pressor range during day-time to increase. This is true only
when the pressor range is expressed as a percentage of the basal
pressure and even then, this increase is not very impressive. In
absolute terms, there is no significant change of the pressor range:
apparently hospitalization prevents blood pressure rising exces-
sively. We do not know, however, whether this is related to the
decrement in the average daily level of blood pressure or simply
because there are fewer stressful events for the patient in the
hospital environment. One could also argue that the constancy of the
pressor range is, in fact, inappropriate, since it should have de-
clined in concert with the average level of pressure. The present
data do not allow us to make conclusions on this point. Clearly,
further studies are needed to determine which mechanisms are involved

in the variability of blood presure and why they remain relatively unaffected by hospitalization.

References

1. De Leeuw P.W., Smout A.J.P.M., Hoogma R.P.L.M., Van Soest G.A.W., Punt R. and Birkenhäger W.H. (1981) Clin. Sci.Suppl. 7. (In press)
2. Birkenhäger W.H. and Schalekamp, M.A.D.H. (1976) Control mechanisms in essential hypertension. Elsevier, Amsterdam.
3. Rowlands D.B., Stallard T.D., Watson R.D.S. and Littler, W.A. (1980) Clin. Sci. **58**, 115.
4. Mann S., Millar-Craig M.W., Balasubramanian V., Cashman, P.M.M. and Raftery E.B. (1980) Clin. Sci. **59**, 497.
5. Athanassiadis D., Draper G.J., Honour A.J. and Cranston W.I. (1969) Clin. Sci. **36**, 147.

AMBULATORY BLOOD PRESSURE MONITORING
A REPORT OF 90 CASES
(RELIABILITY OF A NON-INVASIVE METHOD)

G. GERMANO, A. APPOLLONI, M. CIAVARELLA, A. DE ZORZI
AND V. CORSI

IV Medical Pathology, University of Rome, Italy

Summary

It is important to obtain significant data on differences in the
behaviour of arterial blood pressure in healthy and hypertensive
subjects (4-6), because of the increase in experimental research on
the influence of the autonomic nervous system on stroke volume and
peripherical resistances. Several static and dynamic tests have been
standardized in order to evaluate the answers in healthy and pathological subjects, but we consider such answers to be artificial, and
the individual result cannot be separated from the effect of the
individual lability.
   It is important to evaluate the blood pressure profile of an
average 24-hour day in patients under standard conditions: such data
can be obtained with no risk by non-invasive methods.
   We describe here our study (1,2) executed with the help of
one of these ambulatory monitoring instruments, and we consider
several artefacts affecting the performance reliability of this
method.

Material and Method

We analysed 90 patients (age range 28-64 years) from March to October
1980, using the automatic non-invasive instrumentation Del Mar Avionics Pressurometer II for blood pressure ambulatory monitoring. This
system consists of a Holter recording unit, an ausculatory cuff and a
microphone; the Pressurometer automatically inflates and deflates the
blood pressure cuff at preset intervals (every 7.5-15 and 30 minutes), recording the systolic and diastolic blood pressure measurements of an Electrocardiocorder 446. Thus this is a non-invasive
sphygmomanometric method of measurement , based on the identification
of Korotkoff sounds, sub-divided in five phases during the deflation
of the pressure cuff. It is known (7-8) that non-invasive measurements, in comparison with invasive, over-value the systolic arterial
blood pressure in relation to the diastolic, whether recorded at the
fourth or fifth phase, but these variations can be disregarded.
   We used the 660B Electrocardioscanner and the 661 B.P. Trend
Analyser for the data analysis.
   1856 recording hours were obtained from 90 patients, individual
recordings varying from 12 to 26 hours with a mean of 20.52 hours.
The pre-set intervals were different for day and night, 7.5 minutes
during the day, 30 minutes during rest, so as to provide on average
six measurements for each hour of examination (Table 1).

TABLE 1
Summary

Number of patients	90
Total hours recorded	1.856
Hours per patient	20.62
Mean no. readings of arterial blood pressure per hour	6
Expected no. readings of arterial blood pressure	11,136
Expected no. readings A.B.P. per patient	123.7
Readings of arterial blood pressure obtained	8459
Readings of A.B.P. obtained per patient	93.9

In this way, we expected a total of 11,136 blood pressure measurements with a mean of 123.7 measurements for each patient. Every patient maintained a detailed diary of activities and symptoms occurred during the recording time.

Results

On analysis, the data showed that 8459 blood pressure measurements had actually been obtained, with a mean of 93.9 for each patient (Table 2). By analysing the recordings and diaries, we could attribute the 2677 (24%) missing readings, corresponding to 29.8 "missing" measurements for each patient, to the causes listed in Table 2.

We must note that a high percentage (40.1%) of lost data is due to insufficient instruction to the patients. We believe that adequate instruction of subjects is very important to the use of blood pressure monitoring to avoid unusable readings.

Failure due to the operation of the equipment occurred during the initial stages, ie the first 20 recordings.

The artefactual data readings, defined on the basis of Kennedy's

TABLE 2

Incidence and Causes of "Missing" Blood Pressure Measurement
(Most missing data are referable to the first recordings)

Cause	Incidence	
	Number	Percentage
Lack of co-operation by the patient	1076*	40.1
Inadequate contact between P11 and 446	431*	16.1
Assemblage(battery inadequatedly charged)	364*	13.5
Missed reading of spikes by model 671	359*	13.4
Pressurometer malfunction	244*	9.1
Blood pressure cuff	203*	7.5
Total no missing readings	2677	24
No Missing readings per patient	29.8	

(*) two or more causes occurred in some cases

experince as "absolute" artefacts and "suspected" artefacts (these last ones deemed possible but unlikely, because of their deviation from the individual trend pattern (3)), gave 1711 failure measurements occurring for 20.2% of the blood pressure measurements with a mean of 19.0 for each patient and 0.92 for a single recording hour.

Artefacts were mostly absolutes (60.7%) compared with the relative ones (39.2%).

We noticed that the former artefacts occurred during the environmental noise (for example, driving a car in the heavy traffic) while the seconds occurred during sleep (Table 3).

TABLE 3

Incidence of Artefacts (Kennedy's Classification)

Total no artefacts	1711 (20% of lost data points)
No artefacts per patient	19.0
No artefacts per hour	0.92
Suspected artefacts	672 (39.2%)
Absolute artefacts	1039 (60.7%)

Conclusion

Non-invasive ambulatory monitoring of arterial blood pressure gives many possibilities for clinical diagnosis and therapeutic control of hypertensive subjects (6, 9, 10). Being non-invasive and repeatable, it can be used for the study of arterial blood pressure changes and homeostatic mechanism controlling the arterial blood pressure.

The main aim of this study was to assess the specific technical components. We found that many problems occurred during the initial use of this equipment, but after we had recognized the technical limits, including different control and calibration to the various levels, several malfunctions ceased to occur and readings were no longer missed.

Careful selection and instruction of subjects, and their co-operation, are indispensable if artefacts are to be reduced. This is in agreement with the experience of others (3).

Acknowledgements

We wish to thank M. Paolo Reale for his advice and assistance.

References

1.   Germano G., Damiani S., Cassone R., Sturvi I., Ciavarella M., Calcagnini G., Corsi V. (1980) Com. Congresso Italiano di Cardiologia, Firenze.
2.   Germano G., Damiani S., Appolloni A., Ciavarella M., de Zorzi A., Calcagnini G., Corsi V. (1980) Com. Congresso Ital. Med. Interna, Roma.

3. Kennedy H.L., Padgett N.E., Horan M.J. (1979) Ambul. Electrocad.
    1, 13.
4. Littler W.A., West M.J., Honour A.J., Sleight P. (1978) Am.
    Heart J. 95, 180.
5. Millar-Craig M.W., Bishop N.C., Raftery E.B. (1978) Lancet 15,
    795.
6. Perloff D., Sokoloff M. (1978) Cardiov. Med. 3, 655.
7. Raftery E.B. (1978) Brit. J. Pharmac. 6, 193.
8. Rose G. (1965) Lancet 27, 673.
9. Sokolow M., Werdegar D., Kain K.H., Hinman A.T. (1966)
    Circulation, 24 279.
10. Sokolow M., Perloff D., Cowan R. (1973) Clin. Sci. 45, 195.

Discussion

DR. ALLAZ: Were the artefacts included in the missing measurements?
PROF. PINCIROLI: No, they were excluded.
DR. ALLAZ: But, on the whole, there is a lot of non-analysable data
if there is both missing data and artefacts.
PROF. PINCIROLI: I agree that there is.
DR. SPERTI: Is it possible that there is a large amount of artefacts
because an unselected group of patients was chosen? In our experience, the Del Mar Avionics system is totally unreliable, when
used in obese subjects.
DR. GERMANO (translated into English by Sperti): Initially, an
unselected group of subjects was chosen, but after discovering that
the system does not function in obese subjects, only non-obese subjects were chosen in the second part of the study.
DR. GOLDBERG: Going back to Dr. Raftery's first statements, does
Dr.Germano still feel that there is no non-invasive method - does he
think that this non-invasive method is of no use or is it useful?
PROF. PINCIROLI: The usefulness of the system is judged to be positive. We feel that it is particularly important that the non-invasive
method can be used many times in the same subject - for example, for
follow-up studies and so on.

ROUND TABLE DISCUSSION :
HOW SHALL WE DEFINE BLOOD PRESSURE VARIABILITY

In the Chair : D.L. Clement

Panel: G.O. van Maele   Gent, Belgium
           F.D. Stott   Northwick Park, UK
           R. Cowan   San Francisco, USA
           S. Mann   Bristol, UK
           R.H. Mitchell   Belfast, N.Ireland
           D.G. Altman   Northwick Park, UK

DR. CLEMENT: It is important to explain the reason for having a round-table discussion like this. We all know from experience that everytime a paper on blood pressure variability is presented a discussion follows telling that variability should not be expressed or calculated in that way.

In order to try to have some ideas which might hold for a moment, I thought it would be useful to discuss how we define and determine blood pressure variability now. If we could reach even a partial agreement, that would be useful because it could be maintained for some time as a reference, then revised at the next workshop in the light of new ideas expressed.

The only way to start this discussion is to try to have an idea about what all of us do and how we do it. It is of course slightly different according to whether an invasive or a non-invasive method is used, non-invasive methods mostly having only daytime recordings, while the invasive have day and night recordings.

Dr. van Maele will start by describing what we do with the daytime recordings. We can then go slightly further and see how people process the day and night recordings.

METHODS OF PROCESSING
SEMI-CONTINUOUS BLOOD PRESSURE RECORDING

G.O. Van Maele*, D.L. Clement**

*Department of Medical Informatics, ** Department of
Cardiovascular Diseases, University Hospital,
135 De Pintelaan, B-9000 Ghent, Belgium

Introduction

This discussion starts with a short presentation of the data-
processing of blood pressure measurements obtained with semi-
continuous recording devices at the department of cardiovascular
diseases at Ghent, using a Hewlett Packard 2100 vectorcardiogram
analysis computer system.

Blood Pressure Recording

The measurements are obtained either with the "Remler M200"
ambulatory recorder, or with the Arteriosonde type 1217, but recently
the latter was replaced by the Dinamap system.

For each instrument descriptive parameters and graphical
representations are computed and the measurement data are stored in
separate files.

In the case of the portometer, systolic and diastolic blood
pressure plus heart rate are recorded at 30 minute intervals.

The procedure starts in the clinic at about 8 a.m. and after
the adjustment of the portable recorder three clinic pressures are
recorded. Thereafter the patient returns home where his blood
pressure is registered during his normal daily routine and a detailed
diary kept.

Data Processing

The next day, the ambulatory recordings are analysed and the data for
systolic and diastolic pressure plus heart rate are filled into a
record form. Invalid recordings are marked by a dash.

The first program asks for the patient identification data in
an interactive manner, followed by the read-in of the paper tape and
the storage of the measurements into a data file. Each portometer
recording is characterised by a record number.

A second program then performs the statistical and graphical
computations of the stored data. Identification data is divided into
Patient Information and Study Information and is listed together with
the portometer recordings consisting of both clinic and home values
for systolic and diastolic pressures.

The whole set of descriptive parameters for the home values
is computed and printed (Table 1). It can be seen that for systolic
pressure the mean and median are almost the same and are much closer
to the lowest value than to the highest one. Notice also the position
of the modus which is situated at the level of the lowest recording.
From this one can forecast a marked skew towards the higher values.

TABLE 1

Specimen Patient Report

PORTOMETER - DR. D. CLEMENT   RECORD NUMBER : 505

PATIENT INFORMATION   STUDY INFORMATION
-------------------   -----------------
NAME: ....   PHYSICIAN: Dr. D. Clement
NUMBER: 641231 024   DEPARTMENT:
SEX: FEMALE   STUDY CODE: RO
AGE: 16   STUDY NUMBER: 505
RECORDING DATE:10.04.1981   PROCESSING DATE: 04.05.1981 10:26

	SYSTOLIC BP	DIASTOLIC BP
AZ VALUES	102	82
---------	118	74
	114	78
HOME VALUES	112	98
-----------	140	78
	120	74
	126	56
	126	74
	112	60

DESCRIPTIVE VALUES:			
------------------	NUMBER OF VALUES	: 23	23
	MEAN	: 128	72
	VARIANCE	: 286	173
	STANDARD DEVIATION	: 17	13
	STANDARD ERROR	: 3.5	2.75
	COEFF. OF VARIATION	: 13.2	18.2
	MINIMUM	: 112	56
	MAXIMUM	: 188	102
	MEDIAN	: 126	72
	0.02 PERCENTILE	: 112	56
	0.98 PERCENTILE	: 188	102
	MODUS	: 112	72

This output form is followed by a graphical representation of the blood pressure measurements as a function of time (Fig. 1). In addition to systolic and diastolic pressure the mean pressure is also plotted.

Finally histograms are plotted for systolic, diastolic and mean pressure (Fig. 2). The histogram of the systolic pressure shows a significant positive skewness as mentioned above. Similar histogram plots are made for diastolic pressure and mean pressure.

For Arteriosonde and Dinamap recordings the data processing is carried out in the same way and the output form of the computer processing is identical with these of the portometer.

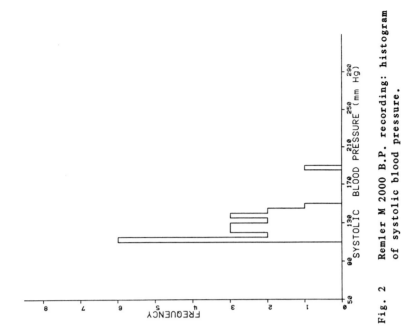

Fig. 1   Remler M 2000 B.P. recording: blood
          pressure in function of time.

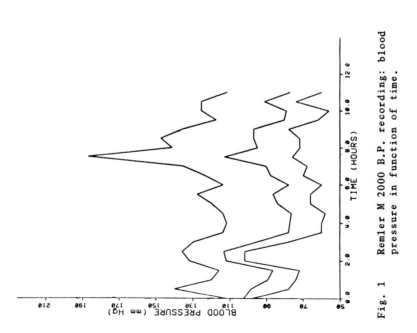

Fig. 2   Remler M 2000 B.P. recording: histogram
          of systolic blood pressure.

Blood Pressure Variability

Currently blood pressure variability is expressed as the standard deviation around the mean. Thus the systolic variability is the standard deviation of the systolic measurements and the diastolic variability is the standard deviation of the diastolic measurements.

When dealing with conditions where the blood pressure is changed, for example by a pharmacological agent, then the coefficient of variation is used instead of the S.D.

DISCUSSION

DR.CLEMENT: To start the discussion I would like Dr. Mann to tell us how he measures blood pressure variability with the 24 hour recordings. Afterwards, we can hear what everyone feels about the subject.
DR. MANN: Perhaps I shall frustrate Dr. Clement in that I do not believe that there is one method of measuring variability, but that there are several all of which are valid because they all look at different questions.

I shall talk aabout a few methods of measuring variability, pointing out those that we use particularly at present.

I believe that the blood pressure response to standard stimuli is a fair method of assessing blood pressure variability, and one that can be compared with others, and also one that is perhaps more standardised than others.

If we have intra-arterial recordings, and are able to take fixed points for each beat, the mean pressure, systolic or diastolic pressures or the heart rate (if that is relevant), we can construct incidence histograms of a fixed period of time from these recordings. We have used these in the past to derive either a variance, or its root (the standard deviation of these periods) to describe variability over a very short period.

To look at variability over different periods of time pooled means can of course be used, means derived over a period of time, be it 1/2 min, 2, 5, 10 mins or 1 hour (as I discussed earlier today), perhaps partially to eliminate artefact and some of the effects of short-term physical and mental activity which might markedly influence the blood pressure variability. As was shown this morning, that is one method which we are investigating at the moment, to describe the variability over a whole 24 hour period.
DR. CLEMENT: In digit numbers, how will you present to us that this is the variability with which you can work for a particular individual, which is shifted to another level if, for example, a drug is given? Can you give us a clear idea about it, just to start the discussion?
DR. MANN: I will stick my neck out and mention the two methods that we have used previously: first Millar Craig, at the last ISAM, presented 6 hourly variance derived straight from the intra-arterial recordings of systolic or diastolic pressure - each individual beat - and, secondly, as a measure of short-term variability I have shown this morning three indices which describe the circadian variation, the standard deviation of the 24 hourly means, the overall amplitude derived from a day/night different from 6 hourly segments of the

curve, and a mean hourly change in blood pressure to look at a slightly shorter-term variability.

DR. CLEMENT: And the mean hourly differences are calculated, and again the standard deviation of the difference?

DR. MANN: No, there is the standard deviation of each hourly mean over the whole 24 hours. The average hourly change is the mean change between each hour and its neighbour. We take the circadian curve that joins hourly points, pull it out like a piece of string, measure the length and divide by 24. That gives the mean change between each hour and its neighbour.

DR. CLEMENT: What is the way the other members of the panel work this out?

MR. COWAN: We have been using the standard deviation, but it has now been called into question because there is some reason to suspect that individual patient's distributions are not normal. However, in 80 to 90% of our patients we found that the distribution curves were normal. However, we may not have been looking at a sufficient number of patients at the higher range.

DR. CLEMENT: So you stick to the standard deviation as it is now?

MR. COWAN: As a measure of intra-daily variability it is the one that we have used, as well as the coefficient of variation.

MR. ALTMAN: May I make two points about standard deviation. First, I do not think it matters whether the distribution is normal. The standard deviation remains a valid measure of the dispersion of the values around the mean.

Secondly, the standard deviation must be highly preferable to using any sort of range because in particular the highest value is quite likely to be artefactual.

DR. MITCHELL: I would like to comment about the statistics. My understanding of signal analysis and statistics does not allow for standard statistics to be applied to something that is an average value which is changing.

DR. STOTT: I agree with Mr. Altman that the problem of non-stationarity of the data is serious. Either we must use a test of stationarity and analyse only the parts which are stationary, or use non-parametric methods of signal analysis.

I am unconvinced that any measures of blood pressure variability which are derived from the analysis of only the blood pressure are of any value, because blood pressure is not an independent variable; it is a function of several other variables. If those other variables remain constant, the blood pressure will remain constant. If they are changing, the blood pressure will change.

Where there is a dependent variable which is a function of a number of independent variables, by looking at the dependent variable only nothing can be inferred. Dr. Mann said one of the most important things that must be done is to look at blood pressure responses to standardised stimuli. To obtain a more comprehensive story, continuous measurements have to be made of other physiological parameters, such as heart rate, cardiac output, peripheral resistance, metabolic rate, work load.

But if we are to be able to take such figures and compare the same patient over a long period, or different patients within a group, or work done on similar patients in different centres, there must be much more standardisation of the conditions of measurement.

DR. MANN: I would like to make a slightly formulated reply to Dr. Stott's statements. While I do that, perhaps he would like to try to think of one physiological measurement that is either totally intrinsic or dependent on only one controlling factor.

The importance of blood presure variability is of physiological importance and of clinical importance. In the clinical world, it is known that by making repeated sphygmomanometer measurements, some patients seem to produce highly variable recordings, whereas others produce rather less variable ones.

The bias due to inaccuracies and errors in measurement have to be eliminated. After that, the clinical question has to be asked whether this variability is important, for example the blood pressure variability itself may influence prognosis in hypertension. Returning to the physiological importance aspect, does it represent a defect in the control system of blood pressure? I showed this morning that there is one, admittedly absolutely major defect in the control system of the blood pressure which not surprisingly produces differences in the indices of variability that can be used.

Secondly, an individual sphygomomanometer reading has to be interpreted by knowing what is the range of variability, qualifying our readings by a knowledge of that range. I do not think that has yet been done.
DR. CLEMENT: I would like to hold Dr. Mann on that point because that is open to a great deal of discussion and to many years' work.

Let us get back to the definition where we started. We have said that something can be done with standard deviation. Dr. Stott said that variability as derived from a blood pressure curve should not be used as an entity because it is dependent on too may mechanisms. In the previous Gent meetings (Blood Pressure Variability, p.43, 1979) it was shown that no clear relationship with sympathetic nervous activity could be shown; there is no other clear cut mechanism shown up to now. When we understand the mechanism of variability, we shall try to measure it better. We have not reached that point, so a way has to be found to work with it now.
DR. MANN: Could standard deviation be accepted as merely a descriptive function of blood pressure variability, allowing for the fact that there may be many mathematical problems attached to it when an attempt is made to make difficult interpretations - but it will at least describe the variability observed in a particular recording.
DR. CLEMENT: It has the benefit of giving us a number with which to work.
DR. STOTT: I think this is very dangerous. Standard deviation is not really very useful unless it is combined with a stationarity test. There is exactly the same variance or standard deviation on the histogram from a blood pressure that shows only one shift over a period of 4 hours and one that shows many shifts of the same amplitude over this period of time, but the physiological meaning is quite different. It is not very difficult to substitute run-length analysis for this - it is documented, it is quite simple and not difficult to do on a computer.
MR. ALTMAN: I think that we must distinguish between taking the standard deviation of data from each individual beat from the sort of histograms that we have seen, and what Dr. Mann has presented, which is taking the standard deviation of 24 hourly mean values, which

quite clearly is a measure of variability in a totally different way.
DR. STOTT: Yes, I agree with that, but I am not sure that the
standard deviation, or variance on 24 hourly means, for instance, may
not be blurring some of the information contained by that technique.

The main thing that the records about which Dr. Mann told us
show, in fact what was first noticed by Sir George Pickering, is that
there is a dramatic difference between the daytime and night-time
pressures even in the hypertensive patients, and even when they are
in bed in hospital.
DR. CASHMAN: Would the Panel clarify whether they feel that
sequential readings taken by a non-invasive method, say, an automatic
cuff, giving one reading a day (after averaging by whatever means),
would constitute independent observations in which standard deviation
might be a legitimate thing to look at? This is in distinction to
what we have been arguing about - which up to now, I think, has been
ambulatory beat-by-beat recordings where all kinds of different problems come in with non-stationarity.
MR. ALTMAN: Yes, reasonably independent observations. However, I do
not like the use of such values to measure the reproducibility of the
system.   There is an interaction of several effects, one of which is
day-to-day variation of a particular subject. Much depends on which
part of the day is being averaged over, if an average is taken. The
daytime values will vary more from day to day than will the night-
time values.
DR. CASHMAN: I wanted to distinguish between the arteriosonde-type
studies about which we have been talking and the intra-arterial
studies, because I think that they are two very different problems.
DR. CLEMENT: Still, mathematically, both situations are rather close
to each other; in the invasive method, the mean of all data from one
hour is calculated; for the non-invasive techniques, also the mean is
calculated but from a lesser number of readings per hour.
DR. CASHMAN: But it is really a question of whether it is thought
that that reading represents the hour.
DR. CLEMENT: Very much so - but that brings us to the same
discussion: if that total hour is averaged by cutting the ups and
downs, putting a mean on it, does that also represent that hour?
DR. CASHMAN: Quite. I think that we have an answer to the second
part of that in the case of ambulatory data, that it does not
represent that hour very well. By implication, there is the same
problem with the automatic cuff systems.
PROF. MALLION: Should invasive measurements be done on one day only
or should they be done for 2, 3 or 4 days because the amounts and
types of physical stress to which patients are submitted are
different from one day to another?
MR. COWAN: I do not know that I can give a definite answer to that
question, but we have some data. We have looked at two consecutive
days for a group of patients and have found that the between-days
correlation for systolic and diastolic pressure is 0.85. However, it
may be interesting that there are significant differences (10 mm Hg
or more) between the means of those two consecutive days in many
patients.
DR. CLEMENT: (intervening) Is that without differences in treatment?
We are talking about, say, placebo ...?
MR. COWAN: Yes. In addition, patients were studied without

treatment on two consecutive occasions that were more widely spaced (one or two years on average). The correlation between the sample taken on the two occasions was much lower, at about 0.3, so there is a major change in the stability of a day's mean that is a function of time.

DR. MANN: May I address this same question of standardisation because it is one of the most crucial questions. First, I would perhaps throw out a challenge and say that it is almost impossible to standardise conditions absolutely, for example, mental activity.

In that context, one of the concepts that I had when I started doing ambulatory monitoring is that basal night-time blood pressure is in any respect more constant than any other measurement of blood pressure.

If we do not take standardised conditions, what about ambulatory conditions? We have shown both on consecutive days and on days about 6 weeks apart, with the administration of placebo being the only difference, that the hourly mean method of deriving a circadian curve produces identical results with no significant differences in patients instructed to go about their normal day's activities.

DR. CLEMENT: The data presented this morning by Dr. van Maele showed that, at least with the Remler device, there is a reproducibility of about 68%.

MR. CROSBY: It seems to me that the question of intra-arterial lines versus hourly cuff measurements, and whether hourly means are taken, really boils down to the classic engineering problem of sampling rates. In many clinical observations the sampling rate is tailored to the activity. For example, if someone is in hospital but not very sick, his temperature might be taken once a day, whereas someone who is very sick might have it taken every half-hour. The amount of data needed depends on how much is going on in the patient.

DR. MANN: I fully accept it, but it is one of the things towards which we have been working in the methods described by Dr. Stott in collaboration with the Imperial College group. Unfortunately, some method of description of the variability is required, and as yet we have been unable to derive one that way, so we have used the more simple methods that people understand - as a merely descriptive tool at present.

DR. SPERTI: In our studies, in order to study the validity of the pressurometer method we have studied the mean of blood pressure values recorded during 20 second periods, taken at 7.45 minute intervals over 24 hours on the Oxford tape. This gives us about 120 readings for each day. The standard deviations obtained by two methods from these 120 readings and from the total Oxford tape are very close, differing only by 10%.

DR. CLEMENT: That brings us to the question of how many points are needed. What do the Panel members think about this?

DR. MANN: The information, as yet only verbal, from Prof. Sayers at the moment is that he seems to think that 10 minute periods during the day will probably remove most of the non-stationarity, with 20 minute periods at night.

DR. MITCHELL: It seems to me that one of our major problems, certainly a problem in our pregnancy studies, has been in defining a normal blood pressure rhythm. In our particular situation we are interested in the differences between the normal and the pre-eclamptic rhythm. If there is a difference that difference will manifest itself not necessarily in a 24 hour rhythm but under controlled conditions in which standard tests are applied, and these tests will be different for a normal person as distinct from an abnormal person.

DR. CLEMENT: It is clear to all of us that if it was possible to know what the mechanism of the spontaneous variations really is, a battery of tests could be set up and we could define, using these tests, what we are trying to define by recording the curve. However, the problem is that the mechanism is unknown.

DR. MITCHELL: But are we going to come back in two years' time and still talk about blood pressure and blood pressure variability when we have not started to look at other mechanisms which may well be controlling blood pressure variability itself?

DR. CLEMENT: What mechanisms are you thinking of?

DR. MITCHELL: I think Dr. Stott has said what we should perhaps be doing; also Dr.Davies in his studies on heart rate. That is one of the parameters which presumably is a function of what is going on. If I remember correctly, he found a considerable amount of variability, beat-to-beat, even though the heart rate was controlled. That is interesting because two years ago we presented some information on pregnancy which demonstrated that as the heart rate variability was changed so the blood pressure variability also changed in a negatively-correlated fashion.

DR. CASHMAN: I get the feeling that we may be converging towards something like 10 or 15 minutes as being the sampling rate which may be both useful and practical from the point of view of automatic cuffs, and also for intra-arterial analysis. Since Dr. Clement is very keen on the idea of standard deviations, could I suggest that a pair of standard deviations should be used; first, the standard deviation of all the values and, secondly, the standard deviation of the difference between one value and the next. This gives some indication whetherthe pattern is a smooth pattern that is followed throughout the 24 hours, or whether it is a very unstable, jagged pattern.

DR. CLEMENT: I like that suggestion. Would Dr. Stott like to comment on that before he gives his solution?

DR. STOTT: As I have said, I am the Devil's advocate and have no solutions, only problems. However, we must over the next two years look at these alternative non-parametric approaches to serial data analysis. In talking about how often to sample, if over the 24 hours there is a blood pressure trend curve like a Gaussian curve, it does not matter much whether sampling is done every beat or every 10 minutes or every half-hour.

DR. CASHMAN: But if, instead of having that, there was a high-frequency square wave all day long, there would be exactly the same interval histogram, and exactly the same distribution, but surely, clinically, that means something very different.

DR. STOTT: That is right, that is exactly what I was saying earlier on. But that comes out automatically if run-length analysis is used. This will give a three-dimensional plot and, according to which way it is projected,it is possible to get back to various simpler things by projecting it on suitable axes.

DR. CLEMENT: The main thing that we are coming to, is that not too many points are needed to define that curve finally. That number will have to be defined in the future. Some discrete points are needed over the day or night, and these points will give us a curve from which it is possible to calculate what we need.

DR. STOTT: I think we can begin to bracket quite accurately what is really needed. In the early days we went to continuous invasive monitoring because it was clear that using any sort of indirect cuff machine, sampling every 15 minutes, it was impossible to know what was being missed. One of the things to emerge from Sayers' analysis is that each beat is not independent of the previous one. If a reading is taken once a minute, nothing is lost. Beat-by-beat measurement is not necessary. The number of degrees of freedom is only about one-hundredth of the number of beats.

Approaching it from the other end, there seems to be little difference in proceeding from hourly means to 15 minute means; which seems to contain all the information that is genuinely independent and useful.

DR. HUNYOR: While I totally agree with Dr. Stott and Mr. Altman, it depends on whether we want to study control mechanisms or to describe clinically-relevant patterns.

Take one case, we had a case rather similar to Dr. Mann's autonomic neuropathy. This lady had a quite remarkable 24 hour course. Each time she sat, stood or sat on the toilet, her blood pressure would sink down. Obviously, with continuous recording we would get a whole catastrophe. There is no doubt that a Remler picture of that would like quite different, but the overall diagnosis and the management would probably be exactly the same.

If we are talking about mechanisms and control problems, I do not think that any of the non-invasive techniques can grapple with those problems. If we are talking about the so-called diurnal circadian rhythms, perhaps the daily fluctuations of catecholamines, steroids and so on, I imagine the non-invasive Remlers and any of the others do very well indeed.

However, there is the second side of the issue, this is to define statistical or mathematical variability of blood pressure so that it can be linked to these mechanisms that we are trying to study. Unless these two are linked, talking about blood pressure variability in its own right, to my mind, has no intrinsic value. However, in clinical terms we do think that the sort of blood pressure which is perfectly flat over a period of time but runs right through the middle of a varying pressure curve, is equally harmful or less harmful for the blood vessels, the myocardium or whatever.

PROF. PINCIROLI: Dr. Stott's comment on dependent variables seems to me important and probably suggests focusing on the distinction between observability and identification. If the convention is accepted that pressure variability is an important symptom for the prognosis of stable hypertension, it is right to look for variability by itself without any particular comment. But if the purpose is to characterise the mechanisms, probably we have to go in a different direction. My suggested is that the number of parameters to be observed should be enlarged; not only blood pressure but also blood flow, heart rate or something else (as has been said many times already).

I want to return to my idea about correcting some blood

measurements with data obtained from an electromyogram. Somebody
said that the state of the muscles may affect the measurements made
by the cuff. It seems to me that measuring the activity of muscle
instead of simply asking the patient about his general state is a
more objective measurement of his state of relaxation.

DR. CLEMENT: At the end of this round-table let me ask each of the
members of the Panel to tell us what we should do in the next two
years. How shall be define variability, as long as there is nothing
better, and what thoughts are there about how many points should be
necessary to define a curve. What are your final comments?

DR. STOTT: At this moment, I am not prepared to make a
recommendation about what I should do for the next two years, I need
rather more time to think about it.

MR. ALTMAN: I• was about to say very much the same. One thing,
though, that must be done is to try some of these different ideas
that have been proposed.

DR. van MAELE: I am not familiar with beat-to-beat variability, not
even with the dependence of the other factors which influence the
blood pressure, but I have nothing against the standard deviation as
a parameter for expressing variation because it is just a descriptive
parameter and has nothing to do with the Gaussian distribution. If I
am asked how to qualify a particular recording, I suggest it should
be done by the median and perhaps by the standard deviation on the
range.

DR. MITCHELL: I should like to see at any rate some of us starting
to look at other parameters which are important. A fair amount of
work has been done, for example, in neonatal monitoring and heart
rate variability. Can that be linked to blood pressure beat-to-beat
variability, for example?

DR. MANN: I think that we should all do it our own way. There is
not a standard method. Different methods of looking at variability
should be explored, tailoring them to the questions that we actually
want them to answer. Finally, we probably should look at comparisons
of different methods of assessment.

MR. COWAN: The primary issue is determining the stability of
variability as a charactertistic of the patient. I can understand
that there are some specialised conditions in which it is known that
the patient will be highly variable from one occasion to another,
but I am unfamiliar with convincing evidence that spontaneous
variability, where there are no observable stimuli, is a
characteristic trait of the patient which may be observed over long
periods of time.

DR. CLEMENT: Let me try to summarise some highlights of this round
table discussion. Several members of the Panel agree that blood
pressure variability can be defined by the standard deviation of the
mean; the main argument against this definition comes from the non-
stationarity of the blood pressure over the time period during which
blood pressure is recorded. The solution to that could be to make a
run-length analysis; however this method is not familiar either to
most investigators or clinicians. Meanwhile, standard deviation has
the best chances to remain the most widely used and easiest
definition of blood presure variability.

       It is very unlikely that, to characterise a patient's individual
blood pressure curve, all numbers from every individual heart beat

are necessary.   Several centres are exploring how many measurements in time should be made to accurately build up the blood pressure curve; measurementsevery 10 minutes during the day and every 20 minutes at night may be sufficient. The answer is probably different according to whether pure clinical information is sought or rather scientific information concerning mechanisms of variability.

Shifts of blood pressure in a time period depend on many, largely unknown, mechanisms. Other cardiovascular parameters, such as cardiac output, heart rate and blood flow through peripheral vessels, should be studied together with blood pressure, and extensively explored. As a result, a battery of stimuli could be set up; the blood pressure response to these stimuli could provide a better approach to an individual's pressure variability than recording a curve in conditions that are hard to standardise.

These points form quite a research programme for the coming years. I hope the next meeting brings us answers to these questions.

PROGNOSTIC IMPLICATIONS OF THE DISPARITY BETWEEN OFFICE AND AMBULATORY BLOOD PRESSURE MEASUREMENTS

R.M. COWAN*, M. SOKOLOW**, AND D. PERLOFF***

*Computer Centre, University of California, San Francisco,
**Dept. Medicine and Cardiovascular Research Institute,
Univerity of California, San Francisco,
***Dept. Medicine, University of California,
San Francisco, USA

Summary

Ambulatory blood pressure measurements were obtained during 12-hour periods of "typical" activity in a prospective study of 650 patients, with uncomplicated hypertension. When these measurements were averaged and compared with averaged readings taken during clinical examinations, it was found that the mean office systolic, diastolic and pulse pressures for the sample were significantly higher than the corresponding ambulatory means. The disparity derived by subtracting the average ambulatory pressure from the average office pressure was significantly greater for systolic than for diastolic pressure. Similarly, the positive correlation between the level of the office pressure and the size of the disparity was greater for systolic than for diastolic measurements. When the sample was sub-grouped into quartiles based on the magnitude of the office-ambulatory disparity in relation to the level of the office systolic pressure, patients in the lowest disparity quartile were found to have a 10-year cumulative morbidity rate of 40 per cent, compared with 20 per cent in the highest quartile.

Introduction

A series of studies originating in this laboratory have attempted to explore the relationship between indirect ambulatory blood pressure measurements and concurrent cardiovascular pathology (1, 2, 3). In general, it has been shown that for any given level of office blood pressure, the higher the ambulatory pressure, the greater the frequency of retinopathy, ECG evidence of left ventricular hypertrophy and prior cardiovascular disease. The present report focuses on the disparity between the office and ambulatory pressures and its association with the subsequent development of cardiovascular-renal disease.

Subjects and Methods

The sample consisted of 650 patients with a diagnosis of essential hypertension, who were referred to the University of California Hypertension Clinic for ambulatory blood pressure assessments. The criteria for inclusion were:

1. A negative history with respect to the cardiovascular-renal events, which comprised the outcome classification (myocardial infarction, angina pectoris, ECG evidence of ischemia or left bundle branch block, coronary insufficiency, cerebrovascular accident, transient cerebral ischaemic attacks, dissecting aneurysm of the aorta, peripheral vascular occlusive disease, uremia, congestive heart failure, severely accelerated hypertension);
2. A minimum follow-up period of two years for patients, who had not experienced a clinical event during he course of the study.

Ambulatory blood pressure measurements were obtained by means of the Remler electronic recording system. Previous reports from this laboratory have provided descriptions of the method and data documenting the close agreement between these ambulatory measurements and simultaneous conventional auscultatory readings (4, 5). Ambulatory readings were obtained at approximately 30-minute intervals during one or two 12-hour periods in which patients engaged in activities of their own choosing, although they were encouraged to make those activities as "typical" as possible. Means and standard deviations for ambulatory systolic and diastolic measurements were calculated. In addition, office systolic and diastolic averages were computed for all pressures recorded during clinic examinations within 90 days of the ambulatory blood pressure assessment. The average ambulatory pressure was subtracted from the average office pressure to provide a measure of disparity. All patients also had ratings of retinal involvement and ECG indications of left ventricular hypertrophy. Retinopathy was coded as positive if the following findings were present: arteriovenous compression and arteriolar narrowing, sclerosis, tortuosity. Left ventricular hypertrophy was coded positive if the ECG shows increased voltage and relatively low or abnormal T-waves.

Results

The sample consisted of 314 males and 336 females. Retinopathy was observed in 18.9 per cent of the sample and left ventricular hypertrophy in 6.9 per cent. The average age at entry was 42.9 (s.d. = 13.7) and the average follow-up interval was 6.1 years. Intervals of 4 years or more were recorded for 69 per cent of the 547 patients with negative outcomes and for 64 per cent of the 103 patients with positive outcomes. Clinical events were classified as follows:

58 coronary disease, 28 cerebral vascular disease, 7 peripheral vascular occlusive disease, 5 congestive heart-failure, 3 renovascular disease secondary to hypertension and 2 "other" forms of vascular disease. Twelve events were fatal: 6 coronary deaths, 4 cerebrovascular accidents and 2 cases of uremia.

The majority (78 per cent) of the ambulatory blood pressure studies were performed in the absence of antihypertensive medication. Table 1 presents the results of paired t-test comparisons of office vs. ambulatory blood pressure measurements. The average office systolic, diastolic and pulse pressures were significantly higher than the corresponding ambulatory measures. Similar comparisons for systolic and diastolic measures are contained in Table 2. Although the office-ambulatory systolic disparity was significantly greater than

TABLE 1

Paired T-Test Comparisons of Office Vs. Ambulatory Measures

	Office		Ambulatory			
	Mean	S.D.	Mean	S.D.	t	p
Systolic	159.8	23.5	144.7	21.9	21.2	< .001
Diastolic	100.3	11.9	91.2	13.7	21.0	< .001
Pulse						
Pressure	59.5	18.4	53.5	16.0	10.8	< .001

TABLE 2

Paired T-Test Comparisons of Systolic Vs. Diastolic Measures

	Systolic		Diastolic			
	Mean	S.D.	Mean	S.D.	t	p
Office-Ambul.						
Disparity	15.1	18.2	9.1	11.0	10.8	< .001
Disparity/						
Office BP (%)	8.9	10.6	8.8	10.9	0.3	n.s.
Standard						
Deviation	12.4	4.3	8.7	2.5	23.9	< .001
Coefficient						
of variation	8.6	2.8	9.8	3.1	-9.4	< .001

the diastolic disparity, no difference was found when the disparity was treated as a percentage of the average office pressure. The ambulatory systolic standard deviation was significantly greater than the ambulatory diastolic standard deviation but, when coefficients of variation were computed from these standard deviations and the assoc-iated means, somewhat greater variability was found in the diastolic measurements.

Correlations between office ambulatory disparity and selected blood pressure variables are shown in Table 3. The correlation between disparity and the level of the office pressure was greater for systolic than for diastolic measurements, but there was no cor-responding difference in the correlations with the average ambulatory pressure. Both disparity measures were unrelated to the associated ambulatory standard deviations and showed weak positive correlations with the coefficients of variation. Both measures of disparity were uncorrelated with age. Although not presented in Table 3, a correla-tion of .62 was found between the systolic and diastolic disparities.

In view of the substantial correlation between disparity and the level of the office systolic presure (Table 3), the sample was di-

TABLE 3

Correlation Coefficients for Office-Ambulatory Disparities

	Systolic Disparity	Diastolic Disparity
Office average	.48	.17
Ambulatory average	-.32	-.34
Ambulatory standard deviation	.03	.05
Ambulatory coefficient of var.	.18	.21
Age	.08	-.08

vided into 4 office systolic intervals. As shown in Table 4, a median disparity of 5mmHg was found for patients with office systolic pressures in the lowest range (<140mmHg). Among patients with systolic pressures in the highest range (>=180mmHg), the median disparity was 6 times as large. Comparing the same intervals, 30 per cent of patients in the lowest range were found to have negative disparities (i.e., ambulatory systolic pressures exceeding the level of the office systolic pressure), whereas only 12 per cent of the patients in the highest interval had negative disparities.

TABLE 4

Relationship of Office-Ambulatory Disparity
to Average Office Systolic

		Median Office-Amb. Disparity			
Office Systolic	N	First Quartile	Median	Third Quartile	Percent Patients with Negative Disparity (Amb.BP > Office BP)
<140	122	-3	5	12	30
140-59	236	1	12	22	23
160-79	171	7	19	29	16
>=180	121	13	30	44	12
TOTAL	650	3	15	26	20

Patients were then classified according to their disparity percentile rank within each office systolic subgroup and comparisons were made for cumulative 10-year morbidity rates estimated by the life-table method (Table 5). Among patients with office systolic pressures averaging below 160mmHg, the rate was 23 per cent for those with the smallest disparities (quartile 1) as opposed to only 8 per cent for those with the largest disparities. Patients with intermediate disparities (quartiles 2 and 3) had morbidity rates which were higher than those of patients with smaller disparities (quartile 4).

TABLE 5

Estimated Cumulative 10-year Morbidity Rates in Relation
to Office-Ambulatory Systolic Disparity

	Average Office Syst.		
Systolic Disparity	<160	>= 160	TOTAL
Quartile 1	23 (91)	41 (74)	40 (165)
Quartiles 2-3	11 (175)	32 (141)	25 (316)
Quartile 4	8 (92)	26 (77)	20 (169)

* Number of patients indicated in parentheses)

Among patients with office systolic pressures of 160mmHg or higher, the percentages were 41 and 26 respectively. Taking the sample as a whole, the cumulative 10-year morbidity rate in the lowest quartile was twice that of the highest quartile (40 vs. 20 per cent).

Discussion

The findings of this study are consistent with our earlier studies of the association between office-ambulatory disparity and concurrent cardiosvascular status, and, in addition, document and antecedent role of disparity in relation to prognosis. Regardless of subsequent treatment (which was not taken into account in the data analysis), the clinical course of these patients was related to blood pressure measurements made at the time of entry into the study. As expected, patients with office systolic pressures of 160mmHg and more had a higher morbidity rate than those with lower pressures. However, within each of these two subgroups, a large office-ambulatory dispar-ity was associated with a more favourable prognosis. In fact, there was little or no difference in morbidity rates between patients in the low-pressure/small-disparity subgroup and those in the high-pressure/large-disparity subgroup (23 per cent and 26 per cent, respectively).

Ambulatory blood pressure measurements evidently can contribute to the assessment of risk in hypertension. On the strength of these findings, we hypothesize that, controlling for office systolic pres-sure, patients with relatively high ambulatory pressures will require more intensive therapy to reduce their morbidity rates to the levels of patients with relatively low ambulatory pressures. In order to develop a more systematic approach to the use of ambulatory record-ings in the management of hypertension, we need additional evidence on how the office-ambulatory disparity is affected by therapy and whether changes in the amount of the disparity influence clinical outcome.

Acknowledgements

This research was supported by grants from the U.S. Public Health Service (HL-18076 and HL-08625) and the Carrie Baum Browning Trust for Heart Research (TWR-54413-0).

References

1.   Sokolow M., Perloff D. and Cowan R.M. (1980) Cardiovascular Reviews and Reports 1, 295.
2.   Perloff D., Sokolow M. and Cowan R. (1981) Biotel. and Patient Monitoring 8, 67.
3.   Sokolow M., Werdegar D., Kain H.K. and Hinman A.T. (1966) Circ. 34, 279. •
4.   Cowan R.M., Sokolow M. and Perloff D. (1980) In: ISAM 1979, Proceedings of the Third International Symposium on Ambulatory Monitoring. (Eds: Stott F.D., Raftery E.B. and Goulding L.) London: Academic Press.
5.   Kain H.K., Hinman A.T. and Sokolow M. (1964) Circulation 30, 882.

BLOOD PRESSURE AND HEART RATE VARIABILITY AT NORMAL AND HIGH BLOOD PRESSURE

M. Di RIENZO, P. CIOFFI, A. PEDOTTI, G. MANCIA*

Centro di Bioingegneria - Fondazione Pro Juventute and
Politecnico di Milano, * Centro di Ricerche Cardiovascolari CNR -
Universita di Milano, Italy

Summary

Since its first application in the late sixties, direct and
continuous blood pressure recording in ambulant human beings has
proved to be a valuable method for:
- investigating phenomena such as behavioural control of
  circulation and blood pressure variability (1, 2, 3, 4)
- improving the diagnosis of hypertension, in particular that of
  borderline hypertension (1, 5, 6)
- providing an optimal evaluation of the efficacy oftreatment
  procedures for hypertension.

In the past few years, a joint project between the Centro di
Ricerche Cardiovascolari, of the Italian National Research Council,
(University of Milano) and the Centro di Bioingegneria, jointly
sponsored by the Pro Juventute Foundation and the Politecnico of
Milano, has involved the monitoring of blood pressure directly and
continuously for 24 hours in a large number of ambulant subjects and
also analyzing the results by suitable computer programmes.

The present report will briefly summarize some of the results
that have so far been obtained. In particular, mention will be made
of:
1. The method for analyzing blood pressure data.
2. The results obtained on blood pressure and heart rate
    variability in normotensive and hypertensive subjects.
3. The relationship between blood pressure and heart rate
    values.

Methods for Analyzing Blood Pressure and Heart Rate Data

The continuous and direct blood pressure recording over a 24-hour
time interval has been performed by the Oxford method, which has been
described in detail in previous studies (2, 7). For safety reasons
in all subjects, the catheter was inserted in a radial rather than a
brachial artery. The blood pressure signal (recorded on a cassette
recorder) was replayed at a speed 60 times the original speed (see
details of the Oxford method) and transferred to a magnetic tape.
The tape was replayed and its output filtered and directed to two
different circuits. The first circuit was is a channel of the A/D
converter, while the second circuit included a device which could
specifically identify the beginning of each pulse wave. The output
signal of this device was connected to a second channel of the A/D
converter. Both signals, namely the pulse pressure wave and the

signal provided by the special device were synchronously sampled at the frequency of 1 kHz. The data were then read by a digital computer (PDP 11/34) which was programmed to provide:

- The average of all values sampled over every 50 ms. interval.
- The maximal and minimal blood pressure values recorded during the 50 ms interval.
- The number of pulse pressure waves that occurred within each 50 ms interval.

The analysis provided values for mean arterial, systolic, and diastolic blood pressure, and heart rate, during each of the time intervals. It should be noted that these intervals could slightly exceed the 50 ms limit because the method of analysis required the use of an integer number of pulse pressure waves. It should also be noted that because the data had been replayed at a speed 60 times faster than the original speed, the 50 ms actually represents 3-second intervals. The values corresponding to these intervals were stored on magnetic discs and used for further analysis (see below).

Blood pressure and heart rate variability in normotensive and hypertensive subjects.

Using the method described above, blood pressure and heart rate variability were examined in 89 subjects of both sexes and various ages, all of whom were hospitalized, but not restricted to bed. In each subject variability was expressed in two different ways.

- From the 3-second values standard deviations were separately obtained for each of the 48 half-hours of the 24-hour recording period. These values were averaged and the results used as an index of variability within half-hour intervals, i.e. a rather 'short-term' variability.
- From the 3-second values, means of the 48 half-hours were also obtained. These means were averaged and their standard deviations were used as an index of variability among half-hours, i.e., a relatively 'long-term' variability (8).

Table 1 shows the short-term and long-term standard deviations in 3 groups of subjects who, on the basis of their 24-hour mean arterial pressure value, could be identified as normotensive, moderate, and severe hypertensive. The hypertension was, in each instance essential in nature. Several results are worthy of comment.

First of all, in each group of subjects, the 'long-term' standard deviation of mean arterial pressure was greater than the 'short-term' one, the difference being statistically significant at $p < 0.05$ when the groups were compared by non paired t-test. Such a trend was also evident when long and short-term heart rate variability were compared in a similar fashion.

Secondly, the standard deviation for mean arterial pressure increased from the normotensive to the hypertensive states (non-paired t-test with $p < .05$) and this occurred when the standard deviation both within and among half-hours were considered. On the otbher hand, the standard deviation for heart rate did not show a similar pattern. The HR value within half-hours showed no signficant difference among the 3 groups, whereas among half-hours it was slightly greater in hypertensive as compared to normotensive individuals,

TABLE 1

BLOOD PRESSURE AND HEART VARIABILITY IN NORMOTENSIVE AND HYPERTENSIVE SUBJECTS

	Mean arterial pressure (mmHg)			Heart rate (b/min)		
	24 hour mean value	SD within half hours	SD among half hours	24 hour mean value	SD within half hours	SD among half hours
Normotensive group (n=22)	88.1 ± 1.7	6.5 ± 0.3	9.5 ± 0.5	75.0 ± 1.8	8.9 ± 0.9	8.7 ± 0.7
M. hypertensive group (n=26)	107.8 ± 0.8	8.1 ± 0.3	12.1 ± 0.7	77.5 ± 1.9	7.9 ± 0.5	10.2 ± 0.6
S. hypertensive group (n=41)	137.9 ± 3.1	9.2 ± 0.4	11.8 ± 0.5	79.5 ± 1.5	8.0 ± 0.6	10.7 ± 0.5

Data shown are the means (± SE) from 3 groups of subjects defined as normotensives, moderate and severe hypertensive according to conventional classification based on cuffmeasurements. For definition of standard deviation (SD) within and among half-hours see text.

Table 2 shows data from the same 3 groups of subjects as the previous table. In this case, however, the blood pressure and heart rate variability are expressed as variation coefficients. It can be seen that as far as mean arterial pressure was concerned, the coefficients were no greater in the hypertensive than the normotensive group. In fact, in the group with severe hypertension the variation coefficients both within and among half-hours were smaller than those observed in the normotensive and the moderate hypertensive. Variation coefficients for heart rate within and among half-hours also did not significantly differ in the 3 groups.

These studies have led us to the following conclusions:

- The tendency for blood pressure to vary about its mean value is greater in subjects with essential hypertension as compared to normotensive subjects. This is the case both for the short and for the relatively long term blood pressure variations that can be identified within a 24-hour time-span.

- The increase in blood pressure variability is proportional to the increase in mean arterial pressure value in the normotensive and in the moderate hypertensive groups. It is less than proportional in subjects with severe hypertension. In other words, in hypertension blood pressure does not show greater percentage variations. In fact, when the hypertensive state is severe, percentage blood pressure variations may be less pronounced.

As we have mentioned earlier, the values that were used to calculate mean arterial pressure variability were derived from the average values sampled within 3-second periods. This implies that the very brief blood pressure variations that might have occurred within these intervals were not taken into account. How this affected total blood pressure variability was examined in 4 subjects. Using the original signal, we progressively increased from 1 to 16 seconds, the time interval over which the data were averaged; the standard deviations of mean arterial pressures were then computed for each of these different intervals.

The results are shown in Figure 1. As it might be expected, the standard deviation showed a progressive reduction from the 1-second to the 16-seconds method of calculation. At 3 seconds, however, the standard deviation was only slightly reduced as compared to the value at 1 second, this being true for all four subjects. Thus, only a minor portion of the variability for mean arterial pressure is lost by our method of analysis. This loss appears to be more than compensated by the advantage of the reduction in the amount of information stored on the mass memory of the computer.

Relationship between Blood Pressure and Heart Rate

A further aspect that was analyzed in our subjects was the correlation of blood pressure and heart rate values within the 24-hours time. The correlation was obtained for each subject by applying the non-parametric test of Smirnoff to the half-hour values. In 74 out of 89 subjects, blood pressure and heart rate were positively correlated. The positive correlation was not limited to the normotensive subjects but was observed in subjects with moderate and severe hypertension as well. Similar results were obtained when standard devia-

TABLE 2

BLOOD PRESSURE AND HEART RATE VARIABILITY IN NORMOTENSIVE AND HYPERTENSIVE SUBJECTS

	Mean arterial pressure			Heart Rate		
	24 hour mean value (mmhg)	VC within half hours	VC among half hours	24 hour mean value (b/min)	VC within half hours	VC among halfhours
Normotensive group (n=22)	88.1 ± 1.7	7.4 ± 0.3	10.8 ± 0.6	75.0 ± 1.8	11.9 ± 0.6	12.3 ± 1.1
M.hypertensive group (n=26)	107.8 ± 0.8	7.5 ± 0.3	11.3 ± 0.7	77.5 ± 1.9	10.2 ± 0.6	13.2 ± 0.8
S.hypertensive	137.9 ± 3.1	6.7 ± 0.3	8.5 ± 0.4	79.5 ± 1.5	10.0 ± 6.1	12.8 ± 0.6

Means ($\pm$ SE) from the same 3 groups of subjects of table 1. In this table, however, variation coefficients (VC) within and among half hours have been calculatedfor each subject the results being averaged for the 3 groups.

WINDOW

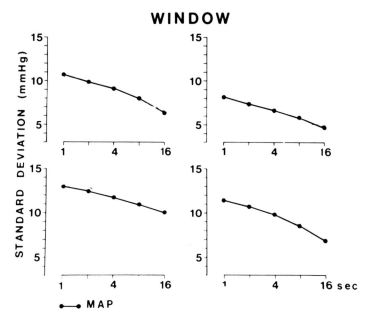

●——● M A P

Fig. 1   Standard Deviation by mean arterial pressure (MAP)
obtained when periods over which data were averaged
(window) were increased from 1 to 16 seconds. Data
from 4 subjects.

tions for heart rate and blood pressure were correlated. These
findings suggest that there   may not be a negative feed-back physiological relationship between heart rate and blood pressure in normal
daily life, at least as far as average half-hour values are concerned. This appears to be the case for both normotensive and hypertensive individuals.

References

1.   Mancia G., Zanchetti A. (1980) Atheroscl. Reviews, **7** 247-254.
2.   Bevan A.T., Honour A.J., Stott F.H. (1969) Clin. Sci. **36** 329-
     344.
3.   Littler W.A., Honour A.J., Sleight P., Stott F.D. (1972)
     Br.Med.J. **iii**, 76-78
4.   Little W.A., West M.J., Honour A.J., Sleight P. (1978) Am.Heart
     J.**95**, 180-186.
5.   Goldberg A.D., Raftery E.G., Cashman P.M.M., Stott F.D. (1978)
     Br. Heart J. **40**, 656-664.
6.   Irvin J.B., Brish H.M., Kerr F., Kirby B.J. (1976), Postgraduate
     Med. Jr., **52** (Suppl. 7). 137.
7.   Stott F.D., Honour A.J., Terry V.G. (1976) Postgraduate Med. JK.
     52, (Suppl. 7), 104.
8.   Mancia G., Ferrari A., Gregorini C., Parati G., Pomidossi G.,
     Bertinierie G., Grassi G., Zanchdetti A.(1980) Cli. Sci., **59**
     401.

NOCTURNAL CHANGES IN BLOOD PRESSURE, HEART RATE AND PRESSOR HORMONES; EFFECT OF ACUTE BETA-BLOCKADE

P.J. WILLEMSE, P.W. de LEEUW AND W.H. BIRKENHÄGER

Dept. of Medicine, Zuiderziekenhuis, Rotterdam,
The Netherlands

Summary

In 10 patients with uncomplicated essential hypertension changes in
blood pressure, heart rate, renin and noradrenaline were followed
during sleep. Five of them received 100 mg of atenolol orally, four
hours before they went to sleep. In both groups of patients, comparable changes in blood pressure and renin occurred, although these
variables were lower in patients, who had taken atenolol. Plasma
renin levels reached a peak value at the trough of blood pressure,
suggesting baroreceptor mediated renin release. Plasma noradrenaline
fell in parallel with blood pressure in untreated as well as in
treated patients. It seems likely, therefore, that withdrawal of
sympathetic tone is an important mechanism in the nocturnal blood
pressure fall.

Introduction

The most conspicuous feature of diurnal variations of blood pressure
is the fall during sleep. Both a decrease in cardiac output and a
decrease in peripheral vascular resistance have been implicated in
this nocturnal fall (1, 2), but the exact mechanism remains unknown.
Also the role of the pressor systems in this pattern is insuffic-
iently understood. In the present study, therefore, we have attempted to relate nocturnal changes in blood pressure to concurrent
changes in the renin-angiotensin system and the sympathetic nervous
system. Since both systems are affected by beta-blocker therapy, we
also assessed the influence of an acute oral dose of atenolol on
these relations.

Patients and Methods

Ten patients with uncomplicated essential hypertension were admitted
to the study. They had all been hospitalized in a metabolic ward for
at least five days. None of them had taken any medication in the
three weeks prior to the study. Sodium intake had been restricted at
55 mmoles per day and checked by 24-hour collections of urine.

On the study day at 14.00 hours, a catheter was introduced into
a brachial artery and connected to a transducer for continuous measurement of intra-arterial pressure. Heart rate was monitored simultaneously from an ECG-recording.

At 16.00 hours and again at 22.00 hours, a blood sample was
taken for determination of active renin and noradrenaline.

Patients usually went to sleep between 22.00 and 23.00 hours. They were separated from other patients in a special ward, to which only the investigators had access. When patients were asleep further blood samples were taken at 01.00 and 04.00 hours of the following day. Immediately after waking (between 06.00 and 07.00 hours) the last sample was drawn.

Patients were divided into two groups. In Group I (n=5), no medication was given, while in Group II (n=5), patients received 100 mg of atenolol per os at about 18.00 hours. Results were analysed with Student's t-test; data are presented as means ± S.E.M.

Results

The nocturnal changes in blood presure, heart rate and pressor hormones for both groups are presented in Figure 1.

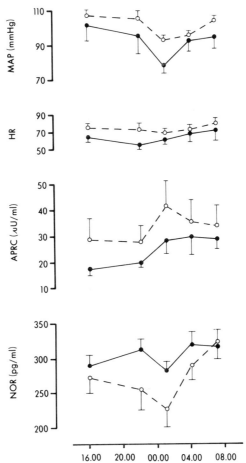

Fig. 1   Changes in mean arterial pressure, heart rate, renin and noradrenaline (mean ± S.E.M) during sleep in patients from group I (open circles) and group (II) (closed circles)

As can be seen there was a pronounced fall in blood pressure with relatively little change in heart rate during the night. Unfortunately, patients from Group II already had slightly lower values for blood pressure and heart rate before they received atenolol, but the differences with Group I were not significant. However, at 01.00 hours, blood pressure fell to a significantly lower level in Group II than in Group 1 (p < 0. 05), whilst heart rate already dropped significantly (p < 0.05) in Group II, within 4 hours after the administration of atenolol. During the night and early morning, heart rate remained lower in Group II, but from 01.00 hours onwards, the difference with Group I was no longer significant.

Renin levels were lower in Group II throughout the study (p < 0.05). However, the behaviour of this hormone during the night was similar in both groups, showing peak levels at the time of the blood pressure nadir.

Noradrenaline levels clearly fell during the night in both patient groups. The fall at midnight coincided with the drop in blood pressure.

Discussion

In view of the preliminary nature of this communication, it is not yet justified to draw firm conclusions.

In particular, this applies to the comparison between Groups I and II. Since only a few patients were studied, it is not surprising that they were not completely matched. However, it seems reasonable to assume that acute beta-blockade does not significantly modify the pattern of blood pressure variability during sleep. If the nocturnal fall in blood pressure would depend solely upon a reduction in cardiac output, one would expect some blunting of the blood pressure changes during beta-blockade. This did not occur in our study; instead, they seemed to be enhanced. However, there is still no certainty about the haemodynamic adaptation to sleep and further studies are needed to clarify the role of the heart in this event.

Changes in plasma renin concentration showed a comparable pattern in Groups I and II, peak levels being found at the time that the blood pressure curve reached a nadir. It may be that larger fluctuations in renin levels would have been observed, if we had sampled more frequently. For instance, with frequent measurements Mullen et al (4) found renin levels to vary with the stage of sleep.

Onset of REM-sleep was associated with a brisk fall in renin. Unfortunately, the authors did not mention blood pressure changes during this period. However, from the study of Khatri and Freis (1969), one might infer that some increase in blood pressure occurred at that time. This in turn could be responsible for suppression of renin. From our results, although less extensive, it is also tempting to speculate that the rise in renin was baroreceptor mediated. Such a mechanism was discarded by Modlinger et al (3), who instead suggested an endogenous (circadian) rhythm of renin, perhaps controlled by the central nervous system. The authors, however, did not provide blood pressure data, although they stated that in 5 out of 6 patients, blood pressure did not fall during the night, while renin levels still rose.

Admittedly, our studies cannot allow us to draw a definite

conclusion, but it seems less likely that a beta-adrenergic mechanism is involved in the early morning rise of renin. The possibility remains that a reduction in alpha-adrenergic tone was resonsible for the increase in renin.

A drop in noradrenaline levels indeed coincided with the nocturnal fall in blood pressure. This may also indicate that the sympathetic nervous system is, at least to some extent, responsible for the observed changes in blood pressure. If this is true, then it is also likely that this mechanism acts through vascular alpha-adrenoceptors, since beta-blockade did not modify the pattern as seen in the untreated subjects.

In summary, our data suggest that the blood pressure fall during sleep is associated with a decrease in sympathetic activity and a rise in renin. During acute beta-blockade, these changes are largely preserved. It seems likely that withdrawal of sympathetic tone by an effect on vascular alpha-adrenoceptors is responsible for the nocturnal drop in pressure. The simultaneous rise in renin levels, most likely is due to stimulation of the renal baroreceptor mechanism, although it cannot be excluded that diminished inhibition of renin secretion by alpha-adrenoceptors is involved.

Acknowledgement

This study was supported by Grant 77080 of the Dutch Heart Foundation.

References

1. Bristow J.D., Honour A.J., Pickering G.W., Sleight P. and Smyth A.S. (1969) Circulation **39**, 48.
2. Khatri I.M. and Freis E.D. (1969) Circulation **39**, 785.
3. Modlinger R.S., Sharif-Zadeh K., Ertel N.H. and Gutkin M. (1976) **43** 1276.
4. Mullen P.E., James V.H.T., Lightman S.L., Linsell C. and Peart W.S. (1980) J. Clin. Endocrinol. Metab. **50**, 466.

BAROREFLEX REGULATION OF BLOOD PRESSURE VARIABILITY

J.V. JONES, J.S. FLORAS, M.O. HASSAN. P. ROSSI,
P.S. SEVER, P. SLEIGHT

Dept. Cardiovascular Medicine, John Radcliffe Hospital,
Oxford and Dept. Clinical Pharmacology,
St. Mary's Hospital, London, UK

Summary

24-hour ambulatory blood pressure recordings were obtained and the
standard deviation around the mean taken as a measure of blood pressure variability. The relationship between this and mental and
physical exercise, plasma noradrenaline, age and baroreflex sensitivity was studied.   Only baroreflex sensitivity was independently related to variability of mean arterial blood pressure.

Introduction

Arterial blood pressure measured either directly or indirectly is
extremely variable. Within the space of a few minutes, the pressure
measured by sphygmomanometer can be widely different. The same is
seen with ambulatory monitoring techniques where blood pressure is
measured on a beat-to-beat basis. Why the blood pressure varies so
much from moment to moment is unknown although many extraneous influences such as fear, excitement, exercise and so on can profoundly
affect the pressure. Recently, there have been several reports on
factors that might influence the variability of arterial blood pressure (1, 2). We also have been performing such studies and in particular, have examined the relationship between blood pressure variability and mental and physical exercise, plasma noradrenaline, age
and baroreflex sensitivity.

Methods

Blood pressure variability was determined from 24-hour ambulatory
monitoring records using the Oxford Medilog System. This has been
described in detail before but, briefly, a flexible teflon cannula,
11 cm. long and internal diameter 0.6 mm., is inserted into the left
brachial artery under local anaesthesia using the Seldinger technique. The cannula is connected to the recording unit by means of a
fine nylon tube about one metre in length. This system records blood
pressure in a linear fashion between 30 and 250mmHg;   its frequency
response of 8-10 Hz makes it adequate for accurate reproduction of
the pressure wave form at rest, but during exercise mean blood pressures are more reliably measured than are systolic or diastolic blood
pressure (3).
    Our subjects were selected on the basis that all of them had
resting supine blood pressures on at least three clinic visits of
over 240mmHg. systolic or 90mmHg. diastolic. They were not admitted

to hospital, but attended at 9.00 a.m. on the day of the study. The arterial line was inserted as was an additional venous line. A period of rest for forty-five minutes followed and then mental (substraction of serial sevens from three hundred) and physical exercise (50 watts for 5 minutes and 75 watts for 5 minutes) tests were performed. Baroreflex sensitivity was determined using the method of Smyth et al (4). At approximately 12 noon, the venous line was removed and the arterial cannula connected to the ambulatory monitoring apparatus and the patient allowed to return home. They attended briefly in the evening for recalibration of the transducer and checking of the system.

The analysis of the ambulatory monitoring data has been described before (5). We use hourly frequency histograms which can be summated to give larger histograms (e.g. of the whole waking period). We also use two minute means of systolic, diastolic and mean blood pressures, which are plotted out to give 720 points on a graph for visual representation of the blood pressure over the 24-hour period.

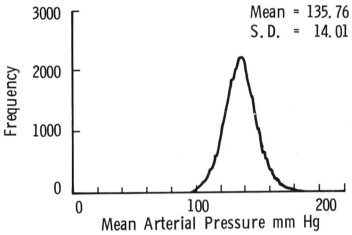

Fig. 1   Frequency histogram of all mean blood pressure recordings during the waking period of intra-arterial ambulatory monitoring in one subject.

The variability of blood pressure can be examined by constructing the frequency histogram and taking the standard deviation as a measure of the variability. These histograms appear to be normally distributed (Figure 1) and therefore, it would seem justified to use the standard deviation in this way. Blood pressure is much lower during sleep and the baroreflex may be reset, therefore, the present results are based on variability as determined from the frequency histograms of blood pressure during the awake period only.

Results

Fifty-six subjects were studied. They ranged in age from 16 to 69 years (mean 44.8 ± 11.1 years). Mean waking arterial pressure in these subjects ranged from 89.5mmHg to 159.5mmHg, with a mean of 118.3mmHg (SD 17.9mmHg) Variability ranged from 8.5mmHg to 20.5mmHg

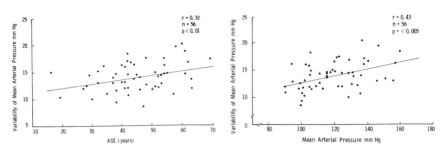

Fig. 2   Relationship between variability of mean arterial blood
(left)   pressure and age in all 56 subjects.

Fig. 3   Relationship between variability of mean arterial pressure
(right)   and mean arterial pressure itself.

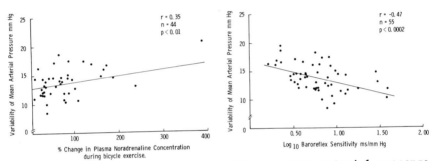

Fig. 4   Relationship between variability of mean arterial pressure
(left)   and % change in plasma noradrenaline concentration during
            bicycle exercise.

Fig. 5   Relationship between variability of mean arterial pressure
(right)   and baroreflex sensitivity.

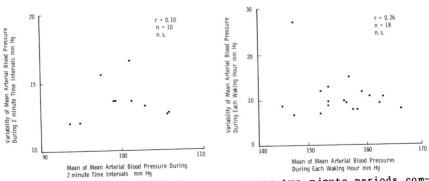

Fig. 6   Variability of blood pressure over two minute periods com-
(left)   pared to the mean pressure over the same short time inter-
            vals.
Fig. 7   Variability of blood pressure over 18 one hour awake periods
(right)   compared to the mean pressure over the same time intervals.

with a mean of 13.8mmHg (SD 2.4mmHg). Variability increased directly with age (r = 0.32, P<0.01) (Figure 2), increasing mean arterial pressure (r = 0.43, P<0.0005) (Figure 3), the relative increase in plasma noradrenaline and blood pressure during exercise (r = 0.35, P<0.01) (Figure 4) and was inversely related to log BRS (r - -0.47, P<0.0002) (Figure 5). Multiple regression analysis revealed log BRS to be the only independent predictor of blood pressure variability (P<0.005). There was no evidence to suggest that variability was increased in borderline hypertension.

Discussion

The coefficient of variation (i.e. standard deviation/mean) has been used by some workers in this field as a measure of blood pressure variability as they have noted, as have we, that standard deviation often increased with increasing mean arterial pressure. However, this approach already assumes that variability increases with pressure increases which, as we also have found, is true but is not as important as baroreflex sensitivity, which itself may allow both mean pressure and its variability to vary.

In order to test the coefficient of variation hypothesis, we examined variability of blood pressure in individual subjects over the short-term (two-minute intervals) (Figure 6) and medium term (one hour periods) (Figure 7) in addition to the longer entire waking period. Over these shorter times, the mean pressure varied from period to period, but variability was found to be independent of the mean pressure under these conditions. After three to seven months of chronic beta blockade, the protocol was repeated in thirty-five of the subjects. Variability did not change although mean arterial pressure fell on average, 19mmHg (P<0.001). The results of the shorter term studies and those with beta blockade suggest that mean arterial pressure and its variability are regulated independently. Diminished baroreceptor buffering of fluctuations in blood pressure appears to lead to increased variability of arterial pressure in hypertension.

References

1. Watson R.D.S., Stallard T.J., Flinn R.M. and Littler W.A. (1980) Hypertension 2, 333.
2. Mancia G., Ferrari A., Gregorini L., Parati G., Pomidossi G., Bertinieri G., Grassi G. and Ranchetti A. (1980) Clin. Sci. 59, 4015.
3. Stott F.D. In: Blood Pressure Variability. Ed. D. Clement. MTP Press, Lancaster, p.55.
4. Smyth H.S., Sleight P. and Pickering G.W. (1969) Circ. Res.24, 109.
5. Sleight P., Floras J. and Jones J.V. In: Blood Pressure Variability. Ed. D. Clement. MTP Press, Lancaster p.61.

BLOOD PRESSURE PROFILES IN GENERAL PRACTICE

G.F. ABETEL

6, Place du Marche CH - 1350 Orbe, Switzerland

Introduction

Private practice is very different from hospital practice, because patients are not selected and are seen for short periods of consultation. Furthermore, ambulatory observation is difficult.

Recent technical approaches allow us to study physiological behaviour outside of medical centres and to improve detection and care. Spatial experiments have proved the interest of such techniques, which are medically applicable in the last few years for continuous cardiac control and more recently in the monitoring of arterial tension (AT).

Significant increase in morbidity and mortality in relation to elevated AT has been demonstrated by epidemiological studies. But treatments remain controversial because of the lack of objective criteria of selection (1, 2, 3, 4, 5).

Research

The WHO defines hypertension (HT) by three blood pressures (BP), equal to or greater than 160/95mmHg, taken at different times.

Froment (6) has proved that two control measurements following a first hypertensive value show a normalization of AT in two thirds of the cases. What happens when the number of AT values is not 3, but 10, 20 or 100 a day?

The first ambulatory profile was made by Bevan in 1968 with an an intra-arterial catheter. He demonstrated the important systolic and diastolic variation over 24-hours. This method has been perfected by the Oxford Group (7). These curves are technically perfect and must serve as a reference for indirect measurements.

But for practical, technical and economical reasons, the practitioner cannot use intra-arterial methods, whence the interest of indirect measures by Riva Rocci cuff linked to a portable electronic system.

Method

All observations were made with a Remler M2000 kindly loaned by Dr. Bernard Indermuhle, Head of the Medical Service of Sandoz Products Company, Switzerland. The quality of this apparatus has been clearly proven by Sokolow et al (8, 9).

More than 300 days of recording (totalling 7500 measurements) have been done to date, all in the sitting position, from 8.0 a.m. to 6.0 p.m. The form of individual profiles and the discrepancy between values recorded in the medical office and those observed in ambulation remain surprising.

For example, a 72-year old woman, since the addition of Cloni-dine to her treatment, complained of inability to read her newspaper after lunch because of vision problems. (AT 105/75, pulse 60). She remains hypertensive in the office (AT 190/110, pulse 80).   The second example is a 28-year old construction-worker, slightly hyper-tensive (AT 145/100, pulse 80), who suffers from headaches which coincide with hypertensive peaks and tachycardia (AT 200/105, pulse 120).

The infrequent problem of higher tension outside the office is another example.

These results are so extravagant, that the first reaction is to question the value of the method.

In order to prove the reliability of the Remler M2000, three morning and three evening measures are made with the Remler shunted to a mercury manometer. The comparison of the six values is made in the evening during the decoding.

Individual concordance is good, only two per cent of patients being discordant. A regression curve based on 883 measures confirms an excellent correlation for systolic and diastolic pressures (Figure 1). An extrapolation can be made for the other values.

Results

The mean daily BP value is the usual method for interpreting a pro-file.

This is a reliable method since the deviation between the median and the mean is negligible. (For 175 profiles, the Sy.X syst. is 2.80mmHg and the Sy.X. diast. 1.48mmHg).

A group of 91 patients, all suspected of HT, was selected on the basis of three occasional measures, taken in the office at about one week interval. Two or three values were pathological. For each case, the mean of the values was compared with the mean of the tension profile (Figure 2).

Two conclusions can be drawn:
1. That in the majority of cases, the ambulatory means seems lower than office means.
2. A tension profile cannot be predicted on the bases of office detection pressures. A regression curve is not possible for systolic or for diastolic pressures.
The tensional behaviour during the day varies in relation to age and treatment. For each decade, aside from the first and second, a drop in AT is observed around 1.0 p.m., which is deeper in the group of treated patients.

The range of variability of systolic arterial tension increases with age. A regression of the systolic range on age shows for non-treated patients a progression from 35 to 50mmHg. Whereas the range for treated patients is remarkable, going from 35 to 75mmHg and in some cases 100mmHg (Figure 3). This could certainly explain some therapeutic accidents.

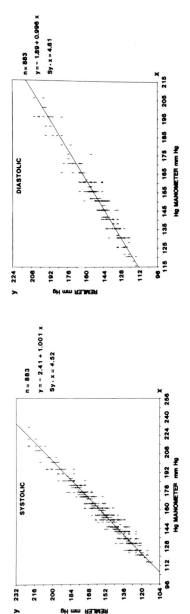

Fig.1 A and B: Regression of Remler on Hg manometer blood pressure for systolic and diastolic pressures

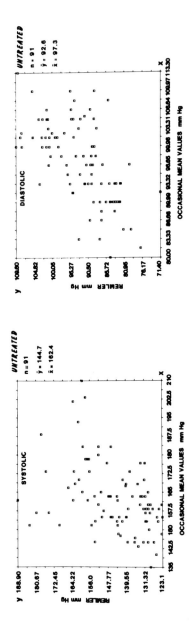

Fig.2 A and B: Correlation between mean of 3 occasional values and mean of Remler profile for systolic and diastolic pressures of untreated subjects

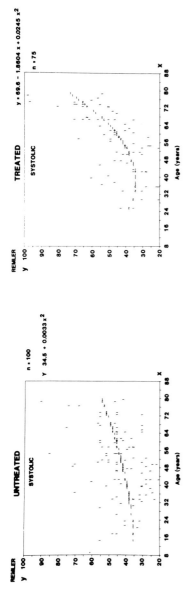

Fig.3 A and B: Regression of systolic range on age for untreated and treated subjects

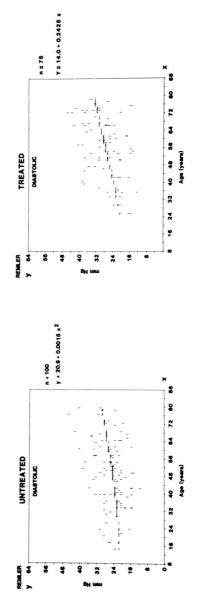

Fig.3 C and D: Regression of diastolic range on age for untreated and treated subjects

Profiles Analysis

It would be useful to establish a conventional system of analysis of
AT profiles in order to carry out long-term epidemiological studies.
The methods available to the practitioner are:
1. Graphic representation of each AT and pulse according to time of
    day.
2. The mean of systolic and diastolic AT.
3. The percentage of AT superior or equal to pre-determined arbitr-
    ary values (for example 160 and 150mmHg systolic, 100 and 90
    diastolic).
4. Systolic and diastolic range.
Armed with these data, the practitioner demands that the statistician
establish reference curves with percentiles.

Conclusions

1. Can HT still be diagnosed according to WHO criteria?
2. No medical office BP values can predict ambulatory tension
    behaviour in the detection period.
3. A drop in BP is observed around 1.0 p.m. from 30 years of age on.
4. The systolic range increases dangerously with age in treated
    patients
5. A standard mode of analyses must be defined for each individual
profile and reference curves with percentiles established.

This study could not have been carried out without the help of my
assistant, Miss A. Bosset, Dr. Ulrich Kreuter, statistican, Dr. Jean-
Charles Bousquet and Mr.Jean-Paul Bonnabry of Sandoz Products, Switzerland.

References

1. Bauer G.E. and Hunyor S.N. (1978) Drugs **15**, 80-86.
2. Walker J.M. and Beevers D.G. (1979) Drugs **18**, 312-324.
3. Management Committee: The Australian Therapeutic Trial in Mild
    Hypertension (1980). The Lancet: 1 1261-1267.
4. Helgeland A. (1980) Am. J. of Med. **69**, 723-725.
5. Carey R.M. and Ayers C.R. (1976) Am. J.of Med. **61**, 811-814.
6. Froment A. (1981) Epidemiologie de l'hypertension arterielle.
    Hypertension arterielle par Ph. Tcherdakoff/Ed. Sandoz, 85-92.
7. Stott F.D. (1978) in: Blood pressure variability (ed. D.
    Clement)   M.T.P. Press, Lancaster, England, 55.
8. Perloff D., Sokolow M. (1978) Card. Med. **6**, 655-668.
9. Sokolow M., Perloff D., Cowan R. (1980) Card. Reviews & Re-
    ports,**4**, 295-3036

DEPENDENCE OF BLOOD PRESSURE VARIABILITY ON SEX, AGE, HEIGHT,BODY-WEIGHT,FAMILY HISTORY OF HYPERTENSION

R.LAURO , E. SANTARELLI, G. REDA, G. PUGLIESE & G. CECCARELLI*

Institute of Medical Clinic II & *General Pathology II,
University of Rome, Italy

Introduction

The purpose of this study was to analyse the dependence of blood pressure (BP) variability on the following parameters: sex, age, height, body-weight, family history of hypertension and menarche.

Methods

The sample consisted of 1600 Rome school-children of both sexes aged 6 to 13 years, sub-divided into groups of 100 according to sex and age. BP was recorded in the school sick-bay using a semi-automatic Royal USM-105 instrument which records diastolic pressure in correspondence of fourth phase Korotkoff sounds and is also able simultaneously to measure the heart rate. During BP measurements children were in a sitting position with the left arm at heart level. After measuring BP, the height and body-weight of each child and the onset of menarche in females were recorded and each child was given a card in order to obtain information from the family doctor on the incidence of hypertension (levels over 160mmHg for SBP and over 95mmHg for DBP, in agreement with the W.H.O.) in the child's relatives. On the basis of these data, each child was attributed a score in relationship to the family history of hypertension, 3 marks ing given in the case of one of the parents being hypertensive and 1 mark in the case of one of the maternal/paternal aunts/uncles or grandparents being hypertensive. Scores of the maternal or paternal family history of hypertension thus ranged between 0 and 5 and scores of the total family history of hypertension (maternal + paternal) between 0 and 10 (Table 1).

BP measurements were performed twice in each child as the strong emotional reaction, usually caused in children by this unusual event, might affect the first value. BP measurements were therefore repeated after an interval of ten minutes.

Comparisons of the values of the two measurements showed a statistically significant difference in both sexes and at all the ages considered; thus, only values obtained from the second measurement were used for subsequent statistical analysis.

TABLE 1

Score Attributed to Each Child in Relation to Family History of
Hypertension (FHH)

Father or mother hypertensive	...	...	...		3 marks		
One uncle/aunt, paternal or maternal, hypertensive		...	...	...	1 mark		
One grandparent, paternal or maternal, hypertensive			...	...	...	1 mark	

Parent	−	−	−	−	+	+	+	+
One uncle/aunt	−	−	+	+	−	−	+	+
One grandparent	−	+	−	+	−	+	−	+
Score of paternal or maternal FHH	0	1	1	2	3	4	4	5

Results

Diastolic blood pressure (DBP) and systolic blood pressure (SBP)
levels for all ages were compared in both sexes.

The hypothesis that DBP in both sexes is equal as far as concerns variance was tested by means of Snedecor's F test which was
always non-significant at the 5% level. The hypothesis of equality
between mean values evaluated by Student's two-sided t test on two
independent samples is rejected only for 13 year-old children (significance at the 1% level) and for 12 year-old children (significance
at the 0.1% level).

As far as concerns SBP, Snedecor's F test is significant at the
5% level only for 12 year-old children, while Student's t test,
confirming the equality between mean values, is significant only for
9 year-old children (at the 1% level) and for 8 year-old children (at
the 5% level) (Table 2).

Analysis of these data therefore demonstrates that sex has a
negligible influence on BP levels.

The dependence of DBP and SBP on age, height and body-weight was
evaluated. First the single characters, then combinations of two of
them and the group of three, were assumed as regressors; the values
of the regressors height and body-weight were grouped in classes of 5
cm. and 5 kg., respectively.

As far as concerns establishing the dependence of BP on the
single characters, two indexes were determined: Pearson's η^2 index
(correlation ratio) and Bravais-Pearson's r index (square correlation coefficient), the latter showing the fraction of BP variability
attributed to the linear dependence on the parameter under consideration; in the event r^2 values are close to η^2 values, it will be
assumed that the dependence of BP on the character is of a linear
nature and it will therefore be useless to employ more complex
curves. η^2 values show that the variability of DBP cannot be
explained by any function of age for more than 21.44% in males and

Table 2

Significance* of difference between variances (evaluated by Snedecor's F test) and mean values (evaluated by Student's two-sided t
test on two independent samples) of males and females for systolic
(SPB) and diastolic (DBP) blood pressure

YEARS	SBP		DBP	
	F test	t test	F·test	t test
6	-	-	-	-
7	-	-	-	-
8	-	+	-	-
9	-	++	-	-
10	-	-	-	-
11	-	-	-	-
12	+	-	-	+++
13	-	-	-	++

* Level of significance: - = non-significant at the 5% level;
                           + = significant at the 5% level;
                          ++ = significant at the 1% level;
                         +++ = significant at the 0.1% level.

19.32% in females or by any function of height for more than 21.05%
in males and 17.63% in females or by any function of body-weight for
more than 24.29% in males and 20.55% in females. Furthermore the
variability of SBP cannot be explained by any function of age for
more than 25.32% in males and 23.66% in females or by any function
of height for more than 29.26% in males and 20.91% in females or by
any function of body-weight for more than 25.48 in males and 18.88%
in females (Table 3a, 3b, 3c).
    The respective complement cannot be explained by the character
under examination and represents an uncertainty margin which can be
explained by means other parameters (sodium intake, etc.) or attributed to casual factors. r^2 values are also so close to the η^2
values as to show the essentially linear nature of the dependence of
BP on the characters assumed as regressors and thus to make use of
more complex curves useless.   As far as concerns evaluating the
dependence of BP on the combinations of two characters (age - height;
age - body weight; height - body weight) and on the group of three
(age - height - body-weight), considering the linear nature of the
dependence, the three regression planes (for the combinations of two
regressors) and the regression hyperplane (for the group of three
regressors) were interpolated by means of the least squares method.
The absence of colinearity among the regressors, which would make the
results unreliable, was previously ascertained by determining the
square multiple correlation coefficient between each regressor and
the other two; the data showed that no index was sufficiently close
to 1 to confirm the existence of a situation of collinearity between
the regressors.   Since the three regression planes and the regression
hyperplane can be interpolated, the respective multiple determina-

Table 3a

η^2 (correlation ratio) and r^2 (square correlation coefficient) values relative to the dependence of systolic (SBP) and diastolic (DBP) blood pressure on age in both sexes.

		η^2	r^2
DBP	♂	0.2144	0.1616
	♀	0.1932	0.1793
SBP	♂	0.2532	0.2496
	♀	0.2366	0.2221

Table 3b

η^2 (correlation ratio) and r^2 (square correlation coefficient) values relative to the dependence of systolic (SBP) and diastolic (DPB) blood pressure on height in both sexes

		η^2	r^2
DBP	♂	0.2105	0.1844
	♀	0.1763	0.1631
SBP	♂	0.2926	0.2768
	♀	0.2091	0.1779

Table 3c

η^2 (correlation ratio) and r^2 (square correlation coefficient) values relative to the dependence of systolic (SBP) and diastolic (DBP) blood pressure on body-weight in both sexes

		η^2	r^2
DBP	♂	0.2429	0.1971
	♀	0.2055	0.1811
SBP	♂	0.2548	0.2159
	♀	0.1888	0.1627

tion coefficients (R^2) were calculated, expressing the fraction of BP variability attributable to the dependence successively considered. The results showed that a fraction of BP variability higher than the characters considered singly cannot be explained either by the combinations of two characters or by the group of three. (Table 4)

Table 4

R^2 (multiple determination coefficient) values relative to the dependence of systolic (SBP) and diastolic (DBP) blood pressure on the combination of two regressors (age-height; age-body-weight; height-body-weight) and on the group of three (age-height-body-weight) in both sexes

Regressors		Age – – Height	Age – –Body-weight	Height –Body-weight	Age – Height – –Body-weight
DBP	♂	0.1917	0.2152	0.2129	0.2167
	♀	0.2035	0.2092	0.1958	0.2147
SBP	♂	0.2905	0.2695	0.2781	0.2909
	♀	0.2403	0.2304	0.1935	0.2408

Total family history of hypertension (maternal + paternal) as regressor was evaluated. The values of the r^2 index (0.0004 in males and 0.0038 in females for DBP; 0.0021 in males and 0.0014 in females for SBP) ws of little importance and excluded the dependence of BP on this character. In order to detect a discriminating action of family history of hypertension on BP levels, as shown by other authors, two groups were considered within the extreme ages (5 and 13 years) consisting of subjects of both sexes with a total family history of hypertension score equal to 0 and ≥ 3 for 6-year old children and equal to 0 and n 5 for 13-year old children. Snedecor's F test and Student's t test were employed on the two independent samples both for DBP and SBP. DBP and SBP were also considered jointly by evaluating the significance of the differences between variance- and covariance- matrices of the two groups (Anderson's test) and the difference bween the two mean vectors (Hotelling's T^2 test). The results showed a statistically non-significant difference between the two groups for 6- and 13-year old children; thus, it can be seen that the character family history of hypertension does not account for BP variability. Two main reasons are probably responsible:

Table 5

r^2 (square correlation coefficient) values relative to the dependence of systolic (SBP) and diastolic (DBP) blood pressure on family history of hypertension in both sexes

	DPB		SBP	
	♂	♀	♂	♀
r^2	0.0004	0.0039	0.0021	0.0014

Table 6

Results of Snedecor's F test (for SBP and DBP), Student's tg test (for SBP and DBP), Anderson's test and Hotelling's T^2 test for 6- amd 13-year old children.

		6-year old	13-year old
Snedecor's F test	SBP	N.S.*	N.S.*
	DBP	N.S.*	N.S.*
Student's t test	SBP	N.S.*	N.S.*
	DBP	N.S.*	N.S.*
Anderson's test		N.S.*	N.S.*
Hotelling's ^{2} test		N.S.*	N.S.*

*N.S. = non-significant at the 5% level.

1.   Effective lack of influence of family history of hypertension on BP levels in the age groups studied, inasmuch as the dependence of BP on this character might occur only later;

2.   Incorrect collection of data due to the indirect approach (through the family doctor) to the child's relatives carried out in order to extend te inquiry not only to the parents, as performed by many authors, but also to the aunts/uncles and the grandparents of the child, in order thus to more completely evaluate the family history of hypertension considering that the disease might not yet have been manifest in account of the young age of the parents.

Results of the combination of family history of hypertension and the best regressor out of age, height and body-weight by means of the calculation of the multiple determination coefficient (R^2) were only slightly higher than the corresponding r^2 relative to the consideration of the best regressor - age, height and body-weight.

For the ages 10, 11, 12 and 13 years in which the sample size both for girls before menarche as well as after menarche was sufficiently large, the dependence of BP values on menarche was evaluated by means of the quartiles tgest. The x^2 test is non-significant at the 5% level except in 11-year old girls and only for DBP (significance at the 5% level) so that it may be concluded that no elements exist by which hypothesize a relationship between BP levels and menarche. On the other hand, using this technique menarche was correlated with height and body-weight; the x^2 was in fact significant at the 5% level for 13-year old girls, at the 1% level for 12-year old girls and at the 0.1% level for 11- and 10-year old girls, as far as concerns height, was non-significant at the 5% level for 13-year old girls, significant at the 5% level for 12-year old girls and at the 1% level for 11- 10-year old girls, as far as concerns body-weight.

Table 7

R^2 (multiple determination coefficient) values relative to the dependence of systolic (SBP) and diastolic (DBP) blood pressure on the combination of family history of hypertension (FHH) and the best regressor out of age, height and body-weight in both sexes.

		R^2	Regressors
DBP	♂	0.2086	FHH + body-weight
	♀	0.1826	FHH + body-weight
SBP	♂	0.2770	FHH + height
	♀	0.2222	FHH + age

Table 8

Significance* of the quartiles (x^2) test on the dependence of systolic (SBP) and diastolic (DBP), height and body-weight on menarche for the ages 10, 11, 12 and 13 years.

Years	10	11	12	13
SBP	-	-	-	-
DBP	-	+	-	-
Height	+++	+++	++	+
Body-weight	++	++	+	-

*Level of significance: - = non-significant at the 5% level
                           + = significant at the 5% level
                          ++ = significant at the 1% level
                         +++ = significant at the 0.1% level

Conclusion

Data emerging from the present investigation show that less than 30% of BP variability was found to depend on age, height and body-weight; furthermore, sex, family history of hypertension and menarche were shown to have no influence on BP variability.

Acknowledgements

The authors were grateful to Professor A. Naddeo, Department of Statistics, Facolta di Economia e Commercio, University of Rome, for performing the statistical analysis of data.